PATHOPHYSIOLOGICAL PHENOMENA IN NURSING

Human Responses to Illness

PATHOPHYSIOLOGICAL PHENOMENA IN NURSING

Human Responses to Illness

THIRD EDITION

Virginia Carrieri-Kohlman, RN, DNSc, FAAN
Professor
Department of Physiological Nursing
University of California—San Francisco
San Francisco, California

Ada M. Lindsey, RN, PhD, FAAN
Dean
College of Nursing
University of Nebraska Medical Center
Omaha, Nebraska

Claudia M. West, RN, MS
Clinical Professor
Department of Physiological Nursing
University of California—San Francisco
San Francisco, California

SAUNDERS
An Imprint of Elsevier Science

SAUNDERS
An Imprint of Elsevier Science

11830 Westline Industrial Drive
St. Louis, Missouri 63146

PATHOPHYSIOLOGICAL PHENOMENA IN NURSING ISBN 0-7216-8453-X

NOTICE

Nursing is an ever-changing field. Standard safety precautions must be followed, but as new research and clinical experience broaden our knowledge, changes in treatment and drug therapy may become necessary or appropriate. Readers are advised to check the most current product information provided by the manufacturer of each drug to be administered to verify the recommended dose, the method and duration of administration, and contraindications. It is the responsibility of the licensed prescriber, relying on experience and knowledge of the patient, to determine dosages and the best treatment for each individual patient. Neither the publisher nor the author assumes any liability for any injury and/or damage to persons or property arising from this publication.

Previous editions copyrighted 1986, 1993

International Standard Book Number 0-7216-8453-X

Executive Publisher: Darlene Como
Senior Developmental Editor: Barbara Watts
Project Manager: Joy Moore
Design Manager: Bill Drone
Cover and Interior Designer: Judy Schmitt

Printed in the United States of America

Last digit is the print number: 9 8 7 6 5 4 3 2 1

Contributors

Eleanor F. Bond, PhD, RN
Professor
Department of Biobehavioral Nursing and Health Systems
University of Washington
Seattle, Washington
Protein-Calorie Malnutrition

Virginia Carrieri-Kohlman, RN, DNSc, FAAN
Professor
Department of Physiological Nursing
University of California—San Francisco
San Francisco, California
Conceptual Approach and Dyspnea

Wanda Crumpton, RN, MSN, ACNP
Acute Care Nurse Practitioner
Little Rock Cardiology Clinic
Little Rock, Arkansas
Dementia

Kennith Culp, RN, PhD
Associate Professor
College of Nursing
The University of Iowa
Iowa City, Iowa
Acute Confusion

Grace E. Dean, RN, MSN
Assistant Research Scientist
City of Hope National Medical Center
Nursing Research and Education
Duarte, California
Anorexia

Lynne A. Farr, PhD
Professor
College of Nursing
University of Nebraska Medical Center
Omaha, Nebraska
Circadian Rhythm Disorders

Joseph J. Gauthier, RN, PhD
Associate Professor of Biology
Biology Department
University of Alabama—Birmingham
Birmingham, Alabama
Infection

Marcia Grant, RN, DNSc, FAAN
Director and Research Scientist
Nursing Research and Education
City of Hope National Medical Center
Duarte, California
Anorexia

Margaret M. Heitkemper, RN, PhD, FAAN
Professor and Chair
Department of Biobehavioral Nursing and Health Systems
University of Washington
Seattle, Washington
Protein-Calorie Malnutrition

Barbara J. Holtzclaw, RN, PhD, FAAN
Professor Emeritus
School of Nursing
University of Texas Health Science Center at San Antonio
San Antonio, Texas
Altered Thermoregulation

Christine E. Kasper, RN, PhD, FAAN, FACSM
Associate Professor and M. Adelaide Nutting Chair
The John Hopkins University School of Nursing
Baltimore, Maryland
Skeletal Muscle Atrophy

Dorothy M. Lanuza, RN, PhD, FAAN
Professor
Niehoff School of Nursing
Loyola University of Chicago
Maywood, Illinois
Circadian Rhythm Disorders

Kathryn A. Lee, RN, PhD, FAAN
Professor
Department of Family Health Care Nursing
University of California—San Francisco
San Francisco, California
Impaired Sleep

Ada M. Lindsey, RN, PhD, FAAN
Dean
College of Nursing
University of Nebraska Medical Center
Omaha, Nebraska
Conceptual Approach and Stress Response

Roxanne W. McDaniel, RN, PhD
Director of Graduate Studies/MS Program
Associate Professor
School of Nursing
University of Missouri—Columbia
Columbia, Missouri
Nausea, Vomiting, and Retching

Christine Miaskowski, RN, PhD, FAAN
Professor and Chair
Department of Physiological Nursing
University of California—San Francisco
San Francisco, California
Pain

Janice D. Nunnelee, RN, PhD, CS/ANP
Clinical Associate Professor of Nursing
University of Missouri—St. Louis
St. Louis, Missouri
Altered Clotting

Gayle Giboney Page, RN, DNSc, FAAN
Associate Professor and Independence Foundation Chair in Nursing Education
Director of PhD Program
The Johns Hopkins University School of Nursing
Baltimore, MD
Stress Response

Mary H. Palmer, RN, PhD, RNC, FAAN
Associate Professor
School of Nursing
University of North Carolina—Chapel Hill
Chapel Hill, North Carolina
Urinary Incontinence

Michele M. Pelter, RN, PhD
Director, Cardiovascular Research
Department of Physiological Nursing
University of California—San Francisco
San Francisco, California
Ischemia

Bethany J. Phoenix, RN, PhD
Assistant Clinical Professor
Department of Community Health Systems
University of California—San Francisco
San Francisco, California
Addiction

Barbara F. Piper, RN, DNSc, AOCN, FAAN
Associate Professor
University of Nebraska Medical Center
College of Nursing
Omaha, Nebraska
Fatigue

Kathleen A. Puntillo, RN, DNSc, FAAN
Professor
Department of Physiological Nursing
University of California—San Francisco
San Francisco, California
Pain

Verna Rhodes, RN, EDS, FAAN
Associate Professor Emeritus
School of Nursing
University of Missouri—Columbia
Columbia, Missouri
Nausea, Vomiting, and Retching

Kathy C. Richards, RN, PhD
Research Health Scientist
Central Arkansas Veterans Healthcare System
Associate Professor
College of Nursing
University of Arkansas for Medical Sciences
Little Rock, Arkansas
Dementia

Marilyn Sawyer Sommers, RN, PhD, FAAN
Associate Dean for Research
Professor
College of Nursing
University of Cincinnati
Cincinnati, Ohio
Alterations in Immunocompetence

Nancy A. Stotts, RN, EdD, FAAN
Professor
Department of Physiological Nursing
University of California—San Francisco
San Francisco, California
Impaired Wound Healing

Michael Stulbarg, MD
Professor of Clinical Medicine
Department of Medicine
University of California—San Francisco
San Francisco, California
Dyspnea

Gretchen Summer, RN, BS, PhD(Cand.)
Doctoral Nursing Student
Department of Physiological Nursing
University of California—San Francisco
San Francisco, California
Pain

Pao-Feng Tsai, RN, PhD
Assistant Professor
College of Nursing
University of Arkansas for Medical Sciences
Little Rock, Arkansas
Dementia

Joan G. Turner, RN, DSN
Professor
School of Nursing
University of Alabama—Birmingham
Birmingham, Alabama
Infection

Claudia M. West, RN, MS
Clinical Professor
Department of Physiological Nursing
University of California—San Francisco
San Francisco, California
Conceptual Approach and Ischemia

Mary Ellen Wewers, RN, PhD, MPH
Professor
The Ohio State University College of Nursing
Columbus, Ohio
Addiction

Preface

The phenomena described in this book are examples of human responses that result from a range of health problems. Some can be considered symptoms, some processes, and some are clinical problems. All are phenomena within the purview of nursing practice and nursing research. The most current knowledge about each phenomenon is presented, offering a basis for developing or examining the knowledge base of nursing practice.

CHAPTER FORMAT

Contributing authors were requested to follow the same outline for the presentation of content about each phenomenon included in this book. This organizational format for content provides a consistent approach used across each chapter. In some chapters, as appropriate for the topic, there is some deviation from the format; however, this consistency in approach has been one of the hallmarks of previous editions of this text.

THIRD EDITION

The strengths of the previous two editions were the inclusion of phenomena commonly encountered by nurses across settings and populations; the state-of-the-art, research-based presentations of knowledge related to these pathophysiological mechanisms; the discussions of measurement and clinical management of these phenomena; and the extensive and timely reviews of the literature related to each phenomenon. Continuing to update the knowledge base underlying these phenomena remains our goal. Knowledge is changing rapidly; for example, what is now known about such topics as dyspnea, immunocompetence, fatigue, and pain has radically altered our understanding of these phenomena, and the newest literature and developments about each phenomena are reflected in this new edition.

Further, we sought to broaden the scope of the book in response to suggestions from reviewers and readers of the previous editions. We recognize, however, the impossibility of including in one volume every important pathophysiological phenomenon of interest to nurses. We have included those that occur frequently in diverse adult clinical populations that are seen in a broad range of health care settings.

Also, in this edition we chose to limit our examination of the phenomena to the adult population because of the difficulty of many authors to explore adequately the phenomena in both adult and pediatric populations. Each chapter, however, includes discussion of developmental risk factors for the phenomenon, which will address the effect of age on the risk of developing the phenomenon.

RELATION TO THEORY AND RESEARCH

Nurse researchers have shown growing support for an inductive approach to theory construction at the beginning, empirical level. Our book supports this empirical level of theory construction. It is important to recognize, however, that the underlying theoretical and empirical bases are not evenly developed for each phenomenon. For some, considerable work has accumulated over a long period; for others, much less is known. Thus, presenting an equivalent volume of research for each phenomenon is not possible. For some phenomena there may be little or no published nursing research, and for others the most exemplary research may not be conducted by nurses. We have, however, incorporated the best examples of research that represent the body of knowledge available for the respective phenomenon.

AUDIENCE

The content and approach of this book make it useful to nurse clinicians, baccalaureate and graduate nursing students, faculty, and researchers. Advanced practice nurses can use the information in this book to help identify these phenomena in adult and older clients across the health-illness continua and to develop, test, and implement clinical nursing therapies to prevent or alleviate these responses. Students and faculty should find this book a thoughtful attempt to create a conceptual foundation from which to teach and learn the science of nursing. Researchers can consider these chapters a baseline of conceptual, research-based information from which to design further investigations, to ask more probing questions, and to continue much needed theory development.

Our intent in the first edition was to stimulate thinking about pathophysiological phenomena and the use of a conceptual approach to organize nursing knowledge. Our purposes now in this third edition are to continue and extend the dialogue on human responses by offering the current knowledge base about 21 pathophysiological phenomena. We hope that readers will continue to benefit from our work and suggest ways in which we can make it more useful in future editions.

Contents

CHAPTER 1

The Conceptual Approach

VIRGINIA CARRIERI-KOHLMAN, ADA M. LINDSEY, & CLAUDIA WEST

The writing of the first edition of this book was prompted by our firm belief in the use of the *conceptual approach* for the study and practice of nursing science. Experiences over the past 15 years have only reinforced our belief in using the conceptual approach for the clinical practice, teaching, and research efforts needed to develop substantive knowledge for the discipline of nursing. The definition of the conceptual approach recommended in this book is the use of a process that deliberately attempts to examine the nature and substance of nursing from a conceptual perspective.[1] Concepts are used as the unifying classification or structure for the teaching, clinical practice, and scientific inquiry of nursing. The selected phenomena are viewed as pathophysiological clinical patient problems. All are human responses or an outcome of illness; some are symptoms, and some are processes. Psychosocial concepts that may influence pathophysiological phenomena are also an integral part of nursing science and are discussed briefly in each chapter as they relate to the pathophysiological phenomenon; however, the focus of this book is on pathophysiological concepts.

The conceptual approach used in this text provides a way of analyzing concepts without creating a set of words that seems "foreign." The language used is commonly understood by all health care professionals and has clinical meaning to them. We have not created a new vocabulary, but rather use generally accepted terminology. The use of a structure and vocabulary that is understood by those active in other disciplines increases the communication and interdisciplinary dialog in the development of content around a selected phenomenon. Research findings can be communicated effectively not only to nurses, but also to others from related disciplines through publications supported and read by other professionals. Adequate pursuit of knowledge about these complex phenomena necessitates multidisciplinary research teams. The conceptual approach facilitates communication among team members while adding to the body of knowledge about the phenomena for the nursing discipline and practice across other disciplines.

The use of a conceptual approach has facilitated the development and teaching of nursing substantive content for curricula and promoted the generation of research questions and research programs relevant to clinical and specialty practice. During the past two decades, nurse investigators using this type of conceptual approach for scientific inquiry have been instrumental in facilitating the dramatic advances in nursing research and have developed a wealth of systematic knowledge relevant to both pathophysiological[2-29] and psychosocial concepts[30-35] that is useful for the study and evaluation of nursing practice.

In clinical practice the conceptual approach means using selected concepts as a framework for assessing the patient's history and physical findings and developing a treatment plan. The conceptual approach helps the nurse to (1) focus on clinical problems encountered across disease categories and populations, (2) become more systematic in making observations about events or conditions that influence the problem, (3) ask questions about relationships among events or conditions that may influence the extent, progression or remission of the clinical problem, (4) collect information about the effectiveness of nursing actions directed toward the clinical problem or phenomenon, and (5) formalize questions that will serve as the basis for studies that may provide the empirical data requisite for influencing nursing practice.

There is a focus on the clinical phenomenon, but within a total care perspective. The phenomenon is viewed in a holistic way. For example, when medical therapy fails to improve a symptom, such as dyspnea or pain, this conceptual approach helps the clinician to think broadly and pursue alternative options, including self-management and behavioral therapies for symptom management. This focus on the symptom in chronic illness has led to changes in systems of care, such as the establishment of pain clinics, sleep disorder clinics, and stress management clinics.

The use of the conceptual approach for education means organizing substantive content around concepts, phenomena, or processes. Discussion of the mechanisms, measurement, and management of these phenomena related to and across different individuals and groups, different illnesses, and various stages of illness provides a framework for course content or an advanced practice specialty curriculum.

In research programs, the conceptual approach is used as a guide for developing nursing science. Concepts and the relationships among other concepts provide the building blocks for testable middle range theories. Research methods used for a program of study may include empirical and phenomenological methods. Qualitative and quantitative measurement can be used for studying the phenomenon. This conceptual approach serves as a template for the identification of variables that may be related or have a cause-and-effect relationship to the concept. Relevant variables may include age, culture, type of illness, trajectory of illness, and different environmental stressors. In the initial descriptive phase, the concept is defined in descriptive studies and, if necessary, instruments are developed and validated to facilitate measurement of the concept. In the next phase of investigation, descriptive, correlational, survey, or cohort designs are used to examine theoretical relationships between the concept and variables that may be linked or related to the concept or phenomenon. It is important to study those variables that theoretically are highly related to the concept and subsequently might be controlled in future studies or are even slightly related and may be creating variability or change in the phenomenon. Finally, using this conceptual approach, interventions that are theoretically thought to cause or affect the concept are examined in quasi-experimental or experimental studies. This process of inquiry is begun at the level appropriate for the amount of multidisciplinary knowledge already determined and communicated. This type of research program, which focuses on the systematic inquiry of a selected concept from description to experimental study, has proliferated over the last two decades. Many of these research accomplishments are represented in the chapters in this book.

FRAMEWORK FOR ORGANIZING CONCEPTS

Nursing scholars continue to emphasize the necessity for developing substantive content (or knowledge base) for nursing practice.[36-38] Developing structures, typologies, and classifications for the knowledge base within the discipline is important if nursing knowledge is to be made specific and visible for individuals in nursing practice.[39] Alternative ways of organizing, identifying, and labeling content for the discipline have been suggested.[36,40,41] The American Nursing Association (ANA) Council on Nursing Research recommended that nursing science encompass the spectrum of human responses to actual and potential health problems.[42] Others have emphasized the need for the study of biobehavioral phenomena and the importance of developing these constructs from a nursing perspective.[43,44] Most agree that the content must be specialty based if it is to be used by practicing clinical nurses and to add cumulatively to a multidisciplinary body of knowledge and to nursing science.[39,45,46]

The categorization of content by concepts in this text provides one method for organizing content that is relevant to the development of in-depth substantive content for the discipline and practice of nursing. Biologically based life processes serve as an overall framework for the categorization and study of the concepts. Life processes are the biological and psychosocial processes that combine to make up the entire individual. They are ever-present, ongoing processes and together are reflected in the total functioning human. The life processes represent an initial delineation and are not mutually exclusive. Selected biological life processes are listed in Box 1-1. Physiological processes provide a framework of study for each phenomenon. A researcher interested in biological science can focus on one or several biological processes. These can be combined with psychosocial processes to provide a more holistic study of the phenomenon. The life processes of regulation, cognition, sensation, protection, and motion are defined in Sections I, II, III, IV, and V, respectively.

USE OF THE CONCEPTUAL APPROACH FOR CURRICULUM PLANNING AND TEACHING

Student Selection and Study of Concepts

Biophysiologically based life processes can be used to organize the theoretical content relevant to nursing care of the chronically or acutely ill patient. In this

BOX 1-1 Selected Biological Processes

Cognition	Generativity
Sensation	Regeneration
Motion	Regulation
Protection	

section we describe the process by which phenomena (human responses or concepts) can be selected and used for teaching in the curriculum. The life processes are used as the higher level of abstraction from which to identify concepts. For example, sensation is a life process; pain and dyspnea are examples of phenomena or concepts classified under this life process.

It is apparent from the list of biological life processes in Table 1-1 that the life processes are at different levels of abstraction than are the human responses or phenomena derived from them. This lack of uniformity in level of abstraction reflects the current state of the formalization of these constructs and/or their biological complexity. To select the phenomena relevant to each life process, individuals from different clinical practice specialties can be involved in the identification of relevant phenomena, concepts, or variables. This initial stage of selection depends on the participants' theoretical knowledge, clinical expertise, and knowledge of the literature. A typical list of words (concepts) that might be generated initially under the life process of sensation is given in Box 1-2. This type of listing can be completed for each life process, with the identification of phenomena that might be emphasized in the curriculum for a certain specialty.

The pathophysiological phenomena may result in disruptions or alterations of these naturally occurring life processes. Our goal in this textbook is to include a number of biophysiological clinical phenomena (human responses) that are of major concern to nurses and for which nurses assume a major role in assessing, monitoring, managing and evaluating. The concepts presented have been selected from an enormous field of possibilities and do not exist as isolated clinical problems but are interrelated. In addition, the importance of a specific clinical concept, human response or outcome will change over time as the scientific frontier is pushed forward and the nature of practice evolves.

Box 1-2 Examples of Words (Concepts) Identified in Relationship to the Life Process of Sensation*

Pain	Sweetness
Stickiness	Comfort
Thirst	Pungency
Hunger	Fatigue
Anxiety	Dyspnea
Special sense deprivation	Perception
	Distress
Itchiness	Hardness
Blindness	Glossiness
Taste	Membrane potential
Deafness	Discrimination
Nausea	Stimulus
Touch	Selectivity
Loudness	Threshold
Receptors	Constancy

*List generated during one faculty meeting.

Within nursing courses, emphasis can be placed on defining physiological processes and mechanisms related to a specific phenomenon; related physiological and psychosocial phenomena; stressors, including medical diagnoses and clinical states; indicator behaviors or manifestations of the phenomenon, including both objective and subjective signs or symptoms; and suggested relevant clinical activities. The focus will depend on the level of the curriculum and the type of course being offered. Pathophysiology courses may compare and contrast physiological and pathological processes causing the phenomenon across disease states, whereas content in clinical courses often focuses on assessment and measurement of the concept and on related risk factors and treatments that can be applied to modulate the phenomenon, such as nausea and vomiting or pain.

Both undergraduate and graduate students might compare and contrast assessment and treatment options for the concept across different disease groups or clinical states using the categories outlined in Figure 1-1, in which the symptom of dyspnea is used as an example of defining and operationalizing one phenomenon. Dyspnea is categorized under the primary life process of sensation. Changes in physiological processes related to dyspnea include, but are not limited to, alterations in receptor stimulation, gas exchange, central perception, muscle force, breathing pattern, respiratory drive, work of breathing, and metabolic load. Selected related physiological and psychosocial concepts include fatigue, hypoxemia, hyperinflation, depression, anxiety, and isolation. Suggested stressors that could be used for further study to compare and contrast the phenomenon among patients include states such as anemia, postoperative states, obesity, pregnancy, deconditioning, and weaning from mechanical ventilation; or medical diagnoses, such as obstructive, restrictive, and vascular pulmonary diseases, cardiovascular diseases, and cancer. Manifestations might include subjective ratings of dyspnea by the patient on a standardized instrument coupled with the observed breathing pattern, objective signs of respiratory distress, and/or the results of various pulmonary

Life Process: Sensation   Key Concept: Dyspnea

Physiological Processes	Related Physiological Concepts	Related Psychosocial Concepts
Altered receptor stimulation	Immobility	Anxiety/panic
Increased respiratory drive	Chronic fatigue	Helplessness
Increased work of breathing	Disability	Depression
Altered ventilatory impedance	Hypoxemia/hypercapnia	Isolation/loneliness
Altered breathing pattern	Dynamic hyperinflation	Loss of role identification
Altered central perception	Increased airway resistance	Changes in lifestyle
Increased metabolic load	Cough	Perception of lack of control
Altered gas exchange	Increased secretions	Loss of energy and vitality
Altered ventilation/perfusion	Sleep disturbances	Loss of concentration
Altered muscle force/strength		
Altered cognition		
Altered mobility		

Subjective Manifestations	Objective Manifestations	Medical Diagnosis	Clinical States
Patient states "short of breath," "can't breathe" or other words that connote he or she is SOB	Rapid respiratory rate Labored breathing Accessory muscle use Audible wheezing	Emphysema Asthma Chronic bronchitis	Postoperative Obesity/cachexia Hypoxemia
Patient rates dyspnea intensity high on NRS, VAS or Borg Scale		Pulmonary fibrosis	Disability
Pt rates dyspnea with ADL on multidimensional scales	Pursed lips breathing	Pneumonia	Hyperinflation
	Restlessness	Pleural effusion	Exercise
	Frozen/immobile position	Pneumothorax	
"Staccato Speech"		Sarcoidosis	Aging
	Diaphoresis/pallor	ARDS	Hyperventilation
	Increased minute ventilation	Primary pulmonary hypertension	"Weaning from ventilator"
	Decreased FEV_1/PEFR	Pulmonary emboli	Kyphoscoliosis
	Decreased MIP/MEP	Congestive heart failure	Anemia
	Hypoxemia/hypercapnia	Lung cancer	Pregnancy

Suggested Activities for Practice and Research

- Use a standardized instrument for measuring dyspnea with a patient who has acute dyspnea and a patient who has chronic dyspnea.
- Compare and contrast physiological mechanisms that are causing shortness of breath in patients with hypoxemic versus ventilatory failure.
- Develop a clinical pathway for a hospitalized patient with acute respiratory failure who is short of breath.
- Differentiate between signs and symptoms of patients with acute and those with chronic dyspnea.
- Develop a checklist of factors causing dyspnea for hospitalized patients with varying diagnoses.
- List self-management strategies reported by patients who have chronic dyspnea that could be taught to others who are short of breath.
- Identify research questions that need to be asked about correlates or treatments for dyspnea.
- Review the literature on the effect of exercise on dyspnea and identify gaps in the literature.

Figure 1-1 Model for examining a phenomenon: Dyspnea. *ADL,* Activities of daily living; *ARDS,* adult respiratory distress syndrome; *FEV_1,* forced expiratory volume in 1 second; *MEP,* maximal expiratory pressure; *MIP,* maximal inspiratory pressure; *NRS,* numeric rating scale; *PEFR,* peak expiratory flow rate; *SOB,* shortness of breath; *VAS,* visual analog scale.

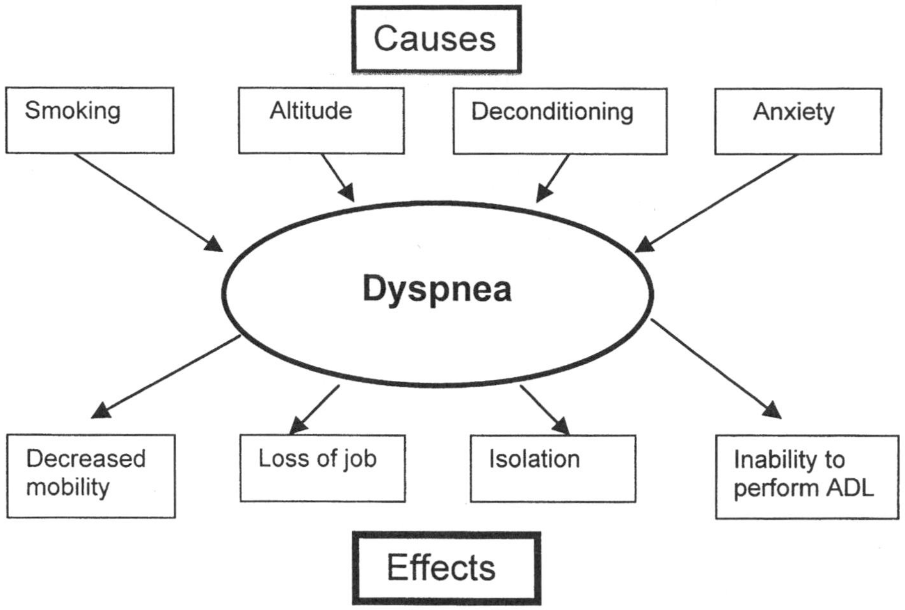

Figure 1-2 Inventory of causes and effects.

function tests. Suggested activities include (1) using a standard instrument to measure dyspnea in patients with acute and chronic shortness of breath, (2) developing a critical pathway for the patient with dyspnea, and (3) identifying self-care management strategies used by patients to teach other patients. These are only examples that can be combined with other activities that the teacher and student develop to further explore the phenomenon; clinically, theoretically, and empirically.

Graduate students who use the conceptual approach may also find it helpful to use the headings in the chapters of this book as an outline. The steps would be as follows: (1) students would define the concept of interest to them; (2) they would examine alternatives for measurement of the concept; (3) they would study related concepts or risk factors that may be manipulated in an effort to improve the pathophysiological phenomenon; and (4) they would study treatments that have been found to affect the concept.

Students in PhD and other doctoral programs can use concepts to generate research questions that are germane to the nursing care of patients and to assist in the development of a theoretical framework or conceptual model to guide their dissertation work related to a phenomenon.

An exercise called an *inventory of causes and effects*[47] can be used to help a graduate student or beginning researcher conceptualize the phenomenon. The concept is placed in the middle of a circle, and those variables known to cause or suspected of causing the phenomenon are diagrammed above, whereas those variables that are the effects or consequences of the phenomenon are depicted as resulting from the phenomenon. In Figure 1-2 the symptom for study, dyspnea, is placed in the middle of the circle. For illustration purposes only, a selected few variables that may cause the concept are depicted in squares above and those that result from dyspnea are depicted in squares below. In the initial phases of thinking about the phenomenon, the variables can be illustrated separately, such as gender, smoking history and isolation, as shown in the illustrated inventory. As the student continues to study additional factors related to the phenomenon, the more numerous causes and effects can be categorized in broader categories such as person, health, or environment. In our experience the depiction of an inventory of variables that cause the concept and those factors that result from the presence of the concept facilitates the student's review of the literature, selection of correlates, treatments that are integral to the study of a phenomenon, and the selection of additional outcomes.

Alternate Ways for Studying Concepts Within Courses

Phenomena may be viewed in one of two ways in the development of courses and teaching of the content: (1) as alterations in one normal life process, or (2) how the phenomenon affects all the life processes. It is helpful to use both approaches. An example of studying the phenomenon as an alteration in one life process is illustrated with the concept of pain under the life process of sensation. Pain is depicted as an alteration in sensation. The physiology and perception of sensations and pathophysiological changes related to pain are studied. Related physiological phenomena may include, but are not limited to, reception, threshold, tolerance to pain, referral of pain, and transmission of impulses. With an understanding of the normal physiological processes of sensation, the student or researcher can subsequently examine related physiological, pathophysiological, and psychosocial concepts, such as pleasure, comfort, analgesia, isolation, anxiety, and depression. Manifestations of pain, the measurement tools to evaluate pain in different settings, and actions to alter the pain experience also may be studied.

An example of the alternate method of viewing the effects of the phenomena across all the life processes is the relationship of pain to all the life processes (e.g., the effects of pain on cognition, affiliation, motion, sensation, and other processes). The approach taken is to examine the pathophysiology or changes in the salient life processes that either result from or contribute to the presence of that phenomenon. Within the discussion of each life process and the changes in them that result from the phenomenon, manifestations that are present as a result of a disruption in the process are examined. Another example of this method is the concept of dyspnea. The effect of dyspnea on each life process might be examined. The researcher would describe changes in the processes of cognition, sensation, regulation, or motion resulting from dyspnea and discuss manifestations of these. Interventions to decrease dyspnea would be studied.

There are advantages to using either approach for teaching concepts. The first alternative may provide more depth of knowledge about the specific human response, whereas the second approach will yield more information about interactions that occur across life processes in relation to the human response. It is recommended that both approaches be used for greater comprehension of each phenomenon. For example, one of the editors has knowledge and expertise in respiratory physiology and nursing care; she has been teaching this content in a graduate program for 25 years. The phenomenon of dyspnea under the life process of sensation is her area of research interest. Examination of the phenomenon across all of the life processes helped her to generate research questions salient to theory development and nursing care of respiratory patients. This human response of dyspnea is relevant across numerous diseases and across age groups and is effected by many psychological and physiological concepts. At the same time it is a clinical symptom frequently encountered by nurses. Other phenomena chosen as representative of human responses seen commonly in cardio-pulmonary specialties include ischemia, fatigue, edema, and pain, all of which could be examined by either of the two approaches. Using life processes in either of these two ways guides the student or professional nurse in thinking conceptually about phenomena related to both health and illness states.

In using this approach for graduate curriculum, selected phenomena can be presented in core lectures and then discussed in specialty seminars with the students. Specialty seminars allow students to focus on the specific human response as it occurs in populations for whom they provide care. For example, the phenomenon "altered immunocompetence" can be presented in lecture, followed by specialty seminars in which the nursing care related to altered immunocompetence in populations with asthma or leukemia or HIV or those receiving chemotherapy treatments would be discussed. These represent topics for nursing seminars in the advanced practice specialty areas of respiratory care and oncology.

We have had more than 15 years of experience with this conceptual approach as a framework for courses for undergraduate, masters, and doctoral students. The use of this approach has provided nursing content for lectures and seminars. In addition, doctoral students have selected conceptual areas that provide both preliminary research questions and the fulfillment of long-term research programs that are adding to the substantive knowledge base for nursing practice.

USE OF THE CONCEPTUAL APPROACH FOR RESEARCH

It is imperative that there be an intentional process of selection of salient clinical problems to provide direction for research for the formulation of questions and hypotheses pertinent to the development of knowledge that can direct practice.[39] Our previous experience had demonstrated the difficulty for faculty, clinicians, and students to generate nursing research questions from published grand theories or broad general clinical specialty content. If there is one dramatic result from the use of the conceptual approach for the past 20 years, it is the impact it has had on facilitating generation of research questions and the development of hypotheses that are relevant to the care of patients in all specialties. The focus on selected phenomena across specialty areas (e.g., pain or alterations in circadian rhythms) also promotes cluster studies resulting in knowledge development with both theoretical and practice implications across specialties for the discipline of nursing.

It has been suggested that middle range theories developed within conceptual areas that are pertinent to the explanation and prediction of phenomena will expedite the development of nursing science.[36,48-50] Middle range theories similar to those discussed throughout the chapters in this book are thought to be more directly relevant than grand theories for addressing practice concerns in a nursing specialty area. Using the conceptual approach supports the development of middle range theories related to one or several related phenomena. Over the past two decades, nurse researchers have expanded and refined definitions of concepts, and developed, refined, or tested instruments to measure these concepts for further study of the phenomenon. They have described concepts across illness groups, ages, and cultures.[13,17,24,51,52] They have conducted correlational studies to identify relationships among the phenomena of interest and demographic, psychosocial, environmental, and biological variables.[53,54] Finally, interventions, both medical treatments and self-care management strategies, have been tested for their efficacy in improving the pathophysiological phenomena as outcomes and related outcomes, such as cost or quality of life.[8,55-57] The study of symptom clusters in selected populations (e.g., pain, sleep, and fatigue in cancer patients) is an evolving focus for nurse researchers who are examining relationships and treatments among more than one concept or symptom.[4] All of these levels of scientific inquiry have helped to build research programs and knowledge bases that ultimately can be used to develop middle range theories for use in practice.

Naturally, the levels of knowledge vary across concepts. For example, there has been increased research focus on the symptoms of pain and fatigue over many diseases and settings. Nurse researchers have been involved in the study of basic physiological mechanisms of pain,[2] the measurement of pain in adults, children, and neonates,[58] different levels and types of pain with certain clinical procedures,[14] and the testing of cognitive behavioral treatments for chronic pain.[56] By contrast, nurses are only beginning to describe disruptions in biological circadian rhythms across illnesses or qualitative descriptions of dyspnea in different diseases or cultures. In the last several years there also has been an impressive increase in national conferences focused on the communication of research findings from studies that have used the conceptual approach, such as those focused on symptoms.[8] Multiinstitutional research initiatives have been funded by the Oncology Nursing Foundation for the study of the symptom of fatigue in cancer patients.[19,59,60]

USE OF THE CONCEPTUAL APPROACH FOR THEORY DEVELOPMENT

This textbook was first published in the 1980s, when there was debate about which nursing models or theories should be used to guide the development of nursing knowledge,[61-63] nursing theories were being critiqued and compared,[64,65] and the central concepts of nursing were being reexamined.[47,66] Although there were grand theories available, the great majority of nurse researchers who were interested in impacting practice drew their concepts and theories from other disciplines.[67,68] These discussions shifted to issues regarding the types of scientific inquiry or methods that should be used to study nursing phenomena.[46,69] There was further delineation of the important concepts within the domain of the discipline and how knowledge should be structured,[40,47,70-72] and analysis and development of concepts and instruments to measure these phenomena, with concurrent deliberation of various methods to teach the concepts.[42,62,71,73]

Discussions in the nursing literature related to the modes of inquiry centered around the use of empirical methods versus phenomenological approaches, qualitative versus quantitative methods, or the "received" and "perceived" view of scientific inquiry.[48,74-76] Currently nurse scientists are using more than one scientific orientation to study human responses, depending on the philosophical beliefs of the researcher, the questions posed, the state of the science, and the type of variables.[69,77]

As suggested by others,[62,69,74] we believe that multiple modes of inquiry are necessary and can be used with the conceptual approach, depending on the question and theoretical level of the concept of interest. The research studies discussed throughout this book provide excellent examples of the use of multiple scientific methods to analyze and develop concepts, propositions, and middle range theories. Diverse multidisciplinary research methods are necessary to begin to understand the complexities of many of these concepts.

During the 1990s, authors continued to suggest alternative ways of organizing, identifying, and labeling content. Meleis[62] proposed that concepts central to the domain of nursing are nursing client, transitions, interaction, nursing process, environment, nursing therapeutics, and health. Kim[71] suggested the client, the client-nurse, practice, and environment as four domains for structuring nursing knowledge. She further identified four classes of client phenomena: essential, developmental, problematic, and health care experiential concepts.

The chapters in this book are all evidence of efforts toward developing knowledge within the patient domain. Concepts from the client-nurse, environment, and practice are presented as correlates that impact the phenomenon. Roy[70] proposed an integrated metaparadigm of nursing science in which she distinguished the understanding of life processes as basic nursing science from clinical nursing science, the diagnosis and treatment of the patterning of life processes. The basic science component included life processes similar to those presented in this chapter. Other major categories of processes included health promotion, developmental, and group processes. She suggested that the burden of operationalizing conceptual categories within these processes rests with individual programs of research. The chapters of this book exemplify nurse researchers' attempts to operationalize conceptual categories. These theorists provided greater specificity for the generally accepted central domains for nursing (i.e., person, environment, health, and nursing).[47] For instance, Kim[71] included infection, confusion, anxiety, and stress as examples of health care experiential phenomena, and the pain experience and stress as client health outcomes within the client-nurse domain.

The nursing diagnosis conference group from which the North American Nursing Diagnosis Association (NANDA) was founded developed a framework that used processes to categorize nursing diagnoses accepted by the group. Descriptive studies have been used to describe variables surrounding diagnoses; however, at the present time this classification remains a nomenclature that is used clinically by some to identify problems.[78] The classification needs further research-generated theory to guide future clinical intervention.[79] Because the human responses discussed in this text have scientific knowledge to support their description, measurement, and related nursing therapeutics, they are viewed as being different from nursing diagnoses and may be at a different level of abstraction. For example, several nursing diagnoses could be identified that would be related to the phenomenon of pain or ischemia.

Another approach using concepts for the development of nursing theory in the 1980s and 1990s has been concept clarification and analysis using a modification of Wilson's techniques[80] of concept analysis, adapted by Walker and Avant.[48] This type of concept analysis is conducted to distinguish between "attributes and nonattributes" of a concept and to determine differences between concepts. Hupcey et al[50] reviewed 24 publications by nurses who have used this technique for theory development with primarily psychosocial concepts that are at a high level of abstraction, such as grief,[31] empowerment,[81] and hope and acceptance.[32] They critiqued the results derived from this method of theory development as lacking substance, comprehensiveness, explanatory power, or ability to transition from one level of theory to another.

The development of middle range theories for nursing began primarily in the 1990s with such theories as Mischel's theory[33] of uncertainty in illness, Pender's model[82] of health promotion and illness prevention, and the theory of unpleasant symptoms published by Lenz and colleagues.[49] Most recently, there has been a renewed call for nurses in the twenty-first century to place an emphasis on middle range theory development.[36] The conceptual approach provides the building blocks for middle range theories that have direct application to practice. Phenomena emanating from actual practice are described, related to other concepts, and then studied in cause and effect studies, thus building a middle range theory. For example, the theory of unpleasant symptoms was derived from clinical observations and the study of similarities and differences between the attributes of the symptoms (concepts) of fatigue and dyspnea.[20]

A dramatic increase in nursing research related to the development of nursing theory for the discipline and practice of nursing took place in the 1990s.[83] The conceptual approach presented in this book has been the basis for many of these research efforts. In part, the conceptual approach has advanced the development of nursing knowledge by a focus on the study of symptoms and helping people to manage symptoms, such as fatigue, sleep disturbances, nausea and vomiting, pain, and dyspnea.[55,84] In the past decade, nurse researchers have contributed extensive scientific knowledge related to symptom perception, correlates that have an impact on perception, measurement, and management strategies to modulate the symptom.[55] All of this knowledge is relevant to the practice of nursing and has contributed to the development of middle

TABLE 1-1 Chapter Subheadings

SUBHEADING	DESCRIPTION
Definition	An operational definition and a clear, succinct orientation to the perspective from which the phenomenon is examined.
Prevalence and Populations at Risk	The magnitude and significance of the phenomenon in a given population (or populations). Individuals who, because of the existence of and/or their responses to personal, health, and/or environmental characteristics and stressors, have an increased predisposition to the occurrence of the phenomenon.
Risk Factors: Environmental, Personal, and Developmental Factors	Factors in an individual's personal history, health, or environment or that occur during the process of aging that predispose him or her to experiencing the phenomenon.
Mechanisms	Pathophysiological processes involved in the development and maintenance of the phenomenon.
Pathological Consequences	Potential detrimental outcomes associated with the phenomenon.
Related Pathophysiological Concepts and Differential Diagnosis	Concepts similar to or occurring with the phenomenon, with illustration of the commonalities and/or differences between them. When appropriate, the history and physical findings that may help to differentiate between different diagnoses and the phenomenon are discussed.
Manifestations and Surveillance	Objective, observable, and/or measurable (direct or indirect) expressions of the phenomenon, including an individual's reported subjective perception. Measurement is the process of evaluating the phenomenon for quantity, quality, or frequency at a given point in time. If appropriate, selected published instruments to measure the phenomenon are discussed. Surveillance is the process of identification and monitoring of selected parameters over time, used to evaluate the status of the phenomenon and the individual's responses.
Clinical Management	Primary objectives and strategies for management of the phenomenon.
Conceptual Model(s)	Exemplary model(s) or theoretical framework(s) that relate the phenomenon to other variables or processes and that are used by nurses to guide their study of and clinical practice related to the phenomenon.
Case Studies	Clinical situations, including manifestations, surveillance, and clinical management, in which the various dimensions of the phenomenon are explored.
Selected Research	Illustrative and significant studies relevant to the phenomenon and its clinical management by nurses.
Questions for Future Study	Areas requiring additional study and/or exemplar questions for further study.

range theories or theoretical propositions to guide the discipline and practice of nursing. Recently Donaldson[38] systematically selected "breakthroughs" in nursing research efforts to generate knowledge from the perspective of the discipline of nursing. Breakthrough research was defined as studies that represented a new realm of scientific knowledge in the discipline of nursing, achieved either per se solum or through reconceptualization of former realms. In addition, and most important to be labeled a breakthrough, the new nursing knowledge had to transcend the discipline of nursing and change the prevailing thinking among other disciplines about the health phenomenon. Programs of research conducted by nurses who have used the conceptual approach were well represented in these selected breakthroughs, including the classical research program of Johnson[85] on pain measurement and management and that of Page,[86] with her demonstration that pain and stress can result in greater tumor metastases (and death) in an animal model (described in Chapter 14, Stress Response).

ORGANIZATION AND CONTENT OF CHAPTERS

Five biological life processes form the broad organizing structure for this book: regulation, cognition, sensation, protection, and motion. The particular phenomena to be included are commonly encountered in populations with acute or long-term illnesses; are alterations in function involving multiple body systems; are seen across the boundaries of age, disease entities, and clinical states; and are those for which nurses have a major role in assessing, monitoring, managing, and evaluating.

A critical and comprehensive examination of the phenomenon in each chapter includes the categories of: definition, prevalence and populations at risk, risk factors, physiological mechanisms, manifestations and surveillance, pathological consequences, related pathophysiological concepts and differential diagnoses, clinical management, conceptual models used to guide the study of the phenomenon, case studies, selected research studies, and questions for future study. These categories are not unlike those suggested by other authors[73,87] and are defined for this text in Table 1-1. Authors of each chapter vary in their use of these divisions, depending on the nature of the phenomenon. When appropriate in some chapters, the differential diagnosis has been included as a guide for taking a patient history and distinguishing between different clinical presentations and physical findings for various diseases that present with the same pathophysiological phenomenon. Case studies illustrate each concept in a given clinical situation. Research from nursing and other disciplines is included to provide the foundation for the conceptual explanation of each phenomenon and to stimulate the generation of exemplar questions for further research. In some chapters, areas requiring additional study are identified. The intent is to provide an approach to study human clinical pathophysiological phenomena that are of major concern in professional nursing practice and to generate a spirit of inquiry that is essential for the continued development of the knowledge base for professional nursing practice.

REFERENCES

1. Carrieri-Kohlman, V., Lindsey, A.M., & West, C.M. (1993). The conceptual approach. In V. Carrieri-Kohlman, A.M. Lindsey, & C.M. West (eds.), *Pathological phenomena in nursing: Human responses to illness* (2nd ed., pp. 1-10). Philadelphia: W.B. Saunders.
2. Gear, R.W., Miaskowski, C., Gordon, N.C., Paul, S.M., Heller, P.H., & Levine, J.D. (1999). The kappa opioid nalbuphine produces gender- and dose-dependent analgesia and antianalgesia in patients with postoperative pain. *Pain 83,* 339-345.
3. Gear, R.W., Miaskowski, C., Gordon, N.C., Paul, S.M., Heller, P.H., & Levine, J.D. (1996). Kappa-opioids produce significantly greater analgesia in women than in men. *Nature Medicine 2,* 1248-1250.
4. Miaskowski, C., & Lee, K.A. (1999). Pain, fatigue, and sleep disturbances in oncology outpatients receiving radiation therapy for bone metastasis: A pilot study. *Journal of Pain and Symptom Management 17,* 320-332.
5. Jacox, A.V., Carr, D.B., Payne, R.B., Berde, C.B., Briebart, W., Cain, J.M., et al. (1994). Management of cancer pain: clinical practice guidelines, No. 9. (AHCPR Pub. No. 94-0592). Rockville, Md.: Agency for Health Care Policy and Research, Public Health Service. U.S. Department of Health and Human Services. Washington, D.C.: U.S. Government Printing Office.
6. Page, G.G., & Ben-Eliyahu, S. (1997). The immune-suppressive nature of pain. *Seminars in Oncology Nursing 13,* 10-15.
7. Breslin, E.H., Roy, C., & Robinson, C.R. (1992). Physiological nursing research in dyspnea: A paradigm shift and a metaparadigm exemplar. *Scholarly Inquiry for Nursing Practice: An International Journal 6,* 81-104.
8. Funk, S.G., Tornquist, E.M., Champagne, M.T., Copp, L.A., & Wiese, R.A. (1989). *Key aspects of comfort: Management of pain, fatigue, and nausea.* New York: Springer.
9. Dalakis, M.C., Mock, V., & Hawkins, M.J. (1998). Fatigue: Definitions, mechanisms, and paradigms for study. *Seminars in Oncology 25,* 48-53.
10. Hart, L.K., Freel, M.I., & Milde, F.K. (1990). Fatigue. *Nursing Clinics of North America 25,* 967-976.
11. Piper, B.F., Lindsey, A.M., & Dodd, M.J. (1987). Fatigue mechanisms in cancer patients: Developing nursing theory. *Oncology Nursing Forum 14,* 17-23.
12. Aaronson, L.S., Teel, C.S., Cassmeyer, V., Neuberger, G.B., Pallikkathayil, L., Pierce, L., et al. (1999). Defining and measuring fatigue. *Image: Journal of Nursing Scholarship 31,* 45-50.
13. Puntillo, K.A. (1990). The pain experiences of intensive care unit patients. *Heart & Lung 19,* 526-533.
14. Puntillo, K.A., White, C., Morris, A., Perdue, S., Stanik-Huitt, J., Thompson, C., et al. (2001). Patients' perceptions and responses to procedural pain: Results from Thunder II Project. *American Journal of Critical Care 10,* 238-251.

15. Humphreys, J.C., Lee, K.A., Neylanm, T.C., & Marmar, C.R. (1999). Sleep patterns of sheltered battered women. *Image: Journal of Nursing Scholarship 31,* 139-143.
16. Lee, K. (1992). Self-reported sleep disturbances in employed women. *Sleep 15,* 493-498.
17. Lee, K.A., Zaffke, M.E., & McEnany, G. (2000). Parity and sleep patterns during and after pregnancy. *Obstetrics & Gynecology 95,* 14-18.
18. Shaver, J., Giblin, E., Lentz, M., & Lee, K. (1988). Sleep patterns and stability in perimenopausal women. *Sleep 11,* 556-561.
19. Nail, L.M., Baresevick, A.M., Meek, P.M., Beck, S.L., Jones, S.L., Walker, B.L., et al. (1998). Planning and conducting a multi-institutional project on fatigue. *Oncology Nursing Forum 25,* 1398-1403.
20. Lenz, E., Pugh, L., Gift, A., Milligan, R., & Suppe, F. (1997). The middle-range theory of unpleasant symptoms: An update. *Advances in Nursing Science 19,* 14-26.
21. McCormick, K.A. (1991). From clinical trial to health policy—research on urinary incontinence in the adult, part I. *Journal of Professional Nursing 7,* 47.
22. Holtzclaw, B.J. (1990). Shivering: A clinical nursing problem. *Nursing Clinics of North America 25,* 977-986.
23. Norris, C.M. (1982). *Concept clarification in nursing,* Rockville, Md.: Aspen.
24. Rhodes, V.A., Watson, P.M., Johnson, M.H., Madsen, R., & Beck, N. (1987). Patterns of nausea, vomiting, and distress in patients receiving antineoplastic drug protocols. *Oncology Nursing Forum 14,* 35-44.
25. Wadle, K.R. (1990). Diarrhea. *Nursing Clinics of North America 25,* 901-908.
26. Gift, A. (1990). Dyspnea. *Nursing Clinics of North America 25,* 955-965.
27. Champagne, M.T., & Wiese, R.A. (1992). Research on cognitive impairment: Implications for practice. In S.G. Funk, EMT, E.M. Tornquist, M.T. Champagne, & R.A. Wiese (eds.), *Key aspects of elder care: Managing falls, incontinence and cognitive impairment* (pp. 340-346). New York: Springer.
28. Farr, L., Keene, A., Samson, D., & Michael, A. (1984). Alterations in circadian excretion of urinary variables and physiological indicators of stress following surgery. *Nursing Research 33,* 140-146.
29. Carrieri-Kohlman, V., & Janson-Bjerklie, S. (1993). Dyspnea. In V. Carrieri-Kohlman, A.M. Lindsey, & C. West (eds.), *Pathophysiological phenomena in nursing: Human responses to illness* (2nd ed., pp. 247-278). Philadelphia: W.B. Saunders.
30. Campbell, J.C., & Humphreys, J. (1993). *Nursing care of survivors of family violence.* St. Louis: Mosby.
31. Cowles, K.V., & Rodgers, B.L. (1991). The concept of grief: A foundation for nursing research and practice. *Research in Nursing and Health 14,* 119-127.
32. Hasse, J., Britt, T., Coward, D., Leidy, N.K., & Penn, P. (1992). Simultaneous concept analysis of spiritual perspective, hope, acceptance and self-transcendence. *Image: Journal of Nursing Scholarship 24,* 141-147.
33. Mischel, M.H. (1990). Reconceptualizaton of the uncertainty in illness theory. *Image: Journal of Nursing Scholarship 22,* 256-262.
34. Meleis, A.I., Sawyer, L.M., Im, E.O., Hilfinger Messias, D.K., & Schumacher, K. (2000). Experiencing transitions: An emerging middle-range theory. *Advances in Nursing Science 23,* 12-28.
35. Abraham, I.L., Neundorfer, M.M., & Currie, L.J. (1992). Effects of group interventions on cognition and depression in nursing home residents. *Nursing Research 41,* 196-202.
36. Jacox, A., Suppe, F., Campbell, J., Stashinko, E. (1999). Diversity in philosophical approaches. In A.S. Hinshaw, S.L. Feetham, & J.L.F. Shaver (eds.), *Handbook of clinical research.* Thousand Oaks, Calif: Sage Publications.
37. Meleis, A.I. (1987). Revisions in knowledge development: A passion for substance. *Scholarly Inquiry for Nursing Practice: An International Journal 1,* 5-19.
38. Donaldson, S. (2000). Breakthroughs in scientific research: the discipline of nursing, 1960-1999. *Annual Review of Nursing Research 2000, 18,* 247-311.
39. Hinshaw, A.S. (1989). Nursing science: The challenge to develop knowledge. *Nursing Science Quarterly 2,* 162-171.
40. Meleis, A.I. (1986). Theory development and domain concepts. In P. Moccia (ed.), *New approaches to theory development.* New York: National League for Nursing.
41. Scholtfeldt, R.M. (1988). Structuring nursing knowledge: A priority for creating nursing's future. *Nursing Science Quarterly 1,* 35-38.
42. Lindsey, A.M. (1990). Identification and labeling of human responses. *Journal of Professional Nursing 6,* 143-150.
43. Cowan, M.J. (1991). Nurse scientists: Research using a nursing and biological Science Model. In: *Nursing research: Global perspectives, 1991 International Council of Nurse Researchers Conference* (p. A411). Kansas City, Mo.: American Nurses' Association.
44. Hinshaw, A.S., Sigmon, H.D., & Lindsey, A. (1991). Interfacing nursing and biologic science. *Journal of Professional Nursing 7,* 264.
45. Walker, L. (1989). The future of theory development: Generic or specialty? Commentary and response. *Nursing Science Quarterly 2,* 118-119.
46. Stevenson, J.S. (1988). Nursing knowledge development: Into era II. *Journal of Professional Nursing 4,* 152-162.
47. Fawcett, J. (1983). *Analysis and evaluation of conceptual models of nursing* (2nd ed.). Philadelphia: F.A. Davis.
48. Walker, L.O., Avant, K.C. (1995). *Strategies for theory construction in nursing* (3rd ed.). Norwalk, Conn.: Appleton & Lange.
49. Lenz, E., Suppe, F., Gift, A., Pugh, L., & Milligan, R. (1995). Collaborative development of middle-range nursing theories: Toward a theory of unpleasant symptoms. *Advances in Nursing Science 17,* 1-13.
50. Hupcey, J.E., Morse, J.M., Lenz, E.R., & Tason, M.C. (1997). Methods of concept analysis in nursing: A critique of Wilsonian methods. In A.G. Gift (ed.), *Clarifying concepts in nursing research.* New York: Springer.
51. Ferrell, B.A., Ferrell, B.R., & Rivera, L. (1995). Pain in cognitively impaired nursing home patients. *Journal of Pain and Symptom Management 10,* 591-608.
52. Carrieri, V.K., Kieckhefer, G., Janson-Bjerklie, S., & Souza, J. (1991). The sensation of pulmonary dyspnea in school-age children. *Nursing Research 40,* 81-85.
53. Puntillo, K.A., Weiss, S.J. (1994). Pain: Its mediators and associated morbidity in critically ill cardiovascular surgical patients. *Nursing Research 43,* 31-36.
54. Janson-Bjerklie, S., Carrieri, V.K., & Hudes, M. (1986). The sensations of pulmonary dyspnea. *Nursing Research 35,* 154-159.
55. Dodd, M., Janson, S., Facione, N., Faucett, L., Froelicher, E.S., Humphreys, J., et al. (2001). Advancing the science of symptom management. *Journal of Advanced Nursing 33,* 668-676.
56. Sindhu, F. (1996). Are non-pharmacological nursing interventions for the management of pain effective—a meta-analysis. *Journal of Advanced Nursing 24,* 1152-1159.

57. Carrieri-Kohlman, V., Gormley, J.M., Douglas, M.K., Paul, S.M., & Stulbarg, M.S. (1996). Exercise training decreases dyspnea and the distress and anxiety associated with it. Monitoring alone may be as effective as coaching. *Chest 110,* 1526-1535.
58. Savedra, M.C., Tesler, M.D. (1989). Assessing children's and adolescents' pain. *Pediatrician 16,* 24-29.
59. Grant, M., Anderson, P., Ashley, M., Dean, G., Ferrell, B., Kawa-Singer, M., et al. (1998). Developing a team for multicultural multi-institutional research on fatigue and quality of life. *Oncology Nursing Forum 25,* 1404-1412.
60. Mock, V., Ropka, M.E., Rhodes, V.A., Pickett, M., Grimm, P.M., McDaniel, R., et al. (1998). Establishing mechanisms to conduct multi-institutional research—fatigue in patients with cancer: An exercise intervention. *Oncology Nursing Forum 25,* 1391-1397.
61. King, I.M. (1988). Concepts: Essential elements of theories. *Nursing Science Quarterly 1,* 22-25.
62. Meleis, A.I. (1991). *Theoretical nursing: development and progress* (2nd ed). Philadelphia: J.B. Lippincott.
63. Newman, M.A. (1981). Theory for nursing practice. *Nursing Science Quarterly 7,* 153-157.
64. Riehl-Sisca, J.P. (1989). *Conceptual models for nursing practice* (3rd ed.). Norwalk, Conn.: Appleton & Lange.
65. Beckstrand, J. (1980). A critique of several conceptions of practice theory in nursing. *Research in Nursing and Health 1,* 175-179.
66. Shaver, J.F. (1985). A biopsychosocial view of human health. *Nursing Outlook 33,* 186-191.
67. Beck, C.T. (1985). Theoretical frameworks cited in *Nursing Research* from January, 1974-June, 1985. *Nurse Educator 10,* 36-38.
68. Mood, L.E., Wilson, M.E., Smith, R., Schwartz, R., Tittle, M., & Van Cott, M.L. (1988). Analysis of a decade of nursing practice research, 1977-1986. *Nursing Research 37,* 374-379.
69. Gortner, S.R., & Schultz, P.R. (1988). Approaches to nursing science methods. *Image: Journal of Nursing Scholarship 20,* 22-24.
70. Roy, C.L. (1988). An explication of the philosophical assumptions of the Roy adaptation model of nursing. *Nursing Science Quarterly 1,* 26-34.
71. Kim, H.S. (1987). Structuring the nursing knowledge system: A typology of four domains. *Scholarly Inquiry for Nursing Practice: An International Journal 1,* 99-110.
72. Orem, D.E. (1985). *Nursing: Concepts of practice* (3rd ed.). New York: McGraw-Hill.
73. Goosen, G.M. (1989). Concept analysis: An approach to teaching physiologic variables. *Journal of Professional Nursing 5,* 31-38.
74. Murdaugh, C.L. (1999). Relationship of research perspectives to methodology. In A.S. Hinshaw, S.L. Feetham, & J.L.F. Shaver (ed.), *Handbook of clinical nursing research* (pp. 61-68). Thousand Oaks, Calif: Sage.
75. Norbeck, J.S. (1987). In defense of empiricism. *Image: Journal of Nursing Scholarship 19,* 28-30.
76. Suppe, F. (1992). Paradigms, socialization and nursing science. In *Proceedings of the 1992 Annual Forum on Nursing. Doctoral Education. Nursing as a human science. Prevailing paradigms and their implications for preparing nurse scientists* (pp. 17-34). Baltimore: University of Maryland.
77. Morse, J.M. (1991). Approaches to qualitative-quantitative methodological triangulation. *Nursing Research 40,* 120-123.
78. Zielstorff, R.D., Tronni, C., Basque, J., Griffin, L.R., & Welebob, E.M. (1998). Mapping nursing diagnosis nomenclatures for coordinated care. *Image: Journal of Nursing Scholarship 30,* 369-373.
79. Whitley, G.G. (1999). Processes and methodologies for research validation of nursing diagnoses. *Nursing Diagnosis 10,* 5-14.
80. Wilson, J. (1969). *Thinking with concepts.* Cambridge, England: Cambridge University Press.
81. Gibson, C. (1991). A concept of empowerment. *Journal of Advanced Nursing 16,* 354-361.
82. Pender, N. (1996). *Health promotion in nursing practice* (3rd ed.). Stamford, Conn.: Appleton & Lange.
83. Hinshaw, A.S. (1999). Evolving nursing research traditions. In A.S. Hinshaw, S.L. Feetham, & J.L.F. Shaver (eds.), *Handbook of clinical nursing research* (pp. 19-30). Thousand Oaks, Calif: Sage.
84. The University of California, San Francisco School of Nursing Symptom Management Faculty Group. (1994). A model for symptom management. *Image: Journal of Nursing Scholarship 26,* 272-276.
85. Johnson, J.E. (1973). Effects of accurate expectations about sensations on the sensory and distress components of pain. *Journal of Personality and Social Psychology 27,* 261-275.
86. Page, G.G., & Ben-Eliyahu, S. (1998). Pain kills: Animal models and neuroimmunological links. In R. Payne, R.B. Patt, & C.S. Hill (eds.), *Progress in patient research and management* (p. 135). Seattle: IASP Press.
87. Kim, M.J. (1988). Physiologic responses in health and illness: An overview. *Annual Review of Nursing Research 5,* 79-104.

SECTION I

Alterations in Regulation

Physiological processes are regulated by exquisitely sensitive controlling and integrating systems; when changes occur, compensatory mechanisms serve to return the processes involved to a normal range of function. The actions of these mechanisms are regulation. When the situational or developmental stressors are sufficiently great or of such prolonged duration that the compensatory mechanisms are unable to bring the processes to a normal range of function, pathological states evolve.

There are numerous examples of this very exquisite regulation of physiological processes. Maintenance of the narrow range of serum calcium; rapid changes in cardiovascular functions when an individual rises to a standing position or exercises; maintenance of blood glucose or pH levels, body temperature, and involuntary changes in respiratory rate or food intake are examples of regulation, that is, maintenance of homeostasis. The myriad complex actions and interactions that occur to keep the individual within a normal range of physiological functioning across systems are generally referred to as *homeostatic mechanisms.*

When the specific changes are identified and the mechanisms involved and the pathological consequences are understood, it then becomes possible to determine what actions or influences nurses may have on alleviating, preventing, or mediating the effects of the consequences and monitoring parameters indicative of the clinical outcome. This kind of nursing practice requires considerable knowledge and ability to comprehend the physiologically and pathophysiologically complex interactions that occur in health and illness.

The six chapters included in this section present phenomena in which alterations in regulatory processes have occurred. These pathophysiological phenomena are alterations in thermoregulation, anorexia, protein calorie malnutrition, circadian rhythm disorders, urinary incontinence, and chemical dependency. These responses are observed frequently in a variety of clinical conditions and across health care settings.

Alterations in thermoregulation may be induced deliberately or may result from disturbances in the thermoregulatory mechanisms. Anorexia reflects alterations in one or more of the physiological processes involved in the regulation of food intake and ultimately in maintaining energy balance. Protein calorie malnutrition results from a variety of alterations, ranging from decreased intake to increased metabolic rate and energy expenditure or from excessive loss of nutrients. Circadian rhythm disorders change an individual's ability to adapt to the external temporal environment and disturb the internal circadian regulation of physiological and metabolic events. Urinary incontinence can be caused by defects in the storage of urine, alterations in urinary elimination, or disturbances in the regulation of both storage and emptying of urine. Chemical dependency, addictions to alcohol, tobacco, and/or street drugs may result from dysfunctional substance use behaviors and lead to alterations in the regulation of many physiological processes.

These particular phenomena were selected as being representative of alterations in regulation. They are seen frequently in a wide variety of health care settings, and they are phenomena for which nurses can have a primary role in identifying, preventing, or alleviating. Nurses also have a primary role in monitoring and documenting the clinical progress of patients with such responses. These professional nursing activities can occur only when nurses have a sufficient comprehension of the phenomena and their attendant complexities. The following chapters provide information that may serve as the basis for professional nursing practice.

CHAPTER

2 Alterations in Thermoregulation

BARBARA J. HOLTZCLAW

DEFINITION

Altered thermoregulation is the impaired ability to regulate body heat and maintain body temperature within a range that is optimal for physiological function. For most persons, body temperature varies no more than 1°C (1.8°F) throughout life, unless there is fever or impaired function. Yet what appears to be an unwavering state involves constant *change.* Change stimulates the highly integrated control mechanisms within several body regulatory systems that influence temperature. The term *dynamic equilibrium* has no more fitting example than thermoregulation. Physical laws of thermodynamics govern the passive transfer of heat throughout the body and to the environment, but physiological mechanisms and behavioral responses drastically influence this process. Heat continuously moves from warmer to cooler regions and is passively lost to the environment by conduction, convection, radiation, and evaporation. Active physiological processes produce heat by metabolic and kinetic activity and conserve heat by shunting circulation away from the body surface. Heat is actively lost by vasodilation and evaporation of sweat. During environmental temperature extremes, behavioral responses conserve or disseminate body heat by changes in body position, physical movement, choice of protective clothing or shelter, and intake of food. Alterations in thermoregulation occur when (1) environmental temperatures overwhelm existing physiological and behavioral resources or (2) disease, injury, or effects of drugs impair one or more physiological mechanisms affecting heat loss, heat generation, or heat conservation.

OVERVIEW OF THERMOREGULATION

A brief review of thermal physiology is helpful in understanding alterations in thermoregulation. Thermoregulatory control centers are located in the brain and are responsive to integrated feedback from thermosensitive receptors in skin, deep body organs, and the central nervous system. The thermoneutral range within which core body temperatures vary without initiating cooling or warming responses is called the thermoregulatory *set-point range.* Deviations above or below thermoneutral levels stimulate control centers that initiate compensatory warming and cooling mechanisms to defend and restore thermoneutral core temperatures. Rising temperatures increase firing rates of heat-sensitive receptors that stimulate cooling responses (vasodilation and sweating). Falling temperatures promote faster firing rates in cold-sensitive receptors and trigger warming responses (vasoconstriction and shivering).

It is tempting to compare the thermoregulatory set-point with a thermostat, but this comparison is far too simplistic a model. Although the set-point range is fairly constant within an individual, there are diurnal variations influenced by hormones and elevated by pyrogens. Ovulatory activity is a well-known modulator of body temperature throughout the menstrual cycle. Complex interrelationships between the thermoneutral range, circadianicity, and biochemical changes are still not completely understood.

As *homeotherms,* or warm-blooded animals, humans are capable of adjusting to or altering their environment. The body maintains the thermoneutral state through parsimonious use and conservation of energy sources. Heat is produced by the body's never-ceasing expenditure of oxygen and nutrients. Cellular metabolism of food, friction produced by contracting muscles and the flow of blood also produces heat. Heat is transferred to the body from solar radiation, contact with warm surfaces, and ingested warm food and drinks. Short-term increases in body temperature may occur during exercise or emotional stress. However, even hyperthyroidism-induced elevations in core body temperature tend to be minimal, because heat is effectively disseminated by increased skin blood flow and sweating. A highly effective system of circulatory shunts redistributes heat to achieve a relatively stable internal temperature when environmental temperatures fall. Vasoconstriction creates a virtual "layer" of nonperfused cutaneous tissue that insulates the underlying organs and vasculature. Shivering generates heat, but muscle contractions promote cutaneous blood flow that enhances heat loss to the environment. This makes shivering ineffective during prolonged cold exposure. Shivering also has high metabolic costs that are three to five times the resting level.[1]

Alterations in Thermoregulation

Thermoregulatory alterations essentially are disorders of heat loss or heat gain (Figure 2-1). Factors inducing these alterations may be environmental, physiological, or a combination of both. Alterations are viewed in this chapter as *hypothermic states, heat illness,* and *febrile responses*. In *hypothermia,* the person is unable to produce or recover sufficient heat to regain that being lost. In heat illness a state of *hyperthermia* exists that reflects an inability to lose heat effectively. Extremes of hypothermia and hyperthermia are characterized by eventual loss of thermoregulatory function:—either from loss of neural conduction by cold or the denaturation of neural protein by heat. This state, called *poikilothermia,* renders the patient incapable of initiating warming or cooling responses, so the body temperature rises or falls toward that of the environment. Elevated temperature in *fever* is the thermal outcome of the febrile response. Thermoregulation remains intact but operates at a higher than normal level.

Measurement of Body Temperature

Continuous monitoring of core temperature with reliable thermometers is indicated for persons at highest risk of temperature alterations. For others, intermittent measurement is usually sufficient, unless there are rapidly developing conditions that could affect thermodynamic states. Newer thermometers that are capable of reading temperatures in the lower range improve detection of accidental hypothermia in clinical settings. *Oral temperature* measurements tend to correlate well with core temperatures during fever, because skin and mucous membranes are well perfused with warm blood. Oral thermometers can only be used if the patient is fully conscious and cooperative; these cannot be used during sleep or stuporous conditions. In hypothermia, hyperthermia, and high fever, the measurement of interest is the *core* or central temperature. Lack of uniformity regarding the term *core* causes confusion, so the measurement site should be designated in reporting values. Of greatest concern is the temperature of the brain, which is at risk during extremely high temperatures. Temperature measurements from the pulmonary artery, esophagus, and tympanic membrane yield close estimates of blood temperature circulating to the brain.

Measurement of *rectal temperature* has long been used to estimate core temperature but carries the hazard of rectal perforation in neonates or restless adults. Soft, pliable thermistor probes or unbreakable electronic thermometers have replaced mercury-in-glass thermometers. Indwelling electronic thermistor probes safely provide continuous measurement in seriously ill patients and provide a good index of *changes* in heat distribution during cooling and rewarming. By contrast, the temperature of the rectum cannot reliably be used to estimate brain and central nervous system temperature. Because the rectum and other regions of the gut derive their temperature from their own blood flow, initial stages of hypothermia, hyperthermia, hypovolemia, and shock may shunt circulation away from the gut to vital centers. *Bladder temperature* can be measured by a thermistor in the indwelling urinary bladder catheter for continuous measurement from the abdominal region. However, this site has many of the same limitations as rectal temperature during hemodynamic and thermal instability.

A core site that approximates temperatures of the heart and arterial blood to the brain is obtained from thermistors in the *pulmonary artery* catheter in persons with hemodynamic monitoring systems. An indwelling electronic *tympanic membrane* thermistor provides another central measure with continuous readings, but this device has the potential for discomfort and perforation with patient movement. Thermistors can be used for continuous *esophageal* and *nasopharyngeal temperature* measurement during surgery and anesthesia, but prolonged use has the potential for trauma to the esophagus or nasopharynx. The accuracy of temperatures from these sites is influenced by the temperature of inhaled gases. Accuracy is improved by placing the esophageal probe in the lower fourth of the esophagus near the heart, but there is an associated risk of tracheoesophageal fistula from prolonged use. Proximity of the esophagus to the heart makes this site inappropriate for patients on cardiopulmonary bypass pumps. Use of *infrared tympanic membrane* thermometers to measure central temperatures is convenient and comfortable for patients who do not require continuous measurement. There is controversy concerning their use in children

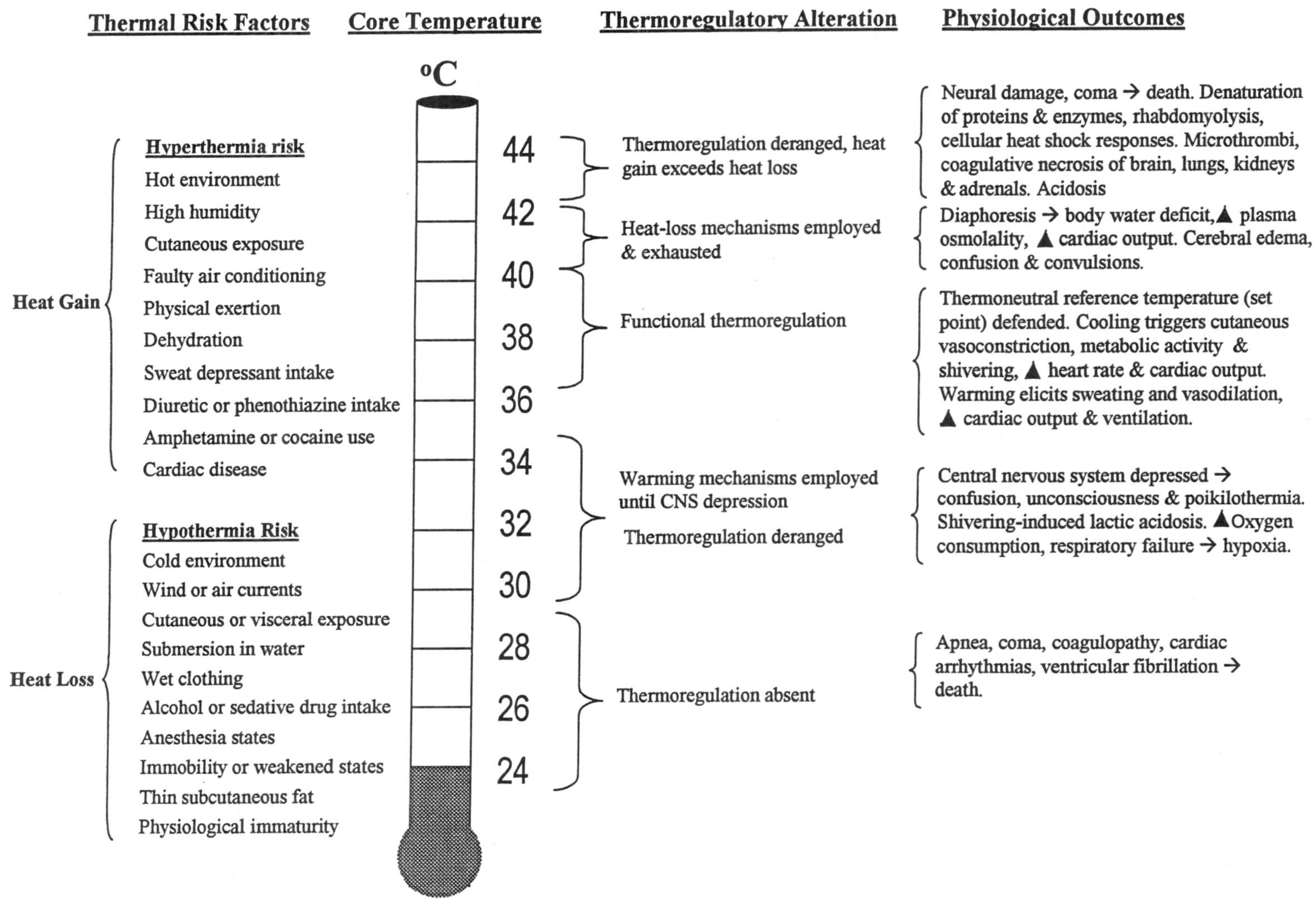

Figure 2-1 Thermoregulatory alterations reflect the body's inability to lose or gain heat sufficiently to match the heat load or deficit. Hypothermia occurs when warming and heat-conserving mechanisms are unable to compete with loss of body heat. Hyperthermia develops when total body heat load overwhelms heat loss mechanisms. Thermoregulatory mechanisms are not altered in fever but defend a higher set-point elevated by a pyrogen.

and the benefits of training personnel in their use.[2-4] Evidence exists that these instruments are less reliable in the upper and lower extremes of measurement needed to monitor a hypothermic or a hyperthermic patient.[5]

Understanding Risks and Dynamics of Altered Thermoregulation

Factors leading to alterations in thermoregulation differ, depending on the health, level of maturation, and environmental situation of the patient. Certain drugs and anesthetic agents will temporarily impair thermoregulatory responses, even in healthy persons. Overwhelming heat and dehydration also threaten persons of apparent good health. Conversely, seemingly mild environmental changes will create thermal stress for the immature infant or the seriously ill adult. In the following sections, hypothermic states, heat illness, and febrile responses will be examined from the perspectives of risk, pathological consequences, manifestations, surveillance, and management.

HYPOTHERMIC STATES: EXTREME INDUCED OR ACCIDENTAL HEAT LOSS

DEFINITION

Hypothermia is a condition of mild to profound heat loss that exceeds the body's ability to maintain the lower limits of normal body temperature (below 35°C [95°F]). *Induced hypothermia* refers to lowering body temperature intentionally for therapeutic reasons. It can be accomplished by surface-cooling with ice packs or cooling blankets, or by means of central heat exchange using a cardiopulmonary bypass pump. Hypothermia is induced in controlled clinical settings but has many of the same risks as does accidental hypothermia. Risks during cooling and rewarming phases are reduced by (1) vigilant monitoring of central and peripheral temperatures, (2) life-support devices to treat emerging cardiac responses and maintain oxygenation, and (3) physical and pharmacological approaches to suppress shivering. Shivering and vasoconstriction during hypothermic cardiac surgery are controlled with drugs and anesthesia. During recovery and rewarming, however, shivering may require use of drugs, ventilatory support, and treatment of acid-base disorders. Surface-cooling procedures are often performed on patients on a clinical unit by nursing staff. Care is needed to prevent shivering and avoid a sudden drift or fall in temperatures to lethal levels.

Accidental hypothermia tends to be the most hazardous hypothermic state, because it usually arises in extremely cold environmental conditions without available treatment. Progressive deterioration of all organ systems quickly leads to death if untreated. The potential for hypothermia exists in less extreme conditions if an individual's capacity for conserving and producing body heat is impaired. Elderly persons, neonates, and those with compromised cardiovascular function fall into this category. Degrees of hypothermia are defined in terms of *duration* (prolonged, acute, and chronic) or *severity* (mild, moderate, and profound). Table 2-1 lists levels and characteristics of each.

PREVALENCE AND POPULATIONS AT RISK

Induced hypothermia is used to treat heatstroke or other hyperthermic states, to reduce cerebral edema in neurological injury, and to lower cellular metabolism and oxygen demand during cardiac surgery. Although the cardiopulmonary bypass pump both cools and rewarms the circulation, rewarming is often incomplete. Heat from warmed blood is lost to previously vasoconstricted regions and lower extremities. Uneven distribution of heat makes the patient vulnerable to shivering and complications of hypothermia for several hours after a bypass procedure.[6]

Accidental or inadvertent hypothermia can occur in healthy persons when they are exposed to low environmental temperatures without adequate protection. People caught unprepared for severe weather during travel, hunting, or camping expeditions are particularly vulnerable. Homeless persons who sleep on cold pavement are frequently found to be hypothermic. Submersion in water for even short periods during boating accidents or flooding conditions can quickly lead to hypothermia.

In clinical situations, hypothermia may be brought about by drugs and anesthetic agents that impair thermoregulatory responses and inhibit behavioral heat conservation. During surgery, loss of heat from open wounds and moist operative surfaces is common. Severely burned patients are at risk because of loss of protective insulation from skin and exposure of denuded surfaces to the air. Immature infants, weak or debilitated adults, and paralyzed patients are at risk, because they are often unable to perceive heat loss, control their environment, or assume heat-conserving positions.

TABLE 2-1 Levels of Hypothermia and Corresponding Clinical Changes

LEVEL	CORE TEMPERATURE	DURATION	ACID-BASE CHANGES	RESPIRATORY AND CARDIOVASCULAR SIGNS	NEUROLOGICAL SIGNS
Mild	34°–35°C (93.2°–95°F)	Acute (few hours) and chronic (days or weeks)	Respiratory and cold diuresis-induced alkalosis and hypocapnia. Rise in metabolic rate five times normal.	Hyperventilation. Peripheral vasoconstriction, increase in BP, HR, and CO. Blood viscosity increases as temperature falls and with cold-induced diuresis causes sludging and coagulopathy.	Sensation of cold, confusion disorientation. Vigorous shivering.
Moderate	30°–34°C (86°–93.2°F)	Acute (few hours)	Respiratory acidosis. At 32°C (89.6°F), 50% fall in CO_2 production and O_2 consumption.	Shallow respirations. BP hard to detect. J wave may appear on ECG. Premature ventricular beats common. At 32°C (89.6°F), prolonged systole lowers HR and CO 30%. Atrial and ventricular dysrhythmias lower HR and CO 50%.	Confusion, stupor, exaggerated tendon reflex and hyperactivity. At 30°C (86°F), pupils dilated, hallucinations and paradoxical undressing. Muscles rigid.
Deep	17°–30°C (62.6°–86°F)	Prolonged (several hours)	Progressive acidosis from pooled circulation and shivering-induced lactic acid.	At 27°–30°C (80.6°–86°F), danger of arrhythmias from cardiac irritability. Below 28°C (82.4°F), atrial fibrillation is common. Death from ventricular fibrillation is possible.	Below 28°C (82.4°F), atrial fibrillation and other arrhythmias are common. Muscle reflexes absent. Muscle rigidity abolished at 26° C (78.8°F).
Profound	<17°C (<62.6°F)	Few to several hours	Combined respiratory and metabolic acidosis. Fall in renal blood flow, and glomerular filtration parallels CO.	At about 10°C (50°F), the QRS disappears on ECG, and only the P wave is visible.	Corneal reflex absent. Disturbed cerebrovascular autoregulation.

BP, Blood pressure; *CO*, cardiac output; *ECG*, electrocardiogram; *HR*, heart rate.

RISK FACTORS

Environmental Factors

Cold climate, in which exposure to high wind, rain, snow, and sleet is possible, and submersion in water are the most obvious environmental factors that cause accidental hypothermia. A less apparent factor is contact with cold surfaces, which conduct heat away from the body. Accident victims who lie on cold pavement for extended periods are particularly at risk for hypothermia. Persons sitting on concrete steps or metal benches and patients lying on cold x-ray or examining tables are also at risk. Submersion in water hastens hypothermia as a result of water's greater thermal conductivity compared with air. All near-drowning accident survivors also must be assessed for hypothermia. The surgical suite is notorious for inducing hypothermia in general surgery patients because of low ambient temperatures, laminar flow of air, and the tendency for instruments and irrigating solutions to cool quickly.

Personal and Developmental Factors

Sedentary or impaired activity increases risk for heat loss to the environment. Alcohol consumption is a common precursor to hypothermia in cold climates. Skin vasodilation and sweating caused by alcohol ingestion causes a false sense of warmth while enhancing heat loss to surrounding air and surfaces. Some drugs, including barbiturates, phenothiazines, and benzodiazepines, promote heat loss. General anesthesia suppresses thermoregulatory activity and promotes hypothermia. Perioperative heat loss has traditionally been considered a consequence of inhibition of vasoconstriction and shivering. A more recent postulate is that general anesthesia widens the interthreshold zone (ITZ), allowing wider fluctuations of body temperature to exist without stimulating thermoregulatory defenses.[7]

Developmental factors that predispose infants and some elderly persons to risk of hypothermia include reduced fatty insulation, weak musculature, and reduced metabolic rate. An infant does not shiver and generates heat by metabolizing fat in brown adipose tissue (BAT). Low-birthweight infants lack body fat for insulation and BAT for heat generation and are less able to curl up into heat-conserving postures. Metabolism of BAT requires oxygen expenditure, so falling body temperatures can increase oxygen consumption to levels causing respiratory distress. The ability to maintain body temperatures in cold temperatures declines in advanced age. Elderly patients tend to become more hypothermic than younger patients during surgery and take longer to rewarm. Many older adults seem less able to sense falling temperatures, and their reduced sensitivity may fail to induce shivering and vasoconstriction.[8]

MECHANISMS

Although the exact mechanisms are still not known, reduced heat generation in older persons is believed to be caused by inefficient autonomic control and reduced peripheral vasoconstriction capability.[9] Other factors may be low basal metabolism and poor food intake. The risk of heat loss and hypothermia is not limited to outdoor exposure; sedentary living, poorly heated homes, and lack of supportive supervision may contribute to conditions conducive to insidious hypothermia in persons with inefficient autonomic control.

PATHOLOGICAL CONSEQUENCES

All body systems are affected by hypothermia, although the most lethal consequences involve the heart. Effects on the nervous system create a particularly deadly feature of hypothermia by causing a paradoxical shift in set-point as a result of severe impairment of thermoregulatory function. This grave pathological sign indicates that all autonomic and thermoregulatory defenses are overwhelmed. The person becomes *poikilothermic* and the body temperature continues to fall.[10] Falling temperatures and declining nerve conduction velocity lead to progressive depression of mental function. When core temperatures reach about 31°C (87.8°F), confusion and stupor, exaggerated tendon reflex, and hyperactivity occur. The heart rate slows and electrocardiographic abnormalities are made worse by poor oxygenation. Premature ventricular beats are common throughout cooling. Changes in the cardiac conduction system in hypothermia are attributed to temperature-dependent kinetics and ion channel conductance in the cardiac action potential. Below 28°C (82.4°F), atrial fibrillation and other arrhythmias, loss of consciousness, and apnea are reflections of altered cardiac conduction and loss of neurological reflexes. At about 10°C (50°F), the QRS complex disappears and only the P wave persists.[9] Hypothermic cooling initially raises blood glucose and insulin levels, although shivering quickly depletes glycogen and induces hypoglycemia.

During initial cooling, osmotic diuresis contributes to sodium and chloride loss and nearly doubles the volume of urine produced. Blood viscosity increases as temperature falls, and body water is lost from cold-induced diuresis. This contributes to sludging and coagulopathy during hypothermia. Although respiratory arrest in accidental hypothermia and near-drowning raises the potential for respiratory acidosis, the ability of the kidneys to regulate acid-base balance is also reduced.

RELATED PATHOPHYSIOLOGICAL CONCEPTS

Dynamic acid-base changes reflect initial alkalosis from hyperventilation and diuresis, followed by progressive acidosis from pooled blood and shivering-induced increases in lactic acid levels.

DIFFERENTIAL DIAGNOSIS

Differential diagnosis of acid-base alterations is made by careful surveillance of arterial blood gases within the context of the history and progress of the hypothermic episode. Metabolic acidosis is most likely to occur during rewarming, when metabolites return to the systemic circulation. It is manifested in rising concentrations of fixed acids, base bicarbonate deficit, and falling arterial pH.

MANIFESTATIONS AND SURVEILLANCE

For those caring for persons at high risk of hypothermia, prevention should be the primary concern. In clinical situations with close monitoring, the first manifestation of hypothermia is usually a fall in core temperature below 35°C (95°F). However, for persons who are exposed to low temperatures in the home or environment, confusion and disorientation may be the first overt sign. As judgment becomes clouded, a person may remove clothing and fail to seek shelter, and hypothermia can progress to profound levels. Surveillance of home-dwelling elderly patients and persons who are rescued from snow or water submersion should include consideration of confusion and disorientation as a possible sign of hypothermia.

Falling core temperatures stage the progression of hypothermia through mild, moderate, deep and profound hypothermia, with each stage affecting vital organ function (see Table 2-1). Shivering activity is a risk factor for lactic acidosis. A shivering severity index (Box 2-1) developed by Abbey and modified by Holtzclaw provides a standardized scale to aid in documentation.[6] As temperatures fall, cardiac arrhythmias become more pronounced. A pathognomonic marker of hypothermia is the humplike *J wave,* also called the *Osborn wave,* seen in lead V_4 at the junction of the QRS complex and S-T segment.[12] The absence of the J wave should not rule out a diagnosis of hypothermia, because it is only detected in about a third of hypothermic patients.

Box 2-1 Shivering Severity Index

Shivering follows cephalad to caudal progression:
- Undetected tremors in masseter muscles
- Visible face/neck contractions
- Visible chest/abdominal contractions
- Extremity contractions/teeth chattering

From Holtzclaw, B.J., & Geer, R.T. (1995). Clinical predictors and metabolic consequences of postoperative shivering after cardiac surgery. In S. Funk, E. Tornquist, M. Champagne, & R. Weise (eds.), *Key aspects of caring for the acutely ill: Technological aspects, patient education, and quality of life* (pp. 226-233). New York: Springer.

Vigilant monitoring of a hypothermic patient is necessary, with comprehensive assessment of neurological activity, oxygenation, renal function, and fluid and electrolyte balance. Continuous digital core temperature readings from hemodynamic monitoring systems are ideal for assessing temperature drift and rapid changes. Indwelling thermistors from body orifices can also provide constant surveillance, and esophageal temperatures closely parallel those of the heart and brain. Rectal and urinary bladder temperatures are less reliable indicators of change, because they tend to lag behind. Whether the patient is being recovered from a hypothermic condition or hypothermia is being induced, the assessment of systemic and tissue oxygenation is paramount. Arterial and venous oxygen saturations are closely monitored, and artificial ventilation is sometimes indicated. Neurological reflexes are observed in conditions of accidental hypothermia to determine its depth and to assess stages of recovery. During intentional or therapeutic cooling, continuous observations of irritability and sedation induced by hypothermia provide early warning signs of undesirable progression. Monitoring urinary output from an indwelling catheter at 15-minute intervals can indicate hypothermia-induced cold diuresis in early stages and later, declining renal function.

CLINICAL MANAGEMENT

Managing Induced Hypothermia After Cardiac Bypass Cooling

After hypothermic cardiopulmonary bypass surgery, hemodynamic instability is aggravated by shivering, temperature drift, and acid-base imbalance. Return of pooled blood from cold unperfused regions brings fixed acids and metabolites that contribute to acidosis. Rapid rewarming is contraindicated to avoid "rewarm shock," in which peripheral vasodilation can significantly decrease systemic vascular resistance.[13] The need for coordinated intensive care during hypothermic rewarming is critical.

Managing Induced Hypothermia During Surface-Cooling

Precautions are necessary to guard against several complications when surface-cooling a patient. Protection of hands and feet and cushioning bony prominences with cotton wadding help to avoid damage from pressure on poorly perfused tissue. Prevention of *temperature drift, afterdrop,* and *shivering* is a significant task during surface-cooling. Drift refers to the tendency for core temperatures to rapidly follow skin temperatures when thermoregulatory reflexes are compromised. Drift contributes to shivering and vasomotor instability. Afterfall or afterdrop is the tendency for core temperatures to continue falling after cooling procedures are discontinued.[10] Drastic cooling stimulates shivering, a response that raises metabolic rate to five times the resting levels. Changes may exceed 1°C (1.8°F) in 15 minutes. Greater control over drift is achieved when the rate of cooling is controlled to allow core temperatures to fall more gradually. When thermoregulatory activity is suppressed, heat continues to flow from the body's deep regions to the cooler periphery. If afterdrop is undetected and untreated, temperatures may fall below 30°C (86°F). If nonpolarizing muscle relaxants are used to suppress shivering by paralysis, additional surveillance is required. Phenothiazines are only marginally effective in reducing shivering and can cause hypotension, tachycardia, and a tendency to core temperature drift. An alternative approach has been shown to reduce shivering during surface-cooling.[11] Three bath towels are placed lengthwise under arms and legs, with the sides drawn up and closed in a temporary "seam" by clips or tape. Tape is also used to close the ends to cover toes and fingertips. These insulating "boots" and "mittens" conserve body heat and protect dominant thermosensory nerve endings on hands and feet, while heat is lost from the trunk to the conductive cooling blanket. The trunk and head are left uncovered. There are fewer thermosensitive nerve endings on the surface of the trunk than in the extremities, so heat is conducted to the cooling blanket without stimulating shivering. By contrast, the skin on the extremities is well endowed with heat loss receptors but remains protected from cooling by insulating wraps.

Managing Accidental Hypothermia

Management of a mildly hypothermic patient involves restoring heat and supporting cardiac, respiratory and thermoregulatory functions. Rewarming options depend on the severity of heat loss. For temperatures above 32°C (89.6°F), the use of passive warming with heated bedclothes, warm convective air blankets, heat lamps or radiant panels, and warmed inhalation gases and intravenous fluids, is usually sufficient. Temperatures below 32°C (89.6°F) require more aggressive therapies, such as respiratory ventilation, drugs to treat shivering and arrhythmias, warmed intravenous fluids, peritoneal lavage, and cardiopulmonary bypass.

A hypothermic person rescued from harsh environmental conditions presents a management dilemma. Although there is an intuitive tendency for caregivers and rescuers to rewarm a profoundly hypothermic patient, there are inherent hazards in doing so. Rapid transport to an intensive emergency center is desirable. At core temperatures of 27° to 30°C (80.6° to 86.0°F), arrhythmias from cardiac irritability are common. Cardiopulmonary resuscitation (CPR) can intensify this danger and should be avoided except in the presence of apnea, ventricular fibrillation, or cardiac arrest. The fact that many persons have survived hypothermia after being found cold and asystolic attests to the cell-conservation powers of low body temperature. Metabolic demand for oxygen is diminished 10% for each degree Celsius fall in body temperature. Once the resuscitation and rewarming efforts begin, they must be continued until the patient has a core temperature of at least 32°C (89.6°F). At this time spontaneous cardioversion is likely, but there is danger of hyperkalemia, acidosis, and ventricular fibrillation. Antiarrhythmic agents, except for bretylium, are often ineffective in the treatment of profound hypothermia.[12] Electrical defibrillation may be indicated.

HYPERTHERMIA AND HEAT ILLNESS: ALTERED HEAT-LOSS MECHANISMS

DEFINITION

Hyperthermia occurs when the body's total heat load exceeds the body's ability to compensate for this excess. The source of the heat excess may be environmentally or endogenously produced.

PREVALENCE AND POPULATIONS AT RISK

The threat of heat disorders exists for all ages, but persons most at risk are those who are elderly and debilitated by chronic illness and those who work or exercise in hot, humid surroundings. Low-birthweight infants who are overheated in isolettes that have faulty thermal control systems are also at risk. The inability to compensate may be caused by physiological impairment or by an extreme of the environmental heat load. In other cases, hypermetabolism can be generated by abnormal muscle contractions and rigidity that produces hyperthermia. Two rare but potentially fatal examples of hypermetabolic conditions that produce uncontrolled heat generation are malignant hyperthermia (MH) and neuroleptic malignant syndrome (NMS).

RISK FACTORS

Environmental Factors

A primary environmental risk factor for heat illness is inadequate ventilation, protection from the sun, and lack of air conditioning. Avoiding overexposure is a primary prevention measure. Secondary prevention includes acclimation of persons to temperature and provision of rest and sufficient water. Tertiary prevention is aimed at early diagnosis and treatment of heat illness before serious disorders develop. High heat and humidity or excessive exercise may deplete body water stores and lead to heatstroke or heat exhaustion. Particularly vulnerable are those who work outdoors in extreme heat while engaged in physical activity, such as digging, firefighting, stonecutting, and military drills. Indoor workers in bakeries, forges, engine rooms, and foundries are also at risk. Each year, persons are affected by heat-related illness from engaging in outdoor sports activities in hot weather. As more adults over age 40 engage in jogging, bicycling, and marathons, the risk of illness resulting from heat intolerance grows.

Elderly persons tend to be less aware of rising environmental temperatures and may fail to take protective measures. They are at higher risk if they live in poorly ventilated homes without air conditioning. If individuals live in unsafe neighborhoods and keep windows and doors tightly closed, temperatures can rise quickly during warm weather.

Personal, Developmental, and Genetic Factors

Personal factors that increase risk of heat intolerance are body water deficit and inability to drink or replace fluid effectively. A person who is partially paralyzed after a stroke may be at risk during extremely warm weather, because he or she cannot reach the water glass or swallow without difficulty. Other personal risk factors include inability to move out of sunlight or to remove warm bedclothes. This is particularly prevalent in infants and elderly persons, who are often overheated in this manner.

Persons with a family history of malignant hyperthermia (MH) may be at risk during surgical procedures. This hereditary disorder is activated when potent inhalation anesthetics and most skeletal muscle relaxants are given.[14] Testing for MH before surgery is possible for those with a known family history, but this information is not always available. For this reason, routine screening and vigilant temperature monitoring throughout surgical procedures and recovery are essential.

MECHANISMS

Environmentally Induced Hyperthermia

The mechanisms of hyperthermia and heat illness are described by Hales[15] as a conflict between homeostatic demands that are cardiovascular and those that are thermoregulatory. The thermoregulatory drive increases skin blood flow and loss of fluid by sweating. These processes reduce central blood volume and initiate the cardiovascular drive to maintain central venous pressure by reducing skin blood flow and volume. Conservation of heat causes core temperatures to rise. Neural dysfunction results from cellular heat shock and thermoregulation becomes impaired. Exertional heatstroke combines the dysfunction of thermoregulation with the complications of coagulopathy and metabolic acidosis.

Hypermetabolic States

The mechanisms involved in MH and NMS, which are drug-related disorders, are hypermetabolic in nature. Both are life-threatening conditions. MH has a hereditary predisposition. Although the patient's muscle has normal structure, function, and appearance, it has an exaggerated response to inhalation anesthetics or depolarizing muscle relaxants. During MH crises, muscle cell membranes become unstable, myoplasmic calcium levels rise, and skeletal muscles develop rigid contractures. In early stages of MH, calcium levels remain relatively low in the myoplasm, so patients may manifest only fever and acid-base disorders. However, as calcium levels rise, severe muscle rigidity develops.[14] These violent muscle contractions generate heat, which may raise temperatures to 44°C (111.2°F). Irreversible neurological damage and death are inevitable without medical intervention. Death may be related to acute pulmonary edema, impaired coagulopathy, and acidosis.

Much less is known about NMS, a disorder with many similarities to MH. Unlike MH, NMS develops more slowly, has no known genetic predisposition. A violent reaction to one administration of a neuroleptic agent does not guarantee reactions to subsequent exposures.[16] Offending drugs include such neuroleptic drug groups as phenothiazines, thioxanthenes, and the butyrophenones. The mechanism of producing hypermetabolic changes lies in a drug's ability to antagonize central dopamine in the hypothalamus and basal ganglia.[17] Dopamine antagonism causes a centrally mediated increase in muscle tone and rigidity.

PATHOLOGICAL CONSEQUENCES

A continuum of pathological events in most heat illnesses leads from mild dizziness to life-threatening neurological damage. Left untreated, a patient with heat exhaustion loses heat-regulating mechanisms and develops heatstroke. *Heat edema* is common among unacclimatized persons entering a hot climate and is secondary to heat-induced vasodilation. *Heat syncope* and orthostatic dizziness arise early in heat injury as a result of volume depletion and postural hypotension. *Heat cramps* are strong and painful tetanic contractions in skeletal muscles of the extremities or the abdomen that result from sodium depletion and hypochloremia. Some rhabdomyolysis, or muscle tissue breakdown, may occur.[18] *Heat exhaustion,* the most common clinical disorder related to exercise in a hot environment, is attributed primarily to insufficient water intake and dehydration, leading to cardiovascular insufficiency. Core body temperature does not usually exceed 40°C (104°F) in heat exhaustion. However, falling blood volume promotes compensatory cutaneous vascular constriction to preserve central circulation. Reduced cutaneous heat loss can drive up core body temperature to precipitate heatstroke.[15] *Heatstroke* occurs when overheating affects the heat-regulating ability of the hypothalamus. It is a lethal and complex disorder characterized by neurological disturbance, anhidrosis and core body temperatures above 40.6°C (105.1°F). At elevations above 42°C (107.6°F), damage from coagulative necrosis of neural tissue may be irreversible. Metabolic acidosis is common during hyperthermia, caused by lactic acid elevations occurring when core temperatures rise to approximately 41° to 41.5°C (105.8° to 106.7°F).[18]

RELATED PATHOPHYSIOLOGICAL CONCEPTS/DIFFERENTIAL DIAGNOSIS

Temperature elevations may occur in hyperthyroidism and adrenocortical insufficiency, but rarely cause temperatures above 40°C (104°F). On the other hand, *thyroid storm,* a condition in hyperthyroidism in which high levels of thyroid hormone increase cellular permeability to sodium, can cause calcium to accumulate in the myoplasm. The resulting hyperthermia and muscle rigidity can be life threatening.[19] Thyroid storm usually occurs when thyrotoxicosis is poorly controlled and a precipitating factor, such as surgery, trauma, childbirth, or withdrawal of antithyroid drugs occurs. Treatment is aimed at (1) reducing serum thyroid hormone levels and blocking their action by means of antithyroid drugs, (2) preventing cardiovascular decompensation and reducing metabolic load by lowering body temperature, and (3) being vigilant for sepsis and other events that may have precipitated the thyroid storm. Body temperature is reduced by the use of cooling blankets, with drugs and insulation to suppress shivering.

MANIFESTATIONS AND SURVEILLANCE

Heat-Related Illness

Heat stress and hyperthermia are on a continuum of development and manifest symptoms differently within varying age groups and health conditions. The very young and very old are highly susceptible to "classical" heatstroke. Infants and small children have not developed maximal sweating capacity and have limited cardiovascular reserve. An elderly person may be taking medications that suppress sweat, cause diuresis, or contribute to hypermetabolism. Classical heatstroke is characterized by absence of sweating, severe respiratory alkalosis, absent or mild lactic acidosis, infrequent rhabdomyolysis, modest hyperuricemia, and a creatinine to blood urea nitrogen (BUN) ratio of 1:10. Hypocalcemia and hypoglycemia are uncommon, and disseminated intravascular coagulopathy (DIC), if present, is mild.[15] Other drugs, such as amphetamines or cocaine, can cause sufficient hyperactivity to induce hyperthermia. The contrast between these manifestations and those seen in healthy young adults, who are more susceptible to "exertional" heatstroke, reflects the differences in cause and outcomes. Heatstroke is the leading cause of death among athletes. Most commonly seen in men, exertional heatstroke is related to physical activity in a hot environment with insufficient intake of water. Sweating is usually present, and respiratory alkalosis is mild. Lactic acidosis is often present, as is acute renal failure. Endotoxin-like outcomes are common and include disseminated intravascular coagulopathy (DIC), petechial hemorrhages, hyperkalemia, hypotension, and acidosis. Coagulopathy contributes to declining oxygenation of vital organs, such as the brain, liver, adrenal glands, and kidneys. Microemboli and coagulative necrosis are seen in postmortem findings.[15]

Monitoring for heat-related illness is directed toward prevention. Health care providers for community, school, and military training programs should be alert for heat illness when exertional activities take place in hot and humid weather. Orthostatic syncope in a hot environment indicates heat-induced cutaneous vasodilation and reduced cerebral circulation. Tetanic and painful muscular cramps from exertional heat stress are caused by salt depletion and tend to occur when the person stops to rest. Hyponatremia, hypochloremia, and low urinary sodium and chloride levels are seen clinically.[19] Provision of oral liquids containing electrolytes, cessation of activity, and rest in a cool environment is aimed at halting progression to more serious heat illness. Monitoring for heat exhaustion requires assessment of body temperature as well as hydration status. Complaints of headache, weakness, fatigue, and impaired judgment are often combined with thirst, nausea, and vomiting. Core temperature is moderately elevated, but usually below 40°C (104°F).[15] Detecting early onset of heatstroke and cooling the person promptly is crucial to averting morbidity and mortality. Hallmarks are dehydration, salt depletion, shock, and respiratory distress. Confusion, personality change, delirium, and coma show progressive nervous system dysfunction. Rectal temperatures rise uncontrollably above 40°C (104°F), making the threat of neural damage imminent. Cooling by means of immersion in ice water, application of a conductive cooling blanket or ice packs, or directing a powerful fan on the wet body surface, are ways body temperature is rapidly lowered. Shaking chills and convulsive fasciculations often accompany aggressive cooling, which increases the risk of temperature drift. For this reason, after treatment is instituted, continual monitoring of rectal temperature by an indwelling thermistor probe is necessary. Treatment is aimed at lowering temperature 2.2° to 3.3°C (3.96° to 5.94°F) per hour. Cooling measures should be discontinued when core temperatures reach 38.9°C (102°F).[19]

Hypermetabolic States

Temperature changes are not the first manifestation of MH and NMS. Instead, the clinical presentation begins with cardiovascular signs and muscle rigidity. The rising temperature is the *consequence* of muscle rigidity and is a late indicator of a pathological condition. For this reason, surveillance must be anticipated in all situations in which anesthetic and neuroleptic drugs are given. In MH the earliest sign is muscle rigidity, beginning with the masseter muscles and often becoming generalized to the extremities. Abrupt sinus tachycardia is a consistent sign, and other arrhythmias occur as hypermetabolic processes, hyperkalemia, acidosis, hypoxemia, and hyperthermia develop. A rapid rise in core temperature is a late sign, with levels rising to 44°C (111.2°F). Flushed skin, profuse sweating, cyanosis, and mottling of skin caused by rising catecholamine levels are classic signs of MH. Rising end-tidal CO_2, despite hyperventilation, is a consistent sign.[16] The patient must be monitored for electrolyte disturbances, which are usually severe. Hyperkalemia results from the increased muscle cell permeability, yet treatment that is too aggressive may lead to hypokalemia and hypocalcemia. Rhabdomyolysis is also a late sign, and as serum myoglobin rises, renal damage occurs. Creatine kinase (CK) rises from values below 170 U/L to levels in the thousands. Acidosis contributes to erythrocyte lysis and microthrombi. Intravascular clotting and consumption of clotting factors play a role in the development of DIC, a major cause of death in MH. Other causes of death include ventricular fibrillation, acute pulmonary edema, renal failure, and cerebral edema. NMS begins with changes in consciousness levels, ranging from abnormal movements and confusion to coma. Cardiovascular lability is reflected in fluctuating blood pressure and pulse, flushing, and profuse sweating. Muscle stiffness resembling "lead pipe" resistance is followed by rising core body temperature in excess of 42°F (107.6°F). Although the same threat of electrolyte disturbance, rhabdomyolysis, DIC, and cardiac arrhythmias seen in MH is present in NMS, the most common cause of death is acute respiratory failure from hypoxia and acidosis.[16] The importance of surveillance in *prevention* of these two rare but potentially fatal disorders cannot be overemphasized. Both are amenable to early treatment, but without early recognition and aggressive definitive treatment, they are fatal.

CLINICAL MANAGEMENT

Treatment of heat-related illness must be aggressive and based on the cause of the condition.

Environmentally induced hyperthermia requires life-support measures and temperature-lowering interventions to avoid progression of cell death and damage to vital organs. Unconscious persons require removal from the thermal stress, tracheal intubation, ventilation to ensure Pa_{O_2} >100 mm Hg and Pa_{CO_2} of <40 mm Hg, and administration of intravenous fluid to correct hypovolemia. Cold normal saline solution in volumes of 6 to 10 L may be required to correct severe fluid deficits. Body temperature can be effectively reduced by placing the patient on a cooling blanket and administering cold intravenous fluids.[16]

Therapies for MH or NMS disorders are specific with pharmacological and supportive care. Dantrolene, a muscle relaxant, is the only known specific therapeutic drug for MH. It is given intravenously in doses of 2 mg/kg, followed by 1- to 2-mg/kg doses at 10-minute intervals. Cooling by surface or invasive methods is indicated to keep core temperatures below 40°C (104°F). Mild cases of NMS are treated pharmacologically with oral dopamine agonists, such as bromocriptine; severe cases may require a nondepolarizing muscle relaxant and dantrolene for 12 to 24 hours, followed by oral dopamine agonist agents.[15] Control of the muscle contractions tends to reduce body temperature, but if temperatures exceed 40°C (104°F), surface-cooling methods should be instituted.

FEBRILE RESPONSES

FEVER OR HYPERPYREXIA

Fever is an abnormally high *controlled* body temperature that occurs as a host response to pyrogens. Unlike hyperthermia, in which *loss* of thermoregulatory control causes the system to overheat, temperatures in fever are regulated, but at a higher level. Molecular mechanisms are involved in elevating and modulating the febrile patient's temperatures at levels that are usually not lethal. Until the early 1970s, fever was known primarily as a thermal phenomenon. Advances in molecular biology show that body temperature elevation is only one of fever's complex manifestations. Two primary dimensions are involved that affect care: *thermal consequences* and *acute phase responses.* Each dimension presents threats or benefits, depending on the individual's preexisting state of health. It is known that a healthy individual receives some host benefits from fever. Studies show that body temperatures of about 39°C (102.2°F) may have immunostimulant and antimicrobial effects that (1) speed migration and secretion of antibacterial substances by neutrophils, (2) enhance the antiviral and antitumor effects of the interferons, (3) stimulate T-lymphocyte proliferation, and (4) reduce plasma iron concentration to suppress bacterial growth.[20]

RISK FACTORS

Inappropriate Aggressive Fever Treatment

Risks related to fever are becoming better understood as their mechanisms are made clearer. Before origins of fever were known, high temperatures were viewed as the cause, rather than the effect, of disease. Aggressive procedures to lower body temperatures caused countless patients undue shivering, distress and energy expenditure. Even today, there is concern that febrile temperatures will rise uncontrollably unless cooling measures are instituted. Newer evidence shows that true fevers tend to be self-limiting and temperatures are kept at safe limits by the body's own fever-lowering "cryogens" and endogenous antipyretics, such as the hormone arginine vasopressin.[20,21] Although it is possible for secondary neural disorders to coexist with fever and cause hyperthermia, true fevers rarely reach harmful levels.

Personal and Developmental Factors

Studies found adults and older children have regulatory mechanisms that tend to limit febrile temperature elevations to 41.1°C (105.9°F).[22] Temperatures that are higher than this are associated with complications of bacteremia, meningitis, or other serious illnesses that impair compensatory controls. Young infants in the first 12 months of life tend to have regulatory mechanisms that limit the level of febrile temperature elevations to 40.0°C (104°F). Infants in the first 2 months of life usually have little or no febrile response to infectious illnesses so any elevation in temperature should be taken seriously.[22] The presence of a rectal temperature of 39°C (102.2°F) in a young infant has as serious diagnostic implications as 40°C (104°F) in an older child.

Febrile responses of elderly adults tend to be of less intensity than those seen in younger persons. This blunted febrile response often allows infection and chronic diseases to go undetected until serious illness develops. Even when they are afebrile, older persons run lower body temperatures than young persons. They also vary more in their average body temperatures (36.0°C/96.8°F to 36.6°C/97.8°F) than do younger persons, who average 36.8°C (98.2°F). The mechanisms of reduced febrile response in old age have been studied primarily in animals, with conflicting reports. One group of studies concluded that aging leads to reduced production of interleukin-1.[23] More recent studies find that cytokine production is not lower, but rather insufficient numbers of β_3-adrenergic receptors are active to effect thermogenesis and mount a fever.[24] How these effects relate to older adults is not clear, but there is convincing evidence that the fever response is blunted in old age. Older patients frequently present with serious infections, but they are afebrile or hypothermic. The presence of any fever, therefore, is serious in an older person. At the same time, the ability to produce a fever has some survival value in elderly patients when confronted with gram-negative bacteremia.[25]

MECHANISMS

Acute Phase Mechanisms

Thermal consequences of fever are preceded by acute phase events that begin with introduction of a pyrogenic substance into the body (Figure 2-2). Pyrogens are not limited to infectious organisms. Nearly any substance can elicit the acute phase response to some extent depending on its amount, site of delivery, its potency and the species and individual sensitivity of the host. Some bacteria and fungi are exogenous pyrogens and induce fever even when they are killed prior to injection. Other microorganisms and inorganic exogenous substances are *antigenic* and trigger release of *endogenous pyrogen* (EP) peptides from monocytes and macrophages of the reticuloendothelial system. These peptides act as cellular messengers, called *cytokines*, and activate widespread systemic proinflammatory reactions. Therefore, whether the pyrogen has arisen exogenously or endogenously, the body's own cytokines are eventually activated. Cytokines known to be involved are interleukin-1 (IL-1α), interleukin-1 beta (IL-1β), interleukin-6 (IL-6), tumor necrosis factor (TNF), interferon alfa (IFN α), interferon beta (IFN β), and macrophage inflammatory protein. Intermediary cytokines and prostaglandins lead to a common pathway to activate impulses to hypothalamic structures. It is no longer considered an acceptable explanation that pyrogenic cytokines flow from the systemic circulation into the hypothalamus.[26] The precise mechanisms by which the large molecules of pyrogenic substances traverse the blood brain barrier into the specialized regions of the brain controlling temperature continue to be studied.[27]

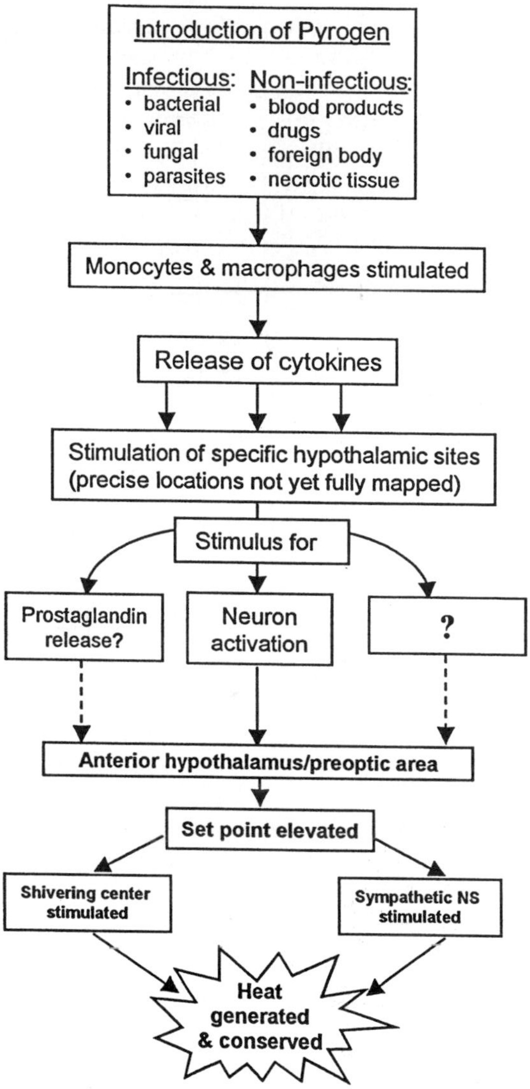

Figure 2-2 A highly simplified diagram of the current views of how fever originates, from introduction of exogenous pyrogen to final pathways that raise the thermoregulatory set-point and trigger warming responses. Still not fully understood are the mechanisms of cytokines that signal transmission across the blood-brain barrier. Broken lines represent postulated linkages and the blank box represents new mechanisms under study.

Thermal Mechanisms

Pyrogenic substances cause thermal alterations by affecting the activity of hypothalamic neurons. The febrile episode is characterized by three distinct phases (Figure 2-3) that reflect the interaction of immunological, neural, musculoskeletal, and circulatory activity. Whether or not cytokines stimulate hypothalamic structures by crossing the blood brain barrier or by liberating mediator substances,

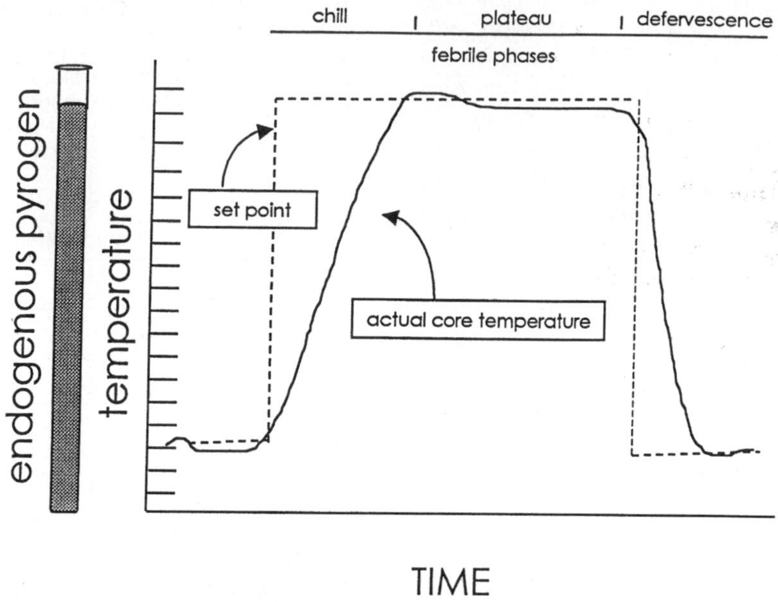

Figure 2-3 The febrile episode.

they are believed to elevate the set-point range. Activity in the preoptic neurons of the hypothalamus induces temperature elevation by inhibiting warm-sensitive neurons and exciting cold-sensitive neurons.[26] Because the set-point has been raised, integrated feedback from the skin and core temperature is sensed as lower than the new set-point. All thermoregulatory mechanisms are intact in fever so this deviation from the thermoneutral range causes the hypothalamus to activate warming responses. Shivering is the primary source of heat during fever, although cellular metabolism is also increased. Friction from oscillating muscle fibers generates heat, consumes oxygen, and contributes to muscle aches during fever. Vasoconstriction conserves the newly generated heat and core temperatures begin to rise. This early period of the febrile episode is called the *chill phase* and is the time during which intervention is particularly effective in reducing the distress and metabolic toll of shivering. Reducing shivering during this period has been shown to keep core temperatures at lower levels. Once the body temperature rises to set-point levels, the stimulus for heat production ceases and a *plateau phase* begins. During this thermal steady-state period, core temperatures and metabolic rate remain high. Shivering and vasoconstriction are not seen, although the patient's increased sensitivity to chilling can induce both responses during the febrile plateau. Finally, when concentrations of the pyrogenic substances fall because of natural or drug effects, warm-sensitive neurons begin to fire appropriately, and the set-point range falls. The discrepancy between the high core temperatures and the new lower set-point creates strong thermoregulatory cooling responses that represent the "break" or *defervescence phase* of the febrile episode.

PATHOLOGICAL CONSEQUENCES

In general, the recent scientific evidence shows that temperature elevation during fever is an adaptive response that enhances host defenses in otherwise healthy humans.[28] The pathological consequences of the febrile response are primarily caused by the effects of cytokines and other proinflammatory mediators that promote loss of appetite, lethargy, sleepiness, malaise, and low serum iron. The complaints of headache, muscle aches, and fatigue during fever are proinflammatory consequences that are better treated with mild analgesics. The effects of temperature elevations are not nearly as stressful and energy depleting as the consequences of severe shivering induced by cooling the febrile patient.

Of particular concern to parents are occurrences of febrile seizures in children. They usually occur between the ages of 3 months and 5 years in 2% to 5% of children in the United States and Western

Europe.[29] True febrile seizures are associated with fever without evidence of intracranial infection or other cause. Sometimes behaviors of the child, such as shivering, breath-holding, syncope, or delirium, may be confused with febrile seizures. There is no evidence that seizure activity is associated with the level of temperature elevation or the rapidity of the temperature rise. Children who convulse during one febrile illness will often tolerate even higher temperatures in subsequent illness.[29] The tendency toward febrile seizures appears to have a hereditary influence, and family history may reveal parents or siblings who were similarly affected while children.[30]

In severe maladaptive expressions of the febrile response, massive inflammation, vascular leakage, and synthesis of a large array of acute phase proteins occur. These tend to be in persons with preexisting compromised organ systems. Another pathological consequence of fever-producing cytokines is seen in persons with HIV infection. Although cellular immunity is suppressed in this disorder, alternate immunological pathways stimulate excessive cytokine production. IL-1, IL-6, and TNF-alpha interactions particularly heighten febrile responses of HIV-infected persons. Catabolic effects of cytokines may actually hasten HIV disease progression by inducing proteolysis, anorexia, wasting, and dehydration.[31,32]

High fevers are often complicated by heavy sweating, during which several liters of water may be lost in a few hours. Because there is an intimate relationship between body temperature and water balance, alterations in one tend to affect the other. Elevations in temperature induced by severe dehydration alone are generally hyperthermic states as a result of impairment of heat loss rather than fever. However, fever and dehydration sometimes coexist. Dehydration can accompany a fever of viral or bacterial origin if the illness or treatment produces diarrhea, vomiting, or diuresis. Loss of fluid volume reduces cardiac output and diminishes the blood flow to skin, which makes the patient less able to lose heat through vasodilation and sweating. Although there is presently no clear evidence that forcing fluids lowers core temperature in euhydrated febrile patients, there is strong scientific rationale for restoring body water in those with fluid deficit.

RELATED PATHOPHYSIOLOGICAL CONCEPTS

Elevated body temperature is often the first recognizable symptom associated with the febrile response. Preoccupation with reducing the temperature is conceptually and clinically counterproductive. Measures to cool the patient are distressful and likely to further stimulate shivering and energy expenditure. A more reasonable concern should be for treating the pyrogenic origin (bacterial, viral or fungal infection, foreign body, blood product, or drug), providing comfort, and preventing energy expenditure and water deficit.

DIFFERENTIAL DIAGNOSIS

Differential diagnosis between fever and hyperthermia is sometimes difficult when hypothalamic injury and infection coexist. Unstable temperatures that drift to either hypothermic or hyperthermic extremes and do not respond to antipyretic drugs are indicative of loss of thermoregulatory control. During fever the temperature tends to be regulated at a higher level and is responsive to antipyretics. Although there is a difference between a dehydration-induced temperature rise and one caused by the pyrogen, the two often become cofactors in serious illness.

MANIFESTATIONS AND SURVEILLANCE

Signs and symptoms of the febrile host response are often felt subjectively by the patient before the temperature rises. Behavioral changes associated with fever are typically depressed activity, lack of attention to usual body care, and anorexia. These same "sick behaviors" can be induced in animals by injecting them with a pyrogen and are related to cytokine activity.[33] Chills, malaise, and irritability precede the temperature elevation. Increase in muscle tension often accompanies the chill phase, and the patient may complain bitterly of extremities feeling cold or numb. Teeth chattering and severe shivering during this phase causes the patient distress. During the plateau phase, the skin becomes warm and mildly flushed, but the patient may wish to remove some of the bed coverings. The danger of recurring chills is high if skin is exposed to ambient air or contact with cold surfaces. During the defervescence phase, patients tend to throw off bedcovers, complain of "burning up," and experience diaphoresis. Sweat often saturates the patient's clothes and bed linens.

The most obvious clinical manifestation of fever is a rising body temperature. Beyond the ability to measure temperatures from a variety of sites, nursing personnel should recognize the relative difference between expected values from the mouth, nasopharynx, tympanic membrane, and rectum

TABLE 2-2 Relationships to Rectal Temperature in the Afebrile State

MEASUREMENT SITE	CELSIUS	FAHRENHEIT
Rectal temperature	37.5°	99.5°
Oral temperature	0.3°–0.5° lower than rectal	98.6°–99°
Esophageal temperature	0.2° lower than rectal	99.1°
Pulmonary artery temperature	0.2°–0.3° lower than rectal	99.0°–99.1°
Tympanic membrane temperature	0.05°–0.25° lower than rectal	99.0°–99.4°
Bladder temperature	0.1°–0.2° lower than rectal	99.1°–99.3°
Axillary temperature	0.6°–0.8° lower than rectal	98.1°–98.4°

From Holtzclaw, B.J. (1998). New trends in thermometry for the ICU patient. *Critical Care Nursing Quarterly 21*(3), 12-25.

(Table 2-2). Although temperatures at these sites tend to rise and fall in synchrony, circulatory shunting causes some regions, such as the rectum, to lag behind. Most clinicians are not proficient in converting from Fahrenheit to Celsius without a conversion chart. Temperature intervals are not the same as Celsius, so conversions involve more than simple addition or subtraction. A 1° change in temperature in Celsius reflects nearly twice the elevation (1°C = 1.8°F) of that in Fahrenheit.

Several factors make measurement of febrile temperatures by oral thermometers less desirable during fever. Measurement of oral body temperature during the chill phase of fever is made difficult by masseter muscle contractions and teeth chattering. Ingestion of cold liquids, particularly in older individuals, may give lower readings for nearly half an hour. Tympanic membrane (TM) thermometers facilitate measurement in children, in older persons, and in persons with severe malaise. A continuing problem is the limitations of TM thermometers for detecting extremes in temperatures; levels around 40°C (104°F) may need to be verified by a reliable electronic rectal thermometer.

CLINICAL MANAGEMENT

The goal of treatment in a patient with fever is not to reduce the body temperature but to manage febrile symptoms. A primary goal is to treat the infectious origin of the fever, if possible, by the use of antibiotics or antimicrobial agents. If the cause is of noninfectious origin, the goal is to halt the pyrogenic exposure. Noninfectious antigens are surprisingly common in patient care, because drugs, blood products, suture materials, or any foreign substance can elicit an antigenic response if it enters the body of susceptible individuals.

Treatment by symptom management for fever consists of suppression of shivering and conservation of energy by insulating the skin; body water restoration by giving palatable oral fluids; and comfort measures with antipyretic/analgesic drugs. *Shivering* should be prevented to conserve the patient's energy and to avoid causing production of more body heat. The work of shivering has been compared with that of shoveling snow or bicycle riding. Shivering stimulus can be reduced significantly by use of the terry cloth extremity wraps described earlier (see section on hypothermia management).

Insulating the extremities during the chill phase avoids stimulating the cold-sensitive neurons that are densely distributed on the hands and feet. Warm socks or down slippers can be used in the home. A light covering over the trunk allows heat to escape from less thermosensitive regions. During the fever's plateau or defervescence, clothing should be removed when wet with sweat. Exposure to drafts can be prevented by having the patient change clothing under the bedcovers. Care must be taken to avoid chilling when the patient ambulates to the bathroom.

Fluids should be offered in whatever form the patient is most likely to take them. During fever, both thirst and appetite are suppressed by circulating cytokines. Room-temperature or warm liquids are less likely to promote chills and are better tolerated. Body water loss from fever can most readily be assessed by comparing body weight before and after a febrile episode. Recognizing that a pint of water weighs 1 pound, a 2-pound loss in a few hours represents a quart of body water. Restoration of fluid when the fever is over is particularly important in children. It is sometimes easier to get children to take gelatin, frozen pops, and fruit juices than to drink water.

Use of antipyretic drugs has changed in recent years with the recognition that the body produces antipyretic substances, such as arginine vasopressin and corticotropin-releasing factor, that reduce core temperatures in febrile patients. Concern for *comfort* is the primary reason for using antipyretic drugs or analgesics. Currently used antipyretic drugs have antiinflammatory and analgesic properties that generally make the patient feel better. Aspirin and other nonsteroidal antiinflammatory drugs (NSAIDs) lower febrile temperatures by blocking the production of and subsequent cytokine mediators from prostaglandins. They are used primarily to relieve the myalgia or headache of fever. The use of aspirin carries the risk of gastric irritation and impairs blood coagulation because of its antiprostaglandin activity. It has also been associated with risk for Reye's syndrome in children. Acetaminophen is a weak prostaglandin antagonist, although it can lower febrile temperatures. It is widely prescribed because it is relatively safe concerning Reye's syndrome in children and is less likely to cause gastric irritation or clotting disorders. Despite these characteristics, acetaminophen should not be considered a harmless drug; overdosage leads to fatal liver toxicity, and some individuals may have idiosyncratic blood dyscrasias and allergies to the product. There is growing use of NSAIDs, such as ibuprofen, indomethacin, and naproxen, for fever. Unfortunately, the use of antipyretics has not been shown to reduce the incidence or recurrence of febrile seizures. The sudden onset of seizures seldom gives sufficient time to give an oral anticonvulsant agent before a seizure occurs. Phenobarbital, primidone, and sodium valproate have been found effective in preventing recurrences.

CASE STUDY

THE PATIENT WITH EXERTIONAL HEATSTROKE

In mid-July, a 20-year-old man was admitted to a southeastern urban emergency department after collapsing during an afternoon Reserve Officers' Training Corps (ROTC) workout at the local university. Rectal temperature was 39.4°C (103°F), heart rate 140, respiratory rate 44, and blood pressure 94/50. His skin was pale and clammy and he remained in a severe stupor. A tracheal intubation was performed, along with insertion of a central venous line and indwelling urinary catheter. There was no urinary output. In light of the high environmental humidity (80%) and temperature (32.2°C [90°F]), an admitting diagnosis was ruled out (RO) cardiac arrhythmia, RO heatstroke. On physical examination, the patient had severe muscle stiffness. Laboratory findings from blood samples indicated hemoconcentration with rising hematocrit and hemoglobin levels; prolonged prothrombin time (PT) and partial thromboplastin time (PTT); hyperkalemia, a mildly decreased serum sodium level; hypocalcemia; hypoglycemia; and markedly elevated BUN and creatinine values. Blood gases revealed a PaO_2 of 150 mm Hg; $PaCO_2$ of 32 mm Hg; a pH of 7.24; HCO_3^- of 13.2 mEq/L; and a base deficit of −13 mEq/L. The PaO_2/FiO_2 ratio was less than 200 mm Hg (33.3 kPa) during mechanical ventilation, and bilateral infiltrates were seen on chest x-ray evaluation. Rhabdomyolysis and myoglobinemia, indicating the breakdown of muscle cells, helped to differentiate between classical and exertional heatstroke. Lactic acidosis and markedly increased creatine phosphokinase (CPK) and aldolase were other features of exertional heatstroke, rather than classical heatstroke. The patient was transferred to the ICU, and treatment included pulmonary ventilation with 100% oxygen, rapid infusion of 6 L of cold normal saline solution (3 L in the first hour), and placement on a surface-cooling blanket with continuous core temperature readings. Extremity wraps of terry cloth toweling were applied to prevent shivering by insulating the hands and feet from the cooling device, while a light cover was placed over the trunk to allow heat transfer. Once the patient's temperature reached 38°C (100.4°F) rectally, the cooling blanket was turned off to prevent afterdrop. Laboratory tests for coagulation defects were performed over the next 24 hours. On the next day, small petechial hemorrhages appeared on his skin and there was still no renal output. Core temperature continued to decrease, until 48 hours after admission it was 37°C (98.6°F) rectally. Scanty urinary output and slow stabilization of vital signs appeared on day 2.

Although the thermal event was successfully reversed by fluid replacement and surface-cooling, and shivering was prevented by insulation of the extremities, the patient did not recover full consciousness. On day 6 he developed an elevated core temperature of 40°C (104°F), signs of endotoxin release, and rising intracranial pressure. A fall in central venous pressure, demonstrated cellular heat shock responses, spherocytosis, and acidosis were indications of disseminated intravascular coagulopathy (DIC). The patient's neural function and condition continued to deteriorate despite aggressive treatment, and death occurred by evening. Postmortem examination revealed coagulative necrosis and cerebral hypoxia as the immediate cause of death, with severe lung, liver, and kidney damage from coagulopathy.

SELECTED RESEARCH

The quest for reliable and accurate methods of detecting temperature elevations continues to dominate nursing research related to altered thermoregulation.[3,34,35] As new devices are introduced to measure temperature, nurses often are the first to test their usability in clinical settings.[36] Of particular interest are temperatures measured at different sites or varying techniques during circulatory and hemodynamic events.[34,37,38] Studies vary in their use of simple correlation or the more meaningful use of Bland-Altmann procedures to determine measures of agreement.[39]

Studies have also explored temperatures that predict critical events, such as shivering.[40,41] Hemodynamic changes that protect the brain from heat were cited as possible factors that made TM thermometers a poor indicator of rising rectal temperatures during exercise-induced hyperthermia.[42]

Significant strides have been made by nurses in studying measures to help infants stabilize body temperatures. The use of skin-to-skin contact, called "kangaroo care," has been particularly successful.[43] Other studies have tested the use of gradients in temperature sites to assess cold stress in infants.[37,38] Some of the earliest nursing research concerning thermoregulatory responses was aimed at preventing shivering during aggressive cooling by surface-cooling. Abbey demonstrated the effectiveness of terry cloth extremity wraps to prevent shivering during hypothermic cooling in two studies.[11,44] The same intervention was found to be effective in studies to prevent drug-induced shaking chills during administration of amphotericin B.[45] Terry towel wraps prevented febrile shivering and were associated with lower temperature elevations in human immunovirus (HIV)-infected persons with infectious fevers. Insulative extremity wraps are also useful when it is necessary to surface-cool febrile patients with acquired immunodeficiency syndrome (AIDS)-related fevers.[46]

Cooling measures were compared in two studies for their ability to lower temperatures without inducing chills. In a study of cooling blankets at four different settings, use of higher settings led to a slower reduction in temperature, but with less shivering and distress.[47] Antipyretics alone were found as effective as more aggressive means for patients not in imminent risk of hyperthermia.[48]

QUESTIONS FOR FUTURE STUDY

Detection, treatment, and symptom management of thermoregulatory alterations continue to provide ongoing questions for study. As advances in medicine and technology help vulnerable groups of patients survive illness, trauma or premature birth, new challenges arise to maintaining thermal balance. The problem of recognizing thermal alterations in the growing elderly population seems of critical proportion. The influence of body temperature on immune function has been demonstrated, yet little is known about how environmental and circadian factors may influence temperatures and outcomes in elderly trauma or surgical patients. The influence of aggressive fluid therapy on well-hydrated febrile patients has not been studied, yet nurses continue to urge patients to "force fluids." Further explorations of relationships between hydration and the production of endogenous antipyretics, such as arginine vasopressin, could help to determine whether these recommendations are prudent.

SUMMARY

The importance of body temperature as a vital sign has long been recognized; however, its implications for assessment and care have only recently been well understood. In healthy persons in temperate climates, a rising body temperature usually heralds an infection or antigenic response to a drug or foreign body. In weak and vulnerable populations, the rise or fall in body temperature must be interpreted more carefully and the implications are more serious. From a low-birthweight infant who sustains significant hypoxia from cold stress to an aging adult who is unaware of impending heatstroke, the need for vigilance surrounding a patient's thermal status is acute.

Prevention is key to eliminating thermal stress, and nurses play an important part in raising clinical and community awareness of potential problems. Newer conceptions about fever's host benefits have helped to focus the care of the febrile patient away from lowering temperature to keeping it within safe limits. Because it is now known that most febrile symptoms are related to cytokine-induced malaise rather than thermal changes, efforts are aimed at promoting comfort and hydration rather than cooling the patient.

New discoveries about how body temperature is maintained and affected by environment and disease will continue to influence nursing care. The informed nurse will also find it imperative to keep abreast of new methods to measure and monitor body temperature and thermoregulatory responses.

REFERENCES

1. Hemingway, A. (1963). Shivering. *Physiological Reviews, 43*, 397-422.
2. Petersen, M.H., & Hauge, H.N. (1997). Can training improve the results with infrared tympanic thermometers? *Acta Anaesthesiologica Scandinavica 41*(8), 1066-1070.
3. Erickson, R.S., & Woo, T.M. (1994). Accuracy of infrared ear thermometry and traditional temperature methods in young children. *Heart & Lung 23*(3), 181-195.
4. Erickson, R.S., & Yount, S.T. (1991). Comparison of tympanic and oral temperatures in surgical patients. *Nursing Research 40*(2), 90-93.
5. Holtzclaw, B.J., Allison, M., Keller, C., & Phillips, R. (1998). The gold standard: Approximating reliability and precision in clinical measures. In *Proceedings, Southern Nursing Research Society 12th Annual Research Conference.*

Fort Worth, Tex.: Southern Nursing Research Society (SNRS).
6. Holtzclaw, B.J., & Geer, R.T. (1995). Clinical predictors and metabolic consequences of postoperative shivering after cardiac surgery. In S. Funk, E. Tornquist, M. Champagne, & R. Weise (eds.), *Key aspects of caring for the acutely ill: technological aspects, patient education, and quality of life* (pp. 226-233). New York: Springer.
7. Sessler, D.I. (1994). Thermoregulation and heat balance: General anesthesia. In E. Zeisberger, E. Schonbaum, & P. Lomax (eds.), *Thermal balance in health and diseases* (pp. 251-265). Basel, Switzerland: Birkhauser Verlagl.
8. Ballester, J.M., & Harchelroad, F.P. (1999). Hypothermia: An easy to miss, dangerous disorder in winter weather. *Geriatrics 54*(2), 51-2, 55-7.
9. Mercer, J.B. (1998). Hypothermia and cold injuries in man. In C.M. Blatteis (ed.), *Physiology and pathophysiology of temperature regulation* (pp. 246-257). River Edge, N.J.: World Scientific.
10. Giesbrecht, G.G., & Bristow, G.K. (1997). Recent advances in hypothermia research. In C.M. Blatteis (ed.), *Thermoregulation: Tenth International Symposium on the Pharmacology of Thermoregulation, Annals of the New York Academy of Sciences, vol. 813* (pp. 663-675). New York: New York Academy of Sciences.
11. Abbey, J.C., & Close, L. (1979). A study of control of shivering during hypothermia. *Communicating Nursing Research 12,* 2-3.
12. Keamy, M.F., & Hall, J. (1992). Hypothermia. In J.B. Hall, B.A. Schmidt, & L.D.H. Wood (eds.), *Principles of critical care medicine* (pp. 848-857). New York: McGraw-Hill.
13. Splittgerber, F.H., Talbert, J.G., Sweezer, W.P., & Wilson, R.F. (1986). Partial cardiopulmonary bypass for core rewarming in profound accidental hypothermia. *American Surgeon 52*(8), 407-12.
14. Heiman-Patterson, T.D. (1991). Malignant hyperthermia. *Seminars in Neurology 11*(3), 220-7.
15. Hales, J.R.S. (1997). Hyperthermia and heat illness: Pathophysiological implications for avoidance and treatment. In C.M. Blatteis (ed.), *Thermoregulation: Tenth International Symposium on the Pharmacology of Thermoregulation.* New York: New York Academy of Sciences.
16. Bristow, G., & Patel, L. (1992). Hyperthermia. In J.B. Hall, B.A. Schmidt, & L.D.H. Wood (eds.), *Principles of critical care medicine* (pp. 858-868). New York: McGraw-Hill.
17. Guze, B.H., & Baxter, L.R. (1985). Current concepts: neuroleptic malignant syndrome. *New England Journal of Medicine 313,* 163.
18. Horowitz, M., & Hales, J.R.S. (1998). Pathophysiology of hyperthermia. In C.M. Blatteis (ed.), *Physiology and pathophysiology of temperature regulation* (pp. 230-242). River Edge, N.J.: World Scientific.
19. Knochel, J.P., & Goodman, E.L. (1997). Heat stroke and other forms of hyperthermia. In P.A. Mackowiak (ed.), *Fever: Basic mechanisms and management* (2nd ed, pp. 437-457), Philadelphia: Lippincott-Raven.
20. Kluger, M.J. (1991). Fever: Role of pyrogens and cryogens. *Physiological Review 71,* 93-127.
21. Cridland, R.A., & Kasting, N.W. (1992). A critical role for central vasopressin in regulation of fever during bacterial infection. *American Journal of Physiology 263,* R1235-40.
22. McCarthy, P.L. (1997). Fever in infants and children. In P.A. Mackowiak (ed.), *Fever: Basic mechanisms and management* (2nd ed, pp. 351-362), Philadelphia: Lippincott-Raven.
23. Inamizu, T., Chang, M.P., & Makinodan, T. (1985). Influence of age on the production and regulation of interleukin-1 in mice. *Immunology 55,* 447-455.
24. Bender, B.S., & Scarpace, P.J. (1997). Fever in the elderly. In P.A. Mackowiak (ed.), *Fever: Basic mechanisms and management* (pp. 363-373). Philadelphia: Lippincott-Raven.
25. Kreger, B.E., Craven, D.E., & McCabe, W.R. (1992). Gram-negative bacteremia IV. Re-evaluation of clinical features and treatments in 612 patients. *American Journal of Medicine 68,* 344-355.
26. Cooper, K.E. (1995). *Fever and antipyresis: The role of the nervous system* (p. 135), New York: Cambridge University Press.
27. Blatteis, C., & Sehic, E. (1997). Fever: How may circulating pyrogens signal the brain? *News in Physiological Sciences 12,* 1-9.
28. Kluger, M.J., Kozak, W., Conn, C.A., Leon, L.R., & Soszynski, D. (1998). Role of fever in disease. In M.J. Kluger, T. Bartfai, & C. Dinarello (eds.), *Molecular mechanisms of fever* (pp. 224-233). Annals of the New York Academy of Sciences, vol. 856. New York: New York Academy of Sciences.
29. Rosman, N.P. (1997). Febrile convulsions. In P.A. Mackowiak (ed.), *Fever: Basic mechanisms and management* (pp. 267-277). Philadelphia: Lippincott-Raven.
30. Rosman, N.P. (1987). Febrile seizures. *Emergency Medicine Clinics of North America 5,* 719-737.
31. Hori, T., Nakashima, T., Take, S., Kaizuka, Y., Mori, T., & Katafuchi, T. (1991). Immune cytokines and regulation of body temperature, food intake and cellular immunity. *Brain Research Bulletin 27,* 309-311.
32. Catania, A., Airaghi, L., Manfredi, M.G., Vivirito, M.C., Milazzo, F., Lipton, J.M., et al. (1993). Proopiomelanocortin-derived peptides and cytokines: Relations in patients with acquired immunodeficiency syndrome. *Clinical Immunology and Immunopathology 66,* 73-79.
33. Dantzer, R., Bluthe, R., Gheusi, G., Cremona, S., Laye, S., Parnet, P., et al. (1998). Molecular basis of sickness behavior. In M.J. Kluger, T. Bartfai, & C. Dinarello (eds.), *Molecular mechanisms of fever* (pp. 132-138). Annals of the New York Academy of Sciences, vol. 856. New York: New York Academy of Sciences.
34. Henker, R., & Coyne, C. (1995). Comparison of peripheral temperature measurements with core temperature. *AACN Clinical Issues 6*(1), 21-30.
35. Schmitz, T., Bair, N., Falk, M., & Levine, C. (1995). A comparison of five methods of temperature measurement in febrile intensive care patients. *American Journal of Critical Care 4*(4), 286-292.
36. Erickson, R.S., Meyer, L.T., & Woo, T.M. (1996). Accuracy of chemical dot thermometers in critically ill adults and young children. *Image: Journal of Nursing Scholarship 28*(1), 23-28.
37. Bliss-Holtz, J. (1989). Comparison of rectal, axillary, and inguinal temperatures in full-term newborn infants. *Nursing Research 38*(2), 85-87.
38. Bliss-Holtz, J. (1991). Determining cold-stress in full term newborns through temperature site comparisons. *Scholarly Inquiry for Nursing Practice 5*(2), 113-123.
39. Bland, J.M., & Altman, D.G. (1986). Statistical methods for assessing agreement between two methods of clinical measurement. *Lancet 1*(8476), 307-310.
40. Earp, J.K., & Finlayson, D.C. (1991). Relationships between urinary bladder and pulmonary artery temperatures: a preliminary study. *Heart & Lung 20*(3), 265-270.

41. Earp, J.K., & Finlayson, D.C. (1992). Urinary bladder/pulmonary artery temperature ratio of less than 1 and shivering in cardiac surgical patients. *American Journal of Critical Care 1,* 43-52.
42. Yeo, S., & Scarbough, M. (1996). Exercise-induced hyperthermia may prevent accurate core temperature measurement by tympanic membrane thermometer. *Journal of Nursing Measurement 4,* 143-151.
43. Anderson, G.C. (1991). Current knowledge about skin-to-skin (kangaroo) care for preterm infants. *Journal of Perinatology 11(3),* 216-226.
44. Abbey, J.C., Andrews, C., Avigliano, K., Blossom, R., Bunke, B., Clark, E., et al. (1973). A pilot study: The control of shivering during hypothermia by a clinical nursing measure. *Journal of Neurological Nursing 5,* 78-88.
45. Holtzclaw, B.J. (1990). Effects of extremity wraps to control drug induced shivering: A pilot study. *Nursing Research 39*(5), 280-283.
46. Holtzclaw, B.J. (1999). Effects of febrile shivering control during HIV-related fever. In *Proceedings: State of the Science Congress: Better health through nursing research,* Washington, D.C.: National Institute of Nursing Research and 19 nursing organizations that support nursing research.
47. Caruso, C.C., Hadley, B.J., Shukla, R., Frame, P., & Khoury, J. (1992). Cooling effects and comfort of four cooling blanket temperatures in humans with fever. *Nursing Research 41,* 68-72.
48. Morgan, S.P. (1990). A comparison of three methods of managing fever in the neurologic patient. *Journal of Neuroscience Nursing 22,* 19-24.

CHAPTER 3

Anorexia

MARCIA GRANT & GRACE E. DEAN

DEFINITION

The ability to sit up and take nourishment is a fundamental human survival need. Food intake is primarily controlled by an individual's desire for food but also has a variety of physiological, psychological, and cultural determinants. When this desire for food (a normal state) is compromised or absent, an individual is said to have *anorexia* (loss of appetite). In its early stages, anorexia usually resolves as the illness abates, and any weight loss is replaced with increased intake.[1,2] Left unchecked, however, anorexia will lead to protein calorie malnutrition (PCM) and weight loss, both of fat and lean muscle mass.

Anorexia may be a transient state, unassociated with significant metabolic change. The existence of anorexia on more than an occasional basis, however, indicates an abnormal state. For the purposes of this chapter, anorexia is defined as an abnormal subjective symptom that involves a loss or lack of appetite for food accompanied by a reduction in food intake. Anorexia may exist as a primary symptom (in eating disorders such as anorexia nervosa) or may be part of a constellation of symptoms (in AIDS, cancer, cholecystitis, and psychiatric illnesses).

The anorexia that accompanies a disease state may be beneficial or deleterious, depending on the duration of the symptom and impact on the person's nutritional status.[3] For example, during an acute infection, anorexia may serve a protective function by preventing the ingestion of micronutrients or macronutrients that would lead to bacterial growth and prolonged infection. Yet the anorexia that accompanies AIDS or cancer may be associated with cachexia, a condition that results in the wasting of body tissues, primarily of fat tissues, but also of lean muscle mass, and can ultimately lead to death.[4,5]

PREVALENCE

Anorexia is one of the most common neurological symptoms observed clinically.[6] However, as a result of the subjective nature of the phenomenon and the wide variety of disorders associated with anorexia, quantitative analysis of the prevalence or frequency of occurrence is extremely difficult.

Malnutrition as an indicator of anorexia is demonstrated by substandard body weight and midarm muscle circumferences and low serum albumin concentrations.[7] The prevalence of malnutrition in free-living elderly persons is approximately 5% to 10%, and significantly higher in hospitalized or nursing home residents (30% to 60%).[7,8] In patients with cancer, malnutrition occurs in approximately 30% to 90%, depending on diagnosis.[9]

In patients with cancer, anorexia is often the presenting symptom.[10,11] The frequency of anorexia in cancer at presentation varies from 15% to 40% and up to 80% in patients with advanced disease.[12,13] Lung cancer patients in particular are vulnerable to anorexia and its resulting weight loss. Approximately 50% of all patients with lung cancer lose weight before their diagnosis. This weight loss is generally considered to be a poor prognostic indicator.[14] Tumor-specific factors, treatment side effects and complications, and psychological factors may all contribute to the development of anorexia in lung cancer.

To accurately identify the frequency with which anorexia and nutritional deficiencies occur in the general patient population, a thorough nutritional history and assessment and measurement of clinical parameters need to be conducted for all patients admitted to a hospital, nursing home, or health care agency. A preliminary evaluation of every patient seen by a provider in a health care facility will increase the likelihood of detecting the presence of anorexia or accompanying nutritional deficiencies.

RISK FACTORS

Almost any patient in any clinical setting is at potential risk for developing anorexia. Factors that contribute to anorexia are extremely diverse, ranging from a disturbance in the hunger-satiety regulatory system to taste abnormalities or to a psychological reaction to disease and treatment. It is not completely understood how anorexia is induced in a specific disease or which factors are predominantly responsible for anorexia in a disease.

Box 3-1 lists diseases and disorders that may lead to the development of anorexia. Many systemic disorders produce significant changes in nutrient intake, absorption, and metabolism that result in altered nutritional status. Increased basal metabolic rate and negative nitrogen balance are common. Alterations in taste acuity, infection, emotional stress, intestinal obstruction, endocrine dysfunction, pain, and fever may precipitate and worsen anorexia. In addition, medications used to treat the chronic diseases listed in Box 3-1 (i.e., analgesics, antibiotics, and digitalis preparations) have side effects that may directly result in anorexia. In addition, many medications (i.e., antidepressants, antihistamines, cancer chemotherapeutic agents, corticosteroids, and NSAIDs) result in side effects such as nausea, stomatitis, and taste changes that secondarily lead to anorexia.

People frequently associate anorexia with the eating disorder anorexia nervosa. This disorder primarily affects previously healthy adolescent females with the ratio of females to males 10:1. Symptoms start with a loss of appetite or refusal to eat that may lead to self-starvation and an emaciated appearance. Both physiological and psychological mechanisms are thought to influence the development of this disease. Anorexia nervosa often goes undiagnosed and untreated, because patients rarely share their symptoms with health care providers.[15]

Eating disorders have reached epidemic proportions in the United States.[15] Patients with suspected eating disorders, such as anorexia nervosa, should be carefully screened for malabsorption syndromes, such as celiac disease, inflammatory bowel syndrome, and early Crohn's disease, because the disease processes are very similar to that of anorexia nervosa. Endocrine disorders also need to be differentiated from anorexia nervosa. Hypopituitarianism or adrenocortical insufficiency is a possible diagnosis in young women with anorexia, weight loss, or amenorrhea. Assessment should include a thorough review of symptoms, including menstrual information, to help formulate differential diagnoses and rule out physical illness.

Among older adults, the major causes of anorexia are pulmonary and cardiac diseases, cancer, dementia, alcoholism, depression, and medications.[16] Over the life span there is a decline in caloric intake, called the *physiological anorexia* of aging.[17] Suspected mechanisms include alterations in the gastrointestinal satiating system, the effect of elevated leptin levels, and a variety of changes in central nervous system neurotransmitters. Aging is also characterized by progressively increasing concentrations of glucocorticoids and catecholamines and decreasing

BOX 3-1 Causes of Anorexia

Endocrine
Addison's disease
Hyperparathyroidism
Panhypopituitarism
Pheochromocytoma

Gastroinstestinal
Gastric carcinoma
Infectious processes
Inflammatory bowel disease

Hepatic
Acute/chronic hepatitis

Biliary
Cholecystitis

Renal
Chronic renal failure
Uremia

Pulmonary
Chronic obstructive pulmonary disease (COPD)
Lung cancer

Cardiovascular
Congestive heart failure (CHF)
Coronary Artery Disease

Immune
AIDS

Hematological
Leukemias
Lymphomas

Neurological
Hypothalamic

Psychiatric Illnesses
Anorexia nervosa
Depression
Substance abuse

Nutritional deficits
Iron
Thiamin
Folate

Others
Connective tissue diseases
Rheumatoid arthritis
Systemic lupus erythematosus

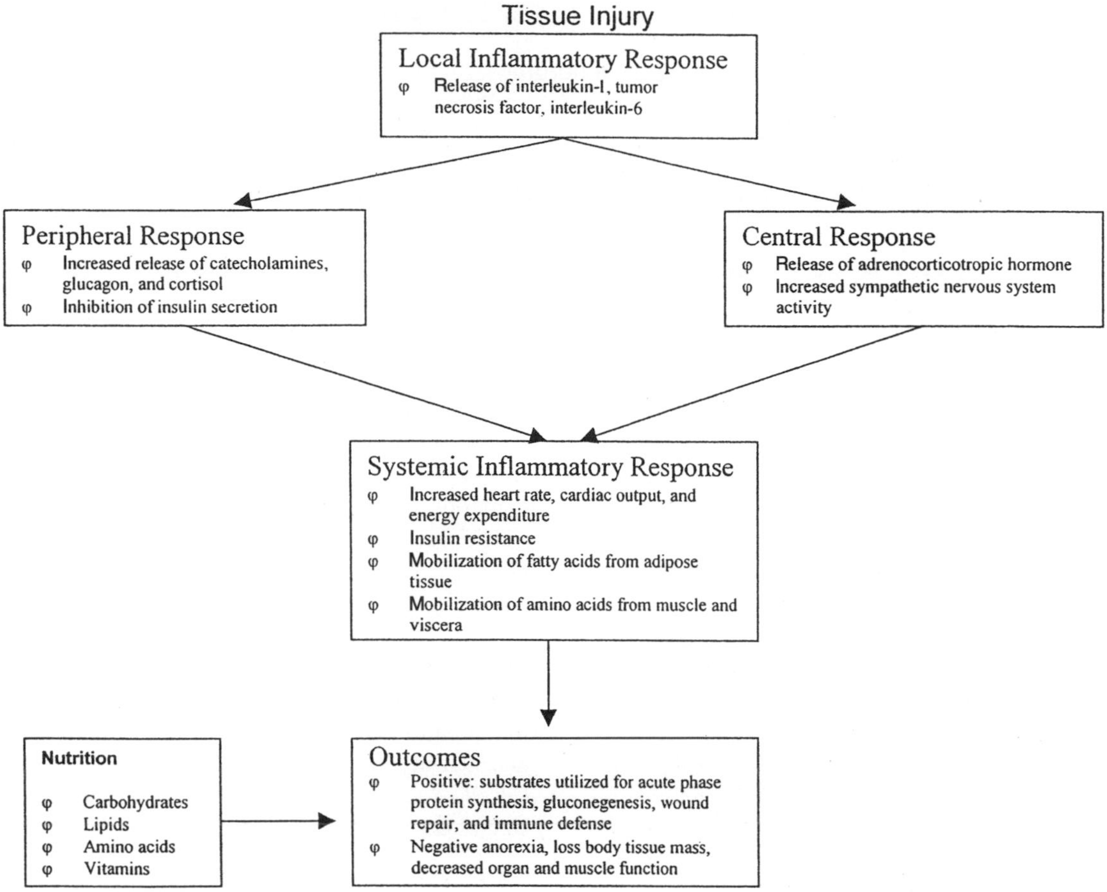

Figure 3-1 **Metabolic response to injury.** Tissue damage causes a local inflammatory response in which inflammatory mediators are released from surrounding tissue and immune cells. If the injury is extensive, these mediators escape localization to produce systemic effects. Changes in the hormonal concentrations in combination with the proinflammatory cytokines interleukin-1, interleukin-6, and tumor necrosis factor increase metabolism and cause the metabolization of fat and amino acids. These are shuttled to the liver and wound to be used as substrate for repair. Nutritional intervention is aimed at promoting the positive aspects of this response and limiting the negative outcomes. However, providing nutrition does not alter the underlying metabolic processes responsible for ongoing tissue catabolism. (From Lennice, T. [1997]. The metabolic response to injury: current perspectives and nursing implications. *Appl Pathophysiology 16*[2], 79-87.)

production of growth and sex hormones, a pattern similar to that seen in patients with chronic stress.[18]

MECHANISMS

Anorexia occurs in response to abnormalities in the hunger-satiety regulatory system. The integration of many neural, chemical, and hormonal influences makes comprehensive study of the regulation of food intake challenging. During pathophysiological processes, modifications in one or more of various components involved in the regulation of feeding will result in anorexia.

Several cytokines and microbial products resulting from infection, injury, inflammation, immunological reactions, toxins, malignancy and necrosis, have been associated with anorexia[19,20] (Figures 3-1 and 3-2). These are described later in the chapter (see Conceptual Models). Cytokines are involved in the acute phase response and cause local and systemic reactions, including anorexia.[21] In addition to pathophysiological processes, cytokines and microbial products used in immunotherapy (e.g., interleukin-1, tumor necrosis factor (TNF), interferon, and bacterial endotoxin) commonly produce anorexia in treated patients. Administration of a particular cytokine may induce secondary release of other cytokines resulting in a multicytokine interaction making it difficult to isolate the true cause of

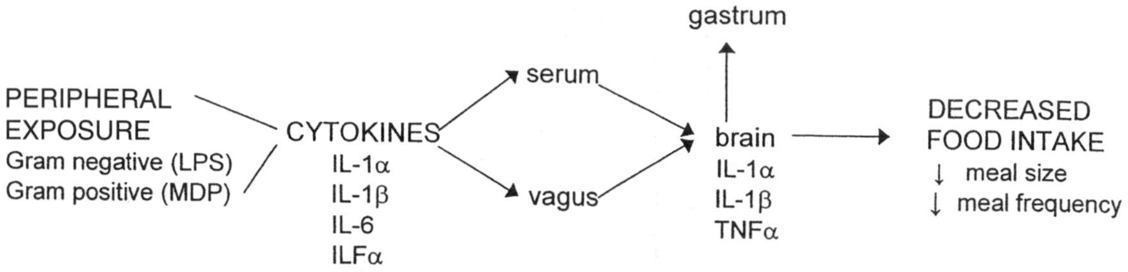

Figure 3-2 Purported pathways by which cytokines (IL-1α, Il-1β, IL-6, TNF-α) affect food intake during infection. (Data from McCarthy, D. [2000]. Cytokines and the anorexia of infection: potential mechanisms and treatments. *Biological Research for Nursing 1*[4], 287-298.)

the anorexia.[22-24] The impact of the route of administration (intravenous, intraperitoneal, or subcutaneous), dose, duration of treatment, and type of cytokine on the degree of anorexia and resulting weight loss requires further investigation.

Recent work on the physiology of feeding behavior has demonstrated that a primary role is assumed by a variety of neuropeptides (i.e., neurotransmitters/hormones in the brain). Central mediators of anorexia appear to be neurochemicals involved in the normal control of feeding, such as serotonin, dopamine, histamine, corticotropin releasing factor, neuropeptide Y, and alpha-melanocyte-stimulating hormone.[25,26] Neuropeptide Y (NPY) is prominent among these neurochemicals. NPY is produced in the hypothalamus. Research has demonstrated that when hypothalamus concentrations and release of NPY are reduced, anorexia is present.[3] When NPY is used to block and reverse the central nervous system anorexic effect of interleukin-1 beta, it has shown promise in reducing anorexia.[27] Further research is needed to understand these interactions so that strategies can be devised with potential therapeutic applications for chronic diseases associated with anorexia.

Another neurotransmitter with a role in the regulation of food intake and thus, in mediating anorexia, is serotonin. The presence of serotonin stimulates the hunger-satiety regulatory center to decrease caloric intake.[28,29] Tryptophan, an essential amino acid, is the precursor of serotonin and is regulated by the intake of carbohydrates and fats. An increase in CNS levels of tryptophan will promote serotonin synthesis, causing early satiety and reduced food intake.[30] Currently researchers are exploring the relationship between concentrations of serotonin in the lateral hypothalamic area and the ventromedial nucleus in an effort to determine the onset mechanism of cancer-related anorexia.[31]

The psychosocial influences on anorexia are as numerous as the physiological factors. Anxiety, whether in reaction to hospitalization, uncertainty of disease and its diagnosis, or change or loss in job status, increases the basal metabolic rate and demands a concomitant increase in food intake if nutritional status is to be maintained. Factors that often accompany illness, such as stress, depression, fear of isolation, or fear of pain, all decrease the desire to eat. In addition to anxiety, the patient may exhibit mood swings, difficulty in concentrating, and insomnia. The loss in weight that accompanies malnutrition may result in a change in body image and self-image. In some cultures, obesity is perceived as a sign of good health, and weight loss is a sign of declining health.[32]

PATHOLOGICAL CONSEQUENCES

Numerous potentially detrimental consequences are associated with prolonged anorexia. Muscle wasting, weakness, depression, increased susceptibility to disease complications, and decreased immunocompetence are a few consequences of anorexia.[16] When anorexia persists, it may result in progressive and concomitant weight loss, creating a cycle of physical deterioration (Figure 3-3). Disruptions in normal metabolic functions, such as starvation not caused by cachexia, results in decreased energy expenditure and alterations in carbohydrate, protein, and fat metabolism. Severe protein loss results in loss of body mass, changes in self-image, fatigue, weakness, anxiety, and depression. Resistance to infection occurs and tissue repair decreases (impaired wound healing) and interferes with the synthesis of enzymes and plasma proteins. A threefold to tenfold increase in morbidity and related mortality rates can exist from undiagnosed and untreated malnutrition.

RELATED PATHOLOGICAL CONCEPTS

The concept of anorexia, although having a unique set of characteristics, must be differentiated from other similar and related concepts. Astute observation and skilled history-taking and recording are

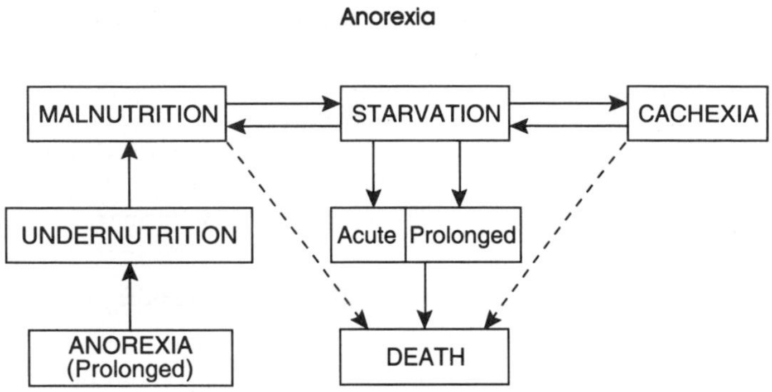

Figure 3-3 **Cycle of physical deterioration in prolonged anorexia.** Undernutrition, inadequate dietary intake and inability to metabolize nutrients normally[62]; malnutrition, insufficient consumption of protein and calories resulting in the progressive loss of lean body mass and adipose tissue; starvation, a clinical state/condition in which the body is deprived of essential nutrients, a manifestation of malnutrition; cachexia, systemic metabolic derangement resulting in progressive wasting. (Data from Blacklow, R. [1983]. Anorexia. In *MacBryde's Signs and Symptoms: Applied Pathologic Physiology and Clinical Interpretation,* 6th ed., Philadelphia: J.B. Lippincott.)

valuable tools used by the clinician in differentiating characteristics of closely related concepts.

A pathophysiological concept closely related to anorexia is nausea, a very disagreeable feeling experienced in the back of the throat and epigastrium and generally accompanied by vomiting. The same stimuli that cause an individual to be anorectic can also cause an individual to be nauseated. Anorexia and nausea, similarly, are ineffective responses associated with a variety of psychophysiological and organic disorders. Psychic stimuli (e.g., strong odors) can trigger anorexia, nausea, and vomiting. Stimulation of the hypothalamus can also trigger anorexia, nausea, and vomiting.[33]

DIFFERENTIAL DIAGNOSIS

Similarly, the stimuli that cause anorexia and nausea are extremely varied and include such clinical states as pregnancy, diabetic ketoacidosis, vascular shock, cardiac diseases, Ménière's disease, and many others. If either anorexia or nausea continues for a prolonged period, malnutrition and weight loss result.

Nausea, like anorexia, may arise from visceral discomfort, treatments, or medications used in illness or therapy; it may also arise from various psychological reactions (e.g., pain, fear, and emotional stress). Also as in anorexia, nausea is a subjective sensation; however, it creates discomfort in both the throat and abdomen. Unlike anorexia, nausea is described as an uncomfortable "tight" feeling in the throat during which an individual feels like vomiting. The feeling is accompanied by a decrease in gastric contractions and spasms of the duodenum.[34] (See Chapter 13 for an in-depth discussion of nausea, vomiting, and retching.)

Anorexia appears to be a factor associated with the circumstances of all episodes of nausea. When nausea is accompanied by anorexia, the motivation to eat is completely extinguished.[35] Any individual who is nauseated has no desire for food.[36] In nausea, thoughts of food and eating are repulsive and may even worsen existing nausea, which may then be followed by vomiting. In anorexia, the desire to eat is absent and there is a general disinterest in food, but the individual may nonetheless still experience the physiological sensation of hunger.

MANIFESTATIONS

Anorexia is primarily a subjective phenomenon but is characterized by objective indicators that are important in assessment. A subjective loss of appetite may be present but may not be noticeable to the individual or to others. When the objective indicators—a decrease in food intake and its consequences—accompany a loss of appetite, a thorough assessment is needed to reveal precipitating factors and address interventions.

Subjective Manifestations

Anorexia is characterized by subjective manifestations that reflect physical, psychological, and social dimensions. Physical characteristics include a loss of appetite and early satiety. The loss of appetite is usually the initial problem and should be described by the patient in relation to the degree of appetite lost as well as the time period involved. The more severe the loss of appetite and the longer the time period involved, the more dangerous anorexia is to the nutritional status and survival of the individual.

Other characteristics of anorexia include the symptom of early satiety, or a feeling of fullness either when usual mealtime occurs, or soon after a meal is started.

Psychological dimensions of anorexia include emotional states, such as depression and anxiety, wherein the patient is experiencing stress, hopelessness, and a loss of motivation. Psychological influence on anorexia also includes food aversions. For example, some patients are unable to tolerate the smell of certain foods such as coffee and hot fat. Food aversions in patients receiving chemotherapy may represent a classic conditioned response, wherein foods ingested immediately before, during, or after administration of chemotherapy are affected.

The social dimensions of anorexia include many factors related to the setting, companions, and types of food. For example, anorexia is common in hospitalized patients who are given unfamiliar foods in an unappetizing setting and without the company of usual eating companions.

Objective Manifestations

Objective indicators of anorexia include a decrease in food intake that is subtle when anorexia is mild or substantial when anorexia is severe. This can lead to other objective indicators, such as weight loss, weakness, and progressive wasting, and can be subsequently dangerous to survival. The period of time over which food intake is decreased is important, because it can be used to predict the seriousness of the situation and how urgently intervention is needed.

A number of other symptoms are associated with a loss of appetite and may represent objective indicators of anorexia. These symptoms should alert the clinician to a high potential for anorexia and the need for regular assessment. Gastrointestinal symptoms that precipitate anorexia include mucositis or pain in the mouth that interferes with the patient's ability to eat. Nausea and vomiting may also lead to anorexia and may be associated with changes in taste and smell, common to cancer patients undergoing chemotherapy or radiation therapy. Dysphagia, or difficulty swallowing, is also associated with a loss of appetite. Several other symptoms are not specific to the gastrointestinal tract but nevertheless interfere with appetite. Pain, when unrelieved, may consume the patient, making it impossible for him or her to eat. Fatigue, a common symptom in many diseases, is associated with loss of stamina and a disinterest in eating. Treatment of any of these syndromes and symptoms may alleviate the anorexia.

BOX 3-2 Symptom Scales That Include Appetite

Symptom Distress Scale[57]
City of Hope QOL Questionnaire[58]
Cella's FACT-G[59]
Profile of Mood States[60]

SURVEILLANCE

Surveillance for anorexia should target patients at risk. Surveillance can be done with a single assessment instrument and expanded when indicated with one that includes a number of related symptoms. Subjective evaluation of anorexia involves having patients rate their appetite intensity on a scale, such as a Likert scale or a numbered scale. Loss of appetite may also be one symptom in a questionnaire or assessment form that includes a number of other symptoms. Examples of symptom scales that include anorexia or appetite are found in Box 3-2. The objective indicators of anorexia include evaluation of food intake, and analyzing that intake for caloric, protein, fat, carbohydrate, and other elements. This analysis may be accomplished by hand or by a computer program. Results are compared to normal requirements for the individual's height and weight and diagnostic condition. Assessment should also include the presence of food aversions. It is not uncommon for patients with cancer undergoing treatment to experience altered taste sensations, learned food aversions, and changes in odor perception.[37]

If the patient describes a loss of appetite, further evaluation should include a thorough nutritional assessment. A routine *baseline* nutritional assessment is required for all hospitalized patients to identify individuals at risk for the presence or development of significant problems. Box 3-3 lists the parameters for

BOX 3-3 Parameters for a Patient at High Risk for Protein-Calorie Malnutrition

A patient is at high risk for protein-calorie malnutrition if one or more of the above parameters is present.

1. A recent 7% to 10% weight loss or an unintentional weight loss of more than 2.2 lb (1 kg) per week
2. Major surgery within the past 6 months
3. Treatment with radiation therapy or chemotherapy within the past 6 months
4. Any illness that has lasted more than 3 weeks within the last 6 months

a patient at high risk for protein-calorie (PCM). The presence of any one of these parameters increases the patient's risk for malnutrition as compared with the normal population. High-risk patients need a thorough nutritional workup. Several nutritional assessment forms with established reliability and validity are available for this evaluation. The Patient-Generated Subjective Global Assessment (PG-SGA) is a well established nutritional assessment that includes the evaluation of weight, food intake, symptoms including appetite, and functional status as defined by the patient, followed by an identification of diseases present, metabolic demand, and physical status as defined by the health professional.[38] The professional then identifies a global assessment of the patient, identifies the metabolic demand present, and performs a physical examination. Scoring results in an overall assessment of nutritional status that can be compared with norms and used to identify appropriate interventions. An advantage of the PG-SGA is its detailed and individualized information. A disadvantage is the time needed for a professional to fill in and score the assessment.

Aspects of the usual medical history are also useful in the assessment of anorexia. If a tumor is present, the type, duration, and location are important aspects. Medications being taken should be noted for possible loss of appetite and related side effects. Other valuable information to document includes any recent surgery, current treatment, an acute disease process, and psychological or socioeconomic factors that affect food intake (e.g., cultural factors, eating companions, assistance with food preparation, and income). Other medical evaluations to include in a nutritional status assessment are a total lymphocyte count and assays for serum albumin, hemoglobin, and hematocrit levels.

Because anorexia is closely tied to other symptoms, when these symptoms occur an anorexia assessment should be initiated and, if needed, a more in-depth nutritional assessment should be performed. These symptoms include pain, nausea and vomiting, depression, anxiety, dysphagia, dyspnea, and fatigue. Assessment of anorexia begins as a simple subjective description but includes an in-depth evaluation of related symptoms and nutritional status, depending on the severity of the appetite loss.

CLINICAL MANAGEMENT

Management of anorexia involves thorough assessment, planned interventions, and reassessment to determine the effectiveness of the interventions. Interventions can be divided into three categories: nutritional support, behavioral approaches, and pharmacological agents.

Nutritional support begins with dietary counseling of the anorexic patient.[39] Analysis of food intake provides information on the number of calories and the distribution of protein, fat, and carbohydrate in the diet. With this information individual dietary counseling can target foods that should be eliminated and foods that should be included to provide adequate caloric and protein intake. Dietary counseling and supplements provide the most economic approach to nutrition support.[40] Usual recommendations for caloric and protein intake to maintain normal weight are found in Table 3-1. When patients are unable to take sufficient calories with usual food, dietary supplements may be ordered. Taste tests of the dietary supplements available should be conducted to plan the most appealing supplement according to the patient's preferences. If swallowing is difficult, supplementation may include either enteral or parenteral nutrition. These invasive approaches are increasingly more expensive in providing nutritional support.[40]

Because anorexia is a multidimensional symptom, many approaches to intervention may prove effective.[41-43] Behavioral approaches focus on meal times and eating; they include serving meals in a comfortable setting, free of disagreeable odors, cheerful surroundings, and the presence of usual meal partners. A decorated tray, a glass of wine, and a comfortable setting may provide sufficient inducement of the patient to increase food intake.[44] Frequent, small meals may result in a greater caloric and protein intake for a 24-hour period. Also helpful is providing up to half of the 24-hour caloric and protein recommendation at breakfast when appetite is usually the highest and satiety is low. Cultural considerations in the selection of food available for the patient are important. Offering culturally diverse foods at a time of decreased appetite is not recommended. Families can be asked to provide favorite foods.

Noting the behavior of family members and caregivers when they help the patient to eat should also be evaluated. When patients lose their appetite and refuse to eat, family members and caregivers may associate this with a decline in health. Chiding the patient can result in an angry patient, even less inclined to eat. Family members and caregivers need to be taught the fine line between encouraging and harassing the patient to eat.

Pharmacological approaches to anorexia include several classes of medications (Table 3-2). Of these,

TABLE 3-1 Recommendations for Normal Caloric and Protein Intake

RULE-OF-THUMB GUIDELINES (VARIES AMONG FACILITIES AND REFERENCES)		
Calories per day	Normal (for adults)	30 cal/kg
	In starvation (because a patient with starvation has a slowed metabolism, his caloric needs decrease)	28 cal/kg
	In elective surgery, mildly increased needs	32 cal/kg
	In polytrauma, significantly increased needs	40 cal/kg
	In sepsis or severe stress, highly increased needs	50 cal/kg
Protein per day	Normal	0.8 g/kg
	With fever, fracture, infection, wound healing	1.5–2 g/kg
	For protein repletion	1.5–2 g/kg
	With burns	1.5–3 g/kg
Protein requirement per day based on albumin level	If albumin is 3.5 g/dl	0.8 g/kg
	If albumin is 2.8–3.5 g/dl	1–1.2 g/kg
	If albumin is 2.1–2.7 g/dl	1.2–1.5 g/kg
	If albumin is <2.1 g/dl	1.5–2g/kg

Data from Dudek, S. (2000). Malnutrition in hospitals: Who's assessing what patients eat? *American Journal of Nursing 100*(4), 36-43.

progestational agents have been studied the most. Studies on megestrol acetate have been conducted in cancer patients and patients with HIV. Improvement in appetite and a lessening of fatigue have been reported. However, no significant change in nutritional status has accompanied these changes.[45-49] Weight gain may occur with higher doses of megestrol, but this weight gain results mostly from a gain in fat deposits.[50]

Prokinetic agents have been used to decrease anorexia by improving early satiety and gastrointestinal motility. Medications that have been tried include metoclopramide and cisapride. These agents are most effective when the anorexia is opioid induced.[51] Cannabinoids have been reported to increase appetite when used in patients with advanced cancer and in AIDS patients.[52] Two forms, dronabinol and nabilone, have been tested with effects on appetite having a duration of up to 24 hours.[53] Smoked cannabis preparations (marijuana) have not shown consistent results, probably because of the difficulties of controlling dose, inhalation duration, the volume inhaled, and individual preferences.[53] Glucocorticoids can affect appetite through a number of mechanisms. They can suppress tumor necrosis factor production, cause euphoria, and inhibit prostaglandin metabolism, all of which can result in a decrease in anorexia. Side effects of glucocorticoids, however, are significant and can diminish the enthusiasm for using this class of medications.[53] Anabolic agents have been identified as a possible class of medications for treatment of anorexia. However, studies are few, some are old, and side effects from these drugs are also considerable.[53] Thus their use has not been extensive.

Another group of medications used for treating anorexia is the cytokine inhibitors. These have been studied primarily in patients with AIDS; the drugs produced significant increases in appetite and weight gain. Side effects include rashes, sedation, constipation, neuropathic symptoms, and neutropenia.[54] Testing outside of the AIDS population is limited.

Although pharmacological approaches to treating anorexia are extensive, few have been effective across disease categories, and many have undesirable side effects.[28] Future studies of these and different agents are needed. Additional interventions are needed to manage related symptoms or syndromes that indirectly effect anorexia.

Anorexia may occur as part of a syndrome and may be alleviated if the syndrome is managed. For example, a loss of appetite and loss of weight usually accompany depression.[42] Treatment of the depression may restore the appetite. Body-image disturbances can be associated with anorexia but vary,

TABLE 3-2 Pharmacological Options in Anorexia/Cachexia Syndrome

MEDICATIONS AND COMMON DOSING	EFFECTS AND/OR INDICATIONS	SIDE EFFECTS AND OTHER CONSIDERATIONS
Progestational agents, especially megestrol acetate 480–800 mg PO qid in liquid suspension	Improve appetite and reduce nausea/ vomiting and taste alterations; most useful for patients expected to live for weeks or months	Fluid retention, menstrual irregularities, and tumor flare in patients with breast cancer; contraindicated in patients with thrombophlebitis; sudden discontinuation can induce hypertension, thromboembolism, vaginal bleeding, peripheral edema, hyperglycemia, Cushing's syndrome, and adrenal dysfunction
Prokinetic agents, especially methoclopramide 10 mg PO tid	Early satiety from delayed gastric emptying or gastric paresis	Dystonic reactions (trismus, torticollis, facial spasm, oculogyric crisis, anxiety), akathisia, and tardive dyskinesia (involuntary chewing, vermicular tongue movements)
Corticosteroids (e.g., dexamethasone) 4–8 mg q AM	Improved sense of well-being; most useful in patients with limited life expectancy or when rapid effect is needed	Euphoria, other mood changes, fluid retention, gastrointestinal irritation
Cannabinoids (e.g., dronabinol) 2.5–5 mg PO q3-6h; some patients prefer to smoke marijuana rather than take oral medications as a source of cannabinoid	Improves appetite and decreases nausea; when smoked with others, serves as a social event	Sedation, euphoria, difficulty concentrating; older patients may have unpleasant feelings from cannabinoids

From Kemp, C. (2001). Anorexia and cachexia. In B.R. Ferrell & N. Coyle (eds.), *Textbook of palliative nursing* (pp. 101-106). New York: Oxford University Press.

depending on the underlying pathophysiological process. For example, a patient with anorexia nervosa has a multidimensional, neurological problem, which includes a body image that always appears fat to that individual. By contrast, a patient with cancer who is losing weight may be very concerned about the change in body image to a thin, wasting body. For each of these patients, treatment of the anorexia may be needed before the body image actually changes. For cancer patients undergoing diagnosis, or during a period of recurrence, anxiety accompanied by anorexia is frequently present. When the anxiety is alleviated, the anorexia may improve.

CONCEPTUAL MODELS

Several conceptual models provide information on various aspects of the anorexia process. Figure 3-1 describes the metabolic response to injury and outlines how tissue injury can lead to anorexia. In this model, cytokines released from the local area of tissue damage stimulate both central and peripheral responses that lead to increases in heart rate, cardiac output, and energy expenditure. Accompanying these changes are mobilization of fatty acids and amino acids that can provide substrate material for tissue repair but can also result in anorexia, loss of tissue mass, and organ and muscle dysfunction. Figure 3-2 further describes pathways by which cytokines bring about a decrease in food intake. Figure 3-3 illustrates the long-range effects of chronic anorexia, wherein catastrophic consequences may result. The nutritional consequence of persistent anorexia is severe undernutrition. The longer the situation persists, the more severe the reaction, eventually leading to death.

Figure 3-4 is a conceptual model that defines the multidimensional nature of the redundant-food model, which includes physiological, psychological, and sociocultural factors that decrease appetite and food intake. In this model the influencing factors are related to cancer and cancer treatment. Within the center of the model, anorexia is depicted as including a decreased ability to eat, a decrease in appetite, and a decrease in food intake. Consequences of anorexia are identified as nutritional losses, and subsequently losses in functional status, treatment

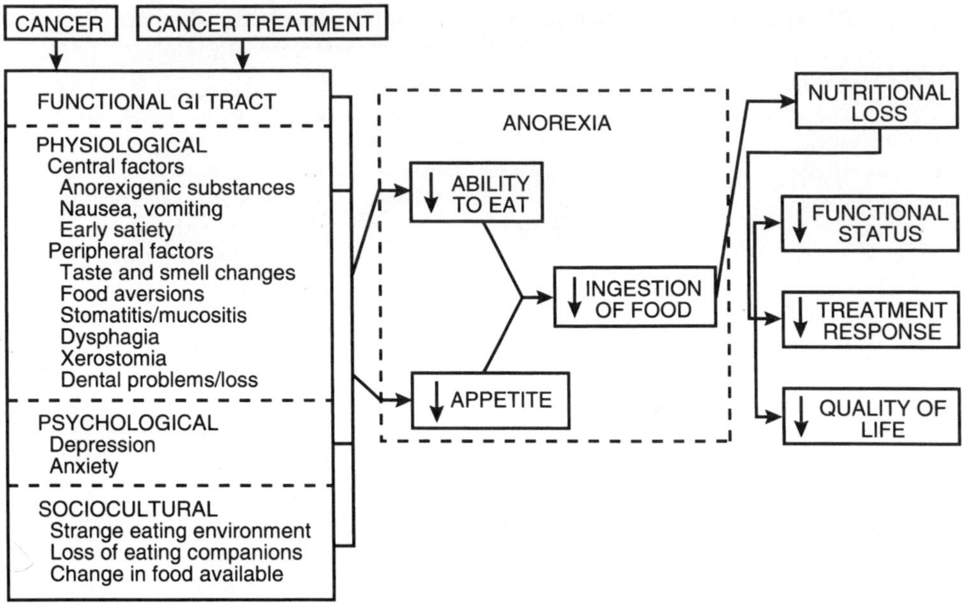

Figure 3-4 **Alterations in regulation.** Anorexia during cancer and cancer treatment.

response, and quality of life. This broad model can be used to design and test interventions to prevent anorexia during cancer and cancer treatment.

CASE STUDIES

CASE STUDY: THE PATIENT WITH HEAD AND NECK CANCER

JA, a 48-year-old man with advanced nasal melanoma, was receiving experimental treatment at a comprehensive cancer center. The therapy, cyclophosphamide (Cytoxan) followed by 5 days of interleukin-2, caused flulike reactions and significant anorexia. His primary tumor had eroded into his left maxillary sinuses and into his maxilla, distorting his face outward. As a result, he had no discernable sense of smell and constant oozing of blood into his mouth. He lost 30 pounds in 2 months.

JA's wife was his constant companion and primary caregiver. During the next 2 months, she tempted him with all his favorite foods (pureed), cajoled him with milk shakes and other supplements between meals, and obtained an appetite stimulant, megestrol (Megace), from his physician. Still he lost weight.

JA was referred for a dietary consultation. Because his gastrointestinal tract was functioning normally, enteral nutrition via a nasogastric (NG) tube was recommended. JA was still working as an executive and negotiated to receive his feedings entirely during the night. He was fitted with a gastrostomy tube after a month of NG feedings. He adapted to nighttime feedings readily, and slowly, over several months, began to gain weight. A diminished appetite returned, but he was unable to eat enough to discontinue the gastrostomy tube. His cancer continued to grow. He eventually succumbed to his disease after more than a year on experimental therapies.

SELECTED RESEARCH

Currently research on anorexia has primarily occurred in three areas—mechanisms of anorexia, pharmacological interventions, and descriptive studies of various populations. Research on mechanisms, which has focused on cytokines, has increased dramatically in the last few years. These research efforts have provided descriptions on the ways in which increases in various cytokines lead to anorexia.[19,20,22,24] Studies using anorexia-oriented models are examples of this area of research.[19,20]

Lennie's research[19] focused on the area of inflammation-induced anorexia and tissue catabolism. Using a rat model, she compared the response to acute inflammation in two groups of rats with limited food access: one with weights reduced by 6% (within normal weight) and the other with weights reduced by 12% (a level clearly below that of normal weight). Half of each group was allowed access to additional food within 1 day after the inflammatory insult. The other half of each group was allowed access to additional food 6 days after the inflammatory insult (the time when anorexia was not expected to be present any longer). The normal-weight rats who were allowed unlimited access to food on the day following the inflammatory insult displayed the most severe anorexia. Results support the perspective that during an acute inflammatory response, redundant protein-energy regulatory mechanisms that interfere with appetite appear to be functional but operate in a way proportional to the time since the inflammatory response.

Another study focused on the problem of maintaining or increasing caloric intake when patients report anorexia, abdominal fullness, nausea and early satiety.[55] Using an anorectic tumor-bearing rat model, these researchers hypothesized that rats fed a liquid diet would result in a greater caloric intake than in rats fed solid food. Results did not support the expectations and illustrated no significant differences between the two groups. Delayed gastric emptying does not necessarily occur in this tumor-induced anorexia model. Further research is needed on the effects of other dietary and nutritional manipulations.

This research provides the beginning basis for describing why anorexia occurs in various disease states, such as trauma (inflammatory response) and cancer. It has also provided some rationale for the testing of various medications in treatment of anorexia. Several classes of drugs have been tested, with various drug doses, testing periods, and with several disease models (primarily cancer and AIDS). These studies (reviewed earlier) have resulted in some successes in improving appetite with little impact on improvement of nutritional status, especially a gain in lean body mass or muscle tissue.[50]

Other studies have focused on descriptions of anorexia in various populations.[14,56]

Sarna et al[14] described the relationship of nutritional intake (a measure of anorexia) to weight change, symptom distress, and functional status in 28 progressive lung cancer patients. The occurrence of nausea, hunger, symptom distress, and appetite disturbance was expected to result in weight loss. Results did not support this expectation, illustrating inconsistent relationships over the 6-month study period. Weight change was not directly related to intake, and symptom distress and symptoms (hunger, nausea, and appetite disturbance) showed subtle fluctuations and inconsistent relationships with food intake. Findings support the need for further study to differentiate the relationship of anorexia to nutritional changes. Results also illustrate the necessity for individual clinical assessment of anorexia and related planning for dietary counseling and interventions. The testing of various interventions may need to await additional descriptive findings.

Patients with lung cancer, a population that presents a clear model of anorexia, were selected for a study of nutritional assessment indicators.[56] In this retrospective study of 93 non–small cell lung cancer patients from the time of diagnosis to death, medical records were examined for relationships between weight change, cancer-related symptoms, and nutritional assessment, intervention and evaluation. Assessment of weight change and appetite were usually found in the chart review, and appeared to part of normal patient care. However, these assessments led to interventions only 60% of the time, and only 44% of those interventions were evaluated for effectiveness. Findings illustrate the low priority of nutrition assessment in clinical care as well as the challenge of using chart data to describe anorexia. What little research has been accomplished to date leaves opportunities for a variety of research studies described next.

QUESTIONS FOR FUTURE STUDIES

Anorexia is a multidimensional problem, with little known about its mechanisms, pathophysiology, or appropriate interventions. The phenomenon is still incompletely understood, and descriptions and mechanisms of anorexia in defined populations are needed. Initial assessment and long-term evaluation require methods that are valid, reliable, and clinically simple to implement. The only area of intervention in which initial research has been conducted is that of pharmacological interventions for anorexia using various products.

Studies of behavioral interventions and their effectiveness are also needed. Is there value in carrying out dietary counseling? How effective is dietary counseling? What methods are available to track and analyze dietary intake? What are the cultural and family influences on anorexia, and is it effective to encourage families to bring home-cooked food to the patient? Research questions that persist range from basic science questions on mechanisms to nursing research questions on approaches to caring for the patient with anorexia. Clearly, much work is needed to gain a better understanding of anorexia.

REFERENCES

1. Bristrian, B. (1999). Clinical trials for the treatment of secondary wasting and cachexia. *Journal of Nutrition 129* (Suppl), 290S-294S.
2. Tisdale, M. (1997). Biology of cachexia. *Journal of the National Cancer Institute 89*(23), 1763-1773.
3. Plata-Salaman, C.R. (1996). Anorexia during acute and chronic disease. *Nutrition 12*(2), 69-78.

4. Ottery, F., Walsh, D., & Strawford, A. (1998). Pharmacologic management of anorexia/cachexia. *Seminars in Oncology 25*(2 Suppl 6), 35-44.
5. Ungvarski, P.J., Angell, J., Lancaster, D.J., & Manlapaz, J.P. (1999). Adolescents and adults: HIV disease care management. In P. Ungvarski & J. Flaskerud (eds.), *HIV/AIDS: A guide to primary care management* (pp. 131-193). Philadelphia: W.B. Saunders.
6. Plata-Salaman, C.R. (1998). Cytokines and anorexia: A brief overview. *Seminars in Oncololgy 25*(1 Suppl 1), 64-72.
7. Abbasi, A., Rudman. (1994). Undernutrition in the nursing home: Prevalence, consequences, causes and prevention. *Nutritional Review 52,* 113-122.
8. Vellas, B., Lauque, S., Andrieu, S., Nourhashemi, F., Rolland, Y., Baumgartner, R., et al. (2001). Nutrition assessment in the elderly. *Current Opinion in Clinical Nutrition and Metabolic Care 4*(1), 5-8.
9. Grant, M., & Ropka, M.E. (1996). Alterations in nutrition. In R. McCorkle, M. Grant, M. Frank-Stromberg, & S.B. Baird (eds.), *Cancer nursing: A comprehensive textbook* (pp. 919-943), Philadelphia: W.B. Saunders.
10. Laviano, A., Renvyle, T., & Yang, Z.J. (1996). From laboratory to bedside: New strategies in the treatment of malnutrition in cancer patients. *Nutrition 12*(2), 112-122.
11. Langstein, H., & Norton, J. (1991). Mechanisms of cancer cachexia. *Hematology/Oncology Clinics of North America 5*(1), 103-123.
12. Nelson, K., Walsh, D., & Sheehan, F. (1994). The cancer anorexia-cachexia syndrome. *Journal of Clinical Oncology 12,* 213-225.
13. Von Roenn, J., & Knopf, K. (1996). Anorexia/cachexia in patients with HIV: Lessons for the oncologist. *Oncology 10*(7), 1049-1056.
14. Sarna, L., Lindsey, A., Dean, H., Brecht, L., & McCorkle, R. (1993). Nutritional intake, weight change, symptom distress, and functional status over time in adults with lung cancer. *Oncology Nursing Forum 20*(3), 481-489.
15. Ressler, A. (1998). "A body to die for": Eating disorders and body-image distortion in women. *International Journal of Fertility and Women's Medicine 43*(3), 133-138.
16. Chapman, K., & Nelson, R. (1994) Loss of appetite: Managing unwanted weight loss in the older patient. *Geriatrics 49*(3), 54-59.
17. Morley, J. (2001). Anorexia, body composition, and aging. *Current Opinion in Clinical Nutrition and Metabolic Care 4*(1), 9-13.
18. Yeh, S., & Schuster, M. (1999). Geriatric cachexia: The role of cytokines. *American Journal of Clinical Nutrition 70*(2),183-197.
19. Lennie, T. (1997). The metabolic response to injury: Current perspectives and nursing implications. *Applied Pathophysiology 16*(2), 79-87.
20. McCarthy, D. (2000). Cytokines and the anorexia of infection: Potential mechanisms and treatments. *Biological Research for Nursing 1*(4), 287-298.
21. Giacosa, A., Frascio, F., Sukkar, S., & Roncella, S. (1996). Food intake and body composition in cancer cachexia. *Nutrition 12*(1 Suppl), S20-S23.
22. Yang, Z., Koseki, M., & Meguid, M. (1994). Synergistic effect of rhTNF-α and rhIL-lα in inducing anorexia in rats. *American Journal of Physiology 267,* R1056.
23. Van der Meer, M., Sweep, C., Pesman, G., Borm, G.F., & Hermus, A.R. (1995). Synergism between IL-1 beta and TNF-alpha on the activity of the pituitary-adrenal axis and on food intake of rats. *American Journal of Physiology 268*(4 Pt 1), E551-557.
24. Papanicolaou, D.A., Wilder, R.L., Manolagas, S.C., & Chrousos, G.P. (1998). The pathophysiologic roles of interleukin-6 in human disease. *Annals of Internal Medicine 128*(2), 127-137.
25. Chance, W., Balasubramaniam, A., & Fischer, J. (1995). Nueropeptide Y and the development of cancer anorexia. *Annals of Surgery 221,* 579-587.
26. Langhans, W. (2000). Anorexia of infection: Current prospects. *Nutrition 16*(10), 996-1005.
27. Sonti, G., Ilyin, S., & Plata-Salaman, C. (1996). Neuropeptide Y blocks and reverses interleukin-1 beta-induced anorexia in rats. *Peptides 17*(3), 517-520.
28. Edelman, M., Gandara, D., Meyers, F., Ishii, R., O'Mahony, M., Uhrich, M., et al. (1999). Serotonergic blockade in the treatment of the cancer anorexia-cachexia syndrome. *American Cancer Society 86*(4), 684-688.
29. Meguid, M., Muscaritoli, M., & Beverly, J. (1999). The early cancer anorexia paradigm: Changes in plasma free tryptophan and feeding indexes. *Journal of Parenteral and Enteral Nutrition 16*(Suppl), 56S-59S.
30. Tait, N. (1996). Anorexia-cachexia syndrome. In S. Groenwald, M. Froggel, M. Goodman, & Yarbro, C.H. (eds.), *Cancer symptom management* (pp. 171-196). Sudbury, Mass.: Jones & Bartlett.
31. Meguid, M.M., Fetissov, S.O., Varma, M., Sato, T., Zhang, L., Laviano, A., et al. (2000). Hypothalamic dopamine and serotonin in the regulation of food intake. *Nutrition 16*(10), 843-857.
32. Kemp, C. (2001). Anorexia and cachexia. In B.R. Ferrell & N. Coyle (eds.), *Textbook of palliative nursing* (pp. 101-106). New York: Oxford University Press.
33. Billen, B.M.K., & Daniels, G.H. (1998). Neuroendocrine regulation & diseases of the anterior pituitary and hypothalamus. In A.S. Fauci, E. Braunwald, K.J. Isselbacter, J.D. Wilson, J.B. Martin, D.L. Kasper, L.H. Stephen, D.L. Longo (eds.), *Harrison's principles of internal medicine* (pp. 1972-1998), New York: McGraw-Hill.
34. Rhodes, V. (1990). Nausea, vomiting, and retching. *Nursing Clinics of North America 24,* 885-901.
35. Rock, C.L., Coulston, A.M., & Ruffin, M.T. (1998). Diet therapy. In A.S. Fauci, E. Braunwald, K.J. Isselbacter, J.D. Wilson, J.B. Martin, D.L. Kasper, L.H. Stephen, & D.L. Longo (eds.), *Harrison's principles of internal medicine* (pp. 464-471), New York: McGraw-Hill.
36. Norris, C. (1982). Nausea and vomiting. In C. Norris (ed.), *Concept clarification in nursing* (pp. 81-100). Rockville, Md.: Aspen.
37. Puccio, M., & Nathanson, L. (1997). The cancer cachexia syndrome. *Seminars in Oncology 24*(3), 277-287.
38. Ottery, F. (1994). Rethinking nutritional support of the cancer patient; the new field of nutritional oncology. *Seminars in Oncology 21*(6), 770-778.
39. Whitman, M. (1999).The starving patient: Supportive care for people with cancer. *Clinical Journal of Oncology Nursing 4*(3), 121-125.
40. Tchekmedyian, N. (1998). Pharmacoeconomics of nutritional support in cancer. *Seminars in Oncology 25*(2 Suppl 6), 62-69.
41. Wilkes, G. (2000). Nutrition: The forgotten ingredient in cancer care. *American Journal of Nursing 100*(4), 46-51.
42. Fleishman, S. (1998). Cancer cachexia. In J. Holland (ed.), *Psycho-oncology* (pp. 468-475). New York: Oxford University Press.

43. Anton, M. (1998). Proactive approaches to nutritional care during radiation therapy. *Cancer Prevention International 3,* 165-173.
44. Grant, M., & Kravits, K. (2000). Symptoms and their impact on nutrition. *Seminars in Oncology Nursing 16*(2), 113-121.
45. Bruera, E. (1998). Pharmacological treatment of cachexia: Any progress? *Supportive Care in Cancer 6,* 109-113.
46. Vadell, C., Segui, M., & Gimenez-Arnau, J. (1998). Anticachectic efficacy of megestrol acetate at different doses and versus placebo in patients with neoplastic cachexia. *American Journal of Clinical Oncology* (CCT) *21*(4), 347-351.
47. Simons, J., Schols, A., & Hoefnagels, J. (1998). Effects of medroxyprogesterone acetate on food intake, body composition, and resting energy expenditure in patients with advanced, nonhormone-sensitive cancer. *American Cancer Society 82*(3), 553-560.
48. Gagnon, B., & Bruera, E. (1998). A review of the drug treatment of cachexia associated with cancer. *Drugs 55*(5), 675-688.
49. Neri, B., Garosi, V., & Intini, C. (1997). Effect of medroxyprogesterone acetate on the quality of life of the oncologic patient: A multicentric cooperative study. *Anti-Cancer Drugs 8,* 459-465.
50. Loprinzi, C., Schaid, D., Dose, A., Burnham, M.L., & Jensen, M.D. (1993). Body-composition changes in patients who gain weight while receiving megestrol acetate. *Journal of Clinical Oncology 11,* 152-154.
51. Nelson, K., & Walsh, T. (1993). The use of metoclopramide in anorexia due to the cancer-associated dyspepsia syndrome (CADS). *Journal of Palliative Care 9,* 14-18.
52. Corcoran, C., & Grinspoon, S. (1999). Treatments for wasting in patients with the acquired immunodeficiency syndrome. *New England Journal of Medicine 340*(22), 1740-1750.
53. Nelson, K. (2000). The cancer anorexia-cachexia syndrome. *Seminars in Oncology 27*(1), 64-68.
54. Klausner, J., Makonkawkeyoon, S., & Akarasewi, P., Nakata, K., Kasinrerk, W., Corral, L., et al. (1996). The effect of thalidomide on the pathogenesis of human immunodeficiency virus type I and M tuberculosis infection. *Journal of Acquired Immune Deficiency Syndromes and Human Retrovirology 11,* 247-257.
55. McCarthy, D.O., & Daun, J.M. (1992). The effect of diet consistency on food intake of anorectic tumor-bearing rats. *Research in Nursing & Health 15,* 433-437.
56. Brown, J.K., & Radke, K.J. (1998). Nutritional assessment, intervention, and evaluation of weight loss in patients with non-small lung cancer. *Oncology Nursing Forum 25*(3), 547-553.
57. McCorkle, R., Young, K. (1978). Development of a symptom distress scale. *Cancer Nursing 1,* 373-378.
58. Ferrell, B.F., Dow, K.H., & Grant, M. (1995). Measurement of quality of life in cancer survivors. *Quality of Life Research 4,* 523-531.
59. Cella, D. (1993). The functional assessment of cancer therapy scale: Development and validation of the general measure. *Journal of Clinical Oncology 11,* 570-579.
60. McNair, D.M., Lorr, M., & Droppleman, L.F. (1971). *EITS manual for the profile of mood states.* San Diego, Calif.: Educational and Industrial Testing Service.
61. Dudek, S. (2000). Malnutrition in hospitals: Who's assessing what patients eat? *American Journal of Nursing 100*(4), 36-43.
62. Blacklow, R. (1983). Anorexia. In *MacBryde's signs and symptoms: Applied pathologic physiology and clinical interpretation* (6th ed., pp. 62-65). Philadelphia: J.B. Lippincott.

CHAPTER

4 Protein-Calorie Malnutrition

ELEANOR F. BOND & MARGARET M. HEITKEMPER

Protein-calorie malnutrition (PCM) generally occurs as a result of disease and/or treatment in developed countries. In developing nations and during famine conditions, the condition can be endemic. Most commonly, PCM is the result of a diet deficient in calories and proteins. In some cases, disease-related increases in caloric demand or problems related to nutrient absorption cause or exacerbate PCM. Clinical studies demonstrate that in hospitalized patients, PCM adversely affects length of stay, morbidity, and mortality. PCM is thought to affect recovery in many types of illness and injury.[1,2] However, correction of nutritional and metabolic deficiencies does not always improve the patient's clinical course.

DEFINITION

PCM is the condition that results when an individual consumes insufficient protein and calories or there is insufficient protein intake with adequate caloric intake. The Institute of Medicine defines PCM as the presence of clinical indications of inadequate intake such as wasting, or biochemical indications such as low serum levels of albumin or other protein.[3] If protein intake is adequate but caloric intake is insufficient, dietary proteins are oxidized as fuel and not utilized in the synthesis of body protein: the patient suffers from PCM despite adequate protein intake. Infection, inflammation, wound-healing, fever, and shivering can increase the body's demand for energy and protein; these conditions can cause PCM in individuals who were previously adequately nourished if intake is not increased to match the demand. When nutrient consumption is insufficient, concurrent micronutrient deficiencies are common.

This chapter focuses on the metabolic consequences of protein and caloric deficit. PCM is also called *protein-energy malnutrition.*

RISK FACTORS

Factors causing PCM include insufficient consumption of calories and protein, hypermetabolism, and malabsorption of nutrients. Certain environmental, personal, and developmental factors place individuals and populations at increased risk to experience these conditions and in turn to experience PCM.

Environmental Risk Factors

Environments with increased risk of PCM include impoverished areas and regions in which infectious diseases are endemic. Clinical institutions have high rates of PCM, yet often the problem goes undetected.

Poor socioeconomic status and unhygienic conditions pose risks for PCM. When poor socioeconomic conditions exist, individuals are more likely to shift to a diet of vegetable protein, which has a lower biological value than animal protein. There may be a deficiency of quality protein or total protein in the diet. Other conditions contribute to PCM among low-income groups: poverty is associated with increased occurrence of infectious disease and infection; infectious diseases or infections in turn increase metabolic rate and calorie/protein need, leading to PCM. Gastrointestinal (GI) infections in particular exacerbate PCM. In addition to the metabolic demand for more calories, anorexia and vomiting lead to decreased consumption of calories; diarrhea can impair absorption. In areas in which parasitic GI infections are endemic, PCM is common as a result of impaired absorption of nutrients.

Hospitals and other institutional care environments pose a risk for PCM. When admitted to hospitals, many older adults (20% to 50% of elderly patients admitted) are already undernourished; McCormack[4] reviewed the literature on the incidence in the older population. A patient's nutritional status often deteriorates during hospitalization as a result of undernutrition, anorexia, medications, and the metabolic response to disease and treatment. In a classic hospital study, Bistrian et al[5,6] described a significant incidence of undernutrition in hospitalized patients. This description was critical to the later development of strategies to enhance caloric intake using such techniques as total parenteral nutrition, peripheral nutrition, and enteral nutrition.

Despite advances in nutritional interventions, PCM continues to occur in hospitalized and institutionalized patients. In a recent prospective study of hospitalized elderly patients who were not terminally ill, Sullivan et al[2] demonstrated that more than 20% had an average daily intake that was less than 50% of their calculated maintenance caloric requirement. Neither canned supplements nor nutritional support were effectively applied in this university-affiliated institution. Although the severely undernourished patients did not differ from the overall group with respect to admission acuity of illness, they had significantly worse outcomes: higher in-hospital and 90-day mortality rates. Also, the undernourished patients had lower serum levels of albumin, prealbumin, and cholesterol at the time of discharge.

Covinsky et al[1] had similar findings. They studied 369 patients over the age of 70 admitted to a tertiary care setting. There were significant relationships between nutritional status and clinical outcomes. Using the Subjective Global Assessment, a tool that employs both history and physical assessment findings, they found that those who were severely malnourished were more likely than well-nourished patients to die within 1 year of discharge, to be dependent in activities of daily living (ADL) at 3 months after discharge, and to spend time in a nursing home during the 1-year follow-up. The inferior outcomes were not the result of greater illness acuity, comorbidity, or functional dependence at the time of admission. Other researchers have reported that PCM is underdiagnosed and is associated with longer length of stay and higher mortality rates.[7]

These findings have considerable practical and public health significance.[8] Admission screening in hospitals and long-term care facilities can identify patients who have or who are at risk for nutrition-related complications.[9,10] Ongoing nutritional status determinations will help to define a patient's nutritional status, because needs and intake vary during treatment.

PCM is also common in nursing homes. Multiple factors potentially contribute to PCM in this setting: lack of qualified staff to provide personal care to patients, including nutrition; improper positioning or lack of positioning of residents or food trays during meals; undiagnosed or unrecognized dysphagia; forced or rapid feeding of residents; and residents being served meals in bed.[11]

Less is known about the incidence of PCM in the community setting. Evidence indicates that place-bound older adults are vulnerable to undernutrition, as evidenced by low serum albumin levels.[4,12]

Personal Risk Factors

Individual risk factors for PCM include impaired physical or mental health and diminished functional ability. Additional individual risk factors include poor dentition, problems with swallowing, polypharmacy, alcoholism or substance abuse, depression, eating disorder, and recent hospital discharge.[13] Genetic predisposition and advanced or young age are individual risk factors. (These will be discussed in later sections.)

PCM is common in patients with serious physical illness, particularly burns, fractures, cancer, sepsis, respiratory distress, cardiovascular disease, renal disorders, liver disease, and pathological conditions of the GI tract. The reasons for undernutrition are complicated, often involving both diminished intake and enhanced caloric need. Anorexia is common with many illnesses (see Chapter 3). Illness often diminishes a person's ability to acquire or consume food. The metabolic response to physiologically traumatic events contributes to PCM and differs from the response to unstressed starvation. Trauma, burns, and sepsis markedly increase the body's metabolic and catabolic rates. *Hypermetabolism* is an increase in the resting energy expenditure. *Hypercatabolism* is a loss of protein stores resulting from increased proteolysis. Hypermetabolism and hypercatabolism tend to be proportionate to the severity of trauma or injury. PCM occurs whenever individual need exceeds intake. In addition to increased metabolism resulting from infection, surgery, burns, and fractures, draining wounds and fistulas can result in excess protein loss and contribute to malnutrition.

GI diseases that limit intestinal nutrient digestion and absorption can lead to malnutrition. Neurological disorders that limit the ability to chew and swallow can affect nutritional status. Chronic cardiovascular disease that restricts sodium intake and energy level can also affect appetite and subsequent nutrient intake. A variety of medications can influence appetite as well as GI function and thus alter nutrient intake and absorption.

Mental illness or other causes of altered functional ability, such as dementia, drug or alcohol abuse, depression, and other mental disorders lead to PCM. Diminished functional capacity can lead to an individual's inability to obtain and prepare food and inadequate consumption of food. Depression is commonly associated with appetite disturbance. Studies have demonstrated that excessive alcohol ingestion will result in disturbed metabolism of most nutrients.[14] Although alcohol intake can lead to hypoglycemia, chronic abusers of alcohol are usually glucose intolerant, possibly as a result of an inhibition of glucose-stimulated insulin secretion. Overall, long-term ethanol intake also leads to negative nitrogen balance and an increased protein turnover. In addition, alcohol alters lipid metabolism, resulting in inhibition of lipolysis.

PCM can occur in cachexia and wasting syndromes. These conditions are the result of the body cell mass loss associated with illness, injury, or disease. In 1997, Roubenoff et al[15] proposed that cachexia occurred in conjunction with cytokine-mediated response to injury or disease. Proinflammatory cytokines, such as tumor necrosis factor (TNF-α) and interleukin-6 (IL-6), may mediate changes in both metabolic rate and appetite. On the other hand, wasting is characterized by loss of body cell mass as a result of semistarvation. Both cachexia and wasting can occur in the same patient.

Genetic Risk Factors

The past decade has seen an exponential growth in our knowledge of genes and body composition. However, studies have focused primarily on genetic risk factors for obesity (overnutrition) and have used predominantly animal models. Several genes have been identified that when mutated can have profound effects on body weight.[16] Individuals with genetic lactase insufficiency are at risk for diarrhea and malnutrition. It has been suggested that among persons consuming similar deficient diets, genetic differences in metabolic enzymes may predispose some to PCM.[17] There is a need for much more work in the identification of genetic factors that alter individual risk for developing PCM or its consequences.

Developmental Risk Factors

Persons at both ends of the age spectrum are particularly vulnerable to problems of PCM.

Infants. Infants, in particular, low-birthweight and premature infants, have reduced protein and energy stores. In addition, specific nutrient deficits may influence outcomes. For example, low-birthweight infants have a prolonged impairment of cell-mediated immunity that can be partly restored by providing extra amounts of dietary zinc.[18] Recent studies have focused on optimal feeding strategies to enhance nutritional intake and reduce such complications as necrotizing enterocolitis in the vulnerable infant population.[19,20]

Children. Children are vulnerable to PCM, which is particularly common among children of impoverished families and in children with a preexisting serious illness, such as end-stage renal disease or cystic fibrosis. In a 1998 report, the World Health Organization (WHO) estimated that worldwide, 27.4% of children under 5 years of age had malnutrition-related growth retardation.[21] Parasitic infections and diarrheal diseases can exacerbate problems related to lack of sufficient food.

Older Adults. Nutritional deficits are seen in at least one third of elderly persons in industrialized societies.[18] Elderly individuals are at risk for undernutrition because of isolation; bereavement; sensory, motor, or mental impairment; chronic diseases and functional disabilities; and economic limitations.

MECHANISMS

When the body is deprived of food, there is an orderly progression of adaptive metabolic responses mediated by hormonal changes. These responses initially maintain serum glucose to meet the energy demands of functioning tissue while preserving body protein stores. Eventually, protein stores are compromised, and alternate fuels such as ketone bodies replace glucose as the primary metabolic substrate. When the acute metabolic demands of illness are superimposed on PCM, adaptation to PCM is altered.

Unstressed Starvation

During starvation, initial hormonal and metabolic changes maintain serum glucose to meet the demands of the brain, renal medulla, hematopoietic tissue, and other metabolically active tissue. Early in a fast, the arterial glucose level falls slightly, resulting in diminished release of the anabolic hormone insulin. There is an increase in the counterregulatory catabolic hormone glucagon. An increased glucagon-to-insulin ratio stimulates glycogenolysis. Glycogenolysis is the process in which liver and muscle glycogen stores are mobilized to produce glucose. These stores are depleted after 12 to 24 hours, depending on the calories needed.[22]

Following glycogen depletion, amino acids (primarily from muscle and visceral tissue proteins) are oxidized to produce glucose via gluconeogenesis. Falling insulin levels evoke lipolysis, although protein is the primary source of calories for 5 to 10 days. Because the body does not have excess protein stores, this stage involves loss of lean body mass and can result in loss of function. Serum proteins (e.g., albumin) are relatively spared at the expense of somatic and visceral protein. Nitrogen is produced during protein breakdown and can be detected primarily as urea in the urine; losses of up to 12 g of nitrogen per day are typical during the first week of starvation.[23] Generally, the first week of total starvation will evoke a 4- to 5-kg loss in body mass.

As fasting continues, lipolysis increases, and free fatty acids become the primary fuel. Ketones and ketoacids are synthesized from the free fatty acids. The brain cannot utilize free fatty acids, but ketoacids can cross the blood-brain barrier and serve as a fuel alternative to glucose in the brain. The process of switching to ketone production and metabolism is known as *ketoadaptation.* As ketones become the predominant fuel, protein breakdown slows but does not stop. Mobilized amino acids are used to synthesize protein, particularly albumin. Urinary nitrogen losses diminish to 3 to 5 g daily. Insulin levels remain low. Metabolic rate slows. Lipid metabolism releases more calories than protein or glucose metabolism. Thus less tissue mass is broken down, and weight loss slows. Hypoalbuminemia develops only after 1 to 3 months. In nonstressed starvation, when serum proteins are metabolized, nitrogen excretion increases again. Death is imminent. This progression of metabolic events might be seen in a patient with anorexia nervosa.

If the starving person is consuming only glucose (as in a patient receiving intravenous dextrose solutions or in an impoverished patient consuming a low-calorie carbohydrate diet) or is consuming proteins of low biological value, this enhances insulin secretion, which slows lipolysis. Adipose tissue is preserved. Amino acid mobilization slows; albumin synthesis slows; hypoalbuminemia occurs earlier.

PCM in Stress States

PCM during stress states is profoundly different from simple nonstressed starvation, with different effects on fuel metabolism and body composition. In general, fuel needs are enhanced and substrate stores are mobilized and exhausted more quickly. Lipolysis produces free fatty acids, but ketone production from free fatty acids is lower. Protein, not fat, remains the major fuel. Nitrogen losses can be very high, as much as 35 g daily. Hypoalbuminemia occurs much earlier.

Under physiological stress conditions, such as trauma, burns, major surgery, infection, and inflammation, a number of neuroendocrine factors contribute to an increased metabolic rate, ultimately leading to PCM. Stressful conditions result in the activation of the hypothalamic-pituitary-adrenal axis, ultimately resulting in the release of cortisol from the adrenal cortex. Cortisol increases protein catabolism, mobilizes amino acids from muscle, and enhances hepatic glucose production. Activation of the sympathetic nervous system component of the autonomic nervous system results in epinephrine release from the adrenal medulla and norepinephrine release from sympathetic nerve endings. These catecholamines enhance the metabolic rate, increase liver glucose release, and enhance lipolysis. Insulin intolerance develops. Gluconeogenesis increases. Lipolysis increases, because this process too becomes insulin resistant. Free fatty acid output rises, fat oxidation increases, and hyperglycemia and acidosis ensue.

In trauma-related sepsis, cytokines are released from macrophages and lymphocytes. Major cytokines in trauma-sepsis include TNF-α and IL-6. These cytokines cause anorexia. They may contribute to the increased metabolic rate in stressed starvation.

Because of these metabolic derangements, nutritional support is a challenge. The increased caloric demand may come at a time when it is difficult for the patient to eat. Calories provided as glucose can enhance the release of insulin and slow adaptation to ketone fuels. Calories provided as protein tend to be utilized for protein synthesis, not oxidized as fuel. If ketoadaptation is prevented, calories provided as lipids are not utilized as fuel.

RELATED PATHOPHYSIOLOGICAL CONCEPTS

Marasmus refers to a clinical condition resulting when caloric intake is insufficient. There is wasting of muscle tissue, loss of adipose tissue, and in children, stunted growth. The hair is typically sparse, thin, and dry; the skin is typically thin and dry. *Kwashiorkor* is seen when both calories and protein are insufficient. Kwashiorkor also results in stunted growth in children; however, in kwashiorkor the subcutaneous tissue is preserved. The liver becomes fatty, and there is hypoproteinemia associated with edema. It is common to see a mixed form of the two conditions, sometimes called *marasmic kwashiorkor.* Cachexia follows food deprivation in the presence of stress and proinflammatory cytokines, such as TNF, IL-1, IL-6, and IL-8. Cachexia is sometimes referred to as *cytokine-induced malnutrition.*[24] Cachexia generally involves anorexia, decreased physical activity, tissue wasting, and weight loss in such diseases as cancer, HIV and AIDS, advanced cardiac disease, and major infections.

PATHOLOGICAL CONSEQUENCES

PCM affects all body systems. There are nervous system, endocrine, skeletal muscle, cardiovascular/hematologic, respiratory, renal, GI, immune, and wound-healing changes.

Nervous System Consequences

The relationship between neuronal functioning and PCM is unclear. Although PCM might alter brain growth, neuronal myelination, and neurotransmitter production, the long-term nervous system consequences of PCM have not been delineated; correlations between nutrition and intelligence or behavior are not clear.[25] The duration of nutritional deprivation, type of nutritional rehabilitation, and psychosocial support affect nervous system development and are difficult to separate from the direct effects of malnutrition in the brain, especially during development.

Dietary caloric restriction has been proposed as a preventive strategy for Alzheimer's disease; this approach has resulted in increased resistance to degeneration in experimental rodent models.[26] There is much need for epidemiological and empirical work in this area.

Endocrine Consequences

Hormonal changes are an integral part of adaptation to PCM, as described earlier. Summarizing the main endocrine changes, insulin, insulin-related growth factors, thyroid hormone, and gonadotropin levels are decreased. Glucocorticoid levels are increased. The result is increased glycolysis, increased lipolysis, increased mobilization of amino acids, preservation of visceral proteins, diminished storage of glycogen, fat, protein, and slowed metabolism.

Skeletal Muscle Consequences

PCM is associated with pathological conditions of the musculature. Skeletal muscle function is impaired[27]; muscle mass, strength, and endurance are reduced in PCM.[28] A functional and biopsy examination of skeletal muscle of patients with PCM caused by anorexia nervosa revealed diminished maximum force of voluntary contraction, atrophy of type 2 (fast twitch) fibers, and abnormal metabolic changes with exercise.[29] The morphological changes were not related to overexercise, known to be a problem in patients with anorexia nervosa. Patients with PCM develop muscle weakness. It is often difficult to separate the effects of deconditioning from the effects of protein or calorie deprivation.

Cardiovascular and Hematological Consequences

Cardiac muscle, vascular, and hematological responses are altered with PCM. Children with severe PCM have decreased cardiac muscle mass and impaired ventricular function; both improved with refeeding.[30] These changes dictate caution in saline fluid administration during early refeeding so as to not overstress the weakened heart.

Changes also occur in vascular reflexes, with patients having more orthostatic sensitivity. As with other changes, these effects may be a direct result of PCM or may be caused by the postural and inactivity changes that typically accompany PCM.

A reduction in hemoglobin concentration and red cell mass is common in PCM. Reduced hematopoietic activity spares amino acids for synthesis of other proteins. In one study, administration of iron, vitamin B_{12}, and folate failed to stimulate red cell or hemoglobin increases; however, protein administration stimulated red cell and hemoglobin production.[31]

Respiratory Consequences

The relationship between nutrition and respiratory function is complex and not fully elucidated. Although patients with PCM have respiratory complications, provision of nutrition does not consistently improve outcomes. In some patients with respiratory problems, caloric restriction and weight loss are associated with clinical improvement.

PCM is associated with changes in lung parenchyma similar to morphological changes associated with COPD. Air spaces are enlarged and surface area for gas exchange is diminished.[32,33] Respiratory muscle function is altered; diaphragmatic mass, strength, and endurance are reduced.[27,28] Prolonged PCM is associated with diminished lung volumes and maximal voluntary ventilation.[28] Metabolic decreases in carbon dioxide production are likely to be associated with a diminished respiratory rate.

Nutritional support has been suggested as a management approach for patients during weaning from mechanical ventilation; protein depletion may be associated with increased risk of postoperative pneumonia and a longer hospital stay in patients receiving ventilation therapy.[34] However, no definitive studies have demonstrated improved weaning outcomes based on nutritional support. Concern exists that gastric feeding may be associated with increased risk of nosocomial pneumonia in patients receiving mechanical ventilation. However, in a small randomized trial, when nutrients were delivered into the small intestine, pneumonia rates and other outcomes were similar.[35]

Although starvation can hasten death, weight loss can improve functional status in some types of respiratory patients. In patients with COPD, PCM is associated with higher mortality rates and inferior respiratory function; in surgical patients it is associated with reduced respiratory function and postoperative respiratory complications. In some ambulatory COPD patients, nutritional repletion is associated with improved respiratory muscle function, but not in all cases; it is not clear whether improved respiratory muscle function results in improved functional exercise capacity or quality of life. A recent meta-analysis demonstrated that among stable COPD patients, supplemental nutritional support did not improve lung function or exercise capacity.[36] Weight reduction in obese patients with asthma improves lung function, symptoms, morbidity, and health status.[37]

Renal Consequences

PCM is associated with structural and functional changes in the kidneys. Kidney mass and protein content diminish proportional to changes in body mass.[38] Glomerular filtration and creatinine clearance are decreased.[39] The neurohormones of stress are associated with salt and water retention in the kidney. Thus a patient with stressed-related PCM tends to preserve the circulating blood volume until the serum protein levels drop and often develops a slight water excess.

Gastrointestinal Consequences

In PCM, intestinal mass and protein content diminish proportionately more than the loss of body mass.[40] The epithelium is altered, with loss of some mucosal integrity.[41] There is impaired absorption, possibly related to loss of brush border enzymes.[42] There are decreased gastric, pancreatic, and biliary secretions and low enzyme and conjugated bile acid concentrations.[43] Enteral feeding is more effective than parenteral nutrition in restoring the integrity of gastrointestinal mucosa[44] and is generally preferred if available.[45]

Gastric emptying is slowed during PCM. Cytokines are important mediators linking neural, immune, and endocrine systems. Nurse scientists interested in understanding the pathophysiology of symptom distress associated with disease have examined peripheral cytokine levels. For example, McCarthy[46] described the impact of TNF-α on gastric emptying and appetite in an effort to understand the effects of cancer and inflammation on weight loss. Such studies are critical to our understanding of mediators linking disease with symptom experiences.

In the liver, hepatocyte structure is relatively well preserved during PCM.[47] Drug metabolism is altered (generally reduced) due to the effect of protein deficiency on the cytochrome P450 system and NADPH-dependent electron transport.[48] Thus patients with PCM may require lower doses of some medications. Drugs that are protein bound may require reduced dosing as well, due to lower serum protein levels.

Immune Consequences

PCM contributes to increased morbidity and mortality through impairment of host defense mechanisms and reduced immune (e.g., macrophage) function. Nutrition is a critical determinant of immune responses and malnutrition is the most common cause of immunodeficiency worldwide. PCM is associated with a significant impairment of cell-mediated immunity, phagocyte function, complement system, secretory immunoglobulin A antibody concentrations, and cytokine production.[18] McCarter et al[49] examined alterations in macrophage intracellular signaling associated with impaired host defense capabilities. Mice were randomized to either control (regular diet) or protein-free diets (PCM) and pair-fed for 1 week. Following endotoxin stimulation, peritoneal macrophages from PCM mice produced significantly less TNF-α and IL-6 than control mice; they had significantly less cell-associated IL-6 when compared with macrophages from control mice. Similarly, macrophages from PCM mice had a significant reduction in mRNA levels for both TNF-α and IL-6. Other macrophage intracellular signaling mechanisms, such as calcium flux and tyrosine kinase phosphorylation were also altered by PCM. The cause of PCM-induced defects in macrophage function and intracellular signaling remain unknown but may be related to the neuroendocrine response to PCM. Deficiency of single nutrients also results in altered immune responses: this is observed even when the deficiency state is relatively mild. Micronutrients (zinc, selenium, iron, and copper) and vitamins (A, C, E, B_6, and folic acid) have important influences on immune responses.

Wound Healing

Wound healing requires adequate nutrition to meet the energy demands of tissue repair while controlling infection. Current recommendations to support wound healing are 1.5 to 3.0 g protein/kg of body weight/day (depending on the extent of the wound), plus 100 to 600 g carbohydrate/day, and ⅓ of the total daily nonprotein calories supplied as fat.[50] It is known that both mild and severe caloric deficiencies impair healing, as measured by hydroxyproline content of test wounds.[51] Significantly, Windsor et al[52] demonstrated that inadequate food intake over the prior week similarly diminished the hydroxyproline content; this impairment was not related to long-term nutrition status, such as protein or fat stores. Hence preoperative or pretrauma nutrition status may be as important as postoperative or posttrauma status and should be evaluated in caring for surgical or trauma patients. Nutritional repletion both before and soon after wounding is needed for wound healing.

DIFFERENTIAL DIAGNOSIS

Patients with PCM are often seen initially for other reasons and report or are noted to have a history of weight loss. The challenge for the clinician is to recognize the problem and devise a plan to address the problem before the patient's vulnerability progresses to severe debilitation. Patients should be screened for changes in appetite, diet, weight, and sources of nutrient loss. Once recognized, the problem should be aggressively addressed.

MANIFESTATIONS AND SURVEILLANCE

Common techniques for assessment of the patient at risk for PCM include dietary, anthropometric, biochemical, and functional indices of nutritional status, as reviewed next. There is no consensus as to the best method for the accurate assessment of nutritional status. Each technique has potential for inaccuracy. Some of the approaches are expensive or impractical. Some techniques are influenced by nonnutritional factors.[53] Clinicians sometimes use multiple measures to determine nutritional status.

Dietary Assessment Methods

A dietary assessment includes history information related to food intake patterns. Data collection can be retrospective or prospective. In a retrospective diet history, the interviewer prompts the subject to recall and describe all food and beverages consumed over a period of time, usually the prior 24 hours. This method might be aided by the use of food models or measuring devices. An alternative approach is to ask the patient how often and in what proportion certain categories of foods are consumed. Because retrospective methods depend on memory, they are not suitable for patients with short-term memory loss. The method is as accurate as the patient's estimation of portion sizes. The method relies on the assumption that the day described is typical and on the patient's willingness to accurately describe diet intake.

Prospective methods involve keeping a food record. Ideally, this includes weighing the food before it is consumed. Most food diaries require substantial effort from the patient and rely on his cooperation. The patient who is not adequately nourished may be incapable of keeping accurate records. Alternative prospective methods such as video-recording or direct observation of food consumption are costly and obtrusive.

Both prospective and retrospective methods of analyzing the diet provide information on food intake. Neither method takes into account problems with absorption of food. Diet records can be validated with information from other observers. It may be helpful to note whether the patient is experiencing hunger.

Foods noted on the patient's dietary history can be compared with food composition tables to determine dietary components. Most food composition data are based on U.S. Department of Agriculture (USDA) compilations. These do not always identify a brand name for prepared foods. While the data are generally adequate to analyze typical diets in industrialized countries, often information on food composition from developing countries is fragmented or missing.

The calculated dietary intake is then compared with the patient's dietary needs. The most accurate method to measure caloric need is with a metabolic cart. The metabolic cart detects respiratory gases and measures oxygen consumption and carbon dioxide production. From these values caloric consumption can be calculated. However, a metabolic cart is cumbersome and expensive; it requires calibration and an experienced user. A less costly alternative is to estimate the patient's caloric need. A common approach is to calculate caloric need using the Harris-Benedict equations, illustrated in Box 4-1,[54] modified to account for caloric demands related to illness and activity.

Protein need is usually based on the 2002 recommendations of the Food and Nutrition Board of the Institute of Medicine.[55] Generally, approximately 0.8 g protein/kg of body weight/day is recommended for adults, with larger amounts recommended in

BOX 4-1 Calculation of Caloric and Protein Needs

Step 1a: Calculate Basic Energy Expenditure (BEE) using Harris-Benedict Equation[54]

Men: BEE = 66 + (13.7 × BW) + (5.0 × height) – (6.8 × age)

Women: BEE = 655 + (9.5 × BW) + (1.8 × height) – (4.7 × age)

Note: BW = Body weight, expressed in kg; height in centimeters; age in years.

Step 1b: Calculate Energy Expenditure (EE) by modifying BEE consistent with activity and metabolic demands

Activity corrections

Sedentary: EE = BEE × 130%
Moderate: EE = BEE × 150%
Strenuous: EE = BEE × 200%

Metabolic corrections

Nonstressed hospitalized patients: EE = BEE × 120%
Catabolic patients: EE = BEE × 150% to 200%
Fever: EE = BEE × [(Number of degrees Celsius of temperature elevation × 13%) + 100%]
Burns: EE = BEE × 140% to 200%
Trauma: EE = BEE × 140% to 200%
Hyperthyroidism: EE = BEE × (110% to 200%)
Hypothyroidism: EE = BEE × (75% to 100%)

Step 2a: Calculate Approximate Daily Protein Requirement

Daily Protein Requirement = (0.8 to 2.0 g/kg BW)

Step 2b: Modify Daily Protein Requirement According to Clinical Circumstances

Choose value toward upper limit of the daily protein requirement range with growth, pregnancy/lactation, repletion following malnutrition

Choose value at or below the daily requirement range for liver or renal failure (e.g., 0.35 g/kg)

children and pregnant or lactating women. These recommendations are calculated based on the amount of protein producing zero nitrogen balance, increased by two standard deviations so as to include 97.5% of the population. The calculations are based on the assumption that caloric intake is adequate and that protein is of high quality and readily digestible.

Anthropometric Methods

Anthropometric measures provide an estimate of nutrition status. Included in this category are height, weight, midarm circumference, and skinfold thickness measurements and related calculated values. There is no anthropometric measure that is considered completely accurate.[55] Measurement error can occur unless the examiner pays careful attention to calibration. A multitude of physical factors, such as edema and variations in clothing, can influence the sensitivity of these measures. Standardized weight and height tables based on insurance company data are used to estimate nutritional status. However, such tools, when they were developed, were based primarily on data from young to middle-aged white adults. In general, anthropometrics tend to provide better information about changes over time within an individual than as a one-time measure of nutritional status.

One of the simplest methods to assess overall nutritional status is body weight (BW) measurement. In ambulatory care settings, BW loss guidelines, including greater than 5% in 1 month or 10% in 6 months, have been used to denote potential health or nutrition problems. BWs are often compared with calculated ideal BW (IBW). For calculation purposes the IBW for women is 100 lb for the first 5 feet in height, plus 5 lb for each inch over 5 feet. In men IBW is 106 lb for the first 5 feet, plus 6 pounds for each inch above 5 feet. The current body weight (CBW) is divided by the IBW to calculate the patient's percent of IBW[57]:

$$\%IBW = CBW/IBW \times 100$$

IBW does not take body build into account. Most adults are not at their IBW; thus expressing weight as the percentage of usual weight can be useful.

The body mass index (BMI) is another indicator of overall body weight status. It is calculated using actual body weight (in kilograms) and height squared. The range accepted as normal in adults is approximately 20 to 27 kg/m^2, corresponding to approximately the 10th to 75th percentile of a healthy population. PCM is suspected when the BMI falls below 20 kg/m^2 and definitive when below 17 kg/m^2 in adults.[58]

Triceps skinfold thickness (TSF) reflects body fat stores. It is measured in the upper arm halfway between the inferior border of the acromiun process and the tip of the olecranon process of the nondominant arm. Midarm muscle circumference (MAMC) reflects lean muscle mass. It is measured at the same level as the TSF. It is calculated as:

$$\text{Circumference} - (3.14 \times \text{TSF})$$

Both TSF and MAMC are less reliable in older adults because of skin changes (e.g., loss of elasticity, decreased subcutaneous fat) associated with aging and are not reliable in disease states associated with increased total body water (e.g., heart failure and renal failure). Standard reference tables are derived from data on healthy adults.

Bioelectric impedance (BIA) is used to measure fat-free mass. The principle underlying this technique is that there are differences in electrical conductivity between fat and fat-free mass. Advantages to this technique include that it is noninvasive, relatively inexpensive and requires little patient participation. However, BIA has been recommended for population based studies rather than as a guide for nutritional therapies for individual patients. Its use is limited in patients with significant fluid and electrolyte imbalances and in those with edema or dehydration.

Biochemical Laboratory Data Methods

Biochemical measurements of PCM include serum measures of plasma proteins, such as albumin, transferrin, and prealbumin. Serum levels of these proteins reflect the dynamic balance among synthesis, distribution, and degradation. Hepatic synthesis is affected by substrate availability (thus proteins can indicate nutrition status), but also by hepatic function. Thus the markers must be interpreted in the context of the patient's clinical condition.

Serum albumin level is commonly used in nutrition screening. It is a useful screening test when the patient is admitted to the hospital to detect chronic PCM. A low serum albumin level at the time of hospital or nursing home admission correlates with other makers of poor nutrition and predicts a poor surgical outcome,[59] less likelihood of survival,[60] and increased cost and length of stay.[61,62] Traditionally, the accepted criteria for undernutrition is a level less than 3.5 g/dl; however, somewhat higher levels have been associated with adverse outcomes.[63] Reuben et al[64] noted higher mortality rates in older adults with more modest decreases in serum albumin level (<3.8 g/dl). Albumin has a half-life of 18 to 20 days. It is unlikely that nutritionally related mechanisms will cause the level to drop acutely. Acute drops in serum albumin level are likely to be caused by protein loss via leaky capillaries or wound drainage; hemodilution also lowers serum albumin and all serum proteins. Albumin levels drop by as much as 1.0 to 1.5 g/dl with acute catabolic illness.[65] Serum albumin level is a poor marker of nutritional repletion.

Transferrin has a shorter half-life than albumin (8 to 10 days); thus it is potentially more useful as a marker of acute malnutrition. Fletcher et al[66] found that transferrin levels correlated with nitrogen balance. Roza et al[67] found that transferrin level correlated with body composition but did not rise with 2 weeks of adequate nutrition repletion. Decreases in serum transferrin levels are associated with an increased mortality rate in elderly patients in nursing homes.[4] Transferrin levels are distorted by the same factors that lower serum albumin: serum extravasation or dilution can lower the levels. Transferrin levels are increased with iron deficiency, pregnancy, hepatitis, and with the use of certain antibiotics and oral contraceptives. Hence it is not an ideal indicator of acute nutrition-related changes, and care must be taken when one is evaluating their significance.[10]

Prealbumin is increasingly used as a nutrition status marker. It has a short half-life, 1 to 2 days and thus is a better marker of successful refeeding. In a group of healthy, obese women, prealbumin levels decreased with calorie or protein restriction, then increased within 72 hours of refeeding.[68] Prealbumin level is distorted by liver dysfunction, dilutional problems, and serum extravasation.

Functional Methods

Functional measures of PCM are somewhat useful in population studies but are problematic in ill patients. In an early study, Klidjian et al[69] used a variety of biochemical and functional measures of PCM. Of the measures used, hand grip strength most sensitively predicted postoperative complications. Electromyographic measurements of muscle fatigue can indicate PCM. The latter method has the advantage that one can stimulate an extremity electrically, not requiring the cooperation of the patient.

Malnutrition adversely affects the immune system. Thus skin tests for anergy (failure to mount an inflammatory response) are another type of functional nutrition status marker. Harvey et al[70] found that improved skin response to common antigens was useful in predicting improved prognosis. However, steroids and general anesthesia suppress skin test responses. Skin testing requires interpretation 24 to 72 hours later.

Recommendations for Nutrition Assessment in Clinical Practice

It is important to detect PCM in patients, but given the complexity and cost of nutritional assessment, it is unrealistic to plan to perform comprehensive nutritional assessment in all patients. It is useful to have screening protocols that will identify patients who merit more comprehensive study. A screening tool sufficient to detect gross deficiencies should include information about diet (appetite, history of poor or altered intake, and unusual dietary restrictions), anthropometry (height, weight, and weight changes), clinical condition (diagnoses associated with nutritional risk), physical assessment data (muscle atrophy, cachexia, and edema), and laboratory data (albumin, hematocrit level, and white blood cell count). When the screening tool detects an increased risk for PCM, patients should be referred for more comprehensive nutritional assessment. Comprehensive assessment is likely to include more detailed dietary analysis, comprehensive anthropometric information (such as skinfold measurements and BIA), and additional laboratory data (such as prealbumin, transferrin, and serum chemistries).

CLINICAL MANAGEMENT

Clinical management of PCM involves nutritional support (i.e., providing the patient with the needed nutrients). In some cases nutrition support has demonstrated efficacy.[71] Although in many cases the efficacy of nutrition support is unproven, it is intuitively reasonable to anticipate that patients will have improved clinical outcomes if they are well nourished.

Clinical management begins with assessing the nutritional risk factors. Management involves careful assessment, including the patient's ability to secure food, functional status, appetite, mood state, dental status, chewing and swallowing abilities, medications that interfere with appetite, absorption and metabolism, and disease-related dietary restrictions. When factors limiting protein-calorie intake are identified, the appropriate plan can be made to nourish the patient. Then one calculates or measures the patient's daily caloric and protein needs and develops a plan to deliver nutrition and reassess the outcome. The Harris-Benedict equation[54] is commonly used to calculate caloric need.

Nutritional support can be safely administered to most patients because of the refinement of enteral and parenteral techniques. It is recommended that patients be fed via the gastrointestinal tract if it is functioning. Generally, enteral feeding is less expensive with better clinical outcomes than parenteral routes.[73,75] Studies suggest that enteral feeding may protect the integrity of the gut mucosa,[78] preserve brush border enzyme activity,[78] and improve immune responses.[79,80]

Enteral feeding is sometimes not tolerated in patients with a functioning GI tract because of diarrhea or gastric retention. In these cases smaller volume feedings or diluted feedings might be better tolerated. Kudsk et al[75] concluded that the use of the enteral route is more important than the composition of the diet. Altering the diet composition or diluting the diet may make liquid feedings more tolerated.

Parenteral feeding can be useful as an adjunct to enteral feeding or as a primary method of feeding if the enteral route is not available (e.g., in the case of bowel obstruction, intractable diarrhea or vomiting, peritonitis, pancreatitis, short bowel syndrome, and ileus). There is no uniformly recommended formulation. Emerging evidence indicates that glutamine supplementation (0.2 to 0.5 g/kg/day) in parenteral formulations is linked with improved outcomes in selected groups of patients. Studies have shown that glutamine is safe, and can be associated with improved nitrogen balance,[81] decreased infections,[82] decreased number of days of mechanical ventilation,[84] reduced length of hospital stay,[82,85] and reduced expenses.[82,83] Most enteral formulations include some glutamine; there is a need for studies of parenteral glutamine supplementation.

If the patient has severe PCM, precautions are needed. The patient may have life-threatening conditions, such as fluid and electrolyte imbalances, infections, hemodynamic alterations, severe anemia, hypothermia, or hypoglycemia. These conditions would merit immediate attention. WHO has prepared guidelines for administration of oral rehydration salt solution consisting of potassium, magnesium, zinc, and copper to be given in combination with food or mixed with glucose in an isotonic solution.

After life-threatening problems are corrected, the goal is to gradually restore nutritional balance. This often involves frequent, small, liquid feedings. The fluid is administered orally if possible, initially in small quantities, for a total of about 70 to 100 ml/kg of body weight.

Patients receiving nutritional support, especially parenteral feeding, should be evaluated periodically for serum electrolyte and glucose concentrations, liver function, and nitrogen balance. Body weight should be monitored; generally gain of more than 1 kg/week suggests the patient is retaining fluid. Complications of parenteral nutritional range from electrolyte disorders to life-threatening sepsis.

CONCEPTUAL MODEL

A conceptual model, based on a human response framework to guide clinical decision making, is illustrated in Figure 4-1. This paradigm is based on the human response model.[87] The model integrates the risk factors, some of which the care provider might

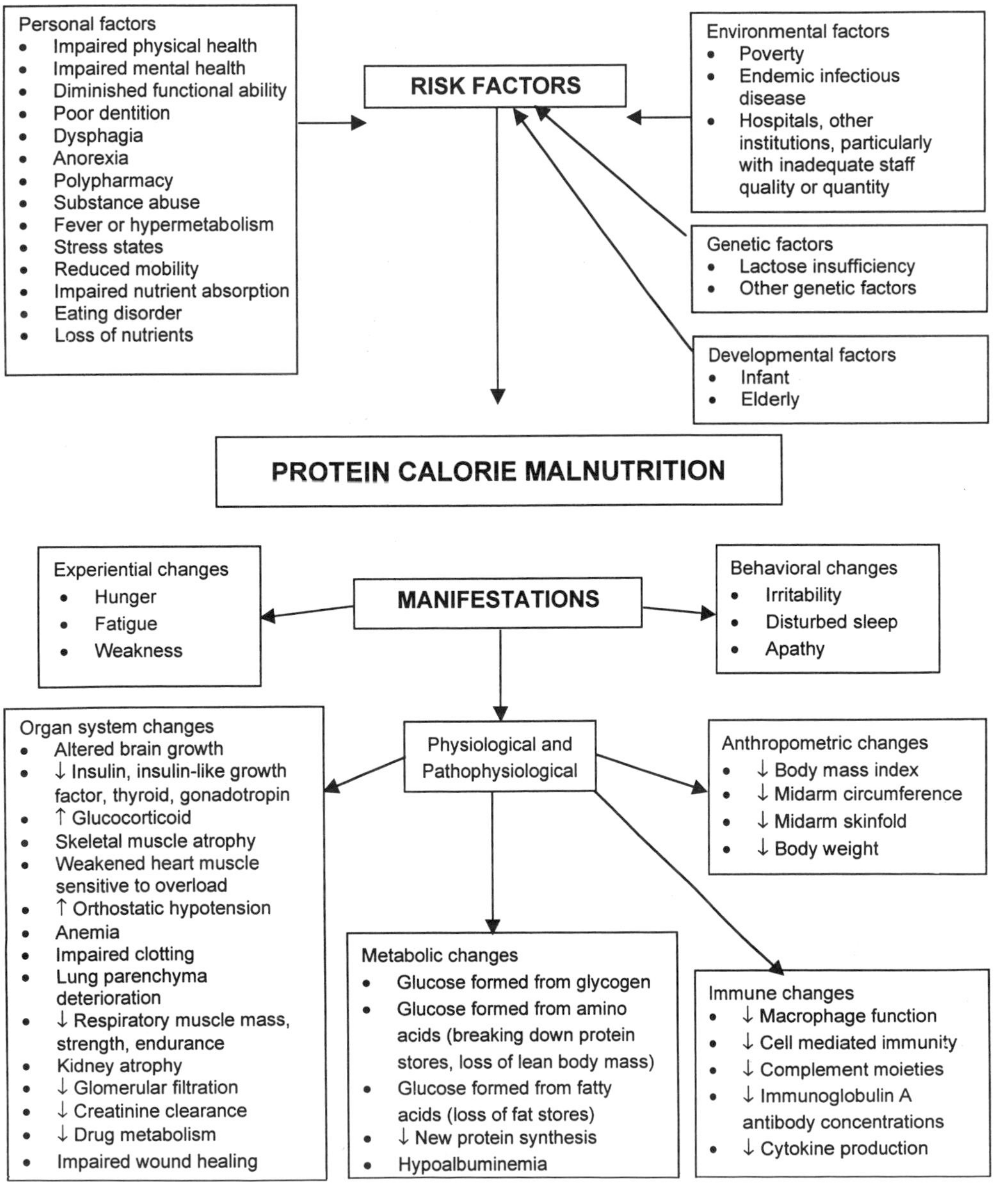

Figure 4-1 The human response conceptual model applied to clinical assessment and management of individuals vulnerable to PCM.

minimize. The model summarizes many manifestations of PCM.

CASE STUDY

CASE STUDY: PCM

Manifestations

PF is an 82-year-old man with a medical history of atrial fibrillation, hypertension, syncope, pacemaker implantation, heart failure, pulmonary edema, chronic renal failure, anemia, dementia, and substantial recent weight loss. His son has brought PF to the geriatric clinic because of complaints of shortness of breath. PF's medications included digoxin, hydralazine, diltiazem, furosemide, aspirin, and carvedilol. PF lives with his wife in a two-story home with essential rooms on the first floor. The wife had a stroke several years ago and is not able to care for PF. The patient states that he does the shopping and cooking. However, the son states that this is no longer true, and that he and his siblings provide food several times weekly. The children have urged PF to accept more help, but he refuses.

Physical examination reveals a thin, cachetic-appearing edentulous male. His clothes appear oversized and a wrist watch dangles (suggesting recent weight loss). His height is 5'9" (175 cm), weight 132 lb (59.7 kg); this represents a weight loss of 8 lb in the last month and 23 lb in the last 4 months (based on data from prior clinic visits).

His review of systems reveals the following data. His Mini-Mental Status Exam score is 16/30, suggesting significant cognitive impairment. He is not able to state the date, time, or place. He has poor item recall (0/3) at 3 minutes, even with prompting. The patient lacks insight into his deficits, stating, "I am in disgustingly good health." His heart rate is 96 beats/min, his pulse is irregularly irregular, and no murmurs are noted. His blood pressure is 150/84; there is no significant change in heart rate and blood pressure with change of posture. No jugular venous distention is noted. There is no peripheral edema. The respiratory rate is 24/min. Coarse breath sounds are auscultated bilaterally at the basal 25% of the lung. The abdomen status is benign, without tenderness.

During nutritional assessment, the patient reports preference for a diet high in meat, spicy foods, and ice cream; he adds salt to most foods. The patient states he does not believe that he has renal disease or hypertension; he does not follow any deliberate dietary modifications. He states that he had no breakfast, but the son reports that he ate well 2 hours before.

Using the Harris Benedict equation for men,[54] PF's caloric need is calculated as 1440 calories/day, as follows:

$$\text{BEE} = 66.5 + (13.7 \times 59.7\ \text{kg}) + (5.0 \times 175\ \text{cm}) \times (6.8 \times 82\ \text{yr}) \text{ or } 1200 \text{ calories}$$

$$\text{TEE} = 1200 \text{ calories} \times 1.2 \text{ activity factor for ambulatory subjects} = 1440 \text{ calories/day}$$

Using the recommendations of the Cochrane Renal Group,[88] some protein restriction is likely to delay the progression of renal failure; thus 0.35 gm/kg of body weight is recommended (21 g/day).

His laboratory test results reveal the following values: serum albumin 4.2 g/dl (normal value in adults [NVA], 3.5 to 5.0 g/dl), transferrin 244 mg/dl (NVA, 250 to 450 mg/dl), total iron-binding capacity (TIBC) 310 μg/dl (NVA, 250 to 410 μg/dl), hematocrit 29.9% (NWA 45% to 52%), hemoglobin 9.6 g/dl (NVA 13 to 18 g/dl). His urine is 5+ for protein.

Surveillance

The patient was admitted to an inpatient unit to refine his medication regimen, manage the heart failure, and improve the nutritional status. While he was hospitalized, the goal was to provide a diet that would maintain body weight after he lost an estimated 1 to 2 kg of retained fluid. Monitoring included daily observation of food consumption, intake and output, and body weight. He was inspected for signs of dependent edema and jugular venous distension; his chest was auscultated for worsening breath sounds. Serum transferrin was monitored weekly. In all cases, because the patient is not a reliable observer, his reports were validated with direct observation of caloric intake.

Clinical Management Across Settings

While PF was in the hospital, the nutrition goal was to maintain current weight while bringing heart failure and hypertension under control. He was placed on a 1500 kcal, 21 g protein, 2 g sodium diet with controlled potassium (because patient has chronic renal failure), integrating the patient's request for spicy and sweet foods. Because the patient is not a reliable reporter of his intake, eating, his caloric intake was measured at each meal. The family was urged to visit during meal times and encourage the patient to eat. Prepared food was supplemented with liquid diet midafternoon and in the evening. The patient was fit with dentures. After eliminating other causes of anemia, it was concluded that the anemia was caused by the severe progressive renal disease and the patient was started on erythropoietin.

Home Management

The goal was that the patient gain weight slowly. He was placed on a diet of 2 g sodium, controlled potassium, 21 g protein, and 2000 kcal. Meals-On-Wheels service was requested, to be supplemented with liquid feeding. The patient was to be visited three times weekly by a visiting nurse (to measure weight) and three times weekly by a physical therapist. The patient was scheduled to return to the clinic every 2 weeks for monitoring of weight, hematocrit level, and clinical status. The family was encouraged to continue visiting at mealtime to monitor food consumption. The family was urged to prepare for placement of PF and his wife in an assisted living facility.

QUESTIONS FOR FUTURE STUDIES

There is a need to develop and validate clinical tools for identifying patients with or at risk for PCM in hospitals, nursing homes, and home settings. Existing reference standards (e.g., BMI and TSF) are based on measurements in healthy people. Needed are reference standards that are applicable to elderly, ill, and young persons. Information about the way reference standards change with illness is needed, as well as how those changes can be used to guide care and alter clinical outcomes.

Research is needed to devise and validate more accurate and efficient ways of predicting a patient's calorie and protein need, so that clinicians can plan intake to match the need. Existing equations are efficient to use but are accurate only in a healthy young adult. Metabolic cart measures of caloric consumption are more accurate but are not available in homes nor in long term care facilities. Needed are accurate methods to use in children, the elderly, the sick, the stressed.

There is a need to develop methods to ensure that people in a variety of venues are adequately fed. What interventions are most effective in preventing PCM in nursing home residents? What interventions work in community or hospital settings or in schools? For patients with diminished appetites, what combinations of interventions to improve appetite and provide nutrition are most effective? Does exercise have a positive effect on appetite in those at risk for PCM?

There is a need for more detailed scientific delineation of the mechanisms and consequences of PCM. What role does the sympathetic nervous system and the hypothalamic-pituitary-adrenal axis play in mediating immune responses to malnutrition? A variety of clinical trials have demonstrated changes in certain nutritional markers with provision of nutrition. There is need to examine the impact of nutrition on more global clinical outcomes.

SUMMARY

PCM is very common, particularly in elderly and chronically ill persons. PCM is linked with poor clinical outcomes. Studies demonstrate that nutritional repletion is associated with improved nutritional markers. Nutrition can be safely administered to most patients via enteral or parenteral routes, with enteral routes generally preferred. Clinical trial evidence is needed that nutrition repletion is linked with improvement in global outcomes.

REFERENCES

1. Covinsky, K.E., Martin, G.E., Beyth, R.J., Justice, A.C., Sehgal, A.R., & Landefeld, C.S. (1999). The relationship between clinical assessments of nutritional status and adverse outcomes in older hospitalized medical patients. *Journal of the American Geriatric Society 47,* 532-538.
2. Sullivan, D.H., Sun, S., & Walls, R.C. (1999). Protein-energy undernutrition among elderly hospitalized patients: A prospective study. *Journal of the American Medical Association 281,* 2013-2019.
3. Institute of Medicine. (2000). *The Role of Nutrition in Maintaining Health in the Nation's Elderly.* Washington, D.C.: National Academy Press.
4. McCormack, P. (1997). Undernutrition in the elderly population living at home in the community: A review of the literature. *Journal of Advanced Nursing 26,* 856-883.
5. Bistrian, B.R., Blackburn, G.L., Hallowell, E., & Heddle, R. (1974). Protein status of general surgical patients. *Journal of the American Medical Association 230,* 858-860.
6. Bistrian, B.R., Blackburn, G.L., Vitale, J., Cochran, D., & Naylor, J. (1976). Prevalence of malnutrition in general medical patients. *Journal of the American Medical Association 235,* 1567-1570.
7. Potter, M.A., & Luxton, G. (1999). Prealbumin measurement as a screening tool for protein calorie malnutrition in emergency hospital admissions: A pilot study. *Clinical and Investigative Medicine 22,* 44-52.
8. Friedmann, J.M., Jensen, G.L., Smiciklas-Wright, H., & McCamish, M.A. (1997). Predicting early nonelective hospital readmission in nutritionally compromised older adults. *Journal of Clinical Nutrition 65,* 1714-1720.
9. Himes, D. (1999). Protein-calorie malnutrition and involuntary weight loss: The role of aggressive nutritional intervention in wound healing. *Ostomy/Wound Management 45,* 46-55.
10. Thomas, D.R. (1997). The role of nutrition in prevention and healing of pressure ulcers. *Clinics in Geriatric Medicine 13,* 497-511.
11. Kayser-Jones, J., Schell, E. (1997). The effect of staffing on the quality of care at mealtime. *Nursing Outlook 45,* 64-72.
12. Ritchie, C.S., Burgio, K.L., Locher, J.L., Cornwell, A., Thomas, D., Hardin, M., & Redden, D. (1997). Nutritional status of urban homebound adults. *American Journal of Clinical Nutrition 66,* 815-816.
13. Edington, J. (1999). Problems of nutritional assessment in the community. *Proceedings of the Nutrition Society 58,* 47-51.
14. Bunout, D. (1999). Nutritional and metabolic effects of alcoholism: Their relationship with alcoholic liver disease. *Nutrition 15,* 583-589.
15. Roubenoff, R., Heymesfield, S.B., Kehayias, J.J., Cannon, J.G., & Rosenberg, I.H. (1997). Standardization of nomenclature of body composition in weight loss. *American Journal of Clinical Nutrition 66,* 192-196.
16. Schalling, M., Johansen, J., Nordfors, L., & Lonnqvist, F. (1999). Genes involved in animal models of obesity and anorexia. *Journal of Internal Medicine 245,* 613-619.
17. Phadke, M.A., Khedkar, V.A., Pashankar, D., Kate, S.L., Mokashi, G.D., Gambhir, P.S., Bhate, S.M. (1995). Serum

amino acids and genesis of protein energy malnutrition. *Indian Pediatrics 32,* 301-306.
18. Chandra, R.K. (1997). Nutrition and the immune system: An introduction. *American Journal of Clinical Nutrition 66,* 460S-463S.
19. Schanler, R.J., Shulman, R.J., Lau, C., Smith, E.O., & Heitkemper, M.M. (1999). Strategies for premature infants: Randomized trial of initiation and method of feeding. *Pediatrics 103,* 434-439.
20. Shulman, R.J., Schanler, R.J., Lau, C., Heitkemper. M.M., Ou, C., & Smith, E.O. (1998). Early feeding, feeding tolerance, and lactase activity in preterm infants. *Pediatric Research 133,* 645-649.
21. WHO website on nutrition: http://www.who.int/nut/
22. Rothman, D.L., Magnusson, I., Katz, L.D., Shulman, R.G., & Shulman, G.I. (1991). Quantitation of hepatic glycogenolysis and gluconeogenesis in fasting humans with 13 C NMR. *Science, New Series 254*(5031), 573-576.
23. Krzywicki, H.J., Consolazio, C.F., Matoush, L.O., & Johnson, H.L. (1968). Metabolic aspects of acute starvation. *American Journal of Clinical Nutrition 21,* 87-97.
24. Beisel, W.R. (1995). Herman Award Lecture: Infection-induced malnutrition—from cholera to cytokines. *American Journal of Clinical Nutrition 62,* 813-819.
25. Winick, M. (1987). Long term effects of kwashiorkor. *Journal of Pediatric Gastroenterology and Nutrition 6,* 933-935.
26. Mattson, M.P. (2000). Emerging neuroprotective strategies for Alzheimer's disease: Dietary restriction, telomerase activation, and stem cell therapy. *Experimental Gerontology 35,* 489-503.
27. Arora, N.S., & Rochester, D.F. (1982a). Effect of body weight and muscularity on human diaphragm muscle mass, thickness, and area. *Journal of Applied Physiology 52,* 64-70.
28. Arora, N.S., & Rochester, D.F. (1982b). Respiratory muscle strength and maximal voluntary ventilation in undernourished patients. *American Review of Respiratory Disease 126,* 5-8.
29. McLoughlin, D.M., Spargo, E., Wassif, W.S., Newham, D.J., Peters, T.J., Lantos, P.L., et al. (1998). Structural and functional changes in skeletal muscle in anorexia nervosa. *Acta Neuropathologica (Berl) 95,* 632-640.
30. Phornphatkul, C., Pongprot, Y., Suskind, R., George, V., & Fuchs, G. (1994). Cardiac function in malnourished children. *Clinical Pediatrics 33,* 147-154.
31. Vitari, F.E. (1981). Primary protein-energy malnutrition: Clinical biochemical, and metabolic changes. In R.M. Suskind (ed.), *Textbook of pediatric nutrition* (pp. 189-215), New York: Raven Press.
32. Kerr, J.S., Riley, D.J., Lanza-Jacoby, S., Berg, R.A., Spilker, H.C., Yu, S.Y., et al. (1985). Nutritional emphysema in the rat: Influence of protein depletion and impaired lung growth. *American Review of Respiratory Disease 131,* 644-650.
33. Sahibjami, H., & Vassalo, C.L. (1979). Effects of starvation and refeeding on lung mechanics and morphometry. *American Review of Respiratory Disease 119,* 443-451.
34. Windsor, J.A., & Hill, G.L. (1988). Risk factors for postoperative pneumonia. The importance of protein depletion. *Annals of Surgery 208,* 209-214.
35. Kearns, P.J., Chin, D., Mueller, L., Wallace, K., Jensen, W.A., & Kirsch, C.M. (2000). The incidence of ventilator associated pneumonia and success in nutrient delivery with gastric versus small intestinal feeding: A randomized clinical trial. *Critical Care Medicine 28,* 1742-1746.
36. Ferriera, I.M., Brooks, D., Lacasse, Y., & Goldstein, R.S. (2000). Nutritional support for individuals with COPD. *Chest 117,* 672-678.
37. Stenius-Aarniala, B., Poussa, T., Kvarnstrom, J., Gronlund, E.L., Ylikahri, M., & Mustajoki, P. (2000). Immediate and long term effects of weight reduction in obese people with asthma: Randomized controlled study. *British Medical Journal 320*(7238), 827-832.
38. Goodman, M.N., Lowell B., Belur E., & Ruderman, N.B. (1984). Sites of protein conservation and loss during starvation. *American Journal of Physiology 246,* E383-E390.
39. Train, V.M., & Sath, B.T. (1973). Effect of starvation on renal function. *Lancet 2,* 620-622.
40. McManus, J.P.A., & Iselbacher, K.J. (1970). Effect of fasting versus feeding on the rat small intestine: Morphological, biochemical, and functional differences. *Gastroenterology 59,* 214-221.
41. Hooper, A.F., Wannemacher, R.W. Jr., & McGovern, P.A. (1968). Cell population changes in the intestinal epithelium of the fat following starvation and protein depletion. *Proceedings of the Society of Experimental Biology and Medicine 128,* 695-698.
42. Kim, Y.S., McCarthy, D.M., Lane, W., & Fong, W. (1973). Alterations in the levels of peptide hydrolases and other enzymes in brush-border and soluble fractions of rat small intestine mucosa during starvation and refeeding. *Biochimica et Biophysica Acta 321,* 262-273.
43. Pitchumoni, C.S. (1973). Pancreas in primary malnutrition disorders. *American Journal of Clinical Nutrition 26,* 374-379.
44. Alverdy, J., Chi, H.S., & Sheldon, G.F. (1985). The effect of parenteral nutrition on gastrointestinal immunity. *Annals of Surgery 202,* 681-690.
45. McQuiggan, M.M., Marvin, R.G., McKinley, B.A., & Moore, F.A. (1999). Enteral feeding following major torso trauma: From theory to practice. *New Horizons 7,* 131-146.
46. McCarthy, D.O. (2000). Tumor necrosis factor alpha and interleukin-6 have differential effects on food intake and gastric emptying in fasted rats. *Research in Nursing & Health 23,* 222-228.
47. Sherlock, S., & Walshe, V. (1948). Effects of undernutrition on man on hepatic structure and function. *Nature 161,* 604-629.
48. Basu, T.K. (1983). The effect of protein malnutrition and ascorbic acid levels on drug metabolism. *Canadian Journal of Physiology and Pharmacology 61,* 295-301.
49. McCarter, M.D., Naama, H.A., Shou, J., Kwi, L.X., Evoy, D.A., Calvano, S.E., & Daly, J.M. (1998). Altered macrophage intracellular signaling induced by protein-calorie malnutrition. *Cell Immunology 183,* 131-136.
50. Whitney, J.A., & Heitkemper, M.M. (1999). Modifying perfusion, nutrition, and stress to promote wound healing in patients with acute wounds. *Heart & Lung 28,* 123-133.
51. Haydock, D.A., & Hill, G.L. (1986). Impaired wound healing in surgical patients with varying degrees of malnutrition. *Journal of Parenteral and Enteral Nutrition 10,* 550-554.
52. Windsor, J.A., Knight, G.S., & Hill, G.L. (1988). Wound healing response in surgical patients: Recent food intake is more important than nutritional status. *British Journal of Surgery 75,* 135-137.
53. Baxter, J.P. (1999). Problems of nutritional assessment in the acute setting. *Proceedings of the Nutrition Society 58,* 39-46.

54. Harris, J.A., & Benedict, F.G. Standard basal metabolism constants for physiologists and clinicians; a biometric study of basal metabolism in man. Philadelphia: J.B. Lippincott. 1919.
55. Food and Nutrition Board, Institute of Medicine. (2002). *Dietary reference intakes for fiber, fat, protein, and amino acid macronutrients.* Washington, D.C.: National Academy Press.
56. Charney, P. (1995). Nutrition assessment in the 1990s: Where are we now? *Nutrition in Clinical Practice 10,* 131-139.
57. Evans-Stoner, N. (1997). Nutritional assessment: A practical approach. *Nursing Clinics of North America 32,* 637-650.
58. Shenkin, A., Cederblad, G., Elia, M., & Isalsson, B. (1996). International Federation of Clinical Chemistry. Laboratory assessment of protein-energy status. *Clinica Chimica Acta 253,* 55-59.
59. Hickman, D.M., Miller, R.A., Rombeau, J.L., Twomey, P.L., & Frey, C.F. (1980). Serum albumin and body weight as predictors of postoperative course in colorectal cancer. *Journal of Parenteral and Enteral Nutrition 4,* 314-316.
60. Rudman, D., Feller, A.G., Nargraj, H.S., Jackson, D.L., Rudman, I.W., & Mattson, D.E. (1987). Relation of serum albumin concentration to death rate in nursing home men. *Journal of Parenteral and Enteral Nutrition 11,* 360-363.
61. Anderson, C.F., & Wochos, D.N. (1982). The utility of serum albumin values in the nutritional assessment of hospitalized patients. *Mayo Clinic Proceedings 57,* 181-184.
62. Reilly, J.J., Hull, S.F., Albert, N., Waller, A., & Bringardener, S. (1988). Economic impact of malnutrition. A model system for hospitalized patients. *Journal of Parenteral and Enteral Nutrition 12,* 371-386.
63. Del Savio, G.C., Zelicof, S.B., Wexler, L.M., Byrne, D.W., Reddy, P.D., Fish, D., & Ende, K.A. (1996). Preoperative nutritional status and outcome of elective total hip replacement. *Clinical Orthopaedics and Related Research 326,* 153-161.
64. Reuben, D.B., Moore, A.A., Damesyn, M., Keeler, E., Harrison, G.G., & Greendale, G.A. (1997). Correlates of hypoalbuminemia in community-dwelling older persons. *American Journal of Clinical Nutrition 66,* 38-45.
65. Patyek, J.A., & Blackburn, G.L. (1984). Goals of nutrition support in acute infections. *American Journal of Medicine 76,* 81-87.
66. Fletcher, J.P., Little, J.M., & Guest, P.K. (1987). A comparison of serum transferrin and serum albumin as nutrition parameters. *Journal of Parenteral and Enteral Nutrition 11,* 144-147.
67. Roza, A.M., Tuitt, D., & Shizgal, H.M. (1984). Transferrin-a poor measure of nutrition status. *Journal of Parenteral and Enteral Nutrition 8,* 523-528.
68. Shetty, P.S., Jung, R.T., Watrasiewicz, K.E., & James, W.P. (1979). Rapid turnover transport proteins: An index of subclinical protein-energy malnutrition. *Lancet 2*(8136), 230-232.
69. Klidjian, A.M., Foster, K.J., Kammerling, R.M., Cooper, A., & Karran, S.J. (1980). Relation of anthropometric and dynamometric variables to serious postoperative complications. *British Medical Journal 281,* 899-901.
70. Harvey, K.B., Moldawer, L.L., Bristian, B.R., & Blackburn, G.L. (1981). Biological measures for the formulation of a hospital prognostic index. *American Journal of Clinical Nutrition 34,* 2013-2022.
71. The Veterans Affairs Total Parenteral Nutrition Cooperative Study Group. (1991). Perioperative total parenteral nutrition in surgical patients. *New England Journal of Medicine 325,* 525-532.
72. Szeluga, D.J., Stuart, R.K., Brookmeyer, R., Utermohlen, V., & Santos, G. (1987). Nutritional support of bone marrow transplant recipients: A prospective, randomized clinical trial comparing total parenteral nutrition to an enteral feeding program. *Cancer Research 47,* 3309-3316.
73. Moore, F.A., Feliciano, D.V., Andrassy, R.J., McArdle, A.H., Booth, F.V., Morgenstein-Wagner, et al. (1992). Early enteral feeding, compared with parenteral, reduces postoperative septic complications: The results of a meta-analysis. *Annals of Surgery 216,* 172-183.
74. Alexander, J.W., MacMillan, B.G., Stinnett, J.D., Ogle, C.K., Bozian, R.C., Fischer, J.E., et al. (1980). Beneficial effects of aggressive protein feeding in severely burned children. *Annals of Surgery 192,* 505-517.
75. Kudsk, K.A., Croce, M.A., Fabian, T.C., Minard, G., Tolley, E.A., Poret, H.A., et al. (1992). Enteral versus parenteral feeding: Effects on septic morbidity following blunt and penetrating abdominal trauma. *Annals of Surgery 215,* 503-513.
76. Moore, E.E., & Jones, T.N. (1986). Benefits of immediate jejunostomy feeding after major abdominal trauma—a prospective, randomized study. *Journal of Trauma 26,* 874-881.
77. Moore, F.A., Moore, E.E., Jones, T.N., McCroskey, B.L., & Peterson, V.M. (1989). TEN versus TPN following major abdominal trauma—reduced septic morbidity. *Journal of Trauma 29,* 916-923.
78. Guedon, C., Schmitz, J., Lerebours, E., Metayer, J., Audran, E., Hemet, J., et al. (1986). Decreased brush border hydrolase activities without gross morphologic changes in human intestinal mucosa after prolonged total parenteral nutrition of adults. *Gastroenterology 90,* 373-378.
79. Kudsk, K.A., Li, J., & Renegar, K.B. (1996). Loss of upper respiratory tract immunity with parenteral feeding. *Annals of Surgery 223,* 629-638.
80. Li, J., Kudsk, K.A., Gocinski, B., Dent, D., Glezer, J., & Langkamp-Henken, B. (1995). Effects of parenteral and enteral nutrition on gut-associated lymphoid tissue. *Journal of Trauma 39,* 44-52.
81. Stehle, P., Zander, J., Mertes, N., Albers, S., Puchstein, C., Lawin, P., et al. (1989). Effect of parenteral glutamine peptide supplements on muscle glutamine loss and nitrogen balance after major surgery. *Lancet 1,* 231-233.
82. Ziegler, T.R., Young, L.S., Benfell, K., Scheltinga, M., Hortos, K., Bye, R., et al. (1992). Clinical and metabolic efficacy of glutamine-supplemented parenteral nutrition after bone marrow transplantation: A randomized, double-blind, controlled study. *Annals of Internal Medicine 116,* 821-828.
83. Byrne, T.A., Persinger, R.L., Young, L.S., Ziegler, T.R., & Wilmore, D.W. (1995). A new treatment for patients with short-bowel syndrome: Growth hormone, glutamine, and a modified diet. *Annals of Surgery 222,* 243-255.
84. Lacey, J.M., Crouch, J.B., Benfell, K., Ringer, S.A., Wilmore, C.K., Maguire, D., et al. (1996). The effects of glutamine-supplemented parenteral nutrition in premature infants. *Journal of Parenteral and Enteral Nutrition 20,* 74-80.
85. Schloerb, P.R., & Amare, M. (1993). Total parenteral nutrition with glutamine in bone marrow transplantation and other clinical applications (a randomized, double-blind study). *Journal of Parenteral and Enteral Nutrition 17,* 407-413.

86. WHO/UNICEF. (2001). *Expert Consultation on Oral Rehydration Salts (ORS) Formulation.* New York: UNICEF HOUSE.
87. Heitkemper, M.M., & Jarrett, M.J. (1997). Research issues in nutrition support. *Nursing Clinics of North America 32,* 755-766.
88. Fouque, D., Wang, P., Laville, M., & Boissel, J.P. (2000). Low protein diets delay end-stage renal disease in non-diabetic adults with chronic renal failure. *Cochrane Database of Systematic Reviews 2000 2,* CD001892.

CHAPTER

5 Circadian Rhythm Disorders

DOROTHY M. LANUZA & LYNNE A. FARR

Rhythmicity is a functional property of all living matter, from a single cell to a complex living organism. Virtually all physiological processes in the body are rhythmic; the period of the rhythms varies in length from milliseconds to daily, monthly, and yearly. The circadian (i.e., approximately 24-hour) rhythm is the periodicity most often investigated in human beings. Selected variables and the time of their peak values (i.e., acrophases) in relation to the sleep/wake cycle are shown in Figure 5-1.[1]

Circadian rhythms are believed to be adaptive mechanisms that enable individuals to adjust to the changing temporal structure of the environment.[2-5] For example, plasma cortisol levels begin to rise shortly before or just after the time of an individual's usual awakening, preparing the person to meet the challenges of the day.[6] It has been suggested that in the healthy state, rhythms are in synchrony[7] and that illness[8-12] and aging[13-16] may be associated with circadian rhythm disorders.

To understand circadian rhythm disorders, we must know rhythm terminology. A biological rhythm is a repetitive, regularly occurring, cyclical change in a physiological process or behavioral function of a living organism. The maximal value of a rhythm is called the *peak;* the time when the peak value occurs is the *acrophase;* the minimum value is the *trough;* the rhythm-adjusted mean is the *mesor;* and the difference between the mesor and the peak or trough represents the rhythm's *amplitude.* The time for completion of one cycle is considered the period of a rhythm and is measured from peak to peak or trough to trough. The cycle is the shortest part of a rhythm that continuously repeats itself. Figures 5-2 and 5-3 illustrate these terms.

Rhythms are generally classified according to the frequency of their cycle as ultradian, circadian, and infradian rhythms. Rhythms with a periodicity of approximately 24 hours (i.e., 20 to 28 hours) are called *circadian.*[17] Rhythms that are shorter than 20 hours are classified as *ultradian* rhythms (e.g., sleep stage cycles), and longer than 28 hours are classified as *infradian* rhythms (e.g., menstrual cycle).[18]

Free-running rhythms are internal rhythms that are no longer synchronized to the 24-hour day by environmental time cues and follow their own non-24-hour periodicity. Thus free-running rhythms result in desynchronization and loss of temporal organization. Transient rhythm desynchronization indicates a temporary phase shift of less than 24 hours among temporally related rhythms to an earlier or later time along a time axis.[3,19] By contrast, spontaneous rhythm desynchronization occurs when two or more rhythms that had similar or inverse time patterns demonstrate a steady state of continuously changing phase relationships of more than 24 hours (i.e., 36 hours).[19]

Rhythms may be exogenous or endogenous. A rhythm that develops in response to external, environmental, periodic stimuli (e.g., the ebb and flow of tides) is called an *exogenous* rhythm. By contrast, genetically determined *endogenous* rhythms originate within the organism and are self-sustaining, even in the absence of external time cues. Rhythmic body temperature, plasma cortisol, and urinary excretion patterns, are examples of endogenous rhythms. Box 5-1 lists characteristics of endogenous rhythms. Entrainment refers to the synchronization of an endogenous rhythm's phase or cycle length with the periodicity of environmental stimuli.[20] The stimulus that is the dominant factor in determining the entrainment of a rhythm is called a *synchronizer* or *Zeitgeber.* The light/dark cycle is the most important Zeitgeber for animals. Alternation of rest and activity because of work and social interaction is thought to be the most important Zeitgeber for human beings.[21] However, light/dark cycles are also important environmental synchronizers.[22]

DEFINITIONS

Circadian rhythm disorders are abnormalities in the circadian timekeeping system. When the circadian

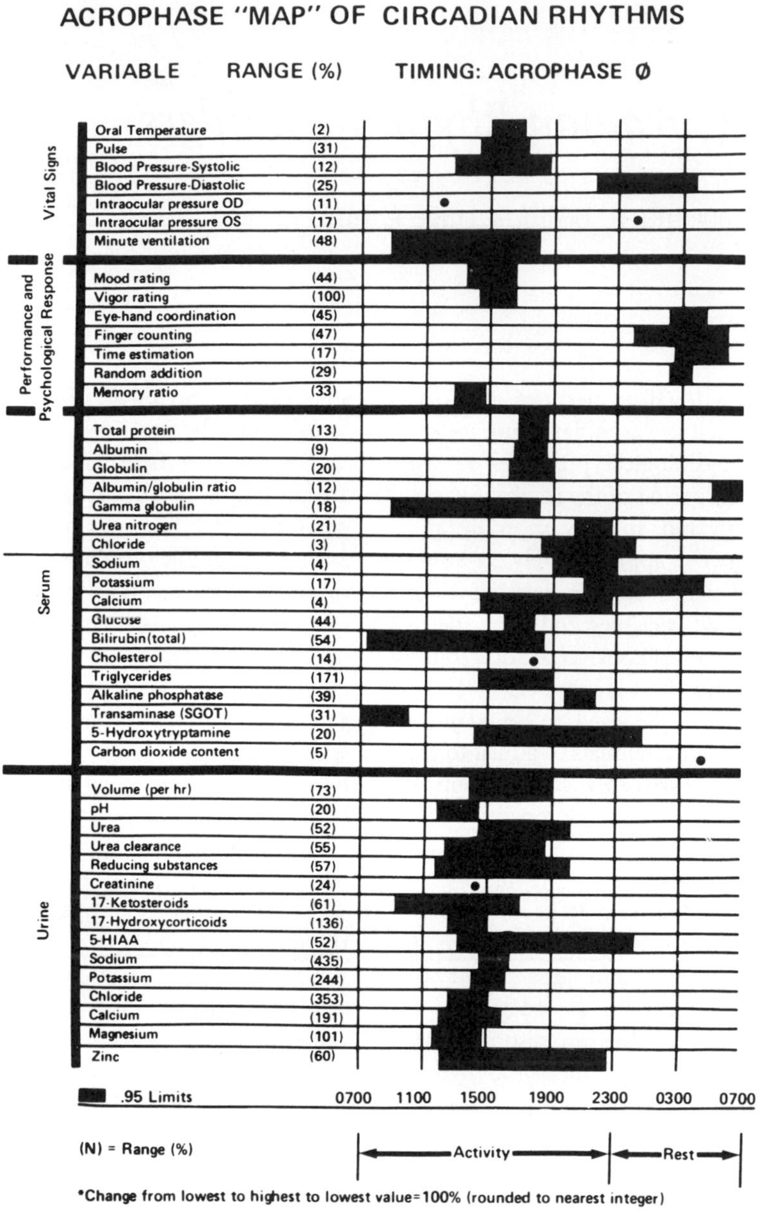

Figure 5-1 **A composite of circadian rhythm data adapted from Halberg (1977) and Kanabrocki et al (1973). The darkened area represents the time when the variable's peak response (acrophase) occurs within a 95% confidence interval. *OD,* Right eye; *OS,* left eye.** (From Kabat, H.F. [1981]. Circadian rhythms and drug dosing. In C.A. Walker, C.M. Winget, & K.F.A. Soliman [eds.], *Chronopharmacology and chronotherapeutics* [p. 10]. Tallahassee: Florida A&M University Foundation. With permission.)

system malfunctions, rhythm disorders can be classified as (1) disorders of phase relations (timing), (2) disorders of amplitude (magnitude of change), and (3) disorders of entrainment (synchronization).[3] These disorders hinder an individual's ability to adapt to the external synchronizers and disturb the internal circadian sequencing of physiological and metabolic events, possibly contributing to the development of disease.[3]

PREVALENCE AND POPULATIONS AT RISK

The prevalence of disorders of the circadian system depends on the category of the rhythm disorder.

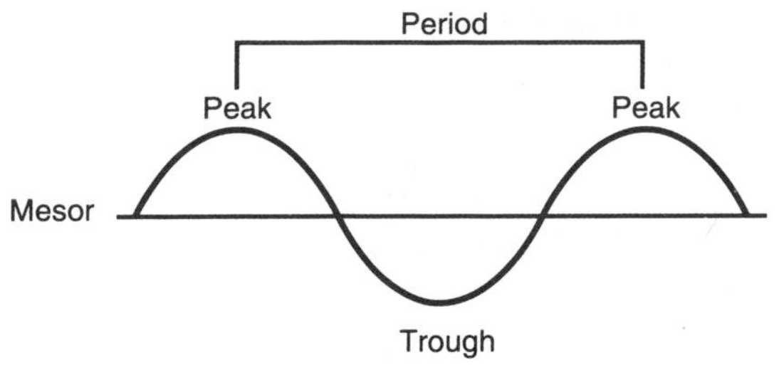

Figure 5-2 A cycle is the shortest part of the rhythm that continuously repeats itself. The period is measured from peak to peak or trough to trough. The mesor is the rhythm-adjusted mean.

Disturbances of the sleep/wake cycle are the most obvious indications of circadian system disorders and are frequently reported by individuals who experience rhythm desynchronization.

SITUATIONAL STRESSORS

The majority of the situational stressors associated with circadian disorders affect the phase or amplitude of the rhythm. For example, phase and/or amplitude disorders are found in shift work; transmeridian jet travel; isolation from environmental time cues; affective disorders; illness[23-26]; head injuries; and surgery,[27,28] including solid organ transplantation.[29,30]

CLINICAL STATES AND DIAGNOSES

Phase Relation Disorders

Internally desynchronized rhythms (transient and spontaneous) are examples of rhythm phase disorders. Rhythms are considered desynchronized when the temporal relationship between two or more rhythms is disrupted. The most common form of desynchronization is transient internal desynchronization.

Transient Internal Rhythm Desynchronization. The cause of transient rhythm desynchronization may be an abrupt change in the sleep/wake cycle as a result of shift work, transmeridian jet travel, or living in an environment with minimal or inadequate external time cues (e.g., in an intensive care unit).[3,31] Initially the individual's internal body rhythms are in synchrony or coupled, but they are out of synchrony with the external temporal environment. While the individual's rhythms are in the process of adapting to the new 24-hour sleep/wake pattern, they become temporarily internally desynchronized or uncoupled. Characteristics of desynchronized rhythms are listed in Box 5-2.

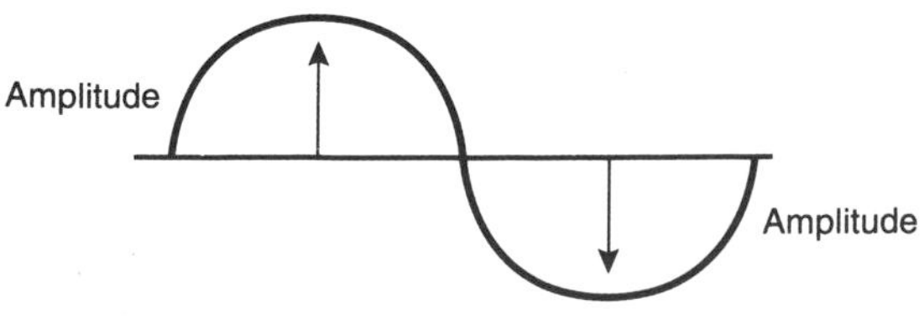

Figure 5-3 The amplitude of a rhythm is the difference between the mesor and the peak.

BOX 5-1 Characteristics of Endogenous Circadian Rhythms

- Regularly occurring oscillating process with a periodicity of approximately 24 hours (i.e., 20–28 hours)
- Genetically inherited
- Endogenous and self-sustaining
- Promote adaptation to the temporal environment
- Influenced by many factors (e.g., environment, social)
- Synchronized by a multioscillator system
- Entrained to the 24-hour day by environmental time cues (Zeitgebers)
- Ubiquitous; found in all living organisms
- Found at all levels of organization, from cells to the whole organism
- Sensitive to light intensity
- Can be measured objectively and subjectively
- Predictable

BOX 5-2 Characteristics of Transient and Spontaneous Desynchronized Rhythms

- Rhythm desynchrony (i.e., a change in the phase relationships between two or more temporally related rhythms)
- Change in rhythm entrainment to the 24-hour day
- Multidimensional effects (i.e., physiological, cognitive, psychological, and behavioral effects)
- Universal; could affect anyone under certain conditions; vulnerable populations at increased risk include: very young, very old, neurotic individuals, people exposed for long periods of time to environments with little or no temporal cues (e.g., ICU patients), transmeridian jet travelers, shift workers, and individuals whose circadian pacemakers are injured or altered
- May lead to pathophysiological and/or psychological consequences

Shift Work. There are a growing number of shift workers. As of May 1997, there were 25 million (27.6%) full-time workers in the United States with flexible shift work schedules.[31] Rotating- and night-shift work causes a person to suddenly change to or from being day-active and sleeping at night to being night-active and sleeping during the day. Shift work can decrease sleep quality and quantity; approximately 60% to 70% of shift workers report having sleep-related problems and feelings of fatigue.[32-34] A shortening of sleep length by approximately 2 to 4 hours has been reported for night-shift workers.[35,36]

Shift Work and Health. Despite the impact shift work has on sleep/wake rhythms, controversy exists as to its effect on workers' general health. For the short term, most shift workers are considered to be as healthy as day workers. However, there is growing interest in the long-term effects of shift work on health.[37-40] There is concern that the sleep disturbance associated with shift work may eventually lead to the development of chronic fatigue and psychoneurotic syndromes.[41] Boggild and Knutsson[42] reviewed 17 shift work studies and concluded that vulnerable shift workers had a 40% increased risk of cardiovascular disease mortality and morbidity as a result of the effects of desynchronized rhythms on diet, sleep, sociotemporal patterns, and associated behavioral changes, such as increased smoking. There is also a higher prevalence of chronic gastritis, peptic ulcer, and colitis among shift workers.[41] Following abrupt changes in activity/rest cycles and sleep loss, metabolic changes occur, such as increased insulin resistance,[43,44] increased production of plasma triglycerides,[45] and delayed melatonin rhythms.[46] Furthermore, the efficacy of pharmacological treatment of diabetes, asthma, hormonal disorders, and other conditions requiring precise timing of medication administration may be hindered in shift workers because of the disruption of the circadian variation of absorption, metabolism, and excretion.[41]

Shift maladaptation syndrome is the term applied to the symptoms of individuals who cannot successfully adjust to shift work.[34,47,48] This subpopulation of individuals is unable to adapt to changing sleep/wake patterns, and exacerbation of medical conditions often occurs, such as respiratory impairment, cardiovascular disease, and epilepsy.[42,47-49]

Factors Affecting Shift Work Adaptation. Attitude, personality, and chronotype (Horne and Ostberg's morningness-eveningness preference),[51] the direction of shift, the season of the year, and the social context associated with the shift work are thought to influence adaptation to shift work.[50,51] While it is proposed that sleep difficulties of shift workers increase with age, research findings are equivocal and further investigation is needed.[32,52-55] Several investigators[56,57] have suggested that a person's chronotype is the best predictor of adjusting or coping with shift work.

Productivity and Safety. In addition to the effects on health, there are major concerns about the effects of shift work on workers' performance and safety.[58] Several types of performance rhythms, such as serial search, verbal reasoning,[59] and vigilance patterns[60] have been found to be temporally associated with body temperature rhythms. Normally low body temperature levels are associated with low activity and performance levels and sleep onset, whereas higher body temperatures are associated with increased alertness, activity, and performance levels. When shift rotation occurs, the synchronization among these rhythms is lost.[61] An individual's body temperature rhythm is lowest at the time of usual sleep, peaks in late afternoon or early evening, and declines to minimal levels at night. An illustration of the circadian rhythm of temperature for a day-active individual is shown in Figure 5-4.[62,63]

The nighttime reduction in shift workers' productivity and safety is thought to be caused by lack of adjustment to the night shift, efforts to work after inadequate sleep, and working while performance capabilities are at a low ebb.[59] Following shift changes, it may take days to weeks for body temperature patterns to become resynchronized with

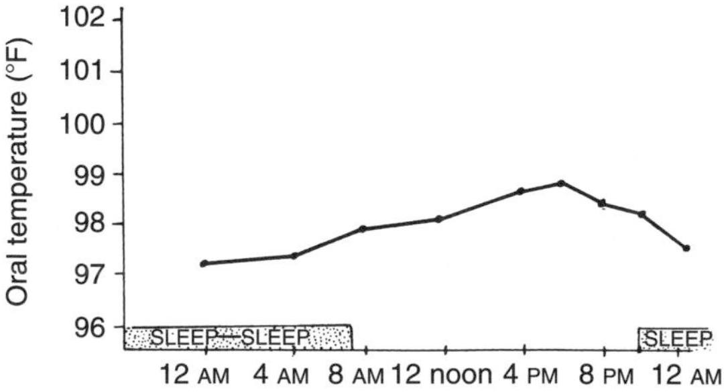

Figure 5-4 **Circadian rhythm of oral temperature of a healthy, day-active individual. The circadian rhythm pattern of temperature tends to rise in the morning, reaching a peak between noon and early evening, then begins to fall, reaching a trough between 2 and 5 AM.** (From Lanuza, D.M. [1976]. Symposium on biological rhythms. *Nursing Clinics of North America, 11*, 584. With permission.)

activity patterns. Incomplete adaptation of a worker's circadian rhythms has been observed even in individuals working permanent night shifts.[64] Therefore, as expected, the incidence of performance errors, delays, and single-vehicle accidents is higher between 3 AM and 5 AM than at any other time of day.[65-68] In fact, it has been suggested that the shift work schedule may have been a factor in the Three Mile Island accident,[69] the Chernobyl incident[72], the Bhopal incident,[59] and the Exxon Valdez accident, because all occurred between midnight and 5 AM.[39]

Jet Lag. Jet lag occurs when a traveler rapidly crosses multiple time zones, usually four or more.[70,71] The symptoms of jet lag are quite similar to those associated with shift rotation and are believed to result primarily from the conflict between the traveler's endogenous circadian rhythms and the external time cues of the new 24-hour time zone.[71,73] Jet lag symptoms may be more severe in persons with morning rather than evening chronotypes and in older rather than in younger individuals. Crossing more time zones and traveling in an eastward direction also increase severity.[70,74] Eastward flights shorten the person's day, resulting in phase advances, whereas westward flights lengthen the person's day, resulting in phase delays.[75,76] Although it takes several days for a transmeridian traveler's physiological functions (e.g., body temperature, sleep, and appetite) to adjust to the new temporal environment, psychological and behavioral alterations adjust more rapidly. Approximately 30% of transmeridian travelers adjust easily, while a similar percentage have a very difficult time adjusting.[77]

Patients in Intensive Care Units. Persons exposed over an extended period to an environment that is deficient in temporal structure and time cues are susceptible to rhythm desynchronization.[21] An intensive care unit (ICU) is an example of an environment with inadequate temporal cues as a result of fairly constant lighting, activity, and noise levels throughout the 24-hour day. Severity of illness, medications, and treatments (e.g., continuous respiratory therapy, parenteral infusions, and/or surgery) also increase the risk of desynchronization.[21] Several studies have shown that circadian rhythms of numerous physiological functions are altered or suppressed in patients with brain lesions or head injury,[12,78,79] patients who underwent surgery,[27,80-85] and/or patients in an ICU.[86] Sleep loss together with desynchronized rhythms may play a role in the development of the syndrome called *ICU delirium* in critical care settings.[21,87]

Spontaneous Internal Rhythm Desynchronization

Absence of Time Cues. In an attempt to determine whether rhythms were endogenous and self-sustaining, early rhythm studies were conducted in environments as free as possible from the influences of Zeitgebers, such as light/dark alternations, atmospheric changes, and external time cues. Studies conducted on human subjects who were living in caves or specially constructed apartments have shown that the rhythms of most physiological variables persist. However, they free-run at frequencies slightly longer or shorter than 24 hours when they are no longer entrained by environmental Zeitgebers.[19] When free-running occurs, the rhythms of body core temperature, rapid eye movement (REM) sleep, plasma cortisol levels, and urinary potassium excretion become desynchronized from the rhythms of rest/activity, skin temperature, slow wave sleep, plasma growth hormone, and urinary calcium excretion[88,89] (Figure 5-5). Thus to prevent spontaneous internal rhythm desynchronization, environmental time cues must be maintained. This is especially important in environments in which

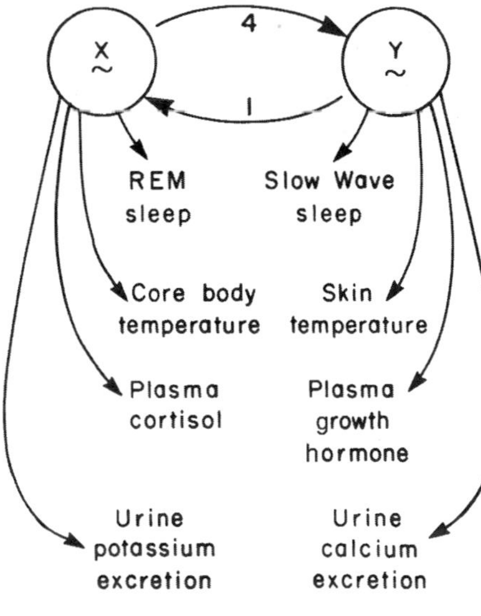

Figure 5-5 Separate pacemakers, X and Y, drive two groups of rhythms. Pacemaker X drives REM sleep, core body temperature, plasma cortisol, and urine potassium excretion. Pacemaker Y influences slow-wave sleep, skin temperature, plasma growth hormone, and urine calcium excretion. The coupling force generated by X is postulated to be approximately four times greater than that of Y on X. (From Moore-Ede, M.C. [1983]. The circadian timing system in mammals: Two pacemakers preside over many secondary oscillators. *Federation Proceedings, 42,* 2803. With permission.)

time cues are absent or inadequate because of the continuous lighting, noise, and activity, such as ICUs.

Phase Disorder Insomnias

Two examples of phase-relation disorders are advanced sleep phase syndrome (ASPS) and delayed sleep phase syndrome (DSPS). Both are circadian disorders of the timing and phase of the circadian clock and both result in sleep disruption. These two disorders have different clinical presentations. Of the populations with sleep problems, the more common DSPS affects approximately 10% of adults, 7% of adolescents, and 0.7% of elderly persons.[90-92] Both ASPS and DSPS are seen in blind individuals whose rhythms are desynchronized.[93]

Delayed Phase Disorder Syndrome. Individuals with DSPS have difficulty adjusting to variations in their bedtime and awakening patterns, because they have a very limited ability to achieve large phase-advances of their sleep/wake cycle.[3,94] Sleep initiation is delayed to socially undesirable times, often early in the morning. These individuals have no problem remaining asleep once sleep occurs.[91,92,94] Because a DSPS patient's normal sleep period is longer, early waking is difficult.

DSPS is treated by resetting the patients' circadian clock by sequentially phase-delaying their sleep around the clock by going to bed later and later until the desired circadian schedule is achieved.[94] Other methods to treat this condition include bright light therapy and melatonin.[95,96] However, the advance or delay potential of these latter interventions depends on the phase of the endogenous circadian clock and the time of day when they are administered.[97-99] Vasopressin has been used successfully to decrease ASPS patients' tendency to awaken early[100] and to increase the time spent in slow wave sleep (SWS).[100,101]

Advanced Sleep Phase Syndrome. By contrast, the chief complaint of persons with ASPS is premature waking in the early morning and difficulty maintaining sleep. To make up the sleep lost in the early morning, persons with ASPS take frequent naps. This is often observed in elderly persons[102] and in blind individuals who are not well synchronized by other cues, such as social activities.[93]

If ASPS and DSPS individuals do not need to adhere to strict sleep schedules or are allowed to take daytime naps, individuals of both types can maintain the same amount of sleep as individuals with normal sleep patterns.[103,104] In institutionalized elderly with ASPS, total sleep is also similar when naps and sleep at night are both counted.[103,105] However, waking early reduces the amount of time the elderly spend in deep, restful, slow wave sleep (SWS).[106] During weekends and vacations, when adherence to a strict sleep schedule is not required, patients with DSPS report no difficulty sleeping.[92,94] A genetic basis for ASPS and DSPS has also been suggested.[107,108]

Affective Disorders. Advanced and delayed circadian rhythms have been implicated in the pathogenesis of affective disorders. Pincus[109] stated that specific abnormalities in circadian phase are among the most consistent findings in biological psychiatry. Manic-depression (bipolar depression) and endogenous depression (unipolar depression) have been postulated to include abnormalities in circadian rhythm timing and phase control, such as the phase-advancement of internal oscillators. This results in early morning awakening, a diurnal pattern of depressive symptoms, and seasonal recurrences.[9,110-113]

Decreases in the amplitude of cortisol,[114,115] melatonin,[115] thyroid-stimulating hormone,[116] sleep,[117] and temperature[118] rhythms have been demonstrated in patients with endogenous depression. Bunney and Bunney[119] proposed that alterations in genes that control circadian timing provide the basis for advancing and delaying circadian cycles in depression. However, it is not clear whether damping of the temperature rhythm amplitude in affective disorders is caused by the illness or a masking effect.[120,121] The term *masking effect* refers to alterations produced in the rhythm of a variable as a result of changes in environmental conditions, such as physical activity and timing of sleep.[121]

Several hypotheses have been proposed to explain the relationship between circadian rhythms and affective disorders, such as the advanced phase hypothesis, the internal desynchronization hypothesis, the delayed phase hypothesis,[120] and the circadian dysregulation theory.[122] These hypotheses all postulate that sleep and other circadian rhythms are out of phase with each other.

The advanced phase hypothesis proposes a phase advance of circadian rhythms that trigger the early morning awakening, the daily fluctuations in moods, and the seasonal recurrences of affective symptoms in patients with depressive conditions.[113] The internal desynchronization hypothesis suggests that the loss of coordination between the peaks of two rhythms, one of which is free-running, triggers an affective illness episode.[123] The delayed phase mood hypothesis postulates that circadian rhythms have abnormalities in their phase relationships so that they are phase delayed in relation to sleep.[111] Finally, the circadian dysregulation hypothesis suggests that depression is characterized by a loss of rhythmicity as a result of blunting or new frequency components.[122] Additional research is needed to resolve the different theories.

Shift Work, Jet Lag, and Affective Illness Similarities. Researchers have expressed considerable interest in investigating the similarities in symptoms, such as sleep and appetite disturbances and feelings of malaise, that occur as a result of shift work, jet lag, and affective illness.[10,112] Although the intensity of the symptoms is usually greatest in individuals with affective disorders, several of the treatments for these conditions are similar. Shift workers and individuals with jet lag share some similarities with people with affective disease; however, they differ in two major ways. First, shift workers and individuals with jet lag can clearly attribute their symptoms to a cause (i.e., an abrupt change in their sleep/wake cycle), whereas persons with affective disease may not know why they feel the way they do.[10,112] Second, circadian rhythms of shift workers and individuals with jet lag are initially internally synchronized, but out of synchrony with the external environment. By contrast, the various hypotheses proposed for affective illness suggest these individuals experience symptoms as a result of abnormal internal circadian rhythmicities. Could it be that individuals who experience distress from shift work and jet lag do so only after their internal rhythms develop abnormal phase relationships? Healy and Waterhouse[112] noted that further investigation is needed of the factors and social events that contribute to vulnerability to distress from shift work, jet travel, and affective illness.

Disorders of Rhythm Amplitude. Diminutions in amplitude have been reported in the elderly,[16,124,125] in patients with endogenous depression,[114-116,118] and in populations living near the Arctic Circle, who experience prolonged periods of continuous darkness or daylight.[126] Other potential causes of low rhythm amplitudes include injury to or failure of the central biological clock or internal oscillator mechanisms or the variables that they control.[3]

Entrainment Failure. There is a small population of individuals whose endogenous circadian rhythms are not entrained to the environmental 24-hour period.[3] For example, *hypernychthemeral syndrome* is a condition in which affected individuals demonstrate progressively later sleep onsets, resulting in a 24.5 to 26 hour sleep/wake cycle.[92,127] This syndrome is an excellent example of entrainment failure.

AGE AND DEVELOPMENTAL FACTORS

Infants and Children. Body temperature is one of the most stable of circadian rhythms and it is often used as a marker rhythm for the endogenous circadian clock. However, most studies report that infants are not born with a developed circadian temperature rhythm. Immediately after birth, infants' temperature rhythms are not circadian.[128,129] The strongest cycle in infants is actually a shorter ultradian period.[130] An adult-type phase (timing) and rhythmic amplitude is not fully established until children are 5 to 7 years of age.[129,131]

A few studies have reported temperature rhythms in preterm infants. These studies have used skin thermistors with frequent sampling for 24 hours or longer to identify rhythms in infants of 34 to 37 weeks' gestational age, measured at postnatal days 10 to 20.[132] However, as in Hellbrugge and Abe's studies,[129,131] the phase and amplitude of the temperature rhythm were found to be different from those of adults. Circadian temperature rhythms were reported in preterm infants (24 to 34 weeks' gestational age)[133] and in infants (30 to 34 weeks' gestational age, 5 to 10 days after birth),[134] using rectal probes with frequent sampling.[133] Although these investigators have reported finding circadian rhythms in very young children, the majority of the evidence suggests that circadian rhythms develop and increase in strength as infants mature.[129-131] Differences among the findings in these studies may be the result of variation in the length of the sampling interval and the choice of statistical analysis techniques. Light and social cues that are determined by environments such as incubators and ICU environments may also play a role in the developing temperature rhythms of neonates and young children. Another influence on developing rhythms that needs to be examined is the effect of temporal behavior of parents or caregivers during early infancy.[4]

Serum cortisol circadian rhythms have been demonstrated in infants as young as 3 months of age[135] and also at 6 months or older.[136] An adultlike circadian salivary cortisol rhythm has been found in 3- to 6-month-old infants.[137,138]

A few studies of circadian systolic and diastolic blood pressure rhythms of children and adolescents have been reported.[139-142] In a study of children with hypertensive and normotensive parents, only 30% of the children demonstrated a circadian blood pressure rhythm.

Adolescents. Carskadon, Labyak, Acebo, and Seifer[143] measured the endogenous circadian body temperature and melatonin rhythms in 10 adolescent boys using a forced desynchrony protocol. All of the adolescents studied had circadian temperature and melatonin rhythms with periods greater than 24 hours. These investigators proposed that the loss of synchrony between the intrinsic oscillator and external environmental cycles explains the phase-delay reported for teenagers and the tendency of adolescents to delay the time of their going to bed and, subsequently, their time of awakening in the morning. These findings confirmed those of Wolfson and Carskadon,[144] who reported that the patterns of sleep and wake that are seen in childhood are changed dramatically in adolescence. These investigators studied 3120 adolescents between 13 and 19 years of age and found that they slept 40% to 50% less each night than younger children as a result of delayed bedtimes, combined with less flexible awakening times. Learning difficulties were related to fewer hours of sleep. These findings led these researchers to suggest that high school classes be started later in the morning to facilitate student alertness and learning.

The delayed sleep habits of adolescents have been reported in a variety of countries as well as the United States.[145-149] The delayed circadian phase of adolescents is also reflected in their preference for activity later in the day, according to the Horne and Osberg Morningness-Eveningness Questionnaire (MEQ). During puberty, young men and women have reported a preference for activity later in the day.[145,147] A delay in time-of-day preference was paralleled by a similar delay in the circadian peak in core body temperature.[145]

Elderly Persons. Many investigators have suggested that rhythm desynchrony occurs with aging. It has been suggested that sleep disturbance is the result and that desynchrony may underlie the chronic sleep-related problems that tend to increase with age.[150-154] Studies designed to describe the characteristics of rhythms in older animals and human beings have yielded equivocal results. For example, while many researchers have reported earlier acrophase, shorter period length, decreased amplitude, and increased internal rhythm desynchronization with advanced age,[16,23,155-162] Czeisler et al[163] reported that circadian rhythmicity persists in the elderly, with no difference in the period. This most recent statement by Czeisler[163] differs from his early writings,[164] in which he reported finding an association among earlier bedtimes, earlier temperature minimums, and earlier waking times in elderly compared with young subjects, and concluded that age-related changes in temperature rhythms are associated with concurrent changes in the timing and quality of sleep. Thus further research on the effect of aging on circadian rhythms is needed.

In relation to changes in rhythm characteristics with age, phase advances in the elderly have also been reported for cortisol,[124,125] circulating leukocytes and lymphocytes,[165] and activity.[166] By contrast, a phase delay in urinary volume excretion of older individuals has been reported, with subjects voiding a greater amount of urine during the night than during the day.[167]

Theories have been proposed to explain the changes in circadian rhythmicity that occur with age. Hofman[168] suggested that decreased rhythmic stability may be occurring in the suprachiasmatic nuclei (SCN). His theory states that the photic information from environmental light/dark cycles synchronizes the endogenous clock of the SCN by inducing periodic changes in the biological activity of certain groups of neurons. According to Hofman, this is the site of age-related changes. He cites arginine vasopressin (AVP) as the basis for the changes. This is based on its position as one of the most abundant peptides in the human SCN and also on the decreased robustness and reduced amplitude of the AVP rhythm that is observed with advancing age. Numbers of AVP secreting cells are diminished in the SCNs of people older than 80 years of age. This change is even more dramatic in Alzheimer's patients.[168,169]

According to Weinert,[170] many of the age-related changes observed in older mice originate within the SCN and are related to the number of functioning neurons. These decrease with advancing age limiting the SCN's ability to produce stable rhythms and to transmit timing information to other systems within the body.

Gender differences in individuals older than 60 years of age have been noted in several variables, such as temperature[55,166] and blood cortisol.[158] In general, the body temperature of older women has been shown to peak more than an hour earlier than men of comparable ages.[55,166] It was postulated that shorter sleep periods and earlier awakenings reported by older women may be associated with an earlier rise in their body temperature.[55,166] Total cortisol is also reported to be higher in elderly women than in elderly men.[158] These gender differences in temperature acrophase and cortisol mesor warrant serious consideration of gender differences when evaluating circadian rhythm studies and their application to patient assessment and health care.

MECHANISMS

Biological Rhythm

Multioscillator System. Studies on both human beings and animals support the postulate that the circadian system is a multioscillator system (i.e., oscillators, acting as pacemakers, drive the rhythms).[19,89,171,172] The terms *oscillator* and *pacemaker* have been used interchangeably, and the term *biological clock* usually refers to one or more major oscillators. Recently two independent oscillators have been determined in human beings and other mammalian species. These are located in the SCN, which is located in the anterior hypothalamus and the retina. The SCN is the *master regulator* of most, if not all, endogenous rhythms.[173] Less is known about the retinal oscillator's role in the mammalian circadian clock. The SCN appears to interact with other areas of the brain to maintain stable circadian rhythmicity. Among these are the paraventricular nuclei and the pineal gland.

Suprachiasmatic Nucleus Oscillator. The role of the SCN in circadian control has been demonstrated by experiments in which the SCN is destroyed or surgically isolated. Lesions made in the anterior-ventral hypothalamus of rodents were found to disrupt circadian rhythmicity in wheel-running,[174] whereas specific lesions to the SCN of rats abolished several circadian rhythms, such as plasma corticosterone,[172] drinking, locomotor activity,[174,175] and sleep/wakefulness.[176]

Current research on the SCN involves a focus on gene regulator factors, which several investigators believe may elucidate the basis of the circadian clock. Two gene regulator factors that are induced with exposure to light are c-fos and NGFI-A.[177-179] These are the products of immediate early genes that control the later steps in transcription and translation of the SCN DNA. The light stimulus required for induction of c-fos is similar to that required to induce phase changes in endogenous circadian rhythms.

Several neurotransmitters are found in the SCN that appear to play an important part in circadian timing and in transmission of timing information to other parts of the brain and body. The relationship of these neurotransmitters is still under investigation. Among these neurotransmitters are arginine vasopressin (AVP), vasoactive intestinal peptide (VIP), somatostatin, gamma amino buteric acid (GABA), gastrin-releasing peptide, and nitric oxide (NO). Although the names of these neurotransmitters seem inappropriate for an area in the brain, it must be remembered that these substances were first named for the area of the body where they were initially identified.

Retinal Oscillator. The SCN receives photic information (electrical input) from the retinas of the eyes through two pathways. The retinohypothalamic tract (RHT) is the direct visual pathway, whereas the geniculohypothalamic tract (GHT) is an indirect path. The GHT appears to modulate input from the RHT. Light plays a very important role in entraining endogenous rhythms of living organisms to the 24-hour day.[11,22] Investigators have demonstrated that blind humans and other mammals who are blind are able to maintain synchronized circadian rhythmicity when the eyes are intact, even though there is no visual sight. However, removal of the eye prevents the synchronizing information from reaching the brain, resulting in drifting (free-running) rhythms, with periods that are usually longer than 24 hours.[180]

Secondary Oscillators. Investigators[19,171,181,182] have suggested that there are multiple secondary internal circadian oscillators, which are loosely coupled with each other to form a coordinated, hierarchical system driven by two or more major circadian oscillators originating in the SCN. For example, circadian rhythmicities have been demonstrated at the cellular level of several organs, such as the adrenal gland, heart, and liver.[89,183] These rhythms are generated by secondary oscillators within the tissues and synchronized under the influence of a major oscillator.[89]

In an environment without external Zeitgebers, the temperature rhythm assumes a periodicity of about 25 hours and the sleep/wakefulness rhythm may change to a periodicity of 33 hours.[19] This suggests that these rhythms are driven by at least two major independent pacemakers. Rhythm splitting occurs when external environmental cues are lost and the two major pacemakers assume separate periodicities.

Wever[19] developed a protocol called *fractional desynchronization* to investigate the concept of two internal pacemakers. Fractional desynchronization involves shortening or lengthening the period of a group of Zeitgebers. When the critical limit of entrainment of an oscillator to a Zeitgeber is reached, the oscillator will break away and its periodicity will free-run. Body temperature is an example of a rhythm that cannot adjust to an entrainment period of less than 23 hours or more than 27 hours.[181] Under experimental conditions that exposed subjects to days that are longer or shorter than the body temperature's entrainment period, the temperature rhythm would break away and resume its free-running cycle. More recently investigators have used a similar protocol of forced desynchronization to separate endogenous or intrinsic oscillators from their exogenous components and synchronizers.[184-188] In this experimental protocol, individuals are subjected to a number of continuous days that are outside of the ability of humans to entrain (less than 23 hours or greater than 27 hours). Under this regimen, the endogenous and exogenous components of a circadian rhythm separate.[189]

X and Y Oscillators. The pacemaker or oscillator associated with the core body temperature rhythm is postulated to be very strong, because its periodicity is maintained within such a limited entrainment range. The oscillator generating the temperature rhythm has been referred to as *pacemaker X,* while the oscillator associated with the sleep/wake rhythm is called *pacemaker Y* and is thought to be located in the SCN. The latter is hypothesized to be much weaker, because sleep/wake rhythms have a much wider range of entrainment. The coupling strength of pacemaker X is believed to be four times stronger than that of pacemaker Y.[89] Both neural and hormonal factors are believed to link the X and Y pacemaker systems.[89,190] In addition to core body temperature, pacemaker X entrains plasma cortisol, REM sleep, and urine potassium rhythms, whereas pacemaker Y entrains skin temperature, plasma growth hormone, SWS, and urinary calcium excretion (see Figure 5-5).[89] The role of two pacemakers was also supported by Borbély and other investigators who have suggested that sleep is the product of two independent oscillators.[191,192]

RELATED PHYSIOLOGICAL CONCEPTS

Sleep, insomnia, fatigue, and susceptibility rhythms are related to circadian rhythm disorders. Changes in sleep quality and quantity and concomitant experiences of increased fatigue, as discussed earlier, are associated with the internal desynchronization of rhythms associated with shift work, jet travel, and affective illness. If the rhythm desynchronizations are prolonged, insomnia can develop. This section will focus on the related concepts of susceptibility rhythms and chronopathology.

Susceptibility Rhythms

Susceptibility rhythm is the term used to indicate that an organism's response to stressors varies throughout the 24-hour day. The existence of susceptibility rhythms is very relevant to health. For example, many studies have shown that a circadian variation exists for susceptibility to noxious stimuli,[193] endotoxins,[194] and drugs.[195] Although this phenomenon has been studied in both human beings and animals, the reproducibility of results are especially impressive in animal studies, where greater control can be actualized. The morbidity and mortality in mice from physical agents, toxins, or chemicals have been shown to be several times higher at one time of day than another.[196-198] Differences in toxicity thresholds that depend on the time of day that the medications are taken has been shown to occur in human subjects as well.[199-201] If a noxious stimulus, such as noise, is applied shortly after mice awaken, the probability of convulsions occurring is much greater than if the stimulus is applied toward the end of the animals' sleep period.[193] The response of rats to injections of pneumococci also shows a circadian variation, with the greatest survival rates being associated with injections during the highest activity span.[202]

Chronopathology

Knowledge of susceptibility rhythms is used in chronopathology, the study of the time factor associated with symptoms and disease. Although susceptibility rhythms are not as well documented in human beings as in animal models, research in this area is growing rapidly. The following are examples of investigations of susceptibility rhythms in human beings. An investigation of the allergic response of individuals to intradermally injected histamine showed that the mildest skin response to histamine occurred at 11 AM and the most severe response at 11 PM.[203] Another study of allergic nasal reactivity to methacholine showed that healthy children and children with allergic rhinitis had a significantly higher response at 6 AM than in the evening.[204]

A circadian variation in the occurrence of conditions and/or symptoms have been shown for asthma, cardiovascular events, allergic rhinitis, arthritis, peptic ulcer disease, migraine and depression, to list a few.[205] To illustrate susceptibility rhythms, research related to patients with asthma and cardiovascular events will be discussed.

Asthma. Peak expiratory flow rate (PEFR) varies throughout the day in healthy individuals without respiratory problems, and this variation is increased in people with asthma.[206] The incidence and intensity of asthmatic symptoms is greatest between 2 AM and 7 AM, with fewer symptoms being reported during the day[207] and during nighttime sleep.[208] Dyspnea is greatest on awakening, about 7 AM, and lowest about 3 PM. Peak expiratory flow varies in a complimentary inverse manner.[206,209] Nighttime increases in airway resistance, pulmonary resistance, bronchial reactivity to irritants, airway inflammation, and vagal tone, accompanied by decreases in bronchodilator substances such as catecholamines and cortisol and beta-adrenergic tone, have been suggested as an explanation.[208-212] Sleep, supine position, and sleep-related changes in lung volume and circulation are also proposed to play a role in the nocturnal worsening of asthma.[213]

Cardiovascular Events. The circadian variation of several physiological systems are thought to influence the occurrence of cerebrovascular and cardiovascular events in vulnerable individuals. Circadian peaks in plasma levels of cortisol, catecholamines, renin-angiotensin, and hemoglobin, as well as increases in vascular tone, platelet aggregation, and blood pressure occur before or within a few hours of awakening and arising[214-216] (Figure 5-6). By contrast, fibrinolytic activity is lowest early in the activity period. Peak platelet aggregation and low fibrinolytic activity leads to a hypercoagulable state[215,217,218] (see Figure 5-6). These circadian rhythm changes place vulnerable individuals at increased risk for ischemia episodes, myocardial infarction, stroke, and sudden cardiac death[214,215,217,219,221] (Figures 5-6 and 5-7).

Evidence indicates that a population circadian rhythm exists for the occurrence of myocardial infarctions.[219,220,222] The most extensive data (N = 8900) on the time of onset of myocardial infarction pain, published by WHO and based on information from 19 European countries, showed that the peak incidence occurred between 8 and 11 AM.[223] These findings were confirmed by Muller et al,[224] who found that the subjective report (N = 2999) of the onset of myocardial pain had a peak incidence between 6 AM and noon. An objective method, using serial plasma cardiac creatine-kinase MB levels (N = 703) to determine the onset of

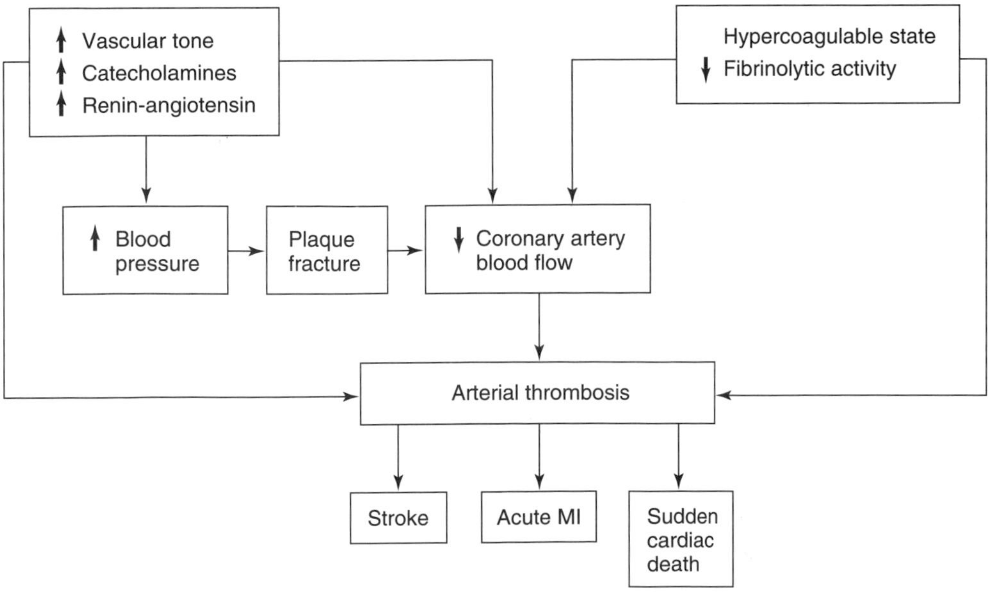

Figure 5-6 Mechanisms influencing temporal patterns of cardiovascular events that may lead to the development of arterial thrombosis and possibly acute MI, stroke, or sudden cardiac death. (From Lanuza, D.M., & Dunbar, S. [1993]. Circadian rhythms: Implications for cardiovascular nursing and drug therapy. *Journal of Cardiovascular Nursing, 8*, 68.)

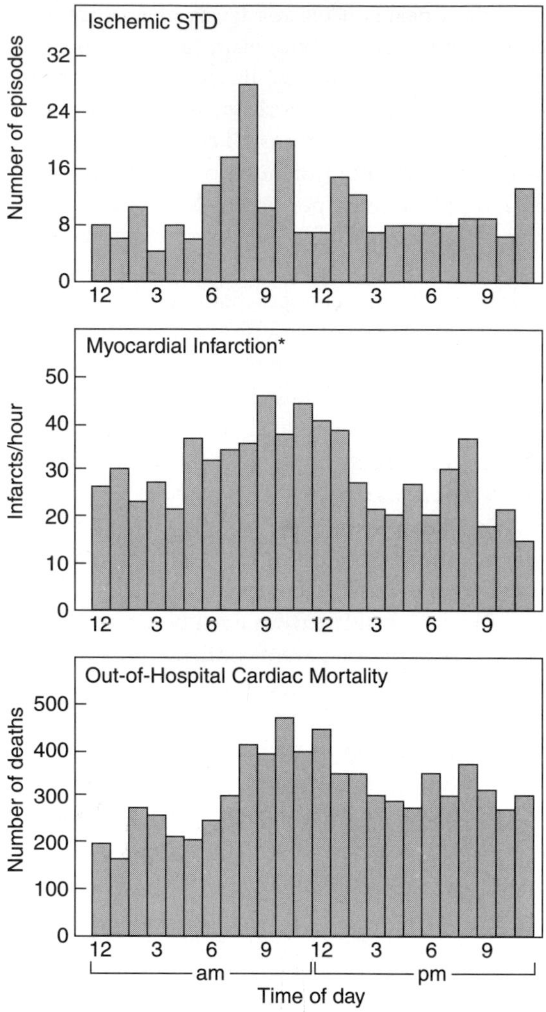

Figure 5-7 **The 24-hour distribution of myocardial ischemia episodes detected by ambulatory monitoring (*top*) is displayed along with the hourly patterns for onset of myocardial infarction (*middle*) and out-of-hospital cardiac death (*bottom*). The peak frequencies in all three pathological conditions occur in the morning hours after awakening.** (From Rocco, M.B., Nabel, E.G., & Selwyn, A.P. [1987]. Circadian rhythms and coronary artery disease. *American Journal of Cardiology [Suppl A]*, 15 C.)

myocardial infarction showed a peak incidence occurring between 5 AM and 2 PM. Interestingly, patients with Prinzmetal's variant angina experienced more angina and ST-segment elevations when they underwent a treadmill test between 5 and 8 AM than when they performed a more strenuous and longer treadmill exercise in the afternoon.[224]

Differential Diagnosis

Knowledge of circadian variations of physiological variables and response to medications is important for differential diagnosis. Because respiratory and cardiovascular chronopathology examples were given earlier, the following discussion will focus on these systems and the influence of circadian rhythms on differential diagnosis.

Inclusion of circadian knowledge in health care and nursing practice is important. For example, in asthmatic individuals the marked circadian rhythmicity of airway patency is a factor to be considered in pulmonary function tests and reversibility tests of airway diseases because the results will be greatly affected by the time of day the tests are performed. Pulmonary function, as indicated by FEV_1 and PEFR measurements, is greatest in the middle of the individual's awake period.[227] A circadian variation also exists in patients' airway responses to bronchodilator beta-agonist aerosol medications: in a diurnally active person, a far greater magnitude of bronchodilation will be seen if this medication is inhaled in the morning rather than in the afternoon.[227] In hypertensive patients, 24-hour ambulatory blood pressure monitoring is increasingly being used to accurately diagnose and differentiate diurnal and nocturnal forms of hypertension and to exclude a diagnosis of the "white coat" phenomenon.[227]

MANIFESTATIONS

Objective Manifestations

Sensitivity to desynchronized circadian rhythms varies among individuals and at different times and under different circumstances within an individual. Objective symptoms associated with desynchronized rhythms include sleep-arousal disorders, such as wakefulness or sleepiness at inappropriate times, changes in sleep/wake patterns, decreases in quantity and quality of sleep, and gastrointestinal irregularity, including hunger or anorexia at inappropriate times, constipation, and peptic ulcers. Continuous monitoring of an individual's vital signs, activity patterns, plasma and urinary hormones, and electrolytes will indicate changes in the phase or the amplitude of the specific rhythm from reported standard patterns. This can be used to detect internal rhythm desynchronization.

Subjective Manifestations

Individuals with desynchronized rhythms may report feelings of fatigue, irritability, general malaise, decreased mental alertness and reaction time, and regular use of medications to induce sleep. They often report feeling inappropriately awake or sleepy, hungry or anorectic, fatigued, and irritable. Their cognitive and physical performance abilities may also decrease.[67,225,226]

SURVEILLANCE AND MEASUREMENT

Understanding normal circadian variation in the patient's physiological variables and being able to assess, predict, and eventually prevent changes that might indicate impending homeostatic instability are important goals of clinical surveillance and clinical rhythm research.

To determine whether patients are experiencing circadian rhythm disorders, one must first assess their "normal" circadian pattern. For example, what are the patient's usual sleep/wake and mealtime patterns? When does the patient feel best and have the best mental and physical performance? Self-report instruments that could be used to assess circadian rhythms include: the Horne and Ostberg Morning-Eveningness Questionnaire,[228] the Torsvall and Akerstedt Scale,[229] and the Composite Morningness Scale.[230] The Composite Morningness Scale is a 13-item self-report tool that uses a Likert-like format to determine whether an individual is a morning chronotype (prefers to arise early and retire early), an intermediate chronotype (in between morning and evening types), or an evening chronotype (prefers to arise later and go to bed later). The authors of the Composite Morningness Scale[230] extracted nine items from Horne and Ostberg's Scale[228] and four items from the Torsvall and Akerstedt's Scale.[229] They then examined the psychometric properties of the "new" Composite Morningness Scale[230] and found that it possessed psychometric properties similar or stronger than the original tools from which the items were extracted. Interitem correlations were positive and moderate to high, ranging from 0.13 to 0.79, and the coefficient alpha for the total scale was 0.87.[230]

Methods used to detect physiological circadian rhythms include continuous telemetry or ambulatory monitoring devices that can be used in hospitals, ambulatory care and community settings. For example, the SpaceLabs ambulatory blood pressure (ABP) device (Model 90202: SpaceLabs, Inc., Tustin, California) measures systolic, diastolic, and mean arterial blood pressure, as well as heart rate and can be programmed to record these parameters at selected time intervals for 24 to 48 hours or longer. It meets the Advancement of Medical Instrumentation's standard.[231] A reliability of 0.96 to 0.98 was reported when this system was compared with conventional ausculatory measurements.[232,233]

Using devices such as the Mini-Motionlogger (Ambulatory Monitoring, Inc., Ardsley, New York) actigraph or the ActiWatch (Mini-Mitter, Co., Bend, Oregon), researchers have also studied activity-rest rhythms and sleep patterns. These battery-operated electronic monitors are relatively simple, non-obtrusive devices that are worn like a wrist watch on the nondominant arm. They measure activity by counting the number of movements of that wrist during a given epoch of time. These loggers have a high level of subject acceptability,[234] as well as documented reliability and validity.[235-237]

In addition, in the hospital setting, temperature graphs may provide information about temperature rhythms. Data collection that involves blood samples can often be obtained from an indwelling arterial or venous catheter or venipuncture. The volume of blood or plasma required for analysis involving hormonal or hematological parameters is low, making multiple analyses of other blood variables possible. In some cases, urine and saliva specimens are appropriate alternatives to using blood for analyzing hormone levels.

In the community setting, ambulatory monitoring devices for temperature, blood pressure, and activity have been used in studies of children and adults. For example, nocturnal labor activity onset has been reported for preterm and term deliveries.[238] Because it is possible for preterm mothers to monitor their uterine contractions with a portable tocodynamometer, the circadian rhythm of uterine contractility can be determined and the effects of scheduling the timing of medications that suppress uterine contractility to coincide with the time of peak uterine contraction activity could be investigated.

Using computer software (e.g., the software included with the SpaceLabs ABP and the motionlogger devices), a gross estimate of a circadian rhythm can be made by a visual examination of the graphs of the data. In addition, statistical packages are available that allow the researcher to analyze the statistical characteristics of a rhythm on a personal computer.

Patients can be taught to monitor their temperature, blood pressure, and keep logs of their activity, meals, sleep (e.g., time of going to bed, time of awakening, quality and quantity of sleep), and moods. Nurses in every setting (e.g., hospitals, nursing homes, and the community), working with any type of patient (e.g., psychiatric, obstetrics, and medical-surgical), in any age group (e.g., neonatal to elderly individuals) can use their knowledge of circadian rhythms to improve the care they provide. For example, a nurse specialist in geriatrics who provided health care to patients in their homes interviewed her patients about their rest/activity patterns and times of feeling most alert and active. She used this assessment of her elderly patients' mental and physical daily rhythms for planning rehabilitation activities with them.[239] She reported that when she modified her usual assessment to include information about her patients' lifestyles and circadian rhythms, scheduling their rehabilitation to fit with their reported circadian rhythm pattern of activity, they demonstrated consistent, sustained improvement.

Methodological Issues

There are many methodological problems associated with rhythm research. When designing circadian rhythm studies it is essential to ensure that the data collection period is adequate. Preferably it should be longer than one 24-hour cycle to capture the circadian rhythm cycle, and the sampling intervals should be frequent enough to detect changes.[240] It is also important to take into consideration potential masking effects.[121,189] For example, the change in body temperature caused by a change in the degree of physical activity may be superimposed on the temperature rhythm and thus affect the findings. When appropriate, statistical methods need to include the ability to detect 24-hour rhythms and rhythms that may be shorter or longer than 24 hours.

Other methodological issues are demonstrated in the area of shift work research. For example, the incidence of morbidity associated with shift work may be greatly underestimated, because workers who experience the most difficulties usually elect not to engage in shift work.[42] Furthermore, the influence of workers' age, the lack of a standard definition of shift work, and the effects of different types of shift work have not been taken into consideration when shift work morbidity has been examined.[42,47]

CLINICAL MANAGEMENT

There are several promising new strategies being proposed or under investigation. These new treatment modalities include chronopharmacology, chronotherapy, and phototherapy.

Chronopharmacology

Susceptibility to the side effects of medications is not the same at all times of day. The study of these rhythms of pharmacokinetics and bioavailability is the field of chronopharmacology. Reinberg and Halberg[241] defined chronopharmacology as the scientific study of biological rhythm dependencies of medication. Chronopharmacology uses information from susceptibility rhythm studies to determine methods of optimizing the effects of medications by manipulating the time that drugs are administered.[195] Chronotherapeutics is closely related to chronopharmacology. While it involves the careful timing of medication administration during the day to coincide with the rhythms of disease activity, it also includes the patient's risk of medical events, and/or the patient's tolerance rhythms to treatments.[227] The ultimate goal of chronopharmacology and chronotherapeutics is to determine the best time to administer the lowest possible dose of a drug or treatment, when it would be most effective, and have the fewest undesirable side effects.

Timing is important in cortisol administration. Studies have shown that the time the drug is administered determines whether the individual's endogenous cortisol levels are suppressed, maintained, or augmented. As reported earlier, the plasma cortisol rhythm for day-active individuals is one in which cortisol levels begin to rise in the latter part of the usual sleep period, reach a peak shortly before or just after awakening, then decline irregularly throughout the day and evening. Minimal levels are reached early in the usual sleep cycle.[6,88] Patients who receive transplanted organs are generally placed on lifetime steroid therapy to augment their endogenous cortisol levels and prevent rejection of the donor organ. Under these circumstances, the goal of treatment is to reinforce the intrinsic adrenocortical activity with negligible suppression by giving a synthetic glucocorticoid, such as prednisone, after the peak secretion of endogenous cortisol in a daily or alternate-day midmorning dose.[242,243] However, if the goal is to suppress adrenocortical activity, the synthetic steroid is given shortly before the time of the endogenous cortisol peak.[195,242] Finally, in situations in which the goal of treatment is replacement because of adrenocortical insufficiency, the steroid should be given in a way that mimics the natural endogenous rhythm; that is, it is administered in two unequal doses, with approximately two thirds given in the morning on awakening and one third before retiring in the evening.[210,244,245]

Treatment of asthma can also benefit from a chronopharmacological approach. Since asthma symptoms occur mainly at night, the administration of medications must be designed so that they achieve their maximal effect in the evening.[212] In asthma patients, Dalonzo et al[246] investigated the effects of the daily administration of specifically formulated theophylline medication in patients prone to nocturnal asthma. In 75% of asthma patients with nocturnal symptoms, administration of theophyline in the evening was more effective in decreasing the nocturnal dip in airflow and reducing occurrence of night time attacks than a four times per day schedule.[243] Circadian effects have also been demonstrated in the control of asthma with corticosteroids.[247]

A chronopharmacological approach can also be used to improve symptom management and enhance outcomes in a variety of medical conditions. For example, the symptoms of rhinorrhea resulting from influenza and cold virus or seasonal and perennial allergic rhinitis vary in severity with time of day.[248] Cough frequency, nose blowing, elevation in sublingual temperature, and decreased alertness were worst in the morning shortly after awakening. They suggest that antihistamine and antiinflammatory therapy would be enhanced by timing them to the pattern of symptoms.

Circadian strategies can also be used to decrease the morning risk of ischemic heart disease by scheduling sustained-released beta-blockers before bedtime; scheduling lipid-lowering medications in the evening to correspond with the circadian rhythm of lipid synthesis; and/or using extended-release medications, such as verapamil (verapamil COER-24) so that 24-hour coverage is achieved with higher levels of the antihypertensive medication available at the beginning of the individual's activity period when the blood pressure surge occurs.[18,219,220,222,249-253]

Chronopharmacology is also implemented in investigations of optimal scheduling of chemotherapeutic agents for cancer patients so they can be given at a time when they can have the most efficient antitumor effect and be least toxic.[254] In a study of side effects, Garufi et al[255] gave floxuridine (FUDR) and leucovorin (L-FA) to cancer patients in a 5-day infusion schedule in which the dose of the drugs followed a sine curve with the maximum dose being administered at 6 PM for 35 courses of therapy at 3-week intervals. Only 2 of 14 patients had mucositis that was severe enough to cause pain on swallowing, dry cracked lips, reddened mucous membranes and edema. Mucositis was less in the other 12 patients. In addition, no severe diarrhea was observed. Similar results were obtained by Levi et al[254] in a multisite, multinational clinical trial of 5-fluorouracil (5-FU), leucovorin (LV), and oxaliplatin (I-OHP). The agent was given in a chronomodulated regimen to treat metastatic colorectal carcinoma. The objec-tive response rate appeared to be approximately threefold, as high as that achieved with current 5-FU–based regimens, and the median survival rate was increased approximately 50%.

Chronotherapy

Chronotherapy is effective in treating DSPS. For example, individuals suffering from delayed sleep-onset insomnia have been treated by phase shifting their rhythms until an acceptable sleep period was achieved.[94,256] Chronotherapy has also been used to treat ASPS.[257] The adverse effects associated with shift rotation can be mitigated by the use of schedules that minimize circadian rhythm disruption. For example, rapid rotation schedules of only 1 or 2 days have been proposed, because the shift exposure to night work is insufficient to allow any rhythm change from the worker's usual sleep/activity pattern.[69,258,259] A major disadvantage of a rapid rotation schedule, however, is that people never adapt to working the night shift, which is problematic in critical professions. Although dedicated "straight" shifts promote better adaptation to the shift work schedule, it is difficult to find a sufficient number of workers willing to work evenings or night shifts only. Another problem arises from the tendency of night workers to shift to a day schedule on their days off.[258] A more realistic chronotherapeutic method of rotating shifts is to do it in a clockwise manner from the day shift to evening shift to night shift and back to the day shift with each shift rotation lasting from 1 to 15 weeks.

Phototherapy

Phototherapy (light therapy) has been shown to be an effective treatment for a variety of circadian disorders. For example, Takohashi et al[260] reported that the circadian pacemaker in human beings could be reset by as much as 12 hours by properly timed exposure to bright light and darkness. The usefulness of bright light therapy to promote adaptation in shift workers and for individuals experiencing jet lag has been a focus of investigation.[261-263] Bjorvatn, Kecklund, and Akerstedt[264] exposed shift workers to 30 minutes of bright light during each of the first 4 nights following a shift to night work and the first 4 nights following a shift back to day activity. Daytime sleepiness was reduced and workers rated their quality of life as better. Treatment with pulses of light has been successful in delaying circadian temperature rhythms and reducing daytime sleepiness.

Baehr, Fogg, and Eastman[265] used intermittent bright light pulses to delay temperature cycles of night shift workers and improve their daytime sleep.

Phototherapy provides an effective treatment for seasonal affective disorder (SAD). Light therapy, alone or in combination with anti-depressant medication, is effective treatment for SAD.[266,267] Time of exposure to bright light is also important for treatment of SAD and depression. Lewy[268] studied depressed patients and a group of matched controls in a crossover experiment and found greater antidepressant effect of light therapy applied in the morning between 6 and 8 AM than light administered in the evening between 7 and 9 PM. In a recent study dawn simulation, in which the light levels were increased slowly over a period of 1.5 hours, were found to be more effective at reducing SAD than was a single 30-minute pulse of bright light.[269]

Phototherapy has also been used to treat depression, panic disorder, obsessive compulsive disorders, and *sun-downing*, a syndrome of confusion and agitation in the evening in persons with Alzheimer's disease.[270] It has also been used to increase the duration of sleep and decrease nighttime awakening in Alzheimer's patients.[271] Clinical practice guidelines have been established for treating DSPS and ASPS with bright light therapy.[272] The phototherapeutic effects of bright light may be related to its inhibitory effect on the neurohormone melatonin. Often melatonin rhythms are not synchronized with the light/dark cycle in individuals with DSPS, in elderly persons,[273] or in blind individuals.[93] Several investigators have suggested that insomnia in older adults may be related to decreased melatonin levels.[274,275] Melatonin has been used in combination with bright light for the treatment of jet lag, depression, bipolar disorder, and SAD and to facilitate adaptation to shift changes by several investigators.[276,277] Although the therapeutic use of bright light is promising, results have been shown to vary between individuals and between laboratories. This may be explained in part by the study of Visser et al,[277] who reported that the part of the retina exposed to the light was critical in the suppression of melatonin.

CASE STUDIES

CASE 1: CIRCADIAN DISRUPTION FOLLOWING SURGERY AND ICU INSOMNIA

Ms. BF, a 55-year-old woman admitted for coronary artery bypass surgery, was anxious and unable to sleep the night before surgery. She reported getting virtually no sleep the night of surgery because of nursing interventions, and very little sleep on her first 2 postoperative days. Ms. BF reported that she was unable to sleep because of pain and the bright lights and noise of the ICU setting. She reported that she has difficulty sleeping in unfamiliar surroundings. Her report of disturbed sleep and pain was confirmed by the charting of the night nurses who were caring for her. However, the nurses reported that Ms. BF seemed reluctant to ask for pain medication. Ms. BF was transferred to a step-down unit on her third postoperative day. She slept on and off that night and throughout the next day. On the fourth postoperative day she appeared to have trouble concentrating and appeared depressed. She stated she felt very tired but still had difficulty sleeping at night because of noise. She also had difficulty participating in her morning physical therapy program. Her appetite was poor, and she found it even harder to eat since the meals were served so early (i.e., 7 AM, 11 AM, and 5 PM). She was used to eating her breakfast at 9 AM, lunch at 1 PM, and dinner at 6:30 PM. Her participation in her morning physical therapy regimen was reported to be minimal.

Ms. BF's sleep history indicated that she was used to going to bed at midnight and awakening at 8 AM. She needed a dark, quiet room to be able to sleep and 8 hours of sleep to feel rested. When asked when she usually felt most mentally and physically alert, she replied, "In the afternoon." The brightness of Ms. BF's room in the ICU and the noise were environmental factors that are under the control of nurses. Her early reluctance to ask for pain medication was related to her misperception that she shouldn't ask for pain medication unless her pain became unbearable. The nurses could have assessed her pain and her knowledge of the importance of requesting pain medication before her pain became severe.

Although it is unknown whether rhythm disturbances were affecting this patient's recovery, significant changes did occur in her sleep/wake pattern. Ms. BF was transferred to a private room on her third postoperative day. She reported that she had very little pain or discomfort. Plans were made so that she would not be bothered before 8 AM so that she could return to her regular wake-up time. The dietician visited the patient and a compromise was negotiated so that the timing of her meals adhered more closely to her usual schedule. The physical therapy department was contacted, and Ms. BF's therapy time was changed to the afternoon. Before discharge 3 days later, Ms. BF reported that she was sleeping much better, was more active, and her appetite had improved.

CASE 2: DELAYED SLEEP ONSET PHENOMENON

JL, a 52-year-old international businessman, was in an automobile accident as a result of falling asleep at the wheel. He was admitted to the hospital with a broken arm and slight concussion. During his history and physical he reported that he had just returned from a trip to Hong Kong and was having a difficult time getting over jet lag. This was his second trip to Hong Kong in 5 months. In fact, for the last several months (since his return from his first trip to Asia), Mr. JL reported that he is unable to fall asleep until 3 or 4 AM. During the week he finds it very hard to wake up and get to work on time. Although he managed, he reported that he feels extremely tired, fatigued, and irritable throughout the day, has trouble concentrating on his work and other things that he needs to attend to. During the weekend, when he doesn't have to wake up early, Mr. JL stated he has no difficulty sleeping (but he still is unable to sleep until 3 or 4 AM) and then often sleeps until noon. While in the hospital, he was given a referral to the sleep disorders clinic, where he was diagnosed as having DSPS insomnia. He underwent a chronotherapeutic phase-shift regimen in which he began a progressive clock-hour delay of three hours per day until a sleep period of from 11 PM to 7 AM was reached. During the therapy, Mr. JL was instructed to maintain a strict lights-on and -off schedule that coincided with the phase-shift program. He eventually established a regular sleep/wake schedule and no longer had difficulties falling asleep at night or waking up in the morning. His concentration improved and he reported that now he no longer felt so exhausted; he felt that he could cope better with everyday demands of life.

IMPLICATIONS FOR PRACTICE

Patients in ICU settings are often placed in situations in which time cues are minimal or absent. The routines and activities may require an abrupt change in the patient's usual sleep/wake patterns and mealtimes. It is thought that these circumstances, as well as the effects of the stressors associated with the hospitalization, could lead to internal desynchronization. Chronotherapy could be used by nurses to try to provide a structured temporal environment for patients experiencing circadian rhythm disorders, such as patients in ICUs and patients with affective illness. Measures that nurses can use to minimize circadian rhythm disorders include the prevention of sleep loss and sleep pattern irregularity and providing time cues such as the maintenance of a regular wake-up schedule, regular eating times, and displaying clocks and calendars.

In his comprehensive study, Smolensky[281] reported the findings of a survey conducted by the Gallup organization in which 320 physicians and 1011 members of the public were questioned to estimate their knowledge of medical chronobiology. Results of this study showed that although 88% of physicians claimed to have at least some familiarity with biological rhythms, most were unable to identify correctly the time of day or night when common medical conditions and events were most likely to occur or worsen. According to Smolensky,[281] American adults also did not know the importance of time-of-day variation in disease. They were not able to give the time of day when asthma, myocardial infarction, or hypertension risk was greatest. This is an important area in which nurses should take the lead by providing information on the optimum timing for ingestion of medications and the timing of other types of therapies to increase their effectiveness and improve outcomes and patient tolerance. Furthermore, nurses need to take the circadian variation of physiological variables into consideration when planning patient care (e.g., patient education, treatments, rest periods, and so on) and interpreting laboratory test results and physiological measurements.

SELECTED RESEARCH

Since its formalization as a discipline in 1963, the study of biological rhythmicity (chronobiology) has been included as an integral part of research in many of the areas of nursing science, biomedical science, physiology, biology, and ecology. The study of chronobiology is growing exponentially. Since 1990, 16,340 studies have been conducted in which circadian rhythms were the main focus or a major part of the study (1425 studies in the year 2000 alone). What these studies illustrate is the range and variability of chronobiology and the chronobiological literature. All kinds of physiological and psychological problems in nursing research and practice are affected by biological rhythmicity. Chronobiology is a critical area in the delivery of health care that cannot be ignored. However, it also offers a tool for developing interventions and strategies to improve patient outcomes and to extend the validity of research results.

It is not possible to review even the most current of these studies here. Many of the important chronobiological studies have been reviewed in the previous sections of this chapter. In reviewing the literature of chronobiology, an interested person might choose to concentrate on a particular area of the science that is important to his or her own research interest. For example, clinical studies that focus on the effects of stressors such as illness, cancer, injury, and surgery on patients' circadian rhythms. Altered circadian rhythms have been reported following different types of general surgery,[81-83,85,279] cardiac pacemaker implantation,[280] coronary artery bypass graft (CABG) surgery, automatic implantable cardioverter/defibrillator (AICD) procedures,[28] and transplant surgery.[29,30] Interestingly, the majority of cardiac transplant patients, maintained their circadian heart rate rhythms while experiencing changes in their blood pressure rhythms.[29] Phase shifts of systolic and diastolic blood pressures were also demonstrated in subjects following lung transplantation.[30]

What these studies illustrate is the range and variability of chronobiology and the chronobiological literature. All kinds of physiological and psychological problems in nursing research and practice are affected by biological rhythmicity. Chronobiology is a critical area in the delivery of health care that cannot be ignored. However, it also offers a tool for developing interventions and strategies to improve patient outcomes and to extend the validity of research results.

QUESTIONS FOR FUTURE STUDY

There are several areas of rhythmicity in which nurse researchers can provide valuable information. For example, circadian rhythms of vital physiological processes such as temperature, heart rate, respiratory rate, cortisol, and other hormones are altered and circadian variation is lost following traumatic events such as elevated brain ventricular pressure,[282] brain lesions,[78] head injuries,[12,79] different types of general surgery,[83,85,279] including coronary artery bypass graft (CABG) surgery,[28] heart transplant surgery,[29] and lung transplant surgery.[30] The influences of environmental stimuli in the ICU on the circadian heart rate variability rhythms of a critically ill patient on ventilators have been studied,[84] but additional work is needed. These investigators have identified episodes of physiological instability that require treatment and interventions to return circadian balance and promote recovery.

Because nurses deliver around-the-clock care, they have many reasons and opportunities to play an important role in biological rhythm research. The number of nurses doing circadian rhythm and sleep research is increasing, but more investigations are needed. Many questions need answers. Some examples of questions for future research include the following:

1. How are patient's circadian rhythms affected by illness?
2. How do the stressors, such as uncertainty of diagnosis, surgery, and pain, associated with hospitalization affect a patient's rhythms?
3. If the patient's rhythms are desynchronized by illness or treatment regimen, does the return to a normal pattern hasten recovery?
4. What interventions help prevent desynchronization of circadian rhythms during the patient's hospitalization, especially in ICUs?
5. Would circadian rhythms of maternal origin for heart rate, respiratory movement, and rest/activity, which are usually detectable in the fetus, be present in situations in which the mother is drug addicted? What effects would the mother's drug use have on the baby's circadian rhythm development?
6. What circadian rhythm changes associated with aging and gender are amendable to interventions?
7. Will using knowledge of the patient's performance (mental and physical) rhythms significantly affect the outcomes of patient education programs and/or physical therapy?

REFERENCES

1. Kabat, H.F. (1981). Circadian rhythms and drug dosing. In C.A. Walker, C.M. Winget, & K.F.A. Soliman (eds.), *Chronopharmacology and chronotherapeutics* (p. 10). Tallahassee: Florida A&M University Foundation.
2. Aschoff, J. (1965). Circadian rhythms in man. *Science 148,* 1427-1432.
3. Moore-Ede, M.C., Czeisler, C.A., & Richardson, G.S. (1983). Circadian timekeeping in health and disease. Part 2. Clinical implications of circadian rhythmicity. *New England Journal of Medicine 309,* 530-536.
4. Recio, J., Miguez, J.M., Buxton, O.M., & Challet, E. (1997). Synchronizing circadian rhythms in early infancy. *Medical Hypotheses 49,* 229-234.
5. Ticher, A., Ashkenazi, I.E., & Reinberg, A.E. (1995). Preservation of the functional advantage of human time structure. *Federation of American Societies for Experimental Biology Journal 9,* 269-272.
6. Lanuza, D.M., & Marotta, S.F. (1974). Circadian and basal interrelationships of plasma cortisol and cations in women. *Aerospace Medicine 45,* 864-868.
7. Felton, G. (1987). Human biologic rhythms. *Annual Review of Nursing Research 5,* 45-77.
8. Luce, C.G. (1970). *Biological rhythms in psychiatry.* (Public Health Service Publication No. 2088). Maryland: National Institute of Mental Health.
9. Wehr, T.A., Sack, D., Rosenthal, N., Duncan, W., & Gillin, J.C. (1983). Circadian rhythm disturbances in manic-depressive illness. *Federation Proceedings 42,* 2809-2814.

10. Healy, D., & Williams, J.M. (1988). Dysrhythmia, dysphoria, and depression: The interaction of learned helplessness and circadian dysrhythmia in the pathogenesis of depression. *Psychology Bulletin 103,* 163-178.
11. Moore-Ede, M.C., Czeisler, C.A., & Richardson, G.S. (1983). Circadian timekeeping in health and disease. Part 1. Basic properties of circadian pacemakers. *New England Journal of Medicine 309,* 469-476.
12. Lanuza, D.M., Robinson, C.R., Marotta, S.F., & Patel, M.K. (1989). Body temperature and heart rate rhythms in acutely head-injured patients. *Applied Nursing Research 2,* 135-139.
13. Moore-Ede, M.C. (1981). Hypothermia: A timing disorder of circadian thermoregulatory rhythms? In R.S. Posos (ed.), *The nature and treatment of hypothermia.* Minneapolis: University of Minnesota Press.
14. Rosenberg, R.S. (1984). Aging and biological rhythms: Complaints of insomnia in the elderly. In E. Hans & H.F. Kabat (eds.), *Chronobiology 1982-1988* (pp. 345-349). Paris: Karger.
15. Smolensky, M.H., & D'Alonzo, G.E. (1988). Biologic rhythms and medicine. *American Journal of Medicine 85,* 34-46.
16. Van Gool, W.A., & Mirmiran, M. (1986). Aging and circadian rhythms. *Progress in Brain Research 70,* 255-277.
17. Smolensky, M.H., Reinberg, A.E., Martin, R.J., Haus, E. (1999). Clinical chronobiology and chronotherapeutics with applications to asthma. *Chronobiology International 16,* 539-563.
18. Smolensky, M.H. (1996). Chronobiology and chronotherapeutics. Applications to cardiovascular medicine. *American Journal of Hypertension 9,* 11S-21S.
19. Wever, R.A. (1979). *The circadian system of man: Results of experiments under temporal isolation.* New York: Springer Verlag.
20. Conroy, R.T.W.L., & Mills, J.N. (1970). *Human circadian rhythms.* London: J&A Churchill.
21. Campbell, I.T., Minors, D.S., & Waterhouse, J.M. (1986). Are circadian rhythms important in intensive care? *Intensive Care Nursing 1,* 144-150.
22. Czeisler, C.A., Kronauer, R.E., Allan, J.S., Duffy, J.F., Jewett, M.E., Brown, E.N., et al. (1989). Bright light induction of strong (type 0) resetting of the human circadian pacemaker. *Science 244,* 1328-1333.
23. Mirmiran, M., Swaab, D.F., Witting, W., Honnebier, M.B.O.M., Van Gool, W.A., & Eikelenboom, P. (1989). Biological clocks in development, aging, and Alzheimer's disease. *Brain Dysfunction 2,* 57-66.
24. Otsuka, A., Mikami, H., Katahira, K., Nakamoto, Y., Minamitani, K., Imaoka, M., et al. (1990). Absence of nocturnal fall in blood pressure in elderly persons with alzheimer-type dementia. *Journal of the American Geriatric Society 38,* 973-978.
25. Eastman, C.I., & Martin, S.K. (1999). How to use light and dark to produce circadian adaptation to night shift work. *Annals of Medicine 31,* 87-98.
26. Witting, W., Kwa, I.H., Eikelenboom, P., Mirmiran, M., & Swaab, D.F. (1990). Alterations in the circadian rest-activity rhythm in aging and Alzheimer's disease. *Biological Psychiatry 27,* 563-572.
27. Lanuza, D.M. (1988). Plasma cortisol changes associated with implantation of the automatic cardioverter/defibrilator [abstract]. *Circulation 78,* 2.
28. Lanuza, D.M. (1995). Postoperative circadian rhythms and cortisol stress response to two types of cardiac surgery. *American Journal of Critical Care 4,* 212-220.
29. Lanuza, D.M., Grady, K., Hetfleisch, M., & Johnson, M.R. (1994). Circadian rhythm changes in blood pressure and heart rate during the first year after heart transplantation. *Journal of Heart and Lung Transplantation 13,* 614-623.
30. Lanuza, D.M., Farcas, G.A., & Patel, M.K. (2000). Changes in lung transplant patients' blood pressure and heart rate mean levels and rhythms [abstract]. *Circulation 102,* 696s.
31. Statistics B.o.L. (1998). *Labor force statistics from the current population survey.* U.S. Department of Labor.
32. Akerstedt, T. (1985). Shifted sleep hours. *Annals of Clinical Research 17,* 273-279.
33. Ostberg, O. (1973). Interindividual differences in circadian fatigue patterns of shift workers. *British Journal of Industrial Medicine 30,* 341-351.
34. Van Reeth, O. (1998). Sleep and circadian disturbances in shift work: Strategies for their management. *Hormone Research 49,* 158-162.
35. Akerstedt, T. (1987). Sleep/wake disturbances in working life. In R.F. Ellingson, N.M.F. Murray, & A.M. Halliday (eds.), *The London symposia* (EEG Supplement pp. 360-363). Amsterdam: Elsevier Science.
36. Smith-Coggins, R., Rosekind, M.R., Buccino, K.R., Dinges, D.F., & Moser, R.P. (1997). Rotating shiftwork schedules: Can we enhance physician adaptation to night shifts? *Academy of Emergency Medicine 4,* 951-961.
37. Thiss-Evenson, E. (1969). Shift work and health. In A. Swensson (ed.) *Proceedings of the international symposium on night shift work* (pp. 81-83). Stockholm, Sweden: National Institute of Occupational Health.
38. Koller, M. (1983). Health risks related to shift work. An example of time-contingent effects of long-term stress. *International Archives of Occupational and Environmental Health 53,* 59-75.
39. Mitler, M.M., Carskadon, M.A., Czeisler, C.A., Dement, W.C., Dinges, D.F., & Graeber, R.C. (1988). Catastrophes, sleep, and public policy: Consensus report. *Sleep 11,* 100-109.
40. Copinschi, G., Van Reeth, O., & Van Cauter, E. (1999). Les rythmes biologiques. Effets du veillissement et de la desynchronisation entre la rythmicite endogene et les conditions d'environnement. *Presse Medicale 28,* 942-946.
41. Costa, G. (1997). The problem: Shiftwork. *Chronobiology International 14,* 89-98.
42. Boggild, H., Knutsson, A. (1999). Shift work, risk factors and cardiovascular disease. *Scand Journal Work Environmental Health 25,* 85-99.
43. Polonsky, K.S., Given, B.D., Hirsch, L., Shapiro, E.T., Tillil, H., Beebe, C., et al. (1988). Quantitative study of insulin secretion and clearance in normal and obese subjects. *Journal of Clinical of Investment 81,* 435-441.
44. Van Cauter, E., Mestrez, F., Sturis, J., & Polonsky, K.S. (1992). Estimation of insulin secretion rates from c-peptide levels. Comparison of individual and standard kinetic parameters for c-peptide clearance. *Diabetes 41,* 368-377.
45. Morgan, L., Arendt, J., Owens, D., Folkard, S., Hampton, S., Deacon, S., et al. (1998). Effects of the endogenous clock and sleep time on melatonin, insulin, glucose and lipid metabolism. *Journal of Endocrinology 157,* 443-451.
46. Barnes, R.G., Deacon, S.J., Forbes, M.J., & Arendt, J. (1998). Adaptation of the 6-sulphatoxymelatonin rhythm in shiftworkers on offshore oil installations during a 2-week 12-h night shift. *Neuroscience Letters 241,* 9-12.

47. Moore-Ede, M.C., & Richardson, G.S. (1985). Medical implications of shift-work. *Annual Review of Medicine 36,* 607-617.
48. Bruugsgaard, A. (1969). Shiftwork as an occupational health problem. In S.A. (ed.), *Proceedings of the international symposium on night and shiftwork* (pp. 9-14). Stockholm, Sweden: National Institute of Occupational Health.
49. Hakkinen, S. (1969). Adaptability to shift work. In A. Swensson (ed.), *Proceedings of the international symposium on night and shift work.* Stockholm, Sweden: National Institute of Occupational Health.
50. Barnes, R.G., Forbes, M.J., & Arendt, J. (1998). Shift type and season affect adaptation of the 6-sulphatoxymelatonin rhythm in offshore oil rig workers. *Neuroscience Letters 252,* 179-182.
51. Reinberg, A., Motohashi, Y., Bourdeleau, P., Touitou, Y., Nouguier, J., Levi, F., et al. (1989). Internal desynchronization of circadian rhythms and tolerance of shift work. *Chronobiologia 16,* 21-34.
52. Kerhoff, G. (1985). Individual differences in circadian rhythms. In S. Folkard & T.H. Monk (eds.), *Hours of work, temporal factors in work-scheduling* (pp. 29-36). New York: John Wiley & Sons.
53. Harma, M., Knauth, P., Ilmarinen, J., & Ollila, H. (1990). The relation of age to the adjustment of the circadian rhythms of oral temperature and sleepiness to shift work. *Chronobiology International 7,* 227-233.
54. Weitzman, E.D., Moline, M.L., Czeisler, C.A., & Zimmerman, J.C. (1982). Chronobiology of aging: Temperature, sleep-wake rhythms and entrainment. *Neurobiology Aging 3,* 299-309.
55. Campbell, S.S., Gillin, J.C., Kripke, D.F., Erikson, P., & Clopton, P. (1989). Gender differences in the circadian temperature rhythms of healthy elderly subjects: Relationships to sleep quality. *Sleep 12,* 529-536.
56. Folkard, S., Monk, T.H., & Lobban, M.C. (1979). Towards a predictive test of adjustment to shift work. *Ergonomics 22,* 79-91.
57. Nachreiner, F. (1997). *Individual and social determinants of shiftwork tolerance.* Finland.
58. Waterhouse, J., Minors, D., & Redfern, P. (1997). Some comments on the measurement of circadian rhythms after time-zone transitions and during night work. *Chronobiology International 14,* 125-132.
59. Folkard, S. (1990). Circadian performance rhythms: Some practical and theoretical implications. *Philosophical Transactions of the Royal Society of London, Series B: Biological Science 327,* 543-553.
60. Colquhoun, W.P. (1971). Circadian rhythms in mental efficiency. In W.P. Colquhoun (ed.), *Biological rhythms and human performance* (pp. 39-107). New York: Academic Press.
61. Wever, R.A. (1984). Toward a mathematical model of circadian rhythmicity. In M.C. Moore-Ede & C.A. Czeisler (eds.), *Mathematical models of the circadian sleep-wake cycle* (pp. 17-79). New York: Raven Press.
62. Kleitman, N., & Ramsaroop, A. (1948). Periodicity in body temperature and heart rate. *Endocrinology 43,* 1-20.
63. Lanuza, D.M. (1976). Circadian rhythms of mental efficiency and performance. *Nursing Clinics of North America 11,* 583-594.
64. Patkai, P., Akerstedt, T., & Pettersson, K. (1977). Field studies of shiftwork: I. Temporal patterns in psychophysiological activation in permanent night workers. *Ergonomics 20,* 611-619.
65. Brown, R.C. (1949). The day and night performance of teleprinter switch board operations. *Occupational Psychology 23,* 1-6.
66. Bjerner, B., Holm, A., & Swensson, A. (1955). Diurnal variation in mental performance. A study of three-shift workers. *British Journal of Industrial Medicine 12,* 103-110.
67. Dinges, D.F. (1995). An overview of sleepiness and accidents. *Journal of Sleep Research 4,* 4-14.
68. Harris, W. (1977). Fatigue, circadian rhythm, and truck accidents. In R. Mackie (ed.), *Vigilance therapy, operational performance, and physiological correlates* (pp. 133-146). New York: Plenum Press.
69. Ehret, C.F. (1981). New approaches to chronohygiene for the shift worker in the nuclear power industry. In A. Reinberg, N. Vieux, & T. Anslauer (eds.), *Night and shift work. Biological and social aspects* (pp. 263-270). Oxford, England: Pergamon Press.
70. Spitzer, R.L., Terman, M., Williams, J.B., Terman, J.S., Malt, U.F., Singer, F., et al. (1999). Jet lag: Clinical features, validation of a new syndrome-specific scale, and lack of response to melatonin in a randomized, double-blind trial. *American Journal of Psychiatry 156,* 1392-1396.
71. Samel, A. (1999). Melatonin and jet-lag. *European Journal of Medical Research 4,* 385-388.
72. Rajaratnam S.M., Arendt, J. (2001). Health in a 24-h Society. *Lancet 22,* 358(9286):999-1005.
73. Gander, P.H., Myhre, G., Graeber, R.C., Andersen, H.T., & Lauber, J.K. (1989). Adjustment of sleep and the circadian temperature rhythm after flights across nine time zones. *Aviation, Space, and Environmental Medicine 60,* 733-743.
74. Reilly, T., Atkinson, G., & Waterhouse, J. (1997). Travel fatigue and jet-lag. *Journal of Sports Sciences 15,* 365-369.
75. Samel, A., Wegmann, H.M., Summa, W., & Naumann, M. (1991). Sleep patterns in aircrew operating on the polar route between Germany and east Asia. *Aviation, Space, and Environmental Medicine 62,* 661-669.
76. Graeber, R.C., Dement, W.C., Nicholson, A.N., Sasaki, M., & Wegmann, H.M. (1986). International cooperative study of aircrew layover sleep: Operational summary. *Aviation, Space, and Environmental Medicine 57,* B10-13.
77. Klein, K.E., Wegmann, H.M., Athanassenas, G., Hohlweck, H., Kuklinski, P. (1976). Air operations and circadian performance rhythms. *Aviation, Space, and Environmental Medicine 47,* 221-230.
78. Dauch, W.A., & Bauer, S. (1990). Circadian rhythms in the body temperatures of intensive care patients with brain lesions. *Journal of Neurology, Neurosurgery, and Psychiatry 53,* 345-347.
79. Okawa, M., Takahashi, K., & Sasaki, H. (1986). Disturbance of circadian rhythms in severely brain-damaged patients correlated with CT findings. *Journal of Neurology 233,* 274-282.
80. Lanuza, D.M. (1989). The effects of two types of cardiac surgery on plasma cortisol levels and its circadian rhythm. In *Proceedings of the 13th Annual Midwest Nursing Research Society Conference: Nursing research: Impact on social issues.* Cincinnati.
81. Farr, L.A., Campbell-Grossman, C., & Mack, J.M. (1988). Circadian disruption and surgical recovery. *Nursing Research 37,* 170-175.
82. Farr, L.A., Gaspar, T.M., & Mann, D.F. (1984). *Desynchronization with surgery.* In E. Haus & H.F. Kabat (eds.), *Chronobiology.* New York: Karger.

83. Farr, L., Todero, C., & Boen, L. (2001). Reducing disruption of circadian temperature rhythms following surgery. *Biological Research in Nursing 2,* 257-266.
84. Felver, L., & Pike, R. (1990). Relationship of heart rate, respiratory rate, and arterial blood pressure rhythms in a mechanically ventilated patient to environmental variables in an intensive care unit. In D.K. Hayes, J.E. Pauly, & R.J. Reiter (eds.), *Chronobiology: Its role in clinical medicine, general biology, and agriculture. Part A. Progress in clinical and biological research.* New York: John Wiley & Sons.
85. McIntosh, T.K., Lothrop, D.A., Lee, A., Jackson, B.T., Nabseth, D., & Egdahl, R.H. (1981). Circadian rhythm of cortisol is altered in postsurgical patients. *Journal of Clinical Endocrinology and Metabolism 53,* 117-122.
86. Campbell, I.T., Bell, C.F., Minors, D.S., & Waterhouse, J.M. (1983). A preliminary study of body temperature rhythms in intensive care [abstract]. *Chronobiologia 10,* 114.
87. Easton, C., & MacKenzie, F. (1988). Sensory-perceptual alterations: Delirium in the intensive care unit. *Heart & Lung 17,* 229-237.
88. Moore-Ede, M.C., Sulzman, F.M., & Fuller, C.A. (1982). A physiological system measuring time. In M.C. Moode-Ede, F.M. Sulzman, & C.A. Fuller (eds.), *The clocks that time us: Physiology of the circadian timing system* (pp. 1-29). Cambridge, Mass.: Harvard University Press.
89. Moore-Ede, M.C. (1983). The circadian timing system in mammals: Two pacemakers preside over many secondary oscillators. *Federation Proceedings 42,* 2802-2808.
90. Ando, K., Kripke, D.F., & Ancoli-Israel, S. (1995). Estimated prevalence of delayed and advances sleep phase syndromes. *Journal of Sleep Research 24,* 509.
91. Anders, T.F. (1982). Biological rhythms in development. *Psychological Medicine 44,* 61-72.
92. Weitzman, E.D., Czeisler, C.A., Coleman, R.M., Spielman, A.J., Zimmerman, J.C., Dement, W., et al. (1981). Delayed sleep phase syndrome. A chronobiological disorder with sleep-onset insomnia. *Archives of General Psychiatry 38,* 737-746.
93. Lockley, S.W., Skene, D.J., Butler, L.J., & Arendt, J. (1999). Sleep and activity rhythms are related to circadian phase in the blind. *Sleep 22,* 616-623.
94. Czeisler, C.A., Richardson, G.S., Coleman, R.M., Zimmerman, J.C., Moore-Ede, M.C., Dement, W.C., et al. (1981). Chronotherapy: Resetting the circadian clocks of patients with delayed sleep phase insomnia. *Sleep 4,* 1-21.
95. Dagan, Y., Stein, D., Steinbock, M., Yovel, I., & Hallis, D. (1998). Frequency of delayed sleep phase syndrome among hospitalized adolescent psychiatric patients. *Journal of Psychosomatic Research 45,* 15-20.
96. Rosenthal, N.E., Joseph-Vanderpool, J.R., Levendosky, A.A., Johnston, S.H., Allen, R., Kelly, K.A., et al. (1990). Phase-shifting effects of bright morning light as treatment for delayed sleep phase syndrome. *Sleep 13,* 354-361.
97. Lewy, A.J., & Sack, R.L. (1997). Exogenous melatonin's phase-shifting effects on the endogenous melatonin profile in sighted humans: A brief review and critique of the literature. *Journal of Biological Rhythms 12,* 588-594.
98. Ando, K., Kripke, D.F., Cole, R.J., & Elliott, J.A. (1999). Light mask 500 lux treatment for delayed sleep phase syndrome. *Progress in Neuro-Psychopharmacology & Biological Psychiatry 23,* 15-24.
99. Shanahan, T.L., Kronauer, R.E., Duffy, J.F., Williams, G.H., & Czeisler, C.A. (1999). Melatonin rhythm observed throughout a three-cycle bright-light stimulus designed to reset the human circadian pacemaker. *Journal of Biological Rhythms 14,* 237-253.
100. Perras, B., Pannenborg, H., Marshall, L., Pietrowsky, R., Born, J., & Lorenz Fehm, H. (1999). Beneficial treatment of age-related sleep disturbances with prolonged intranasal vasopressin. *Journal of Clinical Psychopharmacology 19,* 28-36.
101. Steiger, A., Holsboer, F. (1997). Nocturnal secretion of prolactin and cortisol and the sleep eeg in patients with major endogenous depression during an acute episode and after full remission. *Psychiatry Research 72,* 81-88.
102. Lavie, P. (1989). To nap, perchance to sleep-ultradian aspects of napping. In D.F. Dinges, & R. Broughton (eds.), *Sleep and alertness: Chronobiological, behavioral, and medical aspects of napping* (pp. 99-120). New York: Raven Press.
103. Hoch, C.C., Dew, M.A., Reynolds, C.F., Buysse, D.J., Nowell, P.D., Monk T.H., et al. (1997). Longitudinal changes in diary- and laboratory-based sleep measures in healthy "old old" and "young old" subjects: A three-year follow-up. *Sleep 20,* 192-202.
104. Refinetti, R. (2000). *Circadian physiology.* Boca Raton: CRC Press.
105. Chaperon, C., Farr, L., & LoChiano, E. (1998). *Circadian rhythms and sleep cycles in community-dwelling and institutionalized older adults. In Proceedings of the XXI Midwest Nursing Research Society.* Columbus, Ohio.
106. Lombardo, P., Formicola, G., Gori, S., Gneri, C., Massetani, R., Murri, L., et al. (1998). Slow wave sleep (SWS) distribution across night sleep episode in the elderly. *Aging* (Milan) *10,* 445-448.
107. Jones, C.R., Campbell, S.S., Zone, S.E., Cooper, F., DeSano, A., Murphy, P.J., et al. (1999). Familial advanced sleep-phase syndrome: A short-period circadian rhythm variant in humans [see comments]. *Nature Medicine 5,* 1062-1065.
108. Hohjoh, H., Takahashi, Y., Hatta, Y., Tanaka, H., Akaza, T., Tokunaga, K., et al. (1999). Possible association of human leucocyte antigen DR1 with delayed sleep phase syndrome. *Psychiatry and Clinical Neurosciences 53,* 527-529.
109. Pincus, H. (1997). Neuroanatomical hypotheses derived from neuropathological and imaging investigations (sad and bipolar disorder). In A. Tasman, J. Kay, & J. Lieberman (eds.), *Psychiatry.* Philadelphia: W.B. Saunders.
110. Wehr, T.A. (1990). Reply to Healy, D., & Waterhouse, J.M.: The circadian system and affective disorders: Clocks or rhythms? *Chronobiology International 7,* 11-14.
111. Lewy, A.J. (1990). Reply to Healy, D., & Waterhouse, J.M.: The circadian system and affective disorders: Clocks or rhythms? Chronobiologic disorders, social cues and the light-dark cycle. *Chronobiology International 7,* 15-24.
112. Healy, D., & Waterhouse, J.M. (1990). The circadian system and affective disorders: Clocks or rhythms? *Chronobiology International 7,* 5-10.
113. Goodwin, F.K., Wirz-Justice, A., & Wehr, T.A. (1982). Evidence that the pathophysiology of depression and the mechanism of action of antidepressant drugs both involve alterations in circadian rhythms. *Advances in Biochemical Psychopharmacology 32,* 1-11.

114. Sachar, E.J., Hellman, L., Roffwarg, H.P., Halpern, F.S., Fukushima, D.K., & Gallagher, T.F. (1973). Disrupted 24-hour patterns of cortisol secretion in psychotic depression. *Archives of General Psychiatry 28,* 19-24.
115. Beck-Friis, J., Ljunggren, J.G., Thoren, M., von Rosen, D., Kjellman, B.F., & Wetterberg, L. (1985). Melatonin, cortisol and ACTH in patients with major depressive disorder and healthy humans with special reference to the outcome of the dexamethasone suppression test. *Psychoneuroendocrinology 10,* 173-186.
116. Weeke, A., & Weeke, J. (1980). The 24-hour pattern of serum TSH in patients with endogenous depression. *Acta Psychiatr Scand 62,* 69-74.
117. Beersma, D.G., van den Hoofdakker, R.H., & van Berkestijn, H.W. (1983). Circadian rhythms in affective disorders: Body temperature and sleep physiology in endogenous depressives. *Advances in Biological Psychiatry 11,* 114-117.
118. Avery, D.H., Wildschiodtz, G., & Rafaelsen, O.J. (1982). Nocturnal temperature in affective disorder. *Journal of Affective Disorders 4,* 61-71.
119. Bunney, W.E., & Bunney, B.G. (2000). Molecular clock genes in man and lower animals: Possible implications for circadian abnormalities in depression. *Neuropsychopharmacology 22,* 335-345.
120. Checkley, S. (1989). The relationship between biological rhythms and affective disorders. In J. Aremdt, D.S. Minors, & J.M. Waterhouse (eds.), *Biological rhythms in clinical practice* (pp. 160-183). London: Wright.
121. Wever, R.A. (1985). Internal interactions within the human circadian system: The masking effect. *Experientia 41,* 332-342.
122. Siever, L.J., & Davis, K.L. (1985). Overview: Toward a dysregulation hypothesis of depression. *American Journal of Psychiatry 142,* 1017-1031.
123. Halberg, F. (1968). Physiological considerations underlying rhytmometry with special reference to emotional illness. In J.A. Juriaguerra (ed.), *Cycles biologisques et psychiatrie.* Paris: Georg, Geneve, & Masson.
124. Sherman, B., Wysham, C., & Pfohl, B. (1985). Age-related changes in the circadian rhythm of plasma cortisol in man. *Journal of Clinical Endocrinology and Metabolism 61,* 439-443.
125. Haus, E., Nicolau, G., Lakatua, D.J., Sackett-Lundeen, L., & Petrescu, E. (1989). Circadian rhythm parameters of endocrine functions in elderly subjects during the seventh to the ninth decade of life. *Chronobiologia 16,* 331-352.
126. Lobban, M.C. (1960). The entertainment of circadian rhythms in man. *Cold Spring Harbor Symposia of Quantitative Biology 25,* 325-332.
127. Wollman, M., Lavie, P., & Peled, R. (1985). A hypernychthemeral sleep-wake syndrome: A treatment attempt. *Chronobiology International 2,* 277-280.
128. Rietveld, W.J. (1990). The central control and ontogeny of circadian rhythmicity. *European Journal of Morphology 28,* 301-307.
129. Hellbrugge, T. (1960). The development of circadian rhythms in infants. *Cold Spring Harbor Symposia of Quantitative Biology 25,* 311-323.
130. Zurbruegg, R.P. (1976). Hypothalamic-pituitary-adenocortical regulation: A contribution to its assessment, development and disorders in infancy and childhood with special reference to plasma cortisol circadian rhythm. *Monographs in Pediatrics 17,* Basel: Karger.
131. Abe, K., Sasaki, H., Takebayashi, K., Fukui, S., & Nambu, H. (1978). The development of circadian rhythm of human body temperature. *Journal of Interdisciplinary Cycle Research 9,* 211-216.
132. Updike, P.A., Accurso, F.J., Jones, R.H. (1985). Physiologic circadian rhythmicity in preterm infants. *Nursing Research 34,* 160-163.
133. Mirmiran, M., Kok, J.H., de Kleine, M.J.K., Koope, J.C., Overdijk, J., & Witting, W. (1990). Circadian rhythms in preterm infants: A preliminary study. *Early Human Development 32,* 139-146.
134. Thomas, K.A. (1991). The emergence of body temperature biorhythm in preterm infants. *Nursing Research 40,* 98-102.
135. Vermes, I., Dohanics, J., Toth, G., & Pongracz, J. (1980). Maturation of the circadian rhythm of the adrenocortical functions in human neonates and infants. *Hormone Research 12,* 237-244.
136. Onishi, S., Miyazawa, G., Nishimura, Y., Sugiyama, S., Yamakawa, T., Inagaki, H., et al. (1983). Postnatal development of circadian rhythm in serum cortisol levels in children. *Pediatrics 72,* 399-404.
137. Price, D.A., Close, G.C., & Fielding, B.A. (1983). Age of appearance of circadian rhythm in salivary cortisol values in infancy. *Archives of the Disabled Child 58,* 454-456.
138. Spangler, G. (1991). The emergence of adrenocortical circadian function in newborns and infants and its relationship to sleep, feeding and maternal adrenocortical activity. *Early Human Development 25,* 197-208.
139. Grossman, D.G. (1991). Circadian rhythms in blood pressure in school-age children of normotensive and hypertensive parents. *Nursing Research 40,* 28-34.
140. Halberg, F., Halberg, E., Halberg, J., & Halberg, F. (1984). Chronobiologic assessment of human blood pressure variation in health and disease. In M. Weber & J.M. Drayer (eds.), *Ambulatory blood pressure monitoring* (pp. 13-156). New York: Springer Verlag.
141. Rabarin, J.S., Sothern, R.B., Brunning, R.D., Goetz, F.C., & Halberg, F. (1981). Circadian rhythms in blood and self-measured variables in ten children 9 to 14 years of age. In F. Halberg, et al. (eds.), *Chronobiology. Proceedings of XIII International Conference, International Society For Chronobiology* (pp. 373-385). Milan: Il Ponte.
142. Scarpelli, P.T., Romano, S., Cagnoni, M., Livi, R., Scarpelli, L., Bigioli, F., et al. (1985). The Florence Children's Blood Pressure Study. A chronobiological approach by multiple self-measurements. *Clinical and Experimental Hypertension A7,* 355-359.
143. Carskadon, M.A., Labyak, S.E., Acebo, C., & Seifer, R. (1999). Intrinsic circadian period of adolescent humans measured in conditions of forced desynchrony. *Neuroscience Letters 260,* 129-132.
144. Wolfson, A.R., & Carskadon, M.A. (1998). Sleep schedules and daytime functioning in adolescents. *Child Development 69,* 875-887.
145. Andrade, M.M., Benedito-Silva, A.A., & Menna-Barreto, L. (1992). Correlations between morningness-eveningness character, sleep habits and temperature rhythm in adolescents. *Brazilian Journal of Medical and Biological Research 25,* 835-839.
146. Strauch, I., & Meier, B. (1988). Sleep need in adolescents: A longitudinal approach. *Sleep 11,* 378-386.
147. Ishihara, K., Honma, Y., & Miyake, S. (1990). Investigation of the children's version of the Morningness-Eveningness Questionnaire with primary and junior high school pupils in Japan. *Perceptual and Motor Skills 71,* 1353.

148. Epstein, R., Chillag, N., & Lavie, P. (1998). Starting times of school: Effects on daytime functioning of fifth-grade children in Israel. *Sleep 21,* 250-256.
149. Henschel, A., & Lack, L. (1987). Do many adolescents sleep poorly or just too late? *Journal of Sleep Research 16,* 354.
150. Dement, W.C., Miles, L.E., & Carskadon, M.A. (1982). "White paper" on sleep and aging. *Journal of the American Geriatric Society 30,* 25-50.
151. Lugaresi, E., Zuconni, M., & Bixler, E.O. (1987). Epidemiology of sleep disorders. *Psychiatric Annals 17,* 446-453.
152. Morgan, K., Dallosso, H., Ebrahim, S., Arie, T., & Fentem, P.H. (1988). Prevalence, frequency, and duration of hypnotic drug use among the elderly living at home. *British Medical Journal (Clinical Research Edition) 296,* 601-602.
153. Rumble, R., & Morgan, K. (1992). Hypnotics, sleep, and mortality in elderly people. *Journal of the American Geriatric Society 40,* 787-791.
154. Ouslander, J.G., Buxton, W.G., Al-Samarrai, N.R., Cruise, P.A., Alessi, C., & Schnelle, J.F. (1998). Nighttime urinary incontinence and sleep disruption among nursing home residents. *Journal of the American Geriatric Society 46,* 463-466.
155. Monk, T.H. (1989). Sleep disorders in the elderly. Circadian rhythm. *Clinics in Geriatric Medicine 5,* 331-346.
156. Richardson, G. (1990). Circadian rhythms and aging. In C.E. Finch & E.L. Schneider (eds.), *Handbook of the biology of aging* (pp. 275-305). New York: Van Nostrand Reinhold.
157. Brock, M.A. (1991). Chronobiology and aging. *Journal of the American Geriatric Society 39,* 74-91.
158. Touitou, Y., Sulon, J., Bogdan, A., Touitou, C., Reinberg, A., Beck, H., et al. (1982). Adrenal circadian system in young and elderly human subjects: A comparative study. *Journal of Endocrinology 93,* 201-210.
159. Touitou, Y., Bogdan, A., Haus, E., & Touitou, C. (1997). Modifications of circadian and circannual rhythms with aging. *Experimental Gerontology 32,* 603-614.
160. Touitou, Y., & Haus, E. (1994). Aging of the human endocrine and neuroendocrine time structure. *Annals of the New York Academy of Science 719,* 378-397.
161. Turek, F.W., Penev, P., Zhang, Y., van Reeth, O., & Zee, P. (1995). Effects of age on the circadian system. *Neuroscience and Biobehavioral Reviews 19,* 53-58.
162. Casale, G., & de Nicola, P. (1984). Circadian rhythms in the aged: A review. *Archives of Gerontology and Geriatrics 3,* 267-284.
163. Czeisler, C.A., Duffy, J.F., Shanahan, T.L., Brown, E.N., Mitchell, J.F., Rimmer, D., et al. (1999). Stability, precision, and near-24-hour period of the human circadian pacemaker [see comments]. *Science 284,* 2177-2181.
164. Czeisler, C., Rios, C., & Sanchez, R. (1986). Phase advance and reduction in the amplitude of the endogenous circadian oscillator correspond with systematic changes in sleep-wake habits and daytime functioning in the elderly. *Sleep 15,* 268.
165. Swoyer, J., Irvine, P., Sackett-Lundeen, L., Conlin, L., Lakatua, D.J., & Haus E. (1989). Circadian hematologic time structure in the elderly. *Chronobiology International 6,* 131-137.
166. Lieberman, H.R., Wurtman, J.J., & Teicher, M.H. (1989). Circadian rhythms of activity in healthy young and elderly humans. *Neurobiology of Aging 10,* 259-265.
167. Guite, H.F., Bliss, M.R., Mainwaring-Burton, R.W., Thomas, J.M., & Drury, P.L. (1988). Hypothesis: Posture is one of the determinants of the circadian rhythm of urine flow and electrolyte excretion in elderly female patients. *Age and Ageing 17,* 241-248.
168. Hofman, M.A. (2000). The human circadian clock and aging. *Chronobiology International 17,* 245-259.
169. Swaab, D.F., Fliers, E., & Partiman, T.S. (1985). The suprachiasmatic nucleus of the human brain in relation to sex, age and senile dementia. *Brain Research 342,* 37-44.
170. Weinert, D. (2000). Age-dependent changes of the circadian system. *Chronobiology International 17,* 261-283.
171. Aschoff, J., & Wever, R. (1976). Human circadian rhythms: A multioscillatory system. *Federation Proceedings 35,* 2326-2332.
172. Moore, R.Y., & Eichler, V.B. (1972). Loss of a circadian adrenal corticosterone rhythm following suprachiasmatic lesions in the rat. *Brain Research 42,* 201-206.
173. Turek, F.W. (1998). Circadian rhythms. *Hormone Research 49,* 109-113.
174. Stephan, F.K., & Zucker, I. (1972). *Circadian rhythms in drinking behavior and locomotor activity of rats are eliminated by hypothalamic lesions.* In *Proceedings of the National Academy of Sciences USA.*
175. Fuller, C.A., Lydic, R., Sulzman, F.M., Albers, H.E., Tepper, B., & Moore-Ede, M.C. (1981). Circadian rhythm of body temperature persists after suprachiasmatic lesions in the squirrel monkey. *American Journal of Physiology 241,* R385-391.
176. Ibuka, N. (1979). Suprachiasmatic nucleus and sleep-wakefulness rhythms. In M. Suda & O. Hayaishi (eds.), *Biological rhythms and their central mechanism* (pp. 325-334). Amsterdam: Elsevier.
177. Rea, M.A. (1989). Light increases fos-related protein immunoreactivity in the rat suprachiasmatic nuclei. *Brain Research Bulletin 23,* 577-581.
178. Kornhauser, J.M., Nelson, D.E., Mayo, K.E., & Takahashi, J.S. (1990). Photic and circadian regulation of c-fos gene expression in the hamster suprachiasmatic nucleus. *Neuron 5,* 127-134.
179. Rusak, B., Robertson, H.A., Wisden, W., & Hunt, S.P. (1990). Light pulses that shift rhythms induce gene expression in the suprachiasmatic nucleus. *Science 248,* 1237-1240.
180. Skene, D.J., Lockley, S.W., & Arendt, J. (1999). Melatonin in circadian sleep disorders in the blind. *Biological Signals and Receptors 8,* 90-95.
181. Wever, R. (1975). The circadian multi-oscillatory system of man. *International Journal of Chronobiology 3,* 19-55.
182. Moore-Ede, M.C., Schmelzer, W.S., Kass, D.A., & Herd, J.A. (1976). Internal organization of the circadian timing system in multicellular animals. *Federation Proceedings 35,* 2333-2338.
183. Andrews, R.V., Keil, L.C., & Keil, N.N. (1968). Further observations on the adrenal secretory rhythm of the brown lemming. *Acta Endocrinology* (Copenhagen) *59,* 36-40.
184. Diijk, D., Duffy, J.F., & C.C. (1992). Circadian and sleep/wake dependent aspects of subjective alertness and cognitive performance. *Journal of Sleep Research 1,* 112-117.
185. Boivin, D.B., Czeisler, C.A., Dijk, D.J., Duffy, J.F., Folkard, S., Minors, D.S., et al. (1997). Complex interaction of the sleep-wake cycle and circadian phase

modulates mood in healthy subjects. *Archives of General Psychiatry 54,* 145-152.
186. Hiddinga, A.E., Beersma, D.G., & van den Hoofdakker, R.H. (1997). Endogenous and exogenous components in the circadian variation of core body temperature in humans. *Journal of Sleep Research 6,* 156-163.
187. Gundel, A., & Spencer, M.B. (1999). A circadian oscillator model based on empirical data. *Journal of Biological Rhythms 14,* 516-523.
188. Koorengevel, K.M., Beersma, D.G., Gordijn, M.C., den Boer, J.A., & van den Hoofdakker, R.H. (2000). Body temperature and mood variations during forced desynchronization in winter depression: A preliminary report. *Biological Psychiatry 47,* 355-358.
189. Waterhouse, J., Weinert, D., Minors, D., Atkinson, G., Reilly, T., Folkard, S., et al. (1999). The effect of activity on the waking temperature rhythm in humans. *Chronobiology International 16,* 343-357.
190. Rusak, B., & Zucker, I. (1979). Neural regulation of circadian rhythms. *Physiological Reviews 59,* 449-526.
191. Achermann, P., Dijk, D.J., Brunner, D.P., & Borbély, A.A. (1993). A model of human sleep homeostasis based on eeg slow-wave activity: Quantitative comparison of data and simulations. *Brain Research Bulletin 31,* 97-113.
192. Borbély, A.A. (1998). Processes underlying sleep regulation. *Hormone Research 49,* 114-117.
193. Halberg, F., & Howard, R.B. (1958). 24-hour periodicity and experimental medicine: Examples and interpretations. *Postgraduate Medicine 24,* 349-358.
194. Halberg, F., Johnson, E., Brown, B.W., & Bittner, J.J. (1960). Susceptibility rhythm to *E. coli* endotoxin and bioassay. *Proceedings of the Society for Experimental Biology and Medicine 103,* 142-144.
195. Reinberg, A., Smolensky, M., Labrecque, G., & Hallek, M. (1987). Aspects of chronopharmacology and chronotherapy in children. *Chronobiologia 14,* 303-325.
196. Ohdo, S., Watanabe, H., Ogawa, N., Yoshiyama, Y., & Sugiyama, T. (1996). Chronotoxicity of sodium valproate in pregnant mouse and embryo. *Japanese Journal of Pharmacology 70,* 253-258.
197. Granda, T.G., Filipski, E., D'Attino, R.M., Vrignaud, P., Anjo, A., Bissery, M.C., et al. (2001). Experimental chronotherapy of mouse mammary adenocarcinoma ma13/c with docetaxel and doxorubicin as single agents and in combination. *Cancer Research 61,* 1996-2001.
198. To, H., Kikuchi, A., Tsuruoka, S., Sugimoto, K., Fujimura, A., Higuchi, S., et al. (2000). Time-dependent nephrotoxicity associated with daily administration of cisplatin in mice. *Journal of Pharmacy and Pharmacology 52,* 1499-1504.
199. LeBrun, M., Grenier, L., Bergeron, M.G., Thibault, L., Labrecque, G., & Beauchamp, D. (1999). Effect of fasting on temporal variation in the nephrotoxicity of amphotericin b in rats. *Antimicrobial Agents and Chemotherapy 43,* 520-524.
200. Choi, J.S., Kim, C.K., & Lee, B.J. (1999). Administration-time differences in the pharmacokinetics of gentamicin intravenously delivered to human beings. *Chronobiology International 16,* 821-829.
201. Liu, Z., Fang, S., Wang, L., Zhu, T., Yang, H., & Yu, S. (1998). Clinical study on chronopharmacokinetics of digoxin in patients with congestive heart failure. *Journal of Tongji Medical University 18,* 21-24.
202. Feigin, R.D., San Joaquin, V.H., Haymond, M.W., & Wyatt, R.G. (1969). Daily periodicity of susceptibility of mice to pneumococcal infection. *Nature 224,* 379-380.
203. Reinberg, A., Zagula-Mally, Z., Ghata, J., & Halberg, F. (1969). Circadian reactivity rhythm of human skin to house dust, penicillin, and histamine. *Journal of Allergy 44,* 292-306.
204. Aoyagi, M., Watanabe, H., Sekine, K., Nishimuta, T., Konno, A., Shimojo, N., et al. (1999). Circadian variation in nasal reactivity in children with allergic rhinitis: Correlation with the activity of eosinophils and basophilic cells. *International Archives of Allergy and Immunology 120 Suppl 1,* 95-99.
205. Smolensky, M.H., & Portaluppi, F. (1996). Ambulatory blood pressure monitoring. Application to clinical medicine and antihypertension medication trials. *Ann. N. Y. Acad. Sci. 783,* 278-294.
206. Hetzel, M.R., & Clark, T.J. (1980). Comparison of normal and asthmatic circadian rhythms in peak expiratory flow rate. *Thorax 35,* 732-738.
207. Dethlefsen, U., & Repges, R. (1985). Ein neues Therapieprrinzip bei nachtlichem Asthma. *Medizinische Klinik 80,* 44-47.
208. Syabbalo, N. (1997). Chronobiology and chronopathophysiology of nocturnal asthma. *International Journal of Clinical Practice 51,* 455-462.
209. Reinberg, A., Guillet, P., Gervais, P., Ghata, J., Vignaud, D., & Abulker, C. (1977). One month chronocorticotherapy (dutimelan 8 15 mite). Control of the asthmatic condition without adrenal suppression and circadian rhythm alteration. *Chronobiologia 4,* 295-312.
210. Smolensky, M.H., McGovern, J.P., Scott, P.H., & Reinberg, A. (1987). Chronobiology and asthma. II. Body-time-dependent differences in the kinetics and effects of bronchodilator medications. *Journal of Asthma 24,* 91-134.
211. Jarjour, N.N. (1999). Circadian variation in allergen and nonspecific bronchial responsiveness in asthma. *Chronobiology International 16,* 631-639.
212. Silkoff, P.E., & Martin, R.J. (1998). Pathophysiology of nocturnal asthma. *Annals of Allergy, Asthma, & Immunology 81,* 377-384.
213. Ballard, R.D. (1999). Sleep, respiratory physiology, and nocturnal asthma. *Chronobiology International 16,* 565-580.
214. Rocco, M.B., Barry, J., Campbell, S., Nabel, E., Cook, E.F., Goldman, L., et al. (1987). Circadian variation of transient myocardial ischemia in patients with coronary artery disease. *Circulation 75,* 395-400.
215. Smolensky, M.H., Tatar, S.E., Bergman, S.A., Losman, J.G., Barnard C.N., Dacso, C.C., et al. (1976). Circadian rhythmic aspects of human cardiovascular function: A review by chronobiologic statistical methods. *Chronobiologia 3,* 337-371.
216. Lanuza, D.M., & Dunbar, S.B. (1993). Circadian rhythms: Implications for cardiovascular nursing and drug therapy. *Journal of Cardiovascular Nursing 8,* 63-79.
217. Muller, J.E., Ludmer, P.L., Willich, S.N., Tofler, G.H., Aylmer, G., Klangos, I., et al. (1987). Circadian variation in the frequency of sudden cardiac death [see comments]. *Circulation 75,* 131-138.
218. Rocco, M.B., Nabel, E.G., & Selwyn, A.P. (1987). Circadian rhythms and coronary artery disease. *American Journal of Cardiology 59,* 13C-17C.
219. Cohen, M.C., Rohtla, K.M., Lavery, C.E., Muller, J.E., & Mittleman, M.A. (1997). Meta-analysis of the morning

excess of acute myocardial infarction and sudden cardiac death [published erratum appears in *American Journal of Cardiology* 1998 *81*(2), 260]. *American Journal of Cardiology 79,* 1512-1516.

220. Willich, S.N., Klatt, S., & Arntz, H.R. (1998). Circadian variation and triggers of acute coronary syndromes. *European Heart Journal 19 Suppl C,* C12-23.
221. Peckova, M., Fahrenbruch, C.E., Cobb, L.A., & Hallstrom, A.P. (1998). Circadian variations in the occurrence of cardiac arrests: Initial and repeat episodes [see comments]. *Circulation 98,* 31-39.
222. Cannon, C.P., McCabe, C.H., Stone, P.H., Schactman, M., Thompson, B., Theroux, P., et al. (1997). Circadian variation in the onset of unstable angina and non-q-wave acute myocardial infarction (the TIMI III registry and TIMI IIIB). *American Journal of Cardiology 79,* 253-258.
223. Smolensky, M.H. (1983). Aspects of human chronopathology. In A. Reinberg & M.H. Smolensky (eds.), *Biological rhythms and medicine* (pp. 131-209). New York: Springer Verlag.
224. Muller, J.E., Stone, P.H., Turi, Z.G., Rutherford, J.D., Czeisler, C.A., Parker, C., et al. (1985). Circadian variation in the frequency of onset of acute myocardial infarction. *New England Journal of Medicine 313,* 1315-1322.
225. Ahasan, R., Lewko, J., Campbell, D., & Salmoni, A. (2001). Adaptation to night shifts and synchronisation processes of night workers. *Journal of Physiological Anthropology & Applied Human Science 20,* 215-226.
226. Dinges, D.F., Pack, F., Williams, K., Gillen, K.A., Powell, J.W., Ott, G.E., et al. (1997). Cumulative sleepiness, mood disturbance, and psychomotor vigilance performance decrements during a week of sleep restricted to 4-5 hours per night. *Sleep 20,* 267.
227. Smolensky, M.H., & Portaluppi, F. (1999). Chronopharmacology and chronotherapy of cardiovascular medications: Relevance to prevention and treatment of coronary heart disease. *American Heart Journal 137,* S14-S24.
228. Horne, J.A., & Ostberg, O. (1976). A self-assessment questionnaire to determine morningness-eveningness in human circadian rhythms. *International Journal of Chronobiology 4,* 97-110.
229. Torsvall, L., & Akerstedt, T. (1980). A diurnal type scale. Construction, consistency and validation in shift work. *Scandinavian Journal of Work, Environment & Health 6,* 283-290.
230. Smith, C.S., & Midkiff, K. (1989). Evaluation of three circadian rhythm questionnaires with suggestions for an improved measure of morningness. *Journal of Applied Psychology 74,* 728-738.
231. Baumgart, P., & Kamp, J. (1998). Accuracy of the SpaceLabs Medical 90217 ambulatory blood pressure monitor. *Blood Pressure Monitoring 3,* 303-307.
232. Santucci, S., James, G., Schussel, Y., Steiner, D., & Pickering, T.G. (1993). A comparison of two ambulatory blood pressure monitors-the del mar avionics.
233. O'Brien, E., Mee, F., Atkins, N., & O'Malley, K. (1991). Accuracy of the SpaceLabs 90207 determined by the British Hypertension Society protocol. *Journal of Hypertension 9,* 573-574.
234. Leidy, N., Abbott, R., & Fedenko, K. (1997). Sensitivity and reproducibility of the dual-mode actigraph under controlled levels of activity intensity. *Nursing Research 46,* 5-11.
235. Mason, D., & Tapp, W. (1992). Measuring circadian rhythms. Actigraph versus activation checklist. *Western Journal of Nursing Research 14,* 358-379.
236. Patterson, S., Krantz, D., Montgomery, L., Deuster, P., Hedges, S., & Nebel, L. (1993). Automated physical activity monitoring: Validation and comparison with physiological and self-report measures. *Psychophysiology 30,* 296-305.
237. Chang, A., Kushida, C., Palombini, L., Carrillo, O., Hindman, J., Hong, S., et al. (1999). Comparison study of actigraphic, polymnographic, and subjective perception of sleep parameters. *Sleep 22 (Suppl),* S43.
238. Cooperstock, M., England, J.E., & Wolfe, R.A. (1987). Circadian incidence of labor onset hour in preterm birth and chorioamnionitis. *Obstetrics and Gynecology 70,* 852-855.
239. Hall, L.H. (1976). Circadian rhythms: Implications for geriatric rehabilitation. In C.K. Tom & D.M. Lanuza (eds.), *Symposium on biological rhythms.* Philadelphia: WB Saunders.
240. Monk, T.H., & Fookson, J.E. (1986). Circadian temperature rhythm power spectra: Is equal sampling necessary? *Psychophysiology 23,* 472-479.
241. Reinberg, A., & Halberg, F. (1979). *Chronopharmacology.* Oxford, England: Pergamon Press.
242. DiRaimondo, V.C., & Rorsham, P.H. (1958). Pharmacologic principles in the use of corticoids and adrenocorticotropin. *Metabolism 7,* 5-24.
243. Smolensky, M.H., D'Alonzo, G.E., Kunkel, G., & Barnes, P.J. (1987). Day-night patterns in bronchial patency and dyspnea: Basis for once-daily and unequally divided twice-daily theophylline dosing schedules. *Chronobiology International 4,* 303-317.
244. Beam, W.R., Weiner, D.E., & Martin, R.J. (1992). Timing of prednisone and alterations of airways inflammation in nocturnal asthma. *American Review of Respiratory Disease 146,* 1524-1530.
245. Reinberg, A., Ghata, J., Halberg, F., Apfelbaum, M., Gervais, P., Boudon, P., et al. (1976). Treatment schedules modify circadian timing in human adrenocortical insufficiency. In L.E. Scheving, F. Halbert, & J.E. Pauly (eds.), *Chronobiology* (pp. 168-173). Tokyo: Igaku Shoin.
246. D'Alonzo, G.E., Crocetti, J.G., & Smolensky, M.H. (1999). Circadian rhythms in the pharmacokinetics and clinical effects of beta-agonist, theophylline, and anticholinergic medications in the treatment of nocturnal asthma. *Chronobiology International 16,* 663-682.
247. Pincus, D.J., Szefler, S.J., Ackerson, L.M., & Martin, R.J. (1995). Chronotherapy of asthma with inhaled steroids: The effect of dosage timing on drug efficacy. *Journal of Allergy and Clinical Immunology 95,* 1172-1178.
248. Smolensky, M.H., Reinberg, A., & Labrecque, G. (1995). Twenty-four hour pattern in symptom intensity of viral and allergic rhinitis: Treatment implications. *Journal of Allergy and Clinical Immunology 95,* 1084-1096.
249. Stalenhoef, A.F., Mol, M.J., & Stuyt, P.M. (1989). Efficacy and tolerability of simvastatin (MK-733). *American Journal of Medicine 87,* 39S-43S.
250. Cutler, N.R., Anders, R.J., Jhee, S.S., Sramek, J.J., Awan, N.A., Bultas, J., et al. (1995). Placebo-controlled evaluation of three doses of a controlled-onset, extended-release formulation of verapamil in the treatment of stable angina pectoris. *American Journal of Cardiology 75,* 1102-1106.

251. Muller, J.E., Tofler, G.H., Willich, S.N., & Stone, P.H. (1987). Circadian variation of cardiovascular disease and sympathetic activity. *Journal of Cardiovascular Pharmacology 10,* S104-109.
252. White, W.B., Mansoor, G.A., Pickering, T.G., Vidt, D.G., Hutchinson, H.G., Johnson R.B., et al. (1999). Differential effects of morning and evening dosing of nisoldipine er on circadian blood pressure and heart rate. *American Journal of Hypertension 12,* 806-814.
253. Lemmer, B. (1999). Chronopharmacology and its impact on antihypertensive treatment. *Acta Physiological et Pharmacologica Bulgarica 24,* 71-80.
254. Levi, F., Zidani, R., Brienza, S., Dogliotti, L., Perpoint, B., Rotarski, M., et al. (1999). A multicenter evaluation of intensified, ambulatory, chronomodulated chemotherapy with oxaliplatin, 5-fluorouracil, and leucovorin as initial treatment of patients with metastatic colorectal carcinoma. International Organization for Cancer Chronotherapy. *Cancer 85,* 2532-2540.
255. Garufi, C., Levi, F., Giunta, S., Aschelter, A., Pace, R., Nistico, C., et al. (1995). Chronomodulated 5-day infusion of floxuridine and l-folinic acid in patients with advanced malignancies: A feasibility and tolerability study. *Journal of Infusional Chemotherapy 5,* 134-137.
256. Yamadera, H., Takahashi, K., & Okawa, M. (1996). A multicenter study of sleep-wake rhythm disorders: Therapeutic effects of vitamin B_{12}, bright light therapy, chronotherapy and hypnotics. *Psychiatry and Clinical Neurosciences 50,* 203-209.
257. Moldofsky, H., Musisi, S., & Phillipson, E.A. (1986). Treatment of a case of advanced sleep phase syndrome by phase advance chronotherapy. *Sleep 9,* 61-65.
258. Quera-Salva, M.A., Guilleminault, C., Claustrat, B., Defrance, R., Gajdos, P., McCann, C.C., et al. (1997). Rapid shift in peak melatonin secretion associated with improved performance in short shift work schedule. *Sleep 20,* 1145-1150.
259. Vangelova, K.K., & Dalbokova, D.L. (1998). Variations in 6-sulphatoxymelatonin excretion and oral temperature under a 12-hour shiftwork environment. *Reviews on Environmental Health 13,* 221-226.
260. Takahashi, J.S., & DeCoursey, P.J., Bauman, L., & Menaker, M. (1984). Spectral sensitivity of a novel photoreceptive system mediating entrainment of mammalian circadian rhythms. *Nature 308,* 186-188.
261. Eastman, C.I. (1987). Bright light in work-sleep schedules for shiftworkers: Application of circadian rhythm principles. In L. Rensing, U. van der Haiden, & M.C. Mackey (eds.), *Temporal disorder in human oscillatory systems.* Berlin: Springer Verlag.
262. Daan, S., & Lewy, A.J. (1984). Scheduled exposure to daylight: A potential strategy to reduce "jet lag" following transmeridian flight. *Psychopharmacology Bulletin 20,* 566-568.
263. Czeisler, C.A., & Allan, J.S. (1987). Acute circadian phase reversal in man via bright light exposure: Application to jet-lag sleep research. *Sleep Research 16,* 605.
264. Bjorvatn, B., Kecklund, G., & Akerstedt, T. (1999). Bright light treatment used for adaptation to night work and re-adaptation back to day life. A field study at an oil platform in the North Sea. *Journal of Sleep Research 8,* 105-112.
265. Baehr, E.K., Fogg, L.F., & Eastman, C.I. (1999). Intermittent bright light and exercise to entrain human circadian rhythms to night work. *American Journal of Physiology 277,* R1598-1604.
266. Rosenthal, N.E., Sack, D.A., Skwerer, R.G., Jacobsen, F.M., & Wehr, T.A. (1988). Phototherapy for seasonal affective disorder. *Journal of Biological Rhythms 3,* 101-120.
267. Blehar, M.C., & Rosenthal, N.E. (1989). Seasonal affective disorders and phototherapy. Report of a National Institute of Mental Health-sponsored workshop. *Archives of General Psychiatry 46,* 469-474.
268. Lewy, A.J., Bauer, V.K., Cutler, N.L., Sack, R.L., Ahmed, S., Thomas, K.H., et al. (1998). Morning vs evening light treatment of patients with winter depression [see comments]. *Archives of General Psychiatry 55,* 890-896.
269. Avery, D.H., Eder, D.N., Bolte, M.A., Hellekson, C.J., Dunner, D.L., Vitiello, M.V., et al. (2001). Dawn simulation and bright light in the treatment of sad: A controlled study. *Biological Psychiatry 50,* 205-216.
270. Holsten, F., & Bjorvatn, B. (1997). Phototherapy. An alternative for seasonal affective disorders or sleep disorders. *Tidsskrift for den Norske Laegeforening 117,* 2484-2488.
271. Satlin, A., Volicer, L., Ross, V., Herz, L., & Campbell, S. (1992). Bright light treatment of behavioral and sleep disturbances in patients with Alzheimer's disease. *American Journal of Psychiatry 149,* 1028-1032.
272. Chesson, A.L., Jr., Littner, M., Davila, D., Anderson, W.M., Grigg-Damberger, M., Hartse, K., et al. (1999). Practice parameters for the use of light therapy in the treatment of sleep disorders. Standards of practice committee, American Academy of Sleep Medicine. *Sleep 22,* 641-660.
273. Zisapel, N. (1999). The use of melatonin for the treatment of insomnia. *Biological Signals and Receptors 8,* 84-89.
274. Haimov, I., Lavie, P., Laudon, M., Herer, P., Vigder, C., & Zisapel, N. (1995). Melatonin replacement therapy of elderly insomniacs. *Sleep 18,* 598-603.
275. Myers, B.L., & Badia, P. (1995). Changes in circadian rhythms and sleep quality with aging: Mechanisms and interventions [published erratum appears in *Neuroscience Biobehavioral Reviews* 1996 *20*(2):I-IV]. *Neuroscience and Biobehavioral Reviews 19,* 553-571.
276. Lewy, A.J., Sack, R.L., Miller, L.S., & Hoban, T.M. (1987). Antidepressant and circadian phase-shifting effects of light. *Science 235,* 352-354.
277. Arendt, J., Skene, D.J., Middleton, B., Lockley, S.W., & Deacon, S. (1997). Efficacy of melatonin treatment in jet lag, shift work, and blindness. *Journal of Biological Rhythms 12,* 604-617.
278. Visser, E.K., Beersma, D.G., & Daan, S. (1999). Melatonin suppression by light in humans is maximal when the nasal part of the retina is illuminated. *Journal of Biological Rhythms 14,* 116-121.
279. Farr, L., Keene, A., Samson, D., & Michael, A. (1984). Alterations in circadian excretion of urinary variables and physiological indicators of stress following surgery. *Nursing Research 33,* 140-146.
280. Lanuza, D.M., & Marotta, S.F. (1987). Endocrine and psychologic responses of patients to cardiac pacemaker implantation. *Heart & Lung 16,* 496-505.
281. Smolensky, M.H. (1998). Knowledge and attitudes of American physicians and public about medical chronobiology and chronotherapeutics. Findings of two 1996 Gallup surveys. *Chronobiology International 15,* 377-394.
282. Page, R.B., Galicich, J.H., & Grunt, J.A. (1973). Alteration of circadian temperature rhythm with third ventricular obstruction. *Journal of Neurosurgery 38,* 309-319.

CHAPTER

6 Urinary Incontinence

MARY H. PALMER

DEFINITION

Urinary incontinence, characterized as a disruption in the storage and/or emptying mechanism of the bladder, is "the complaint of any involuntary leakage of urine."[1] Several types of established urinary incontinence have been defined. These include stress, overactive bladder/urge, mixed (a combination of stress and urge), and overflow incontinence.

Stress incontinence, also called *genuine stress incontinence* (GSI), is "the involuntary loss of urine occurring when, in the absence of detrusor contraction, the intravesical pressure exceeds the maximum urethral pressure."[1] In urge incontinence, the loss of urine is "associated with a strong desire to void."[1] The term *overactive bladder* (OAB) has been proposed for the syndrome of urinary frequency, urgency, and urge incontinence. The definition of OAB is a "condition referring to the symptoms of frequency, urgency, and urge or reflex incontinence, either singly or in combination, when appearing, in the absence of local pathological factors explaining these symptoms."[2]

Other terms used to define involuntary urine loss are *enuresis,* "any involuntary loss of urine,"[1] and *nocturnal enuresis,* "incontinence during sleep."[1] Other terms used in conjunction with urinary incontinence are *post-micturition dribble, continuous leakage, unstable detrusor,* and *detrusor hyperreflexia.* The first two terms are self-explanatory; the latter two refer to overactive bladder function.[1] Unstable detrusor means the detrusor contracts either spontaneously or with provocation (i.e., a cough), even when the person is attempting to inhibit micturition. Detrusor hyperreflexia is "overactivity due to disturbance of the nervous control mechanisms."[1]

For lay persons, the term *incontinence* carries several meanings. The *American Heritage Dictionary* defines *incontinent* as follows: "1. Not restrained; uncontrolled; *incontinent rage.* 2. Lacking normal voluntary control of excretory functions. 3. Lacking sexual restraint; unchaste."[3] Given this context, people may be reluctant to use *incontinence* to define their behavior.

Mitteness and Barker[4] found that older adults define urinary incontinence different than health care providers. They learned that if an older person wets a pad that was intended to catch urine, this urine loss was not considered incontinence or an "accident." For most women who lost urine during a sneeze, it was not considered abnormal; rather, it was a "fact of life."

PREVALENCE AND POPULATIONS AT RISK

Approximately 200 million people worldwide are incontinent.[5] The direct costs of urinary incontinence in the United States were estimated at $23.6 billion for the year 1995.[6] Incidence of urinary incontinence refers to the rate of new cases developing during a specific period of time in an at-risk group. This rate gives the probability for a member of a vulnerable group, such as postmenopausal women or hip fracture patients, to become incontinent. Incidence studies help to identify risk factors. Identification of risks can lead to the development of prevention or risk reduction strategies.

Table 6-1 summarizes select studies reporting the prevalence of urinary incontinence in the primary/ambulatory care, acute care, long-term care, and community settings. Different sampling techniques, inclusion criteria, definitions of urinary incontinence, and screening measures are used, limiting the ability to generalize the findings. Lack of documentation in the medical record leads to underreporting of the magnitude of this problem. Unless medical and nursing staff view incontinence as a problem, its existence will not be documented. Another problem in determining the true prevalence of incontinence is its often transient nature. Incontinence may develop as a result of an acute medical condition, such as delirium, immobility,

TABLE 6-1 Urinary Incontinence Prevalence Studies

RESEARCH STUDY	SAMPLE	DEFINITION USED	PREVALENCE
Setting: Acute Care			
Morbidity and Mortality Weekly Report (1991), United States[7]	N = 41,456,685 discharge records	"Involuntary loss of urine so severe as to have social or hygienic consequences."	10.1 per 10,000 population for men and 16.6 per 10,000 for women.
Nakayama et al (1996), Denmark[23]	N = 935 stroke patients	Patients classified as continent when they could "fully control the bladder/bowel and had no accidents."	36% were incontinent on admission, 15% were incontinent upon discharge, and 8% were incontinent at 6-month follow-up.
O'Connor (1996), Australia[24]	N = 637 hospital patients	None stated.	8% incontinent and 14.7% had indwelling catheters by staff report.
Chiarelli & Campbell (1997), Australia[25]	N = 304 women in postnatal ward of teaching hospital; mean age, 28 years; range, 16-43 years of age	"Stress is leakage on such activities as coughing, sneezing, laughing or lifting and urge incontinence is a strong desire to void accompanied by leakage."	Overall, 64% reported stress urinary incontinence during pregnancy. In the month of pregnancy, 57% reported stress with or without urge incontinence and 42% reported urge incontinence with or wihout stress incontinence.
Palmer et al (1997), United States[8]	100 consecutive hip fracture patients	"Involuntary loss of urine sufficient enough to be a problem."	19% were incontinent preoperatively, and the overall incidence of incontinence was 48% in men and 24% in women.
Setting: Primary/Ambulatory Care			
Peacock et al (1994), United States[26]	Medical records of 159 black female patients, 27-86 years of age	International Continence Society definition.	Urge: 33.3%; stress: 31.4%; nonspecific: 11.3%; detrusor overactivity: 36.5%.
Turan et al (1996), Turkey[27]	N = 1250 respondents, women 18 to 44 years of age; primary care	Involuntary loss of urine.	24.5% overall. 6.6% daily.
Wilson et al (1996), New Zealand[28]	N = 1505 postpartum women, 15-45 years of age (mean age, 27.8 years)	Leakage of urine.	34.3% at 3 months' postpartum; 3.3% daily; 8.4% before pregnancy; 27.2% during pregnancy; 7.6% after delivery only.
Groutz et al (1999), Israel[29]	N = 300 nulliparous, primiparous, and grand multiparous women 20-43 years of age	Stress incontinence was "involuntary leakage of urine with coughing, laughing, sneezing, or any other physical effort." Regular incontinence was "involuntary excretion or leakage of urine in inappropriate places or at inappropriate times twice or more a month, regardless of the quantity lost."	42.3% overall developed stress incontinence during their last pregnancy. Prevalence: nulliparous: 28%; primparas: 49%; multiparas: 50%.

Setting: Long-term Care			
Palmer et al (1991), United States[11]	N = 430 subjects, 65 years of age and older; newly admitted nursing home residents	Incontinent during the day.	39% at 2 weeks after admission; 44% 1 year after admission.
Brandeis et al (1997), United States[30]	N = 2014 women = 75.5% 60 years of age and older; all nursing home residents	The presence of at least two episodes of involuntary urinary leakage per week.	49% overall.
Setting: Community			
Nygaard et al (1994), United States[12]	144 college women (mean age, 19.9 years) participating in competitive varsity sports	"Have you ever experienced unanticipated urinary leakage during participation in your sport?"	28% reported urine loss during their sports activities.
Wetle et al (1995), United States[21]	N = 3809 men and women 65 years of age and older	"Difficulty holding urine until they can get to a toilet."	28%
Umlauf & Sherman (1996), United States[31]	N = 1490 men, 52-99 years of age	"Uncontrolled urine leakage of any amount during the month."	29%
Nygaard & Lemke (1996), United States[32]	N = 2025 women, 65 years of age and older	Stress: leak urine when coughing, sneezing or laughing; urge: difficulty holding urine until reaching the toilet.	41% stress; 55% urge at baseline.
Brown et al (1996), United States[19]	N = 7949 women, 69-101 years of age	Leaked urine or lost control of urine.	41% overall and 14% leaked daily.
Davis et al (1997), United States[13]	N = 563 women soldiers; average age, 28.3 years	"Have you ever leaked urine? By leaking urine we mean involuntary loss beyond your control to the extent that it becomes a social or hygienic problem."	30% reported symptomatic urine loss with activity.
Nakanishi et al (1997), Japan[33]	N = 1405 men and women, 65 years of age and older	"Do you wet yourself?"	9.8% overall reported for both sexes.
Goluboff et al (1998), United States[34]	N = 480	Not defined; however, men who did not regularly use pads were considered dry.	Postoperatively, 8% leaked daily; 10.6% had postoperative procedures related to voiding problems; 24% had urgency postoperatively.

Continued

TABLE 6-1 Urinary Incontinence Prevalence Studies—cont'd

RESEARCH STUDY	SAMPLE	DEFINITION USED	PREVALENCE
Setting: Community—Cont'd			
Roberts et al (1998), United States[20]	N = 778 men and women, 50 years of age and older	Assessed by questions: "In the last year, have you had slow leakage or dribbling of urine throughout the day? Have you had leakage of urine when you coughed or sneezed in the last year? In the last year, when urine of leakage has occurred, were you aware of the need to urinate before the leakage occurred?"	Overall age-adjusted prevalence: for women, 48.7%; for men, 24.3%.
Talcott et al (1998), United States[35]	260 men, median age, 65 years of age (range, 41-86)	Self-reports of urine dribbling or leaking and use of absorptive pads and penile clamps.	Postprostatectomy incontinence at 3 months: 24%; at 12 months: 11%. Following radiotherapy, at 3 months: 2%; at 12 months: 2%.
Roberts et al (1999), United States[36]	1540 men and women, 50 years of age and older	"1. In the last year have you had any slow leakage or dribbling of urine throughout the day? 2. Have you had leakage of urine when you coughed or sneezed in the last year? 3. In the last year when leakage of urine occurred, were you aware of the need to urinate (pass your water) before the leakage occurred?" UI: Yes to question 1 or if they answered "usually" or "often" to questions 2 and 3.	Age-adjusted urinary incontinence prevalence in men: 25.6% (95% CI 22.5-28.8). Women 48.4% (95% CI 44.7-52.2).

Hojberg et al (1999) Denmark[37]	N = 8309 women attending routine antenatal care	"Urinary incontinence was defined as involuntary loss of urine within the last year"	8.9% had urinary incontinence in the previous year: 55.2% had pure stress; 7.6% had pure urge; and 26.6% had mixed incontinence.
Palmer et al (1999), United States[14]	N = 1113 fully employed women in an academic setting	"Have you ever lost urine when you were not able to get to the toilet on time? Have you ever lost urine when you were asleep? Have you ever lost urine without meaning to at any time not mentioned above?"	21%
Fultz et al (1999), United States[38]	N = 606 non-Hispanic African-American women, 3385 non-Hispanic white women	"During the last 12 months, have you lost any amount of urine beyond your control?"	23.02% white and 16.17% African-American women reported incontinence.
Stanford et al (2000), United States[39]	N = 3533 men responded (62%) to questionnaire	Level of urine control, frequency of incontinence, use of pads, and extent of any problems with urinary incontinence.	40.2% reported occasional leakage; 6.7% reported frequent leakage; 1.6% no control at 24 months after prostatectomy.
Johnson et al (2000), United States[40]	N = 1776 men and 1674 women; National Survey on Self-Care and Aging	Levels of incontinence specified: none, mild to moderate, and severe. "Do you ever leak urine when you cough, laugh or sneeze? How often do you have difficulty holding your urine until you can get to a toilet? How often do you lose control of your urine completely?"	Men: 11% had mild to moderate and 6% had severe incontinence. Women: 25% had mild to moderate and 12% had severe incontinence.

or infection, and may resolve as the patient's condition improves. The use of chemical and physical restraints can also induce incontinence because the patient loses the ability to access toilet facilities and has an increased dependency on others to meet elimination needs. Point prevalence, though, may be inflated if transient cases are captured during the study period. Better understanding of incidence and remission is needed. Therefore, in the study of the epidemiology of incontinence, specification of time frame and follow-up to determine changes in continence status is critical.

In one large study of acute care patients, investigators using hospital discharge information from Medicare Part A from 1984 through 1987 determined the annual age-standardized rate of incontinence to be 16.6 per 10,000 for women and 10.1 per 10,000 for men. When sex and race were taken into account, white women had the highest standardized rate (16.8), followed by black men (13.6), black women (9.7), and white men (9.6).[7] In another study of patients who had undergone surgical repair of hip fracture, men had a significantly higher incidence of incontinence than women did (48% versus 24%; $p < 0.03$). In patients with dementia, however, the differences between the sexes were not significant (60% versus 55%).[8]

The prevalence of urinary incontinence in nursing home residents in the United States is estimated to be approximately 50%.[9] One international report of prevalence in 441 nursing home residents was 55.1%.[10] Few longitudinal studies have been conducted to determine the incidence of incontinence in the long-term care setting. One study conducted over the first year of admission to the nursing home found urinary incontinence was more prevalent in men than women (68% versus 40%); the incidence of incontinence after the first year of admission to the nursing home was also higher in men (48%) than in women (24%).[11]

Reports of the prevalence of incontinence in the community vary. For example, in young nulliparous women the prevalence of incontinence while engaged in sports (average age, 19.9 years) was reported to be 28%[12]; 28% of military women (average age, 28.3 years) participating in field maneuvers lost urine during physical activity[13]; and 21% of full-time working women in an academic setting (average age of 40 years) reported losing urine at least monthly.[14]

Men who have undergone surgical and radiation treatment for prostate cancer also report urinary incontinence.[15] In one study, 87% of the men reported being incontinent one month after surgery. This percentage decreased to 63% at 6 months after surgery.[16] In another study using Medicare records, 1.3% of the men were incontinent 5 years after receiving radiation treatment for localized cancer. Incontinence rates may differ by surgical procedure.[17] Bishoff et al[18] reported that 79% of perineal prostatectomy patients were incontinent, with 39% wearing protective pads, whereas 85% of retropubic prostatectomy patients were incontinent and 56% wore protective pads.

In a study with a large group of older community-dwelling women (N = 7949), the reported prevalence of urine leakage was 41% overall, with 14% who leaked every day.[19] Because older community-living adults have varying degrees of health and functional status, subgroups may have a higher prevalence of urinary incontinence than the general population of older adults. For example, in adults 50 years old and older, those with fecal incontinence were also more likely to be incontinent of urine.[20] Older adults receiving home care had an overall prevalence of urinary incontinence of 28%.[21]

Incontinence is a prevalent condition across the life span. Little is known, however, about incontinence in different races and ethnic groups. One report indicated white women had higher prevalence of pure genuine stress incontinence than black women.[22]

RISK FACTORS

Environmental Factors

Medications and medical conditions that increase the volume of urine production may precipitate incontinence. Fast-acting diuretics can overload the bladder and shorten the time between onset of the sensation of needing to void and actual voiding. Medications with anticholinergic action have a urinary-retentive effect; overflow incontinence may result especially in vulnerable persons, such as men with benign prostatic hypertrophy (BPH). One side effect of alpha-adrenergic antagonists, beta-adrenergic agonists, and calcium channel blockers is urinary retention.

Ingested alcohol has a diuretic effect; in sufficient amounts, it clouds the consciousness of the individual, thus impairing his or her ability to perceive and act on the need to void. Caffeine, especially in high amounts (i.e., more than 400 mg/day) has been associated with detrusor instability.[41] It has been shown that decreasing the amount of caffeine consumed has been associated with fewer daytime incontinence episodes in women.[42] Current and former smoking has been associated with increased risk for urinary symptoms in men.[43]

Lack of timely access to toilet facilities poses a risk for incontinence. The normal maximal capacity for adult bladders is 500 ml.[44] Once the bladder is filled to capacity, it is difficult to retain urine. Therefore individuals who have restricted access to toilet facilities, cognitive impairments, mobility limitations, or need for physical assistance and extra time to reach facilities are at risk for incontinence.

Personal Factors

Psychological processes, such as depression and anxiety, have been associated with incontinence.[45,46] One mechanism suggested is that anxious women are less tolerant of incontinence than nonanxious women and present with incontinence earlier.[46] Impaired mobility and cognitive function place nursing home residents at significant risk of becoming incontinent during the first year after admission to the facility.[47] Other studies also show a link among incontinence, dementia, and mobility impairments.[8,47-50]

Developmental Factors

Comparisons between children who have not been toilet trained and incontinent old people have been made for years.[51] In 1749 a physician wrote, "Children and old people often piss-a-bed in their sleep, but these come not to the physician to be cured."[52] Even today one can overhear caregivers talking about changing "diapers" on nursing home residents instead of talking about disposable briefs. There are developmental aspects (i.e., pregnancy, menopause) to continence that must be considered in assessment, treatment, and management of urinary incontinence.

In general, children are toilet trained by 3 years of age, with girls toilet trained earlier than boys (2.25 years versus 2.56 years).[53] Variability in the age of toilet training ranges from 0.75 years to 5.25 years. [53] There is an assumption that adults are dry until the onset of old age, but recent studies show urinary incontinence is not solely a geriatric condition. Age alone does not cause urinary incontinence. Women of all ages report episodes of varying severity and impact on work and quality of life,[12-14,19] and many people maintain continence well into old age.[19]

Most women experience lower urinary tract symptoms of frequency and nocturia during pregnancy.[54] Urinary incontinence during pregnancy is a strong predictor of incontinence postpartum.[55] Incontinence is expected to resolve in the postpartum period when pelvic floor muscle exercises are performed. Some women, however, may have developed neuromuscular changes or incurred neuromuscular damage during pregnancy and childbirth that could lead to incontinence.[56] The causal mechanism has not been identified. Low urethral resistance and defective pressure transmission in early pregnancy may continue throughout the pregnancy and postpartum period.[57] In addition, some researchers postulate that the use of forceps may damage the pudendal nerve.[58]

Urine loss during sexual intercourse is sometimes reported.[59,60] Although the mechanism is not clear, deep coital penetration and abdominal pressure are considered risk factors. Increased body mass index has also been proposed as a risk factor for incontinence in women.[14,19,61]

Age-related changes occur in the bladder, including decreased bladder capacity and delayed onset of the awareness of bladder fullness.[45] The consequences may be frequency in voiding and a decrease in time between conscious desire to void and actual voiding. An increase in residual urine after voiding and an increase in the number of involuntary detrusor contractions are also considered aging changes. These changes do not cause incontinence directly, rather they enhance the risk of incontinence. Current research clearly demonstrates that age alone does not cause incontinence.[9]

Urge incontinence is more frequently seen in men and older adults.[62] BPH in men is associated with aging[63]; approximately half of men with BPH that causes obstruction of the outlet of the bladder also have detrusor instability and urgency.[64]

Menopause may be a risk factor for the development of incontinence.[65] Postmenopausal women experience thinning of the vaginal wall and increased vascular frailty. The vaginal wall is vulnerable to infection or trauma without estrogen replacement.[66] The urethra and bladder neck are also estrogen sensitive and may become less efficient in closure and coaptation (i.e., degree of mucosal sealing).

MECHANISMS

Genuine Stress incontinence

Individuals who involuntarily lose urine in the absence of detrusor contraction experience genuine stress incontinence. A small volume of urine is lost as a result of events causing a sudden increase in intraabdominal pressure (e.g., sneezing, coughing, and active exercises). It is generally believed that sphincter abnormalities cause genuine stress incontinence.[67] In women, a change in location of the bladder neck and proximal urethra during abdominal straining can cause lack of structural support and hypermobility of the urethra.[67] The underlying mechanism for stress incontinence may be unequal transmission of abdominal pressure to both the urethra and bladder. Normally the bladder neck and proximal urethra lay above the pelvic muscle, within the abdominal cavity, and there is uninterrupted transmission of increases in intraabdominal pressure with corresponding increases in intraurethral pressure. When the bladder neck and proximal urethra are not supported in a position in which transmission of pressure increases can take place, when the intraurethral pressure is exceeded, urine leakage will occur.[67]

GSI can result from changes in the position of the female pelvic structures, such as prolapse of the bladder into the vagina (i.e., cystocele), uterine prolapse into the vagina, and bulging of the rectum into the vagina (i.e., rectocele), that cause an anatomical deviation of the bladder neck and proximal urethra. In postmenopausal women, atrophic vaginitis and weakening of vaginal tissues resulting from estrogen deficiency are also purported to cause stress incontinence by decreasing coaptation, thus decreasing outlet resistance.[67,68] The mucosal folds that line the urethra create opportunities for urine leakage, but this lining provides the viscosity enabling coaptation. Because contraction of the pelvic musculature aids in the lengthening, support, and compression of the urethra, a weak or lax pelvic muscle would contract less efficiently and thus have a weaker effect on the urethra.[68]

There are differences between men and women in the smooth muscle that composes the bladder neck. The bladder neck smooth muscle in the female urethra follows a longitudinal path in the urethral wall. There is no evidence of a well-defined collar of smooth muscle, such as that which surrounds the male bladder neck and proximal urethra to prevent retrograde ejaculation.[69] Other factors such as elastic tissue, striated muscle, and a vascular component aid in the provision of a functional watertight sphincter in women.[70]

Intrinsic sphincter deficiency (ISD) is considered another cause of stress urinary incontinence. With ISD, the urethral sphincter opens during increased intraabdominal pressure while the urethrovesical junction remains relatively unchanged; therefore there is no descent of the bladder and urethra on straining.[68] Intrinsic sphincter deficiency and urethral hypermobility often coexist.[67]

Urge Incontinence

Urge incontinence involves bladder abnormalities, in contrast to the sphincter abnormalities described in stress incontinence. Figure 6-1 illustrates an involuntary (uninhibited) contraction of the detrusor at the early phase of bladder filling. When there are contractions of a sufficient magnitude that are not inhibited early in the filling cycle, incontinence

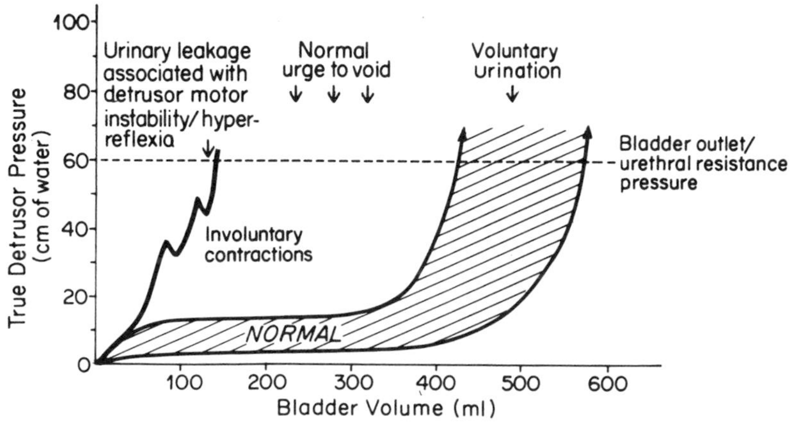

Figure 6-1 **Schematic diagram illustrating normal pressure-volume relationships in the bladder and the urodynamic phenomenon of uninhibited or involuntary bladder contractions—also called detrusor-motor instability or detrusor hyperreflexia.** (From Ouslander, J. [1989]. Incontinence. In R. Kane, J. Ouslander, & I. Abrass [eds.], *Essentials of geriatric medicine* [2nd ed., p. 144]. New York: McGraw-Hill. With permission.)

may occur. Uninhibited contractions may be caused by neurological disorders (detrusor hyperreflexia) or by nonneurological conditions (detrusor instability). Neurological causes are classified as supraspinal neurological lesions or suprasacral spinal lesions. Supraspinal neurological lesions include Parkinson's disease, cerebrovascular accidents, brain tumor, and multiple sclerosis. When a lesion is above the pons, loss of voluntary control could occur.[67] If interruptions occur between the pontine micturition center and the sacral reflex center, suprasacral lesions such as multiple sclerosis or spinal cord trauma, then lack of coordination between emptying of the bladder and relaxation of the urethra can occur. This dysfunction, detrusor-external sphincter dyssynergia (DESD), manifests as involuntary contractions of the striated urethral musculature during an involuntary detrusor contraction.[67]

Defects at the sacral reflex center can have varying effects on micturition. Damage to sympathetic nerve pathways results in different abnormalities than damage to parasympathetic or somatic nerve pathways. Complete parasympathetic lesions leave the bladder areflexic and the result is urinary retention. Sympathetic lesions affect sphincter function. Somatic nerve (i.e., pudendal nerve) damage to afferent and efferent nerve pathways means loss of perianal sensation and ability to contract anal and urethral sphincters. Peripheral neuropathy that disrupts afferent input to the brainstem and cortical center of control (i.e., tabes dorsalis, diabetic neuropathy) leads to diminished conscious control of micturition.

Detrusor instability also occurs in the absence of neurological activity, as when there is an outlet obstruction, local tumor, or infection. An individual experiences frequency and urgency when the parasympathetic response to obstruction, infection, or inflammation in the spinal micturition center exceeds the inhibitory effect of the cortical micturition center. Uninhibited detrusor contractions may also result from deconditioned voiding reflexes.[71] For example, some people resort to frequent voiding and maintaining chronic low bladder volume in an attempt to avoid incontinent episodes. Unfortunately, this practice leads to reduced bladder capacity and, with time, the bladder wall thickens, aggravating the condition of decreased tone and increased instability.[71]

The term *detrusor overactivity* has sometimes been used for urge incontinence in the elderly.[72] No reliable methods of determining the etiology of detrusor contractions in the elderly are available, making treatment decisions difficult. The condition of detrusor hyperactivity with impaired contractility (DHIC) is considered common in the elderly. This condition, which presents as involuntary detrusor contractions with retention, can mimic other voiding dysfunctions such as stress incontinence.[72]

Overflow Incontinence

Overflow incontinence results from two different pathological mechanisms. The first mechanism involves a bladder with normal contractility but with an obstruction at the outlet. This results in overdistention of the bladder. Once the intravesical pressure exceeds intraurethral pressure, urine will dribble out continuously. When an enlarged prostate gland surrounding the bladder neck and proximal urethra occludes the outlet, overflow incontinence may occur. Symptoms of bladder outlet obstruction include hesitancy, decrease in force of stream, nocturia, pain during micturition, frequency, urgency, sensation of incomplete emptying, prolonged voiding time, and small voided volumes.[73] Men with BPH and who are taking prescribed or over-the-counter medications with urinary retention as a side effect are at risk of developing acute urinary retention and thus overflow incontinence. Other causes of outlet obstruction are urethral stricture and fecal impaction.[9] The underlying mechanism of overflow incontinence caused by fecal impaction is unclear.

The second mechanism of overflow incontinence is chronic myogenic decompensation or impaired detrusor contractility. The result is a large flaccid acontractile bladder or underactive detrusor.[67] The same result can occur when neuropathy exists that damages efferent motor pathways to the bladder. A common cause is peripheral neuropathy resulting from diabetes mellitus.[74] Alcoholic neuropathy and lumbar disk herniation are also associated with overflow incontinence.

PATHOLOGICAL CONSEQUENCES

Urinary incontinence is associated with poor self-reported health[40,75] and may share the same risk factors (i.e., lower extremity impairment, sensory impairment) with falls and functional dependence.[76] It is considered a marker or indicator of frailty[40,77] but may not be a risk factor of mortality. Another potential pathological outcome to urinary incontinence is alteration in skin integrity. Adults with concurrent conditions that affect skin integrity such as fecal incontinence, malnutrition, peripheral vascular disorders, dependent edema secondary to inactivity and circulatory disorders, and diabetes mellitus may be at increased risk for developing a localized dermatitis or pressure ulcers.[9]

RELATED PATHOPHYSIOLOGICAL CONCEPTS AND DIFFERENTIAL DIAGNOSIS

Leach and Yip[73] reported that bladder dysfunction is related to the severity of the underlying disease process. A person may present with a combination of different types of incontinence. For example, women, often report mixed symptoms of stress and urge incontinence.[78,79] Identification of underlying mechanisms for incontinence, therefore, is important for the correct diagnosis and use of appropriate interventions. Acute changes in cognitive functioning and level of mobility, the presence of inflammatory processes, and the ingestion of certain pharmacological agents may cause acute onset (transient) incontinence. Resnick and Yalla[80] identified an acronym, DIAPPERS (Delirium, Infection, Atrophic urethritis/vaginitis, Pharmaceuticals, Psychological problem, Excess urine output, Restricted mobility, and Stool impaction), to identify factors that may precipitate acute incontinence. Identification and effective treatment of these conditions should alleviate acute onset (transient) incontinence.

Delirium, often the first sign of an infection in elderly persons, can result in urinary incontinence as a result of a diminished ability to perceive and interpret sensations of bladder fullness. Behaviors exhibited while delirious, confused, disoriented, or excessively restless may lead to the administration of chemical or physical restraints, thus limiting independent access to toilet facilities. A restrained person of any age may become incontinent. Cognitive impairment or dementia has been associated with urinary incontinence.[11,81]

Acute urinary tract infections, including pyuria, sometimes causes urgency and a sense of precipitation. Bacteriuria is a common finding in older adults, but its relationship to the development of urinary incontinence is not clearly understood. Asymptomatic bacteriuria is often transient in nature and traditionally is not treated.[9] However, bacteriuria with symptoms of fever, pain, frequency, urgency, and dysuria must be treated with appropriate antimicrobial agents. Atrophic urethritis or vaginitis, inflammation of the urethra, or vaginitis resulting from estrogen deficiency can be treated with topical or oral hormonal replacement therapy. Medications that increase urine production, alter mental status, or directly affect detrusor function (i.e., relaxation or contractility) can lead to acute onset urinary incontinence.

Restricted or impaired mobility can also lead to transient incontinence. A sudden change in mobility, such as a sprain or fracture of a lower extremity, can lead a normally continent and independent adult to become incontinent until the previous level of mobility is resumed. Imposed bed rest can also contribute to incomplete emptying of the bladder unless a normal voiding position can be assumed.

As mentioned earlier, men with BPH are also at risk for developing overflow incontinence as a result of outlet obstruction. Such medical conditions as hyperglycemia and hypercalcemia may induce polyuria, which in turn can lead to transient incontinence.

Fecal incontinence rarely occurs in the absence of urinary incontinence.[20] Fecal incontinence may be a sign of stool impaction. Individuals with fecal incontinence are at risk for developing pressure ulcers, especially bedridden persons.[82] Therefore, although pressure ulcers may not be a direct result of urinary incontinence alone, fecal and urinary incontinence are prevalent conditions found in impaired populations.

Because treatment depends on an accurate diagnosis, identification of the underlying cause of the involuntary urine loss is crucial. In women, the differential diagnosis of incontinence involves several types: genuine stress incontinence, urge incontinence from detrusor instability, urge incontinence from detrusor hyperreflexia, mixed incontinence, overflow incontinence (less often), and abnormalities of the lower urinary tract.[68] Differential diagnosis in men follows the same pattern, with emphasis on urge and overflow incontinence and stress incontinence following prostatectomy. In frail older adults, detrusor hyperreflexia with impaired contractility (DHIC) requires careful diagnosis to differentiate it from stress incontinence.

MANIFESTATIONS, MEASUREMENT, AND SURVEILLANCE

Manifestations of each type of urinary incontinence should be used in the differential diagnosis. (See those listed in Table 6-2.) People with urinary incontinence, especially women, often do not report incontinence to their physician or other health

TABLE 6-2 Manifestations and Surveillance of Urinary Incontinence

TYPE	MANIFESTATIONS	SURVEILLANCE
Stress	Report involuntary urine loss with a cough, sneeze, laugh, or change in position.	Leakage of urine from full bladder while patient is standing and coughs or strains as if having a bowel movement. Bladder record for at least 2 days showing leakage of urine on physical exertion. Pelvic examination for fascial defects, (i.e., rectocele, cystocele, sphincter tone and mobility), and for inflammation or atrophy. Simple cystometry exhibiting absence of detrusor contractions during leakage.
Urge	Report of need to void comes on too fast and strongly to get to toilet; frequent voiding, loss of urine at sound of water running or when waiting for access to toilet.	Evidence of urinary tract infection, inflammation of bladder wall; uninhibited detrusor contractions during cystometric testing, evidence of neurological lesion at supraspinal, suprasacral levels. Bladder record for at least 2 days showing urine loss with complaints of urgency.
Overflow	Report of incomplete emptying, constant dribbling of urine, pain in abdomen, unaware of urine leaking.	Palpable bladder on abdominal examination; large amount of urine in bladder, evidence of outlet obstruction. Evidence of detrusor underactivity or acontractility during neurological and physical examinations.

care professionals out of a belief that there is nothing to be done or because of the sensitive nature of the subject.[14,83-85] Adults of any age should be asked about their bladder function, especially episodes of incontinence, as part of regular health screening.

Nursing assessment includes making the distinction between transient and established incontinence. The history of an individual with urinary incontinence should include current medications (including over-the-counter preparations and self-prescribed herbal remedies, medical and psychiatric conditions, past surgeries (especially back, abdominal, and pelvic surgeries), a description of urinary symptoms, including their onset, and the frequency and severity of incontinent episodes. Information about antecedent factors and behaviors is also important. Some exemplary questions the nurse might pose include these:

When did the incontinence start?

Was it associated with coughing, laughing, sneezing, or other activity that increased intraabdominal pressure?

Was a diuretic taken?

How much fluid is consumed in a day?

Did the person attempt to delay voiding, and for how long?

Did the person make an effort to get to a toilet?

What environmental factors may have hindered or enhanced access to the toilet?

The effects of incontinence on everyday life and the quality of life should be explored. Questions for the nurse to pose include these:

Does the individual avoid social interactions or limit social outings?

Are intimate relationships affected by incontinence?

The methods the person currently uses to manage incontinence need to be elicited as well as the person's motivation to improve continence status. In institutionalized older adults, the level and quality of interaction between an incontinent older adult and nursing staff should be assessed. Reliable and valid tools are available to measure the psychological effects of incontinence.

The physical examination includes a thorough assessment of the neurological and genitourinary systems. The abdomen is palpated for masses and tenderness. A rectal examination is performed for impaction and masses, the size of the prostate gland in men, and the level of sphincter tone and perineal sensation. Assessment of the level of mobility, manual dexterity, and the mental status is important.

The York Incontinence Perceptions Scale (YIPS), an eight-item rating scale, was developed to detect levels of coping, control, and acceptance of urinary incontinence in adults. It has been tested in older adults.[86] This scale complements the Incontinence Impact Questionnnaire,[87] which measures the affect that incontinence has on different functional and social activities. This instrument was developed for women with incontinence. Instruments to assess quality of life in incontinent men are also available.[88]

The psychological impact of urge incontinence appears to differ from that of stress incontinence.[89] The Urge Impact Scale (URIS-24) was developed to determine the impact of urge incontinence on older adults. It measures the psychological burden, perception of personal control, and self-concept. This tool still needs testing with diverse racial and ethnic groups, but it can provide researchers and clinicians information about the impact of urge incontinence.

A written record of incontinent episodes is important in the assessment of the frequency and severity of incontinence. A bladder record or voiding record makes a permanent document for the date, day, and time of continent voids, time and quantity of involuntary urine loss, activities engaged in at time of the incontinent episode, and fluids ingested throughout the day. For motivated and literate individuals, space should be included on the bladder record for comments about factors that influence or potentially cause the incontinent episode.

The value of the information from bladder records cannot be underestimated. The nurse must compile the information to determine whether a voiding pattern can be detected before implementing a treatment regimen. After treatment begins, the nurse must examine the information from the bladder record to determine the effectiveness of the treatment on the frequency and volume of urine lost. Clinical algorithms have been developed for evaluating incontinence and they can also provide assistance in determining the course of treatment.[9,90-93] The urine should be examined for microscopic hematuria and evidence of infection. A postvoid residual specimen provides information regarding the emptying capacity of the bladder: a residual volume exceeding 100 ml may indicate an obstruction at the bladder outlet or weak detrusor contraction. Blood chemistry analysis includes the determination of urea nitrogen, creatinine, and glucose levels.

The use of urodynamic tests, such as the cystometrogram, urethral pressure profile, leak point pressure, uroflowmetry pressure flow studies, and videourodynamics, to evaluate all incontinent adults has been questioned.[28] However, urodynamic studies are indicated when neurological abnormalities are identified or incomplete bladder emptying occurs with overflow incontinence, and in stress incontinence with associated urethral dysfunction.[73] Urodynamic testing may detect the underlying mechanism in mixed incontinence cases, helping to predict outcomes of treatment and determine reasons for treatment failure.[44]

Ouslander[94] described bedside diagnostic tests to evaluate incontinence in older adults. For example, the individual is asked to void naturally to determine the voided amount and the volume at which the desire to void occurs. A postvoid residual urine specimen is then obtained via catheter. With the catheter in place, the bladder is filled with sterile water or saline solution to determine bladder filling capacity and whether uninhibited detrusor contractions occur. The individual is asked to cough in the supine and sometimes in the standing position after the catheter is removed to observe for urinary leakage. These tests have levels of 75% sensitivity and 95% specificity.[94] The simple cystometrogram is used to determine the filling and storage capacity of the bladder. Transducers used to monitor intravesical pressure and intraabdominal pressure when the bladder is filled detect uninhibited bladder contractions. It has been observed that phasic involuntary contractions often occur in young adults with urge symptoms but with no evident neurological lesion, whereas a single contraction that causes leakage occurs in older adults with cortical dysfunction.[44]

Uroflowmetry is used to evaluate bladder emptying. The rate of urine flow is measured by a strip chart recorder as the person voids into a special apparatus. This test is used to diagnose urethral obstruction.[62]

A voiding cystourethrogram is the test used to evaluate pelvic relaxation in women, postprostatectomy incontinence in men, and urinary retention after abdominal-perineal resection.[73] The presence of spinal abnormalities, cystocele, urethral diverticula, and intraurethral abnormalities, as well as abnormal movement of the urethra during voiding, can be detected with this procedure.

An objective measure of urine loss is the pad test. Preweighed pads are used and changed after a provocative maneuver. This test is helpful, because self-reports of urine loss often do not correlate with pelvic muscle strength.[95] This objective measure of urine loss should be used in conjunction with subjective measures of improvement during intervention phases of research studies and in clinical practice evaluations.

CLINICAL MANAGEMENT

Surgical procedures to repair pelvic organ prolapse in women, relieve bladder outlet obstruction secondary to an enlarged prostate in men, and implant artificial sphincters have been reviewed in the literature.[9,94,96-103]

Primary Prevention

The goal of primary prevention strategies is to maintain continence and to prevent incontinence. Adults should be encouraged to adopt lifestyle changes that promote a healthy bladder. These include drinking at least 6 to 8 glasses of water a day,[104] maintaining ideal body weight, not smoking, using good hygiene habits after elimination, emptying the bladder when the urge is present, and maintaining regular bowel habits. Adequate hydration, dietary fiber, and regular physical exercise are important components to healthy lifestyle behaviors and may decrease the risk of incontinence.

Secondary Prevention

Secondary prevention strategies are designed to improve or cure urinary incontinence with outcomes of continence or improved continence. Because of their noninvasive nature and lack of side effects, behavioral therapies are considered the first line of treatment for stress and urge incontinence.[9] These therapies include scheduled toileting, bladder retraining, contingency management, and pelvic floor muscle exercises with or without biofeedback. Other forms of treatment such as medications can be used in conjunction with behavioral therapies.[105] In institutional long-term care settings, prompted voiding with staff management techniques (i.e., performance feedback and supervision) have been used with success to improve the continence status of elderly residents.[106,107]

Scheduled toileting, also called *habit training,* involves a fixed schedule, traditionally every 2 to 4 hours, for bladder emptying. A bladder record is kept and is modified after the individualized pattern of continent and incontinent voiding is identified. Continence depends on caregivers' diligence in adhering to the schedule of toileting patients. The goal of this intervention is not rehabilitative; rather, it is to keep the individual dry and to prevent complications. This is a frequently used intervention in institutionalized settings with cognitively impaired adults who have been diagnosed with functional or urge incontinence.[108,109]

Bladder retraining, also called *bladder drill* or *bladder training,* involves a variable schedule of voiding. This intervention is suitable for an individual who is motivated and able to understand and interpret body sensations. The person keeps a bladder record and is encouraged to extend the length of time between voidings. This intervention is used to treat urge incontinence through urge inhibition. By increasing the time between voidings, bladder capacity will increase and urgency will eventually lessen. Lifestyle modifications and pharmacological therapy are used before and in conjunction with this intervention.[110]

Pelvic muscle exercises with biofeedback has been used with genuine stress incontinence, urge incontinence, and bladder-sphincter dyssynergia.[111] An individual must be cognitively intact and sufficiently motivated to understand and respond to visual or auditory biofeedback of various physiological parameters of urine control. Usually during a cystometric procedure, the individual watches tracings of bladder and abdominal pressure, bladder contraction, and sphincter and pelvic muscle activity. Physiological responses are changed through a process of operant conditioning in which the individual learns by observing the results of the voluntary efforts made to control bladder and sphincter activity.[112]

Pelvic muscle exercises without biofeedback, also called *Kegel exercises,*[113] are most commonly used to treat genuine stress incontinence in women. Women who are comfortable with the use of this technique learn how to contract the pelvic floor muscle without performing a Valsalva maneuver. Ten-second pelvic muscle contraction, followed by 10-second relaxation, should be performed for 30 to 45 repetitions a day.[114] Women can perform a digital examination to test the strength of the contraction.[114] Because the individual must adhere to the exercise regimen daily, motivation is an integral part of this therapy. Pelvic muscle exercises can be used in conjunction with biofeedback, scheduled voiding, intravaginal weights, or bladder retraining.[115]

Prompted voiding with staff management in the institutional setting involves a series of steps, including regularly scheduled verbal exchanges with incontinent older adults and asking about their current level of dryness and if they need to use the toilet. The staff member also provides physical assistance to the toilet and documents the outcome. An adequate number of direct caregivers is essential. Staff education and changes to the environment are crucial to help staff members to change their own behavior from incontinence containment to proactive actions, such as toileting patients before incontinent episodes occur.[116] Education is necessary, but not sufficient, in changing staff behavior; therefore individual feedback is given to each staff member in the form of verbal or written praise about performance.[106,117-119]

Pharmacological Therapy

Pharmacological treatment may be used alone or in conjunction with behavioral therapies. Medications are used to improve bladder emptying, to inhibit bladder contraction, and to strengthen the bladder outlet (Table 6-3).

Antimuscarinic agents (anticholinergics) are used to treat urge incontinence by inhibiting bladder contractions. Propantheline and emepronium are commonly used, but because of the potential anticholinergic side effects (i.e., blurred vision, changes in mental status, and constipation), they must be used cautiously in older adults. Antimuscarinic medications are contraindicated in persons with narrow-angle glaucoma.[120] Oxybutinin and dicyclomine are also used to treat urge incontinence; in addition to their anticholinergic properties, they may have a relaxant effect on the detrusor, thus increasing bladder capacity. Flavoxate possesses calcium channel antagonistic activity and produces a local anesthetic effect but has no anticholingeric properties. Reports are mixed about its effectiveness in treating detrusor overactivity and urge incontinence.[120]

Genuine stress incontinence can be treated with medications that increase intraurethral pressure. These include alpha-adrenergic agonists and beta-adrenoceptor antagonists. Estrogen also is used to treat stress incontinence in women.[121] Alpha-adrenergic agonists, such as ephedrine and phenylpropanoline, are contraindicated for individuals with hypertension, hyperthyroidism, and cardiovascular disease. Estrogens are contraindicated in women with a history of carcinoma of the breast and thrombophlebotic disease.

Tertiary Prevention

The purpose of tertiary prevention strategies is to provide comfort and to prevent complications. Therefore, after other treatments have failed, collection devices may be the appropriate means to control urine loss. In tertiary treatment, external urine collection devices, external and indwelling catheters, disposable and reusable absorbent pads, and undergarments are used. Indwelling catheters are considered the last resort for incontinence management because of the associated morbidity, (i.e., bacteriuria and increased risk of septicemia).[9] Indwelling catheters, however, are appropriate devices for management when intermittent catheterization is inappropriate[122] (i.e., when accurate monitoring of urinary output, maintenance of skin integrity and/or wound cleanliness, and provision of comfort for terminally ill persons are essential).

Absorbent pads and undergarments are useful as the sole management strategy for intractable incontinence or as adjuncts to other therapies (e.g., pelvic floor muscle exercises). Absorbent products include

TABLE 6-3 Pharmacotherapy for Urinary Incontinence

PRESENTATION	DYSFUNCTION	PHARMACOTHERAPY
Failure to store	Increased bladder activity	Antimuscarinic agents such as propantheline Medications with mixed actions such as oxybutynin, dicyclomine, propiverine, flavoxate
Failure to store	Increased bladder sensation	Topical urethelial analgesic such as pyridium Tricyclic antidepressant, such as imipramine
Failure to store	Decreased outlet resistance	Estradiol, alpha-adrenoceptor agonist
Failure to empty	Decreased bladder activity	Muscarinic agents, such as urocheline
Failure to empty	Decreased bladder sensation	None
Failure to empty	Increased outlet resistance	Alpha-adrenoceptor antagonists, such as doxazosin, terazosin

disposable and reusable briefs, pads, pant liners, and shields. A multitude of incontinence products are available. Assessment of type and severity of incontinence, level of functioning, and personal preferences play a part in determining the product best suited for the individual. A variety of resources are available that describe available continence products.[123-125] These products should only be used after careful assessment. They may be used in conjunction with other therapies, or as a last resort to promote the quality of life of individuals who would not benefit from restorative or rehabilitative interventions. They can never be used solely for the convenience of the staff or as a substitute for human intervention.

CONCEPTUAL MODELS

Urinary incontinence is a prevalent condition affecting people across the life span. Because of its prevalence and impact on health care costs, caregivers, and affected adults, a public health perspective is needed. Multiple risk factors and etiological mechanisms have been identified. A Continence Promotion Model has been proposed[126] (Figure 6-2).

This model includes primary prevention strategies (i.e., keeping continent people continent) as well as rehabilitative and palliative interventions. Removal of factors that place individuals at risk for becoming incontinent receives equal attention from health care providers as do traditional interventions to cure or improve the condition. Desired outcomes for each level of health promotion are also identified in this model. Independent continence indicates that the individual's own attempts are successfully maintaining continence. Dependent continence means an individual is continent as a result of the efforts of the caregiver. Social continence refers to effective incontinence containment that allows the individual to remain in society without stigma.[127] Urine containment and odor control are major elements in social continence strategies. Improved continence refers to individuals who remain incontinent with intervention, but have an increased level of dryness over their baseline condition. Reduction of even one incontinent episode a day may represent improved continence status for some individuals indicating treatment success, whereas it may signal treatment failure for others.

CASE STUDIES

CASE STUDY I

Mrs. L visited a gynecologist at her daughter's insistence. She is a 66-year-old white widow who lives alone in her home of 40 years. She is active in volunteer work at the local community hospital and enjoys spending time with her three grandchildren. Since the birth of her last child 30 years ago, Mrs. L has experienced a small amount of urine leakage without warning when she laughs forcefully, sneezes, or coughs. She has never mentioned this condition to her physician. A gynecologist had not examined her for 14 years, since the onset of menopause. Recently Mrs. L has trouble getting to the bathroom in time. She just started using commercially available undergarments for bladder control, limiting her fluid intake during the day, and toileting herself every hour regardless of feeling the need to void. During a recent shopping trip with her daughter, she wet through her undergarments while attempting to get to the public rest room.

On examination, Mrs. L's abdomen was soft, nondistended, and free of scars. She delivered two children by vaginal delivery when she was 30 and 36 years old. Family history was negative for breast cancer, and Mrs. L's latest mammogram revealed no evidence of malignancy. She also denied history of vascular disease. During the pelvic examination, there was no evidence of a cystocele or uterine prolapse. While Mrs. L was standing, there was a small leakage of urine when she was instructed to cough forcefully. Further examination revealed that the vaginal walls looked pale and there was a white discharge, indicating atrophic vaginitis. There was weak muscle tone when she was instructed to contract during the manual examination of the vagina. The rectal examination was negative for fecal impaction or rectal mass. A postvoid residual measured less than 50 ml. Laboratory tests revealed the serum glucose, urea nitrogen, and creatinine within normal limits. Results of a urine culture were negative.

Mrs. L was instructed to keep a bladder diary for 14 days and to keep a record of her fluid intake. It was recommended that she attempt to drink 6 to 8 glasses of water a day and to avoid caffeinated drinks. Conjugated estrogen to be applied intravaginally was prescribed to treat atrophic vaginitis, and Mrs. L was instructed to perform pelvic floor muscle exercises three times a day with at least 15 to 20 repetitions during each session. An instruction sheet was given to remind her (1) not to tense her abdomen, buttocks, or thigh muscles during the exercises, (2) that each contraction should last 10 seconds, with 10 seconds of relaxation, (3) the exercises ought to be practiced in the lying, sitting, and standing positions, and (4) to check for the correct muscle being exercised by inserting a finger into the vagina and contracting the muscle.

After 4 weeks of regularly performing the exercises and increasing her fluid intake while eliminating caffeinated beverages, Mrs. L noticed a decrease in the number of incontinent episodes, from an average

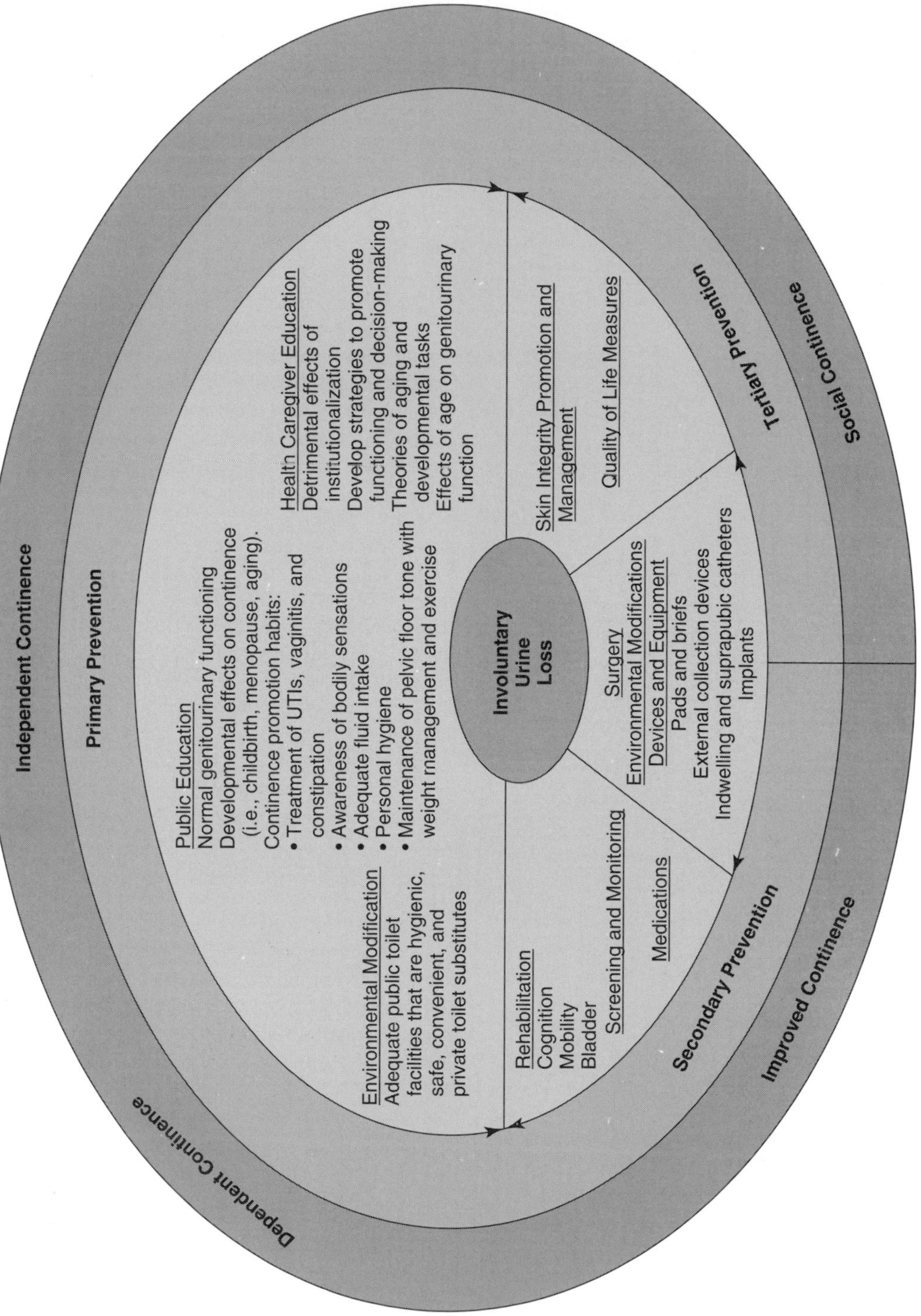

Figure 6-2 Continence promotion model.

of ten episodes a week to five episodes a week. She also found a pattern to some episodes of urine loss: urine was lost when she moved from a sitting to standing position. She was instructed to contract her pelvic floor muscles before changing positions. Also, a bladder retraining schedule was instituted, initially set at every 2 hours, with the anticipation of increasing the interval to 3 or 4 hours, to decrease urgency symptoms. After another 8 weeks, Mrs. L continued to be highly motivated to follow the regimen and was so pleased with the reduction in wetness (i.e., she had only two episodes, with reduced volume, in a month) that she stopped wearing bladder control undergarments.

CASE STUDY 2

Mrs. R is a 79-year-old black, widowed resident of a small rural nursing home. Her feet are deformed from years of neglect and poorly fitting shoes, and she ambulates with great difficulty. She is unable to walk unless she wears shoes with special supports. Mrs. R is cognitively impaired. Her score on the Folstein Mini Mental State Examination[80] is 15, indicating significant cognitive impairment. The staff must frequently reorient her to time and place. She recognizes familiar faces, but she does not retain names. She is cooperative with her care and tries to be independent. Mrs. R is incontinent of urine at least twice a day and at least once during the night. Each time she is incontinent, she is attempting to get to the bathroom. Mrs. R voids in large amounts and is very distressed about being incontinent. Her history is negative for a cystocele or pelvic or rectal surgeries; she is a nulliparous. A urine test for culture and sensitivity was negative for bacteria. Her fasting blood sugar was 100 mg/100 ml, creatinine 5 mg/100 ml, and urea nitrogen 12 mg/100 ml.

The nursing staff wrote a care plan that included a bladder record and a scheduled toileting regimen. After 3 days a pattern of incontinent episodes emerged, and the scheduled toileting regimen was refined to offer Mrs. R assistance to the commode immediately on arising, before retiring at night, and every 3 hours during the day. Environmental modifications included a bedside commode at night and a second pair of shoes that offered support but were easier for Mrs. R to slip on without assistance. Nursing staff members also consistently praised her continent behavior and her attempts at self-toileting. Incontinent episodes diminished to less than twice a week.

SELECTED RESEARCH

Little nursing research was conducted in the United States on urinary incontinence in adults, especially older adults, before the 1970s. Few nursing studies using case-control research designs are available. Reports in the literature are of descriptive studies or clinical trials with small samples. However, more recently nurse researchers have been conducting research related to incontinence, and evidence indicates that nursing interventions are successful in the management of incontinence.[128] In the long-term care setting, anecdotal reports abound that environmental modifications, such as encouraging self-toileting behavior, making toilets accessible, and positive staff attitudes improve continence status.[13,84-85,90-93] The characteristics of incontinent patients in nursing homes have been reported.[6] Incontinent residents generally exhibit higher levels of cognitive and mobility impairment than continent residents.[11,81] Nurses have long used behavioral therapies to manage incontinence in various groups in institutional settings.[96] Many of these interventions focus on modifying the antecedents or the consequences of incontinence.[53] Behavioral therapies differ in administration.[129] Some therapies may be self-managed by the individual, such as pelvic muscle exercise with biofeedback; other therapies are staff managed, especially for individuals with cognitive and mobility impairment.

A randomized controlled trial of a toileting program individualized to an older person's voiding pattern (pattern urge response toileting [PURT]) demonstrated treatment effectiveness peaking at 6 weeks after implementation; 86% of the experimental group had improved continence to some degree. Approximately one third had a 20% reduction in episodes of incontinence.[130] Engel et al[131] augmented a prompted voiding therapy with a staff management component. Individual staff members received feedback from their supervisors regarding their performance of completing assigned toiletings. Bar graphs depicting the percent of completed toileting were shared at biweekly meetings. Letters praising performance or encouraging increased performance were given to the staff member. A 6-month summary letter signed by the director of nursing was placed in the personnel file. These investigators found that behavioral therapy was effective in increasing continence and that individualized feedback was more effective than group feedback. Subsequent research supported these findings.[132]

Mitteness and Barker[4] provided valuable information about the cognitive organization of incontinence by community-dwelling older adults. Elaborate plans were made to avoid detection by peers and others, and little effort was made to seek medical help. Many women viewed incontinence as a hygiene problem rather than a medical one.[133]

Knowledge about the characteristics of incontinent adults in the community continues to grow. The clinical characteristics of 200 incontinent older women included a high proportion with mixed incontinence (27%). Genuine stress incontinence was present in the majority (66%) of the sample, and more than a third of the women had atrophic vaginitis.[134] The exact mechanism of improvement with pelvic muscle exercise and biofeedback and with bladder retraining in community-based older women is unclear. Clinical improvements in terms of decreasing the number of incontinent episodes were found, but there had been no significant improvements in urodynamic parameters (i.e., maximum urethral closure pressure, functional urethral length, and so on).[135]

Further evidence of the effectiveness of pelvic muscle exercises and bladder training has been provided by a multisite study in women's health care settings.[136] Women (N = 1474) were screened for urinary incontinence in ambulatory care settings and women who screened positive for incontinence (N = 842) were offered behavioral treatment. Women who continued in treatment and who were contacted at 4 months for follow-up (N = 132) reported significantly fewer episodes of incontinence and decreased volume of urine loss during these episodes. The impact of incontinence also significantly decreased from baseline in this group. This study provides evidence for the application of evidence-based protocols in nursing practice. There was significant attrition from this and other studies. It may be that women effectively use self-management strategies, often for years before seeking help, and will withdraw from studies when there are competing priorities for time (i.e., work and leisure activities).[137]

Self-care strategies, such as monitoring fluid intake, have been investigated.[138] Women 50 years of age and older (N = 32) were randomized to one of three groups: those who increased fluid intake by 500 ml, those who maintained baseline fluid intake, and those who decreased fluid intake by 500 ml. Because adherence to the protocol was poor (women found it easier to decrease intake rather than increase it), results were insignificant. The researchers noted, however, that women who were contacted (N = 29) for follow-up expressed appreciation in having their awareness heightened about the effect of fluids on their voiding pattern.

Incontinence in cognitively impaired elders in the community has been successfully treated with an individualized scheduled toileting program.[139] Subjects (N = 118; average age, 79.89 years) were randomly assigned to the individualized scheduled toileting program or to the control group. People with moderate cognitive impairment and ability to cooperate with toileting were identified as those most likely to succeed in the toileting program.

The quality of life of incontinent individuals has received significant attention.[140,141] The International Continence Society recommends inclusion of quality of life as an outcome measure in all incontinence research.[142] Chiverton et al[143] reported a revised model of factors that influence the quality of life of incontinent women. They reported that depression was not a mediator for quality of life but that mastery had a direct effect on both depression and quality of life. They proposed that nurses develop and test interventions that increase women's sense of mastery to reduce depression and enhance quality of life. Quality of life has been studied in men after prostate cancer treatment. Men who were treated with surgery had significantly worse sexual and urinary function than those who were treated with radiation. However, the men who underwent surgical treatment had better bowel function than those who received radiation treatment.[144] Men who underwent radical prostatectomy for prostate cancer surgery expressed a need for more detailed information about dealing with postoperative complications (i.e., incontinence and impotence). They were often too overwhelmed with the cancer diagnosis to be able to grapple with preoperative education. They also expressed that there was a lack of professional health care provider support.[145] The lack of attention to incontinence after prostate cancer treatment may be because of the notion that incontinence is a women's issue. Because men do experience incontinence, especially with cognitive impairments[8,11] and after surgical treatment for prostate cancer,[146] more research investigating incontinence in men is needed.

QUESTIONS FOR FUTURE STUDY

Although age alone does not cause incontinence, researchers need to conduct longitudinal prospective studies to develop a clearer understanding of the natural history and development of urinary incontinence in adults. These studies should include developmental aspects, such as pregnancy, childbirth, and menopause.

The short- and long-term efficacy of different therapies, such as pelvic floor muscle exercise, electrical stimulation, and intravaginal cones, in culturally diverse populations has not been clearly determined.[147-153] Ethnic diversity in studies is urgently needed, because incontinence may present differently and require different interventions in various groups. Nurse researchers need to participate in multisite clinical trials and to replicate and extend research studies in various practice settings to develop evidence-based continence practice. For example, it is not clear whether results from studies with institutionalized elderly persons ought to be generalized to frail elders in home care. Most studies have been conducted with white middle-class subjects.

Research-based primary health promotion strategies to maintain continence throughout the life span have yet to be developed or studied, but interest is growing.[154,155] Educational strategies are needed for health care professionals and laypersons to understand the normal changes in the functioning of the urinary system with age and how to access existing treatment modalities for incontinence. Nurses need to devise factual consumer-focused information about urinary incontinence and bladder health. This information needs to be widely disseminated, not only in health care settings but also in places in which women work and reside. Issues of ethical continence care, such as equal access to continence care and respect of patient rights, also need to be explored further.[156]

Concurrent with the increasing awareness of the different types of incontinence and clinical criteria for diagnosis is the need for sensitive and specific assessment tools in the clinical setting. There continues to be a need to incorporate tools to assess voiding patterns and pelvic muscle strength into nursing and other health care professionals' practice.

Research has shown that nurses play a significant role in the assessment and treatment of urinary incontinence.[157-158] Although today there is a better understanding of the causes of incontinence and multiple interventions, more research—especially interdisciplinary research with large diverse samples—is needed. There is evidence that bowel function is related to bladder function[159,160]; therefore consideration of the interrelationships among the pelvic structures and mechanisms is also urged.[161]

It is imperative that nurses play a major role in the identification of individuals at risk for becoming and remaining incontinent and in the development of new techniques and products to meet the hygienic, personal, and social needs of incontinent adults at different stages of their life. Studies with underrepresented groups, such as African Americans, Hispanics, and Asians, are needed to better understand the presentation and impact of this condition. Viewing urinary incontinence with a life span approach to incontinence will advance primary prevention efforts and perhaps in the long-term reduce both the incidence and prevalence of incontinence.

REFERENCES

1. Abrams, P., Cardozo, L, Fall, M., Griffiths, D., Rosier, P., Ulmsten, U., van Kerrebroeck, P., Victor, A. & Wein, A. (2002). The standardization of terminology of lower urinary tract function: Report from the Standardisation Sub-committee of the International Continence Society, *Neurology and Urodynamics 21*(2), 167-178.
2. Payne, C. (1999). Advances in nonsurgical treatment of urinary incontinence and overactive bladder. *Campbell's Urology Updates Attachment 6, 1*(1), 1-20.
3. *American Heritage Dictionary of the English Language* (3rd ed., p. 915). (1992). New York: Houghton Mifflin.
4. Mitteness, L., & Barker, J. (1995). Stigmatizing a "normal" condition: Urinary incontinence in late life. *Medical Anthropology Quarterly 9*(2), 188-210.
5. Abrams, P. (1999). Foreword. In P. Abrams, S. Khoury, & A. Wein (eds.), *Incontinence.* Plymouth, England: Health Publications.
6. Newman, D. (1997). How much society pays for urinary incontinence. *Ostomy/Wound Management 43*(1), 18-25.
7. Morbidity and Mortality Report. (1991). Urinary incontinence among hospitalized persons aged 65 years and older—United States, 1984-1987. July 5, 1991, *40*(26), 433-436.
8. Palmer, M., Myers, A., & Fedenko, K. (1997). Urinary continence changes after hip fracture repair. *Clinical Nursing Research 6*(1), 8-24.
9. Fantl, A., Newman, D., Colling, J., DeLancey, J., Keeys, C., Loughery, R., et al. (1996). Urinary incontinence in adults: Acute and chronic management. Clinical practice guideline. (AHCPR Pub. No. 96-0682). Agency for Health Care Policy and Research. Rockville, Md.: Department of Health and Human Services.
10. Landi, F., Sgadari, A., & Bernabei, R. (1998). Urinary incontinence in nursing home residents. *Journal of the American Geriatrics Society 46*(4), 536-537.
11. Palmer, M., German, P., & Ouslander, J. (1991). Risk factors for urinary incontinence one year after nursing home admission. *Research in Nursing and Health 14,* 405-412.
12. Nygaard, I., Thompson, F., Svengalis, S., & Albright, J. (1994). Urinary incontinence in elite nulliparous athletes. *Obstetrics & Gynecology 84*(2), 183-187.
13. Davis, G., Sherman, R., Wong, M., McClure, G., Perez, R., & Hibbert, M. (1999). Urinary incontinence among female soldiers. *Military Medicine 164*(3), 182-187.
14. Palmer, M., Fitzgerald, S., Berry, S., & Hart, K. (1999). Urinary incontinence in working women: An exploratory study. *Women and Health 29*(3), 67-82.
15. Palmer, M. (2000). Urinary incontinence post-prostatectomy: Magnitude of the problem. *Journal of Wound, Ostomy and Continence Nursing 27*(3), 129-137.
16. Jonler, M., Madsen, F., Rhodes, P., Sall, M., Messing, E., & Bruskewitz, R. (1996). A prospective study of quantification of urinary incontinence and quality of life in

patients undergoing radical retropubic prostatectomy. *Urology 48*(3), 433-440.

17. Lee, W., Schultheiss, T., Hanlon, A., & Hanks, G. (1996). Urinary incontinence following external-beam radiotherapy for clinically localized prostate cancer. *Journal of Urology 152*(11), 1707-1708.
18. Bishoff, J., Motley, G., Optenberg, S., Stein, C., Moon, K., Browning, S., et al. (1998). Incidence of fecal and urinary incontinence following radical perineal and retropubic prostatectomy in a national population. *Journal of Urology 159*(4), 1276-1280.
19. Brown, J., Seeley, D., Fong, J., Black, D., Ensrud, K., Grady, D., et al. (1996). Urinary incontinence in older women: Who is at risk? *Obstetrics & Gynecology 87*(5), 715-721.
20. Roberts, R., Jacobsen, S., Rhodes, T., Reily, T., Girman, C., Talley, N., & Lieber, M. (1998). Urinary incontinence in a community-based cohort: Prevalence and healthcare-seeking. *Journal of the American Geriatrics Society 46*(4), 467-472.
21. Wetle, T., Scherr, P., Branch, L., Resnick, N., Harris, T., Evans, D., & Taylor, J. (1995). Difficulty with holding urine among older persons in a geographically defined community: Prevalence and correlates. *Journal of the American Geriatrics Society 43*(4), 349-355.
22. Bump, R. (1993). Racial comparisons and contrasts in urinary incontinence and pelvic organ prolapse. *Obstetrics & Gynecology 81*(3), 421-425.
23. Nakayama, H., Jorgensen, H., Pederen, P., Raaschou, H., & Olsen, T. (1997). Prevalence and risk factors of incontinence after stroke. The Copenhagen Stroke Study. *Stroke 28*(1), 58-62.
24. O'Connor, T. (1996). Management of urinary continence problems in an acute general hospital. *International Journal of Nursing Practice 2*(1), 47-49.
25. Chiarelli, P., & Campbell, E. (1997). Incontinence during pregnancy. Prevalence and opportunities for continence promotion. *Australian and New Zealand Journal of Obstetrics and Gynecology 37*(1), 1:66-73.
26. Peacock, L., Wiskind, A., & Wall, L. (1994). Clinical features of urinary incontinence and urogenital prolapse in a black inner-city population. *American Journal of Obstetrics and Gynecology 171*(6), 1464-1471.
27. Turan, C., Zorlu, C., Ekin, M., Hancerliogullari, N., & Saracoglu, F. (1996). Urinary incontinence in women of reproductive age. *Gynecologic and Obstetric Investigation 41,* 132-134.
28. Wilson, P., Herbison, R., & Herbison, G. (1996). Obstetric practice and the prevalence of urinary incontinence three months after delivery. *British Journal of Obstetrics and Gynaecology 103,* 154-161.
29. Groutz, A., Gordon, D., Keidar, R., Lessing, J., Wolman, I., David, M., & Chen, B. (1999). Stress urinary incontinence: Prevalence among nulliparous compared with primiparous and grand multiparous premenopausal women. *Neurology and Urodynamics 18,* 419-425.
30. Brandeis, G., Baumann, M., Hossain, M., Morris, J., & Resnick, N. (1997). The prevalence of potentially remediable urinary incontinence in frail older people: A study using the minimum data set. *Journal of the American Geriatrics Society 45*(2), 179-184.
31. Umlauf, M., & Sherman, S. (1996). Symptoms of urinary incontinence among older community-dwelling men. *Journal of Wound, Ostomy and Continence Nursing 23*(6), 314-321.
32. Nygaard, I., & Lemke, J. (1996). Urinary incontinence in rural older women: Prevalence, incidence and remission. *Journal of the American Geriatrics Society 44*(9), 1049-1054.
33. Nakanishi, N., Tatara, K., Naramura, H., Fujiwara, K., Takashima, Y., & Fukuda, H. (1997). Urinary and fecal incontinence in a community-residing older population in Japan. *Journal of the American Geriatrics Society 45*(2), 215-219.
34. Goluboff, E., Saidi, J., Mazer, S., Bagiella, E., Heitjan, D., Benson, M., & Olsson, C. (1998). Urinary continence after radical prostatectomy: The Columbia experience. *Journal of Urology 159,* 1276-1280.
35. Talcott, J., Rieker, P., Clark, J., Propert, K., Weeks, J., Beard, C., et al. (1998). Patient-reported symptoms after primary therapy for early prostate cancer: Results of a prospective cohort study. *Journal of Clinical Oncology 16*(1), 275-283.
36. Roberts, R.O., Jacobsen, S.J., Reilly, W.T., Pemberton, J.H., Lieber, M.M., Talley, N.J. (1999). Prevalence of combined fecal and urinary incontinence: A community-based study. *Journal of the American Geriatrics Society 47*(7), 837-841.
37. Hojberb, K., Salvig, J., Winslow, N., Lose, G., & Secher, N. (1999). Urinary incontinence: Prevalence and risk factors at 16 weeks of gestation. *British Journal of Obstetrics and Gynaecology 106,* 842-850.
38. Fultz, N., Herzog, R., Raghunathan, T., Wallace, R., & Diokno, A. (1999). Prevalence and severity of urinary incontinence in older African American and Caucasian women. *Journal of Gerontology 54A*(6), M299-M303.
39. Stanford, J., Feng, Z., Hamilton, A., Gilliland, F., Stephenson, R., Eley, J., et al. (2000). Urinary and sexual function after radical prostatectomy for clinically localized prostate cancer. *Journal of the American Medical Association 283*(3), 354-360.
40. Johnson, Bernard, Kincaide, J., & Defriese, G. (2000). Urinary incontinence and risk of death among community-living elderly people: Results from the National Survey on Self-Care and Aging. *Journal of Aging and Health 12*(1), 25-46.
41. Arya, L., Myers, D., & Jackson, N. (2000). Dietary caffeine intake and the risks for detrusor instability: A case-control study. *Obstetrics & Gynecology 96*(1), 85-89.
42. Tomlinson, B., Doughert, M., Pendergast, J., Boyington, A., Coffman, M., & Pickens, S. (1999). Dietary caffeine, fluid intake and urinary incontinence in older rural women. *International Urogynecology Journal 10,* 22-28.
43. Koskimaki, J., Hakama, M., Huhtala, H., & Tammela, T. (1998). Association of smoking with lower urinary tract symptoms. *Journal of Urology 159,* 1580-1582.
44. Homma, Y., Batista, J., Bauer, J., Bauer, S., Griffiths, D., Hilton, P., Kramer, G., Kulseng-Hanssen, S., Rosier, P., & Stohrer, M. (1999). Urodynamics. In P. Abrams, S. Khoury, & A. Wein (eds.), *Incontinence.* Plymouth, England: Health Publications.
45. Palmer, M. (1996). Urinary continence: Assessment and promotion. Gaithersburg, Md.: Aspen Publishers.
46. Watson, A., Currie, I., Curran, S., & Jarvis, G. (2000). A prospective study examining the association between the symptoms of anxiety and depression and severity of urinary incontinence. *European Journal of Obstetrics & Gynecology and Reproductive Biology 88,* 7-9.
47. Ouslander, J., Palmer, M., Rovner, B., & German, P. (1993). Urinary incontinence in nursing homes: Incidence, remission and associated factors. *Journal of the American Geriatrics Society 41*(10), 1083-1089.
48. Ouslander, J., Schnelle, J., Uman, G., Fingold, S., Nigam, J., Tuico, E., & Bates-Jensen, B. (1995). Predictors of

successful prompted voiding among nursing home residents. *Journal of the American Medical Association 273*(17), 1366-1370.
49. Schnelle, J., MacRae, P., Ouslander, J., Simmons, S., & Nitta, M. (1995). Functional incidental training, mobility performance and incontinence care with nursing home residents. *Journal of the American Geriatrics Society 43*(12), 1356-1362.
50. Davidson, H., Borrie, M., & Crilly, R. (1991). Copy task performance and urinary incontinence in Alzheimer's disease. *Journal of the American Geriatrics Society 39*(5), 467-471.
51. Smith, P., & Smith, L. (1997). Continence and incontinence: Psychological approaches to development and treatment. London: Croom Helm.
52. Kirshen, A., & Cape, R. (1984). A history of urinary incontinence: Or 400 years of incontinence—are we any drier? *Journal of the American Geriatrics Society 32*(9), 686-688.
53. van Gool, J., Bloom, D., Butler, R., Djurhus, J., Hjalmas, K., de Jong, T. (1999). Conservative management in children. In P. Abrams, S. Khoury, & A. Wein (eds.), *Incontinence.* Plymouth, England: Health Publications.
54. Cardoza, L., & Cutner, A. (1997). Lower urinary tract symptoms in pregnancy. *British Journal of Urology 1* (Suppl), 80, 14-23.
55. Foldspang, A., Mommsen, S., & Djurhuus, J. (1999). Prevalent urinary incontinence as a correlate of pregnancy, vaginal childbirth and obstetric techniques. *American Journal of Public Health 89*(2), 209-212.
56. Gunnarsson, M., & Mattiasson, A. (1999). Female stress, urge, and mixed urinary incontinence are associated with a chronic and progressive pelvic floor/vaginal neuromuscular disorder: An investigation of 317 healthy and incontinent women using vaginal surface electromyography. *Neurology and Urodynamics 18,* 613-621.
57. van Geelan, J., Lemmes, W., Eskes, T., & Martin, C. (1982). The urethral pressure profile in pregnancy and after delivery in healthy nulliparous women. *American Journal of Obstetrics and Gynecology 144*(6), 636-649.
58. Snooks, S., Henry, M., & Setchell, M. (1986). Risk factors in childbirth causing damage to the pelvic floor innervation. *International Journal of Colorectal Disease 1,* 20-24.
59. Vierhout, M., & Gianotten, W. (1993). Mechanisms of urine loss during sexual activity. *European Journal of Obstetrics and Gynecology and Reproductive Biology 52,* 45-47.
60. Barlow, D., Cardoza, L., Francis, R., Griffin, M., Hart, D., Stephens, E., & Sturdee, D. (1997). Urogenital ageing and its effect on sexual health in older British women. *British Journal of Obstetrics and Gynaecology 104,* 87-91.
61. Mommsen, S., & Foldspang, A. (1994). Body mass index and adult female urinary incontinence. *World Journal of Urology 12,* 319-322.
62. Staskin, D. (1986). Age-related physiologic and pathologic changes affecting lower urinary tract function. *Clinical Geriatric Medicine 2,* 701-730.
63. Agency for Health Care Policy and Research. (1995). Prostate disease. Patient outcomes Research Team Final Report. AHCPR Pub No 95-N010, Rockville, Md.: U.S. Department of Health and Human Services.
64. Wells, T., & Diokno, A. (1989). Urinary incontinence in the elderly. *Seminars in Neurology 9*(1), 60-67.
65. Rekers, H., Drogendijk, A., Valkenburg, H., & Riphagen, F. (1992). The menopause, urinary incontinence and other symptoms of the genito-urinary tract. *Maturitas 15,* 101-111.
66. Hammond, C. (1996). Menopause and hormone replacement therapy: An overview. *Obstetrics and Gynecology 87*(Suppl 2), 2S-15S.
67. Blaivas, J., Romanzi, L., & Heritz, D. (1998). Urinary incontinence: Pathophysiology, evaluation, treatment overview, and nonsurgical management. In P. Walsh, A. Retik, E. Vaughan, & A. Wein. *Campbell's Urology* (7th ed.). Philadelphia: WB Saunders.
68. Retzky, S., & Rogers, R. (1995). Urinary incontinence in women. *CIBA Clinical Symposia 47*(3), 2-32.
69. Mundy, A. (1999). Structure and function of the lower urinary tract. In A. Mundy, J. Fitzpatrick, D. Neal, & N. George (eds.), *Scientific basis of urology.* Oxford, England: ISIS Medical Media.
70. Gosling, J. (1979). The structure of the bladder and urethra in relation to function. *Urologic Clinics of North America 6,* 31-38.
71. Wein, A. (1986). Physiology of micturition. *Clinics of Geriatric Medicine 2,* 689-699.
72. Resnick, N., & Yalla, S. (1998). Geriatric incontinence and voiding dysfunction. In P. Walsh, A. Retik, E. Vaughan, & A. Wein (eds.), *Campbells' Urology* (7th ed.). Philadelphia: WB Saunders.
73. Leach, G., & Yip, C. (1986). Urologic and urodynamic evaluation of the elderly population. *Clinics of Geriatric Medicine 2*(4), 731-755.
74. Tewari, A., & Narayan, P. (1999). Voiding dysfunction in men with lower urinary tract symptoms and benign prostatic hyperplasia. In U. Nseyo, E. Weinman, & D. Lamm (eds.), *Urology for primary care physicians.* Philadelphia: WB Saunders.
75. Johnson, T., Kincade, J., Bernard, S., Busby-Whitehead, J., Hertz-Picciotto, I., & DeFriese, G. (1998). The association of urinary incontinence with poor self-rated health. *Journal of the American Geriatrics Society 46*(6), 693-699.
76. Tinetti, M., Inouye, S., Gill, T., & Doucetter, J. (1995). Shared risk factors for falls, incontinence, and functional dependency. *Journal of the American Medical Association 273*(17), 1348-1353.
77. Herzog, A., Diokno, A., Brown, M., Fultz, N., & Goldstein, N. (1994). Urinary incontinence as a risk factor for mortality. *Journal of the American Geriatrics Society 42*(3), 264-268.
78. Cundiff, G., Harris, R., Coates, K., & Bump, R. (1997). Clinical predictors of urinary incontinence in women. *American Journal of Obstetrics and Gynecology 177*(2), 262-267.
79. Seim, A., Eriksen, B., & Hunskaar, S. (1996). A study of female urinary incontinence in general practice. *Scandanavian Journal of Urology and Nephrology 30*(6), 465-471.
80. Resnick, N., & Yalla, S. (1992). Evaluation and management of urinary incontinence. In P. Walsh, A. Retik, T. Stamey, & E. Vaughn (eds.), *Campbell's urology* (6th ed.). Philadelphia: WB Saunders.
81. Skelley, J., & Flint, A. (1995). Urinary incontinence associated with dementia. *Journal of the American Geriatrics Society 43*(3), 286-294.
82. Allman, R., Goode, P., Patrick, M., Burst, M., & Bartolucci, A. (1995). Pressure ulcer risk factors among hospitalized patients with activity limitation. *Journal of the American Medical Association 273*(11), 865-870.
83. Burgio, K., Ives, D., Locher, J., Arena, V., & Kuller, L. (1994). Treatment seeking for urinary incontinence in older adults. *Journal of the American Geriatrics Society 42*(2), 208-212.

84. Cohen, S., Robinson, D., Dugan, E., Howard, G., Suggs, P., Pearce, K., et al. (1999). Communication between older adults and their physicians about urinary incontinence. *Journal of Gerontology 54A*(1), M34-M37.
85. Harrison, G., & Memel, D. (1994). Urinary incontinence in women: Its prevalence and its management in a health promotion clinic. *British Journal of General Practice 44,* 149-152.
86. Lee, P., Reid, D., Saltmarche, A., & Linton, L. (1995). Measuring the psychosocial impact of urinary incontinence: The York Incontinence Perceptions Scale (YIPS). *Journal of the American Geriatrics Society 43*(11), 1275-1278.
87. Wyman, J., Harkins, J., & Choi, S. (1987). Psychosocial impact of urinary incontinence in women. *Obstetrics and Gynecology 70*(3, Part 1), 378-381.
88. Schwartz, E., & Lepor, H. (1999). Radical retropubic prostatectomy reduces symptoms scores and improves quality of life in men with moderate and severe lower urinary tract symptoms. *Journal of Urology 161*(4), 180-186.
89. DuBeau, C., Kiely, D., & Resnick, N. (1999). Quality of life impact of urge incontinence in older persons: A new measure and conceptual structure. *Journal of the American Geriatrics Society 47*(8), 989-994.
90. Thuroff, J., Abrams, P., Artibani, W., Haab, F., Khoury, S., Madersbacher, H., et al. (1999). Clinical guidelines for the management of incontinence. In P. Abrams, S. Khoury, & A. Wein (eds.), *Incontinence.* Plymouth, England: Health Publications.
91. American Medical Directors Association. (1996). Urinary incontinence clinical practice guideline. 1-800-876-2632.
92. National Association for Continence. (2000). Guideline for urinary incontinence in assistive living facilities. Spartansburg, S.C.: The Association.
93. Multiple Sclerosis Council for Clinical Practice Guidelines. (1999). Urinary dysfunction and multiple sclerosis. Paralyzed Veterans of America: Washington, D.C.: www.pva.org.
94. Ouslander, J. (1986). Diagnostic evaluation of geriatric urinary incontinence. *Clinics of Geriatric Medicine 2*(4), 715-730.
95. Brink, C., Wells, T., Sampselle, C., Taillie, E.A., & Mayer, R. (1994). A digital test for pelvic muscle strength in women with urinary incontinence. *Nursing Research 43*(6), 352-356.
96. Jarvis, G., Bent, A., Cortesse, A., McGuire, E., Milani, R., Quartey, J., et al. (1999). Surgical treatment for incontinence in adult women surgery of female lower genito-urinary fistulae. In P. Abrams, S. Khoury, & A. Wein (eds.), *Incontinence.* Plymouth, England: Health Publications.
97. Herschorn, S., Boccon-Gibod, L., Bosch, J., Bruschini, H., Hanus, T., Low, I., et al. (1999). Surgical treatment in men. In P. Abrams, S. Khoury, & A. Wein (eds.), *Incontinence.* Plymouth, England: Health Publications.
98. Barrett, D., Abol-Enein, H., Castro-Diaz, D., Hohenfellner, M., Stohrer, M., & Tanagho, E. (1999). Surgery for neuropathic patient. In P. Abrams, S. Khoury, & A. Wein (eds.), *Incontinence.* Plymouth, England: Health Publications.
99. Ulmsten, U., Johnson, P., & Rezapour, M. (1999). A three-year follow up of tension free vaginal tape for surgical treatment of female stress urinary incontinence. *British Journal of Obstetrics and Gynecology 106,* 345-350.
100. Smith, D., Appell, R., Winters, C., & Rackley, R. (1997). Collagen injection therapy for female intrinsic sphincteric deficiency. *Journal of Urology 157,* 1275-1278.
101. Bartholomew, B., & Grimaldi, T. (1996). Collagen injection therapy for type III stress urinary incontinence. *AORN Journal 64*(1), 75-86.
102. Smith, D., Appell, R., Rackley, R., & Winters, C. (1998). Collagen injection therapy for post-prostatectomy incontinence. *Journal of Urology 160,* 364-367.
103. Kageyama, S., Kawabe, K., Suzuki, K., Ushiyama, T., Suzuki, T., & Aso, Y. (1994). Collagen implantation for post-prostatectomy incontinence: Early experience with a transrectal ultrasonographically guided method. *Journal of Urology 152,* 1473-1475.
104. Saltmarche, A., & Gartley, C. (1997). P97: Prevention of urinary incontinence: A consensus statement. *Ostomy/Wound Management 43*(10), 1-5.
105. Burgio, K., Locher, J., & Goode, P. (2000). Combined behavioral and drug therapy for urge incontinence in older women. *Journal of the American Geriatrics Society 48*(4), 370-374.
106. Palmer, M. (1997). Research in long-term care: What do we know, what can we use? *Ostomy/Wound Management 43*(10), 28-39.
107. Eustice, S., Roe, B., & Paterson, J. (2001). *Prompted voiding for the management of urinary incontinence in adults (Cochrane Review). Update.* Oxford, England: Cochrane Library Software.
108. Snow, T. (1988). Equipment for prevention, treatment, and management of urinary incontinence. *Topics in Geriatric Rehabilitation 3*(2), 58-77.
109. Fonda, D. (1999). Management of incontinence in older people. In P. Abrams, S. Khoury, & A. Wein (eds.), *Incontinence.* Plymouth, England: Health Publications.
110. Mold, J. (1996). Pharmacotherapy of urinary incontinence. *American Family Physician 54*(2), 673-680.
111. Petrilli, C., Traughber, B., & Schnelle, J. (1988). Behavioral management in the inpatient geriatric population. *Nursing Clinics of North America 23*(1), 265-277.
112. Burgio, K., Whitehead, W., & Engel, B. (1985). Urinary incontinence in the elderly. *Annals of Internal Medicine 103*(N4), 372-379.
113. Kegel, A. (1948). Progressive resistance exercises in the functional restoration of the perineal muscles. *American Journal of Obstetrics and Gynecology 56,* 238-248.
114. Dougherty, M. (1998). Current status of research on pelvic muscle strengthening techniques. *Journal of Wound, Ostomy and Continence Nursing 25*(2), 75-83.
115. Nygaard, I. (1996). Nonoperative management of urinary incontinence. *Current Opinion in Obstetrics and Gynecology 8,* 347-350.
116. Stevens, A., Burgio, L., Bailey, E., Burgio, K., Paul, P., Capilouto, E., et al. (1998). Teaching and maintaining behavior management skills with nursing assistants in a nursing home. *Gerontologist 38*(3), 379-384.
117. Agency for Health Care Policy and Research. (1996). Establishing, implementing, and continuing an effective continence program in a long-term care facility. AHCPR Pub. No. 96-0063. Rockville, Md.: Department of Health and Human Services.
118. Roberto, K., Wacker, R., Jewell, E., & Rickard, M. (1997). Resident rights. Knowledge of and implementation by nursing staff in long-term care facilities. *Journal of Gerontological Nursing 23*(12), 32-40.
119. Lekan-Rutledge, D., Palmer, M., & Belyea, M. (1998). In their own words: Nursing assistants' perceptions of

barriers to implementation of prompted voiding in long-term care. *Gerontologist 38*(3), 370-378.
120. Andersson, K., Appell, R., Cardozo, L., Chapple, C., Druitz, H., Finkbeiner, A., et al. (1999). Pharmacological treatment of urinary incontinence. In P. Abrams, S. Khoury, & A. Wein (eds.), *Incontinence.* Plymouth, England: Health Publications.
121. Griebling, T., & Nygaard, I. (1997). The role of estrogen replacement therapy in the management of urinary incontinence and urinary tract infection in post-menopausal women. *Endrocrinology and Metabolism Clinics of North America 26*(2), 347-360.
122. Wagg, A., & Malone-Lee, J. (1998). The management of urinary incontinence in the elderly. *British Journal of Urology 82*(Suppl 1), 11-17.
123. National Association for Continence. (2000). Resource guide (10th ed.). Spartansburg, S.C.: The Association.
124. Continence Products Evaluation Network. (1999). All-in-one disposable bodyworn pads for heavy incontinence. London, England. Medical Devices Agency, www.medical-devices.gov.uk.
125. Newman, D. (1999). *Urinary incontinence.* Los Angeles: Lowell House.
126. Palmer, M. (1994). A health-promotion perspective of urinary continence. *Nursing Outlook 42*(4), 163-169.
127. Fonda, D. (1990). Improving management of urinary incontinence in geriatric centres and nursing homes. Victorian Geriatricians Peer Review Group. *Australian Clinical Review* (Sydney) *10,* 66-71.
128. Dougherty, M., & Jenson, L. (1999). Managing urinary and fecal incontinence. In A. Hinshaw, S. Feetham, & J. Shaver (eds.), Handbook of clinical nursing research. Thousand Oaks, Calif.: Sage Publications.
129. Burgio, K., & Burgio, L. (1986). Behavioral therapies for urinary incontinence in the elderly. *Clinical Geriatric Medicine 2,* 809-827.
130. Colling, J., Ouslander, J., Hadley, B., Eisch, J., & Campbell, E. (1992). The effects of patterned urge-response toileting (PURT) on urinary incontinence among nursing home residents. *Journal of the American Geriatrics Society 40*(2), 135-141.
131. Engel, B., Burgio, L., McCormick, K., Hawkins, A., Scheve, A., & Leahy, E. (1990). Behavioral treatment of incontinence in the long-term care setting. *Journal of the American Geriatrics Society 38*(3), 361-363.
132. Palmer, M., Bennett, R., Mark, J., McCormick, K., & Engel, B. (1994). Urinary incontinence: A program that works. *Journal of Long Term Care Administration 22*(2), 19-25.
133. Peake, S., Manderson, L., & Potts, H. (1999). "Part and parcel of being a woman": Female urinary incontinence and constructions of control. *Medical Anthropology Quarterly 13*(3), 267-285.
134. Wells, T., Brink, C., & Diokno, A. (1987). Urinary incontinence in elderly women: Clinical findings. *Journal of the American Geriatrics Society 35,* 933-939.
135. Elser, D., Wyman, J., McClish, D., Robinson, D., Fantl, A., Bump, R., et al. (1999). The effect of bladder training, pelvic floor muscle training, or combination training on urodynamic parameters in women with urinary incontinence. *Neurology and Urodynamics 18,* 427-436.
136. Sampselle, C., Burns, P., Dougherty, M., Newman, D., Thomas, K., & Wyman, J. (1997). Continence for women: Evidence-based practice. *Journal of Obstetric, Gynecologic, & Neonatal Nursing 26*(4), 375-385.
137. Kincade, J., Johnson, T., Ashford-Works, C., Clark, M., & Busby-Whitehead, J. (1999). A pilot study to determine reasons for patient withdrawal from a pelvic muscle rehabilitation program for urinary incontinence. *Journal of Applied Gerontology 18*(3), 379-396.
138. Dowd, T., & Campbell, J. (1996). Fluid intake and urinary incontinence in older community-dwelling women. *Journal of Community Health Nursing 13*(3), 179-186.
139. Jirovec, M., & Templin, T. (2001). Predicting success using individualized scheduled toileting for memory-impaired elders at home. *Research in Nursing and Health 24*(1), 1-8.
140. Kelleher, C., & Khullar, V. (1997). A new questionnaire to assess the quality of life of urinary incontinent women. *British Journal of Obstetrics and Gynecology 104,* 1374-1379.
141. Burgio, K., & Ouslander, J. (1999). Effects of urge urinary incontinence on quality of life in older people. *Journal of the American Geriatrics Society 47*(8), 1032-1033.
142. Donovan, J., Naughton, M., Gotoh, M., Corcos, J., Jackson, S., Kelleher, C., Costa, P., & Lukacs, B. (1999). Symptoms and quality of life assessment. In P. Abrams, S. Khoury, & A. Wein (eds.), *Incontinence.* Plymouth, England: Health Publications.
143. Chiverton, P., Wells, T., Brink, C., & Mayer, R. (1996). Psychological factors associated with urinary incontinence. *Clinical Nurse Specialist 10*(5), 229-233.
144. Yarbro, C., & Ferrans, C. (1998). Quality of life of patients with prostate cancer treated with surgery or radiation therapy. *Oncology Nursing Forum 25*(4), 685-693.
145. Moore, K. (1999). The early post-operative concerns of men after radical prostatectomy. *Journal of Advanced Nursing 29*(5), 1121-1129.
146. Moore, K. (1999). A review of the anatomy of the male continence mechanism and the cause of urinary incontinence after prostatectomy. *Journal of Wound, Ostomy and Continence Nursing 26*(2), 86-93.
147. Lamhut, P., Jackson, T., & Wall, L. (1992). The treatment of urinary incontinence with electrical stimulation in nursing home patients: A pilot study. *Journal of the American Geriatrics Society 40*(1), 48-52.
148. Susset, J., Galea, G., Manbeck, K., & Susset, A. (1995). A predictive score index for the outcome of associated biofeedback and vaginal electrical stimulation in the treatment of female incontinence. *Journal of Urology 153,* 1461-1466.
149. Kondo, A., Yamada, Y., & Nijima, R. (1995). Treatment of stress incontinence by vaginal cones: Short and long term results and predictive parameters. *British Journal of Urology 76,* 464-466.
150. Nygaard, I., Kreder, K., Lepic, M., Fountain, K., & Rhomberg, A. (1996). Efficacy of pelvic floor muscle exercises in women with stress, urge, and mixed urinary incontinence. *American Journal of Obstetrics and Gynecology 174*(Part 1), 120-125.
151. Burgio, K., Locher, J., Goode, P., Hardin, M., McDowell, B., Dombrowski, M., et al. (1998). Behavioral versus drug treatment for urge urinary incontinence in older women: A randomized clinical trial. *Journal of the American Medical Association 280*(23), 1995-2000.
152. Berghmans, L., Hendriks, H., DeBie, R., Van Doorn, E., Bo, K., & Kerrebroeck, P. (2000). Conservative treatment of urge urinary incontinence in women: A systematic review of randomized clinical trials. *BJU International 85,* 254-263.
153. Weinberger, M., Goodman, B., & Carnes, M. (1999). Long-term efficacy of nonsurgical urinary incontinence treatment in elderly women. *Journal of Gerontology 54A*(3), M117-M121.

154. Fonda, D. (1997). Promoting continence as a health issue. *European Urology 32*(Suppl 2), 28-32.
155. Lightner, D. (1999). Conservative management for urinary incontinence. American Urological Association Update Series, Lesson 15, pp. 114-120, Houston: American Urologic Association, Inc., office of Education.
156. Stanley, R. (1998). Applying the four principles of ethics to continence care. *British Journal of Nursing 7*(1), 45-51.
157. Sampselle, C., Burns, P., Dougherty, M., Newman, D., Kelly, T., Wyman, J. (1997). Continence for women: An evidence-based practice. *Journal of Obstetrics, Gynecology, and Neonatal Nursing 26*(4), 375-385.
158. Roe, B., Doll, H., & Wilson, K. (1999). Help seeking behaviour and health and social services utilisation by people suffering from urinary incontinence. *International Journal of Nursing Studies 36,* 245-253.
159. Pannek, J., Haupt, G., Sommerfeld, H., Schulze, H., & Senge, T. (1996). Urodynamic and rectomanometric findings in urinary incontinence. *Scandinavian Journal of Urology and Nephrology 30,* 457-460.
160. Gordon, D., Groutz, A., Goldman, G., Avni, A., Wolf, Y., Lessing, J., & Menachem, D. (1999). Anal incontinence: Prevalence among female patients attending a urogynecologic clinic. *Neurourology and Urodynamics 18,* 199-204.
161. Wall, L., & DeLancey, J. (1991). The politics of prolapse: A revisionist approach to disorders of the pelvic floor in women. *Perspectives in Biology and Medicine 34*(4), 486-496.

CHAPTER

7 Addiction

BETHANY J. PHOENIX & MARY ELLEN WEWERS

DEFINITION

The term *addiction* has been used to describe many compulsive, problematic patterns of behavior, such as "sex addiction" or "gambling addiction." However, addiction most commonly implies persistent, maladaptive use of psychoactive substances, such as alcohol, tobacco, and street drugs despite negative consequences. The *Diagnostic and Statistical Manual of Mental Disorders,* 4th Edition (DSM-IV),[1] identifies two types of persistent substance use disorders, *substance abuse* and *substance dependence* (Box 7-1). Substance abuse encompasses a range of dysfunctional substance use behaviors. These range from occasional use accompanied by hazardous behavior (e.g., drunk driving) to bingeing. Substance dependence involves use that is more frequent, more compulsive, and accompanied by a wider range of negative consequences. There may also be physical adaptations to heavy substance use, such as tolerance and withdrawal.[1]

Despite clear behavioral differences between substance abuse and dependence, some authors propose that the concept of addiction encompasses both.[2] Others suggest that there is a qualitative change when heavy use becomes dependence.[3] Although research is clarifying some of the persistent brain changes associated with dependence, no clear demarcation point can be established between substance abuse and dependence.

This chapter will include both the categories of substance abuse and dependence, because both involve repeated use of psychoactive substances despite negative consequences. The discussion of pathophysiological processes will rely primarily on research that has used samples of substance dependent individuals.

We will discuss information about addiction to a range of substances. However, particular emphasis will be placed on cigarette smoking as an example of an addictive behavior. The Surgeon General's groundbreaking report in 1988 determined that nicotine is the primary psychoactive agent in cigarette smoke that is responsible for dependence.[4] The DSM-IV includes nicotine dependence as a disorder,[1] because tolerance, withdrawal, and pleasant (euphoriant) effects are produced by tobacco use.[4]

PREVALENCE AND POPULATIONS AT RISK

Addictive behavior is widespread in the United States, although specific prevalence estimates vary widely depending on the criteria used to define addiction. A large population survey done in the early 1980s using criteria from the DSM-III found that 16.7% of American adults had experienced a substance use disorder at some point in their lives—13.5% involving alcohol use, and 6.1% involving other drugs. The survey also found that 6.1% of the population had experienced substance-related problems in the last 6 months (4.8% alcohol, 2.0% other drugs).[5] Approximately 10 years later, a similar epidemiological survey using slightly revised criteria found a 26.6% lifetime rate of substance abuse or dependence (23.5% alcohol, 11.9% other drugs), with 11.3% of the population having had problems in the past year.[6] Both surveys indicate that a high proportion of persons with drug use disorders also misuse alcohol.

Prevalence of cigarette smoking among adults in the United States has remained unchanged throughout the past decade. It was estimated that in 1997, 48 million American adults, or 24.7%, were classified as current smokers (i.e., self-reported use of cigarettes every day or most days).[7] It is estimated that 34.8% of all U.S. high school students use some form of tobacco, with 9.2% of middle school students and 28.4% of high school students categorized as current cigarette smokers (i.e., used within the past 30 days).[8]

In general, rates of substance abuse and dependence are about twice as high in men as in women, although this varies considerably by culture and by substance. Among adults in the United States, male smoking prevalence is slightly higher (27.6%) as

BOX 7-1 DSM-IV Criteria for Substance Dependence and Substance Abuse

Criteria for Substance Dependence

A maladaptive pattern of substance use, leading to clinically significant impairment or distress, as manifested in three or more of the following, occurring at any time in the same 12-month period:

1. Tolerance, as defined by either of the following:
   - Need for markedly increased amounts of the substance to achieve intoxication or desired effect
   - Markedly diminished effect with continued use of the same amount of the substance
2. Withdrawal
3. The substance is often taken in larger amounts or over a longer period than was intended
4. There is a persistent desire or unsuccessful efforts to cut down or control substance use
5. A great deal of time is spent in activities necessary to obtain the substance, use the substance, or recover from its effects
6. Important social, occupational, or recreational activities are given up or reduced because of substance use
7. The substance use is continued despite knowledge of having a persistent or recurrent physical or psychological problem that is likely to have been caused or exacerbated by the substance

Criteria for Substance Abuse

A maladaptive pattern of substance use, leading to clinically significant impairment or distress, as manifested by one or more of the following, occurring within a 12-month period:

1. Recurrent substance use resulting in a failure to fulfill major role obligations at work, school, or home
2. Recurrent substance use in situations in which it is physically hazardous
3. Recurrent substance-related legal problems
4. Continued substance use despite having persistent or recurrent social or interpersonal problems caused or exacerbated by the effects of the substance
5. Symptoms have never met the criteria for Substance Dependence for this class of substance

American Psychiatric Association. (1994). *Diagnostic and statistical manual of mental disorders* (4th ed., text revision). Washington, D.C.: Author.

compared with females (22.1%).[7] However, prevalence of smoking among women is expected to surpass that estimated for men early in the twenty-first century.[9] Smokeless tobacco use is more prevalent in males compared with females (30.7% vs. 4.8%).[10]

Age also affects substance use and abuse. In a meta-analysis of longitudinal studies of drinking behavior, Fillmore et al[11] noted that in most cultures, the quantity of alcohol consumed per occasion is highest in the late teens and early twenties. Notably, among smokers, those aged 18 to 24 and 25 to 44 now have almost identical prevalence estimates (28.7% and 28.6%, respectively).[7] In the past, only smokers aged 25 to 44 had prevalence estimates of this magnitude. This change is disturbing and indicates an increased use of tobacco among younger adults.

When racial and ethnic groups are looked at in the aggregate, differences in rates of addiction are not striking. Native Americans tend to have higher rates of alcohol and drug addiction than others, and addiction rates for Asian Americans and Pacific Islanders tend to be lower.[12] However, there is considerable variation in substance use patterns within ethnic groups based on such factors as socioeconomic status, geographic location, and degree of acculturation.

Smoking prevalence is disproportionately higher among certain minority groups in the United States.[13] Recent estimates range from 15.3% to 39.2%, with Asian Americans and Pacific Islanders reporting the lowest prevalence and Native Americans and Alaska Natives the highest. However, considerable variation exists within ethnic subgroups. For example, among Southeast Asian immigrant men, estimates of 43% have been recently reported. The prevalence of smoking among African American adults in 1994 to 1995 was 26.5%, similar to white adults (25.9%) during the same time interval. The overall smoking prevalence estimate among Hispanic adults during 1994 to 1995 was 18.9%, with males significantly higher than females (22.9% vs. 15.1%).

RISK FACTORS

It is generally agreed that addiction is a heterogeneous phenomenon that is influenced by a variety of factors.[14,15] These include social/environmental, psychological/behavioral, developmental, and biological determinants[16] (Figure 7-1). Risk factors for addiction can be considered in two categories. The first includes risk factors that determine whether an individual will be exposed to heavy substance use, and these risks are primarily social and environmental. The second category comprises

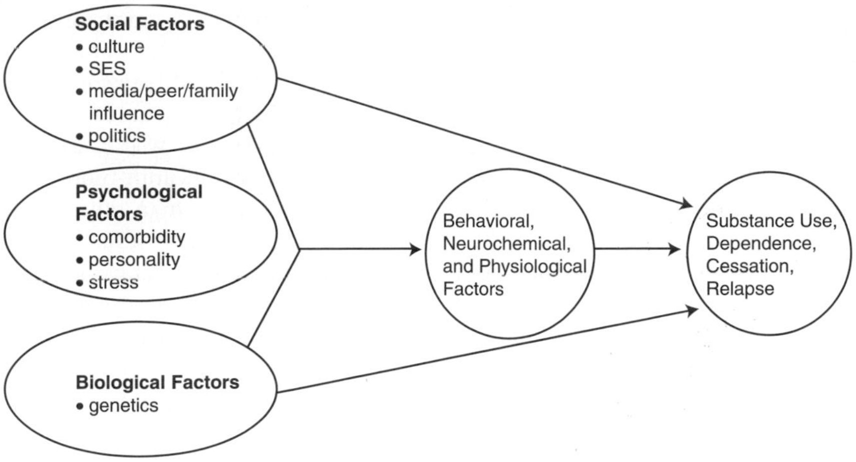

Figure 7-1 Biobehavioral model of addiction. (National Cancer Institute. National Institutes of Health [1998]. Adapted from Anderson, Office of Behavioral and Social Sciences Research. Published in Tobacco Research Implementation Group [1998]. Tobacco research implementation plan. Priorities for tobacco research beyond the year 2000.)

the factors that determine whether persistent use will lead to addiction. These are primarily inherent in the individual and include biological, developmental, and psychological risk factors.

Environmental Factors

Factors in the physical and social environment that determine exposure to addictive substances include substance use patterns in the family and peer group, laws and regulations governing distribution and use of a substance, and economic factors, such as advertising and marketing.

Family and Peer Influences. Social learning governs the development of substance use habits. By observing the behavior of family members and peers, individuals learn what types of psychoactive substance use are socially sanctioned.[17] In addition to role-modeling appropriate or inappropriate substance use behavior, parents and friends may be part of rituals that initiate children into substance use. It has been observed that most smokers are surrounded by family members and friends who also smoke, thus providing strong cues for continued engagement in the behavior.[18,19]

Two contrasting examples illustrate how children's socialization into substance use may either increase or decrease their risk for addiction. In his memoir, *Angela's Ashes*,[20] Frank McCourt describes how Irish boys were brought to the local pub at age 15 by their fathers for a "first pint." Boys were socialized into regular heavy drinking in all-male environments outside the home. Drinking to the point of intoxication was common and socially sanctioned. Like McCourt's father, many of the men in this community experienced problems associated with alcohol abuse and dependence, such as marital conflict and poverty caused by "drinking up their paychecks."

In Jewish families, socialization to alcohol use is typically quite different. Children begin drinking wine with their families. Consumption is minimal, and the wine is drunk in religious rituals with no intent to cause intoxication. Persons raised using alcohol in this way are noted to have a reduced risk of alcohol problems.[17]

In many communities, peer groups surpass families in their influence on substance use behavior. In the United States, adolescents typically begin experimenting with alcohol, cigarettes, and drugs with peers. When with peers, teens are more likely to become intoxicated and to engage in hazardous behaviors.[17]

Education and Socioeconomic Status. Level of educational attainment appears to be an excellent predictor of tobacco consumption. Marked differences in tobacco use initiation, prevalence, and quitting are related to education, with less educated persons having higher levels of initiation and prevalence and lower levels of cessation.[21] It has also been reported that socioeconomically disadvantaged persons in the United States have a higher prevalence of tobacco consumption.[9]

Economic and Legal Influences. Because exposure to a psychoactive agent is a key factor in developing addiction, ready availability of such substances in a community increases the risk of addictive problems. Legal substances such as alcohol and cigarettes are widely distributed and advertised, although legal and regulatory constraints limit their accessibility to minors. Although the production and distribution of illegal drugs is necessarily more clandestine, these substances may nevertheless be widely available in some communities, even to children.

Cost is a potent factor influencing substance use. There is evidence from numerous econometric studies that increases in cigarette prices lead to reductions in smoking.[22] These reductions include both the amount of cigarettes consumed by an individual and the overall prevalence of smoking within the population. In addition, youths and young adults are much more responsive to the price of cigarettes than older adults are.[23] Similarly, decreases in cost can increase use of a drug. Cocaine became widely used in inner-city communities when crack, a much cheaper and more easily consumed form of the drug, was introduced.[24]

Personal Risk Factors

Psychological and Behavioral Influences. Personality testing has failed to consistently identify an "addictive personality." However, it does appear that two broad dimensions of personality, behavioral dysregulation and negative emotionality, increase the risk of substance use disorders.[25]

Addiction may be one of a complex of maladaptive behaviors resulting from an underlying defect in behavioral regulation; other manifestations may include hyperactivity, impulsivity, sensation-seeking, and conduct disorder. The link between impulsive and antisocial behavior and substance abuse is demonstrated by the extremely high rate (83%) of lifetime substance use disorders in persons diagnosed with antisocial personality disorder.[5] Behavioral characteristics such as novelty seeking have been hypothesized as correlates of tobacco use.[26]

The tendency to experience negative mood states, such as depression and anxiety, also has been robustly correlated with substance abuse and addiction.[27,28] The idea that some addicts "self-medicate" persistent unpleasant mood states has been widely discussed in the substance abuse literature. Khantzian's psychodynamic self-medication theory[29] proposes that an addict selects his or her "drug of choice" based on its ability to compensate for defects in the ability to regulate emotions. In addition to influencing the initial development of an addiction, negative mood states have been demonstrated to increase the risk of relapse after substance abuse treatment[27] and smoking cessation.[30]

Not surprisingly, substantial evidence exists that persons with psychiatric disorders are at increased risk of developing substance use disorders. An analysis of Epidemiologic Catchment Area (ECA) data[5] found that persons with any of the psychiatric disorders studied which included mood, psychotic, and anxiety disorders, as well as antisocial personality disorder, were significantly more likely to have a substance use disorder than others in the population. Persons with the most severe psychiatric disorders were the most likely to abuse substances. For example, people with schizophrenia had a rate of substance use disorder 4.6 times as high as that of the general population, and people with bipolar illness were 6.6 times as likely to suffer from addiction.[5]

Psychiatric comorbidity is more common in smokers than in the general population. Regular smoking has been reported to occur more frequently among individuals who had experienced a major depressive disorder than among individuals who had never experienced major depression or among individuals with no psychiatric diagnosis.[31] Further, smokers with major depression were observed to be less successful in achieving long-term abstinence from smoking. In addition, a very high percentage of patients with schizophrenia smoke and many express little interest in cessation.[32]

Reasons for the high rate of psychiatric/substance abuse comorbidity may include physiological factors, such as alterations in neurotransmitter systems that increase vulnerability to addiction. Such alterations may be caused either by psychiatric illness or the medications used for its treatment. Both psychiatric and substance use disorders may be precipitated by similar experiences, such as exposure to abuse or trauma. Addiction may develop as a response to stigma, joblessness, and other social disadvantages related to living with a disabling mental illness.[33]

Genetic Influences

A significant body of evidence implicates genetic influences in the development of addictive disorders. Research on male twin pairs suggests that 60% to 80% of the liability for abuse or dependence of stimulants, sedatives, cocaine, and opiates is inherited.[34] In addition, the genetics of alcohol abuse and dependence has been extensively studied in the United States, Europe, and elsewhere. Heritability of alcohol use disorders is estimated to be approximately 40% to 60% in men (35) and 51% to 59% in women.[36]

First-degree relatives of alcoholics have a substantially greater likelihood of developing alcohol-related problems. Children of alcoholic parents demonstrate three to four times more alcoholism than children of nonalcoholics.[37,38] That this is the result more of genetic influences than of social learning, cultural influence, or other environmental factors common to family members is suggested by the results of twin and adoption studies. Twin studies demonstrate that monozygotic twins have higher rates of concordance in alcoholism diagnoses than dizygotic twins do.[35,36] Alcoholism in a biological parent is a more reliable predictor of alcoholism in adoptees than is alcoholism in the adoptive parent.[39-41]

Because alcoholism is a heterogeneous condition with a multifactorial etiological picture, there are a number of factors thought to be under genetic control that may be responsible for its development. Personality characteristics such as impulsivity are thought to be heritable,[25] as are psychiatric disorders such as bipolar illness,[42] and these factors increase the risk of alcohol use disorders. In addition, studies of factors specific to alcohol use have revealed that offspring of alcoholics are likely to have a less intense response to ethanol and thus can drink more heavily without being conscious of intoxication.[39] In a heavy-drinking milieu, lack of this warning feedback may lead to consistent heavy drinking and the consequent development of alcohol-related problems.

Evidence indicates that smoking behavior also has a genetic component. Studies in twins have determined that monozygotic twins are more similar in terms of smoking than dizygotic twins are.[43,44] Similarly, large cohort studies of twins in Sweden and Finland have estimated that genetics accounts for 53% of the total variance in smoking.[45] Findings from the National Heart, Lung, and Blood Institute Twin Study suggest that a common genetic factor may contribute to the use of tobacco, alcohol, and coffee.[46]

MECHANISMS

The neurobiology of addiction is currently the focus of numerous research efforts, and understanding of this complex phenomenon is developing rapidly. Although some of the mechanisms involved are substance specific, there appears to be processes common to all addictions that lead to persistent changes in brain functioning. Leshner[3] noted that addiction is not just a matter of using a large quantity of drugs: "Addiction is a qualitatively different state because the addicted brain is, in fact, different in its neurobiology from the nonaddicted brain." Although not all of the neurobiological processes involved in addiction have been well explained, there are several processes that appear to explain addicts' apparent "loss of control" over their substance use. These involve multiple brain structures and neurobiological processes.

Brain Reward System

The mesolimbic dopamine system has been identified as a reward pathway in the brain.[3] It consists of a collection of structures extending from the midbrain into the prefrontal cortex (Figure 7-2). The function of this system is to reward behaviors that ensure survival for the individual or the species, such as eating or procreating. These behaviors activate the mesolimbic dopamine system, stimulating dopamine release in the nucleus accumbens, which leads to a feeling of satisfaction or well-being.[3]

All drugs of abuse share the ability to stimulate the mesolimbic dopamine system artificially and produce feelings of satisfaction or euphoria.[3] Conscious enjoyment of these euphoric effects is a powerful reinforcer for continued drug use. In addition, the similarity between the process of drug-related stimulation of the brain reward system and stimulation of this system by survival-related behaviors essentially misleads the preconscious brain to conclude that use of the substance is good for the individual, when in fact it is not. Classical conditioning occurs as the brain reward system is repeatedly stimulated, progressively strengthening the association between substance use with its attendant circumstances and feelings of well-being.[47]

The association of drug use with euphoric effects is considered to be one of the primary mechanisms involved in the *initiation* of a drug habit. However, some authors suggest that the enduring sensitization of dopamine systems seen in addictive use does not mediate pleasure but is instead involved in assigning motivational significance to external stimuli. According to the incentive-sensitization theory of addiction proposed by Robinson and Berridge,[48] dopamine systems become progressively more sensitized and the brain develops an increasingly strong focus on drug-related stimuli: "Thus 'wanting' is gradually transformed into craving, drugs become craved to the relative exclusion of all else, and drug-associated stimuli elicit this craving independent of any pleasure they produce."

The proposition that the euphoric properties of drugs of abuse are separate from their reinforcing properties is supported by several observations. First, some drugs with euphoric properties, such as marijuana and MDMA ("ecstasy"), rarely become the focus of compulsive use. In contrast, nicotine

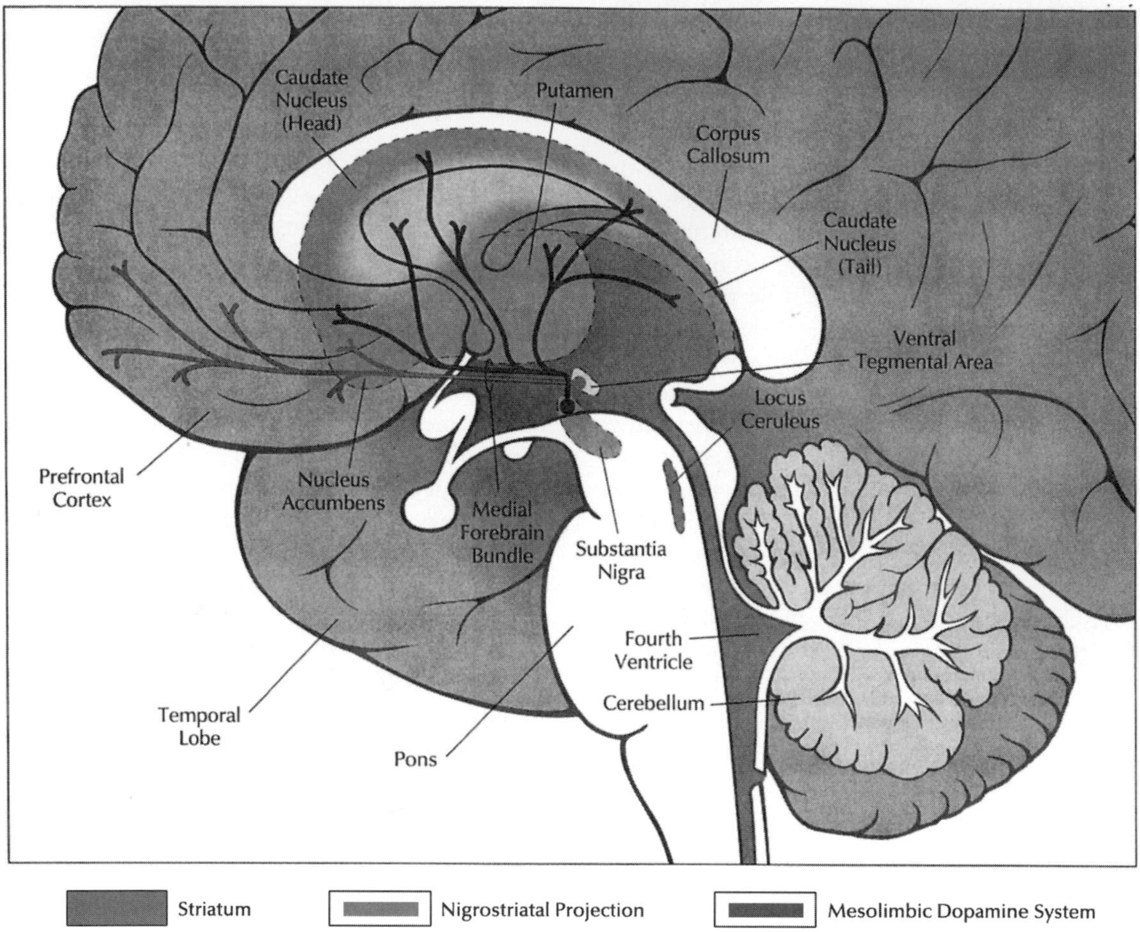

Figure 7-2 **Brain reward pathways. The mesolimbic dopamine system plays an important role in producing pleasurable responses to natural rewards, such as food and sex. Abused drugs produce a surge of dopamine release in the nucleus accumbens, which is thought to contribute to euphoric drug effects.** (From Leshner, A.I. [1997]. Drug abuse and addiction are biomedical problems. *Hospital Practice* [Special Report], 3.)

is a decidedly addictive drug, but produces little euphoric or "high" effect, relative to other drugs of abuse.[49] Second, addicts frequently report that they continue compulsive drug use long after it has ceased to be pleasurable, and indeed, has become associated with many aversive consequences.[50]

Negative Affect

In addition to the drug-associated learning that connects substance use to positive affects, addiction may lead to long-term changes that inhibit the ability to experience pleasure.[51] Accommodation to intense artificial stimulation of the brain's pleasure centers by substances of abuse leads to a decrease in the ability to enjoy normally pleasurable stimuli, creating negative affect in the absence of the drug. This dysphoria occurs not only in acute withdrawal states (e.g., "crash" after a cocaine binge), but may persist even after long periods of abstinence. Koob[51] noted that this is due not only to changes in the mesolimbic dopamine system, but to changes in neurotransmitter systems involving serotonin, GABA, and endorphins.

Pomerleau and Pomerleau[52] described a biobehavioral model of smoking explaining the relationship between nicotine and the dysphoric states that accompany deprivation, often leading to a resumption of smoking. The model suggests that nicotine provides strong reinforcement to continue smoking, via neuroregulatory mechanisms that improve mood and relieve dysphoria. Based on the biobehavioral model of smoking, and as applied to relapse, smokers may be at increased risk for resuming the behavior because they have learned to "cope" with dysphoric states, or negative affect, by smoking. When anxiety-producing situations occur during tobacco abstinence, smokers may resume the behavior because of the strong reinforcement properties that nicotine provides, via the release of neuromodulators (e.g., dopamine, serotonin) known to improve mood states.

Drug-Induced Cortical Changes

In addition to the acute and long-term positive reinforcing effects of drug use and the persistent anhedonia, or diminished ability to experience pleasure, that occurs when the brain is deprived of drugs to which it has become accustomed, repeated drug use causes changes in the brain's cortex. The use of PET scans has demonstrated that cocaine use causes decreased glucose metabolism in parts of the frontal cortex that persist over 3 months.[53] Parts of the cortex that are inactivated by cocaine use (i.e., the orbitofrontal cortex and cingulate gyrus), are involved in controlling repetitive behavior. Abnormalities in these cortical areas also are seen in individuals with obsessive-compulsive disorder, and may account for the compulsive repetition of behaviors for which there is no conscious motivation.[54] Persistent inactivation of the cortex by drug use may contribute to the compulsive, driven quality of substance use that is no longer even pleasurable.[50]

Maltzman[55] made a similar case that chronic alcohol use leads to inactivation and atrophy of the frontal lobes of the brain. Because foresight, planning, and other executive functions of the brain are centered in the frontal lobes, dysfunction of these areas leads to inability to anticipate the consequences of one's actions and make appropriate plans, and failure to override impulses from other brain areas. In addition, the frontal lobes play an important role in modulating emotions and assigning motivation, therefore, frontal lobe dysfunction can lead to derangements in mood and motivation.

In summary, the pathophysiology of addiction appears to involve a cascade of drug-related changes in brain functions. Initially, the activation of brain reward circuitry leads to a strong association between drug use and feelings of euphoria and well-being. Repeated stimulation of mesolimbic dopamine systems involved in assigning motivational significance eventually leads to compulsive desire for drugs independent of any pleasurable effects. Simultaneously, repeated artificial stimulation of the brain reward system resets the threshold for experiencing pleasure. Addicts have difficulty experiencing pleasure in response to natural pleasurable events, and experience negative affect in the absence of drugs. Some of the brain circuitry involved in memory, as well as parts of the brain's frontal cortex responsible for executive functions such as evaluating, planning, and decision-making, experience reduced activity and are less able to override powerful drives toward drug use.

Childress et al[56] drew parallels between the alterations seen in addicted brains on PET scans and the experience of addicted individuals:

> The lack of hippocampal activation during craving suggests the subordination of explicit (factual) memory to an amygdala-driven emotional state. The developing brain signature of cue-induced craving is thus consistent with its clinical phenomenology: the drug user is gripped by a visceral emotional state, experiences a highly focused incentive to act, and is remarkably unencumbered by the memory of negative consequences of drug taking.

PATHOLOGICAL CONSEQUENCES

In addition to the distortions in brain functioning detailed above, addiction can lead to numerous pathological consequences in other body systems, depending on the substance involved and the route of administration. For instance, when needles are shared to inject drugs such as cocaine or heroin, blood-borne diseases such as hepatitis and HIV can be spread. Heart and lung damage is caused by a cascade of events that are triggered with cigarette smoking and results in emphysema and coronary heart disease. Box 7-2 provides a list of some of the more common sequelae of addiction.

RELATED PATHOPHYSIOLOGICAL CONCEPTS

Physiological dependence, demonstrated by *tolerance* and *withdrawal,* is usually part of addiction and may characterize individuals with a more severe clinical course.[57] This is not true for all substances—for example, marijuana typically produces very little tolerance and no consistent withdrawal syndrome has been identified.[1] It is also true that persons can experience physiological dependence without the behavioral dyscontrol characteristic of addiction. For instance, postsurgical patients treated with narcotic pain medications may develop tolerance and experience withdrawal if these medications are withdrawn too abruptly without developing drug craving or using the medications in larger amounts than intended.

Tolerance

Tolerance is the need for a markedly increased amount of the addictive substance to achieve intoxication that develops with continued use, or the substantial decrease in effect from using the same amount.[1] Although the exact neural mechanisms involved vary from substance to substance, in general, tolerance represents a process in which compensatory neurophysiological changes offset the primary action of the particular substance of abuse. For instance, alcohol produces its depressant effect by disrupting the function of glutamate, the brain's major excitatory neurotransmitter. Chronic interference with the function of glutamate, and associated inhibition of the neurotransmitters serotonin, dopamine, norepinephrine, and gamma-aminobutyric acid (GABA), lead to compensatory up-regulation or supersensitivity of postsynaptic receptors.[58] As applied to cigarettes, acute pharmacodynamic tolerance occurs rapidly during smoking and appears to be related to nicotine's occupancy of its receptors, which is related to nicotine concentrations in the blood.[59]

BOX 7-2 Pathological Consequences of Addiction by Substance or Route of Administration*

Alcohol
Liver damage/cirrhosis
Esophageal varices
Gastritis
Pancreatitis
Impotence/sexual dysfunction
Fetal abnormalities
Withdrawal seizures
Peripheral neuropathy
Dementia
Suicide

Tobacco
Cancers, especially lung, head and neck, bladder, pancreas
Chronic bronchitis
Emphysema
Cardiac disease, especially coronary artery disease and hypertension
Impotence
Low-birthweight infants, spontaneous abortion
Peripheral vascular disease

Intravenous Drug Use
HIV infection
Hepatitis B and C
Subacute bacterial endocarditis
Wound infections
Necrotizing fasciitis
Overdose death

Stimulants (Cocaine and Amphetamine)
Paranoid psychoses
Violent behavior
Cerebral vascular accident
Myocardial infarction

*Partial list.

Withdrawal

Withdrawal occurs when blood or tissue concentrations of a substance rapidly decline in a person who has had prolonged heavy use of that substance and produces symptoms opposite to the action of the drug. With alcohol, tolerance produces a situation in which postsynaptic neurons become supersensitive to the effects of neurotransmitters. When ethanol is no longer present to produce the accustomed interference with neurotransmission, postsynaptic neurons are excessively stimulated. This produces signs of autonomic hyperactivity, such as sweating, tachycardia, hypertension, and tremors, and can produce CNS symptoms such as agitation, delirium, and seizures.[60]

A nicotine withdrawal syndrome has been well described[1] (Box 7-3). The syndrome is variable in terms of character, severity and duration.[61] Symptoms have been reported to occur within the first

BOX 7-3 DSM-IV Criteria for Nicotine Withdrawal

A. Daily use of nicotine for at least several weeks
B. Abrupt cessation of nicotine use, or reduction in the amount of nicotine used, followed within 24 hours by four (or more) of the following signs:
   1. Dysphoric or depressed mood
   2. Insomnia
   3. Irritability, frustration, or anger
   4. Anxiety
   5. Difficulty concentrating
   6. Restlessness
   7. Decreased heart rate
   8. Increased appetite or weight gain
C. The symptoms in Criterion B cause clinically significant distress or impairment in social, occupational, or other important areas of functioning.
D. The symptoms are not due to a general medical condition and are not better accounted for by another mental disorder.

American Psychiatric Association. (1994). *Diagnostic and statistical manual of mental disorders* (4th ed., text revision), Washington, D.C.

24 hours postcessation,[61] are most prominent during the first 3 to 5 days after quitting[62] and can persist for 14 days and longer.[63]

MANIFESTATIONS

The manifestations of addictive behavior are extremely various, depending on the substance of abuse, route of administration, and stage of the disorder. The effects of alcohol and cocaine on the central nervous system are discussed briefly below, although both substances cause additional wide-ranging alterations in body systems. Although crises such as a traumatic injury while intoxicated, drunk driving arrest, or workplace problems related to substance use may reveal substance-related problems, physical signs of addiction often do not appear until late in the disorder.[64]

Cocaine is a stimulant that may be smoked, snorted, or injected. The drug can cause vasoconstriction and vasospasm, which may potentially lead to myocardial infarctions, cerebrovascular accidents, or sudden death. Sustained deficits in brain perfusion may lead to persistent compromise in neuropsychological functioning. Alteration in brain dopamine systems may lead to psychotic symptoms, particularly paranoia, and periods of severe depression when the intoxicating effects of cocaine have worn off. The association of cocaine use with increased sexual activity, often with multiple partners, results from the drug's ability to stimulate sexual interest and excitement. Disturbances in appetite often result in severe weight loss.[65]

Alcohol, consumed in beverages, is a central nervous system depressant. People with histories of heavy drinking may experience blackouts, acute anterograde amnesia for events occurring during an episode of intoxication.[66] Alcoholic hallucinosis, or auditory hallucinations that occur in a clear state of consciousness in the absence of other alcohol withdrawal symptoms, is another potential complication of alcohol addiction.

The combination of toxic effects of alcohol on brain tissue and nutritional deficiencies associated with alcoholism can lead to more persistent neurological abnormalities. Wernicke's encephalopathy, an acute neuropsychiatric syndrome presenting with confusion, ataxia, and abnormal eye movements, results from severe thiamine deficiency. If untreated, Wernicke's encephalopathy can progress to Korsakoff's psychosis. This syndrome is misnamed, since it is characterized by persistent memory disturbances, confabulation, and personality deterioration, and does not present with psychotic symptoms.[67] Continued heavy drinking can lead to cerebellar degeneration and dementia.[66]

MEASUREMENT

Routine substance abuse screening for all patients is recommended in primary care settings.[64] A number of screening tests are available for this purpose, including the Alcohol Use Disorders Identification Test (AUDIT); the Michigan Alcoholism Screening Test (MAST), which also comes in short and geriatric versions; and the Problem Oriented Screening Instrument for Teenagers (POSIT). Perhaps the best-known screening test for alcoholism is the CAGE, which can be adapted to include drugs (Box 7-4). The Center for Substance Abuse Treatment[64] also recommends asking patients if they have used street drugs more than five times in their lives. A positive answer indicates a need for further screening.

If substance abuse or dependence is suspected, a more thorough assessment should be done. Detailed assessment of substance use should include all drugs used, route of administration, quantity and frequency of use, circumstances of use, and associated high-risk behavior, such as drunk driving or unsafe sex. Sequelae or consequences of use should also be assessed, including legal complications, impaired role functioning, family discord, and physical and psychological problems. The Addiction Severity Index (ASI) is the instrument most commonly used in research and clinical practice to assess patterns of substance use and associated problems. The ASI is a structured clinical interview that collects

BOX 7-4 The CAGE Questionnaire Adapted to Include Drugs (CAGE-AID)

- Have you felt you ought to **cut down** on your drinking or drug use?
- Have people **annoyed** you by criticizing your drinking or drug use?
- Have you felt bad or **guilty** about your drinking or drug use?
- Have you ever had a drink or used drugs first thing in the morning to steady your nerves or get rid of a hangover **(eye-opener)?**

One positive answer indicates a need for further evaluation.

Mayfield, D., McLeod, G., & Hall, P. (1974). The CAGE questionnaire: Validation of a new alcoholism screening instrument. *American Journal of Psychiatry, 131*, 238–246.

information in seven areas potentially affected by substance use to yield a score of severity of addiction.

Given the tendency of addicted persons to deny or minimize the problems associated with their substance use, the assessment process should occur over a period of time and include information from multiple sources. Collateral sources may include family members or other treatment providers, if permission is obtained from the patient. Laboratory tests, such as blood or urine toxicology, can establish drug or alcohol use, and liver function tests may reveal organ damage due to substance use.

The most common approach to identifying tobacco use is asking about current consumption patterns. Self-reported current smoking is generally defined as daily use, or use that occurs on most days.[68] Selected groups may be at risk for underreporting and include persons with smoking-related diseases, pregnant women, adolescents and those in cessation treatment.[69] Although biochemical measures of tobacco smoke exposure are available, the more sophisticated assays for nicotine and cotinine (i.e., the major metabolite of nicotine) are usually reserved for research studies.[70] In clinical practice, expired air carbon monoxide (CO_a) analysis can be performed and is a reliable, noninvasive and inexpensive method of assessing smoking status.[71] Disadvantages of CO_a analysis include its relatively short half-life and the inability to detect smokeless tobacco use.[72] To assist with misclassification because of CO's relatively short half-life, it is recommended that CO_a assessment be performed in the afternoon to permit an accumulation of CO in the body.

Another frequently used specialized smoking measure is the Fagerstrom Test for Nicotine Dependence (FTND) (Figure 7-3), a six-item paper and pencil tool that assesses nicotine dependence.[73] Two specific FTND items, the time to first cigarette of the day and number of cigarettes smoked per day, are especially useful. Nicotine replacement therapy,

1. How soon after you wake up do you smoke your first cigarette?

   ___ Within 5 minutes (3 points)
   ___ 6-30 minutes (2 points)
   ___ 31-60 minutes (1 point)
   ___ >60 minutes (0 points)

2. Do you find it difficult to refrain from smoking or using tobacco products in places where it is forbidden, (e.g., church, at the library, in the cinema, etc.)?

   ___ Yes (1 point) ___ No (0 points)

3. Which cigarette would you hate most to give up?

   ___ First one in the morning (1 point) ___ All others (0 points)

4. How many cigarettes/day do you smoke?

   ___ 10 or less (0 points)
   ___ 11-20 (1 point)
   ___ 21-30 (2 points)
   ___ 31 or more (3 points)

5. Do you smoke more frequently during the first hours of waking than during the rest of the day?

   ___ Yes (1 point) ___ No (0 points)

6. Do you smoke if you are so ill that you are in bed all day?

   ___ Yes (1 point) ___ No (0 points)

Total score of greater than 7 indicates nicotine dependence.

Figure 7-3 Fagerstrom Test for Nicotine Dependence (FTND). (Heatherton, T.F., Kozlowski, L.T., Frecker, R.C., & Fagerstrom, K.O. [1991]. The Fagerstrom Test for Nicotine Dependence: A revision of the Fagerstrom Tolerance Questionnaire. *British Journal of Addiction 86,* 1119–1127.)

in the form of 4 mg gum, is generally recommended for those attempting cessation who are categorized as highly nicotine dependent (greater than 7).[74]

Nonjudgmental interviewing techniques, such as using neutral language and normalizing substance use, increase the validity of patient reports and are likely to produce less resistance. An empathetic interviewing style that highlights incongruity of patient goals with continued substance use but acknowledges ambivalence toward change has been shown to be more effective than a confrontational style in increasing motivation to change substance use patterns.[75]

CLINICAL MANAGEMENT

When the assessment indicates a need for substance abuse treatment and the patient is willing to accept treatment, a plan for clinical management can be developed. A plan for substance abuse treatment should consider the intensity of treatment, types of treatment available, and need for treatment of associated conditions.

Treatment Intensity

For persons with substance abuse or high-risk use, brief interventions (one or two sessions) have proved effective in reducing substance-related problems. Such interventions include specific feedback about the harms or potential harms involved with the individual's particular pattern of substance use, advice about what kind of behavior change is necessary, and a range of choices for achieving such change.[76]

For persons requiring more intensive addiction treatment, the American Society of Addiction Medicine[77] has developed patient placement criteria that take into account such factors as motivation for treatment, withdrawal potential, relapse potential, and presence of comorbid medical or psychiatric conditions. These criteria specify four levels of addiction treatment: outpatient; intensive outpatient/partial hospitalization; medically monitored intensive inpatient; and medically managed inpatient treatment. Tobacco cessation treatment is typically conducted in an outpatient setting, although inpatient programs have been developed for those with severe nicotine dependence.[78]

Types of Treatment

Detoxification is often the first step in treatment of a severely dependent individual. The goals of detoxification are to clear the patient's system of the substance of abuse, to alleviate the physical and psychological discomforts of withdrawal, and to prepare the patient for the next phase of treatment.[79] Although most detoxification can be done on an outpatient basis, persons addicted to substances with a potentially hazardous withdrawal syndrome (alcohol, sedative/hypnotic drugs) may require inpatient care. Medications used for detoxification may either be those with actions similar to the drug of abuse (e.g., benzodiazepines for alcohol withdrawal) that can be gradually tapered to allow the nervous system to adjust to the absence of the drug or may medicate specific withdrawal-related discomforts (e.g., hydroxyzine for anxiety).

Pharmacological. Several different types of medication may be used as an ongoing part of addiction treatment. Functions of these medications include: producing an aversive response; substituting another drug in the same class with fewer negative effects; blocking or decreasing the reinforcing properties of the drug and decreasing craving; or treating comorbid conditions.

Disulfiram (Antabuse) has been used for many years as an adjunct to alcoholism treatment. Disulfiram interferes with alcohol metabolism in the liver, causing an accumulation of acetaldehyde, a toxic breakdown product. Patients who drink while taking disulfiram develop headache and nausea, and may become seriously ill if they continue to drink. Disulfiram may cause damage to the liver or peripheral nerves, and may precipitate psychoses in persons with psychotic illness.[64]

For persons addicted to opiates, longer-acting opioids such as methadone or l-alpha-acetylmethadol (LAAM) can be substituted for heroin. Methadone and LAAM are administered orally and absorbed more slowly, so they do not produce the same "rush" of intoxication followed by craving and withdrawal. Because these medications can be administered daily (methadone) or three times a week (LAAM), persons maintained on them do not have to spend most of their day procuring and consuming heroin, and are able to focus on other important life goals. Buprenorphine, a partial opiate agonist, produces an effect similar to heroin, but after a point, higher doses produce no greater effect. Buprenorphine also blocks the effect of heroin if it is taken concurrently.[80]

Medications used to decrease the reinforcing properties of drugs include opiate antagonists naltrexone and nalmefene.[81] These drugs block the psychoactive effects of heroin, and are sometimes used to prevent relapse in abstinent individuals likely to be exposed to opioids, such as health professionals. Naltrexone has also been demonstrated to decrease relapse to heavy drinking in persons treated for alcohol dependence, probably by reducing the activity of endorphins, natural opioids that are stimulated by drinking.[82] Acamprosate, a drug that prevents excitatory neurotransmitter activity in a way similar to that of alcohol, has been successful in decreasing craving and preventing relapse in alcohol dependent individuals.[83]

An additional important component of pharmacotherapy for addiction involves the treatment of comorbid psychiatric conditions that may precipitate relapse. Many substance-dependent individuals experience symptoms of anxiety and depression during their first weeks and months of abstinence. Although these symptoms may be related to withdrawal and will resolve spontaneously, treatment should be initiated if the symptoms are severe, or the patient has a clear history of significant symptoms of anxiety or depression not related to substance use. Because of their abuse potential, benzodiazepines are not recommended for long-term treatment of anxiety in recovering addicts. Buspirone (Buspar) does not cause dependence and may be an effective alternative for anxiety treatment.[64] Several classes of antidepressants have shown some efficacy in preventing relapse to cocaine use,[80] and some studies have demonstrated reductions in alcohol consumption in alcoholics treated with selective serotonin reuptake inhibitors (SSRIs).[83] Although effective treatment of depression in substance-dependent individuals clearly reduces their risk for relapse by relieving negative affect, it is still unclear whether the effect of these medications on neurotransmitter systems produces some additional anticraving effect.

Nicotine. The management of smoking cessation also includes pharmacotherapy, especially in the form of nicotine replacement, which reduces the withdrawal symptomatology that accompanies cessation.[84] Nicotine replacement therapy assists the smoker while undergoing adjuvant behavioral counseling, or while learning to cope with not smoking. According to the Agency for Healthcare Research and Quality (AHRQ) Treating Tobacco Use and Dependence Clinical Practice Guideline, nicotine replacement is recommended as a major element of treatment, primarily in the form of gum and transdermal patch.[85] Nicotine nasal spray and the nicotine inhaler have also been evaluated and are available for use in therapy.[86,87] An investigation that examined the efficacy of nicotine replacement combination pharmacotherapies has indicated that the use of multiple drugs during the course of cessation treatment improves efficacy.[88] In addition, nonnicotine medications, such as the antidepressant bupropion hydrochloride, have been recently observed to be effective alone, as well as in combination with the nicotine patch, for treatment of smoking cessation.[89]

Psychosocial. Although medications can be helpful in treating addictions, psychosocial and behavioral interventions remain the mainstay of treatment for most drugs of abuse. These interventions aim to modify the patterns of associative learning resulting from drug use, and to strengthen cortical control over a process that has become largely driven by the limbic system. Psychosocial interventions may be used with individuals, families, or groups.

A variety of psychosocial approaches are used to treat addiction, and no one form of psychosocial treatment has been found to produce consistently superior results. Many treatment programs use an eclectic approach that incorporates elements of several different approaches. For purposes of this discussion, treatments will be grouped into cognitive/behavioral approaches and the Twelve Step approach used by groups such as Alcoholics Anonymous (AA). Treatment for nicotine dependence primarily focuses on cognitive/behavioral models, with little emphasis on a Twelve Step approach.

Cognitive and behavioral treatments (CBT) for addiction generally have several goals: to change distorted cognitions about substance use; to change the behavioral reinforcers for substance use; and to teach skills necessary for achieving and maintaining abstinence. In recent years, harm reduction approaches have deemphasized the importance of abstinence as an immediate outcome, focusing instead on immediate reduction of high-risk behaviors associated with substance use, such as needle-sharing and unsafe sex.[90]

Motivational Enhancement Therapy[91] is a primarily cognitive approach that aims to foster motivation to change substance use patterns. One of the key components of this approach is assessment of both the costs and the benefits of continued substance use. This technique focuses attention on the consequences of use that may be denied or minimized, as well as identifying needs currently met by substance use that may be better served by other activities.

Functional analysis that identifies thoughts, feelings, and circumstances before and after substance use is a cognitive technique common to many treatment approaches. This analysis helps to identify high-risk situations and "triggers" for drug use. The information obtained is used to help patients avoid risky situations, or plan alternative behaviors in advance.[92]

Skills training is another significant component of CBT approaches. Training includes not only skills specific to avoiding relapse, such as drink refusal and coping with craving, but also more general coping skills, such as stress management and assertiveness. The lack of a repertoire of mature skills for coping with painful affects and interpersonal difficulties may contribute to addicts' use of substances to manage these problems.[92]

Changing reinforcement contingencies is an important behavioral component of CBT. This may involve cooperation by family members, employers, or other significant individuals, such as probation officers, to provide negative consequences for using drugs and positive rewards for continued abstinence. In some programs, money or vouchers are used to reward individuals when urine toxicology specimens are drug free.

In contrast to CBT, approaches that regard substance abuse as a maladaptive learned behavior that can be modified, AA and other Twelve Step groups regard alcoholism and drug addiction as a disease that cannot be cured, but can be controlled by following a program of moral and spiritual renewal. Participants are encouraged to regularly participate in Twelve Step fellowship meetings, find a more experienced member as a sponsor, and "work the steps" found in the AA "Big Book." In contrast to the CBT approach, which is quite structured and identifies specific skills to be learned, the "steps" of AA are abstract and require individualized interpretation (e.g., Step 4: "Made a searching and fearless moral inventory of ourselves").[93]

Although CBT and Twelve Step approaches may differ in philosophy and emphasis, they share some common functions and are not incompatible. Several AA aphorisms are similar to CBT concepts—for instance, AA's "people, places, and things" is similar to the CBT concept of "high-risk situations,"[92] and the AA acronym HALT (hungry, angry, lonely, tired) identifies unpleasant feeling states that can precipitate relapse. Persons being treated with CBT may be encouraged to attend Twelve Step meetings to increase social support for abstinence or to help deal with drug craving.

CASE STUDIES

CASE STUDY 1

Alan is a 42-year-old married white man who was recently hired as the vice-president of a small biotechnology company. During a routine history and physical for new employees, the nurse practitioner (NP) learns that Alan previously received intensive outpatient treatment for alcoholism after his divorce from his first wife. He abstained from drinking for about 2 years after treatment but began drinking "socially" about 18 months ago. Since assuming his present job, his drinking has escalated to the point at which he is not only drinking five or six shots of whiskey at night after work, but also has two or three drinks at lunchtime, and at least once a week he has a shot of whiskey to "help me get going" in the morning. In the past 2 weeks he has noted difficulty getting to sleep and staying asleep and will sometimes have a shot of whiskey to get back to sleep. He has made several attempts to cut down, but states, "I feel like I can't handle the pressure at work without a few drinks." Although he is drinking substantial amounts, he feels he rarely becomes intoxicated. Alan denies use of any other drugs.

Alan works very long hours and feels that job-related stress has been a major contributor to his increased drinking. He denies that his work performance has suffered, although he says that his secretary gave notice last week after he sarcastically criticized her work. Alan also acknowledges that he has been short-tempered with his wife and two young children. His wife is very concerned about his drinking and has threatened to leave him if he doesn't get some help. Three weeks ago, the car Alan was driving rear-ended another car, causing some automobile damage but no injuries. Alan denies that his drinking had anything to do with this accident.

Alan is slightly overweight and appears tired and a bit restless. On physical examination, his liver is slightly enlarged and tender. Laboratory test results are normal, except for gamma-glutamyl transferase (GGT), which is elevated.

The NP discusses these findings with Alan and notes that his current alcohol intake is well over the two drinks per day maximum for men recommended by the National Institute on Alcohol Abuse and Alcoholism. His current problems with drinking include marital and family conflict; sleep difficulties; problems with co-workers; a recent motor vehicle accident; and liver function changes. These problems, as well as development of tolerance (less effect from alcohol consumed) and his unsuccessful attempts to cut down, indicate a diagnosis of alcohol dependence. The NP recommends outpatient treatment.

Alan is ambivalent about accepting treatment. He recognizes that "my drinking may be getting a little out of control" and is anxious to avoid a second divorce, but he feels it is very important that the project he is currently leading at work succeed and does not think he can sustain his work performance if he stops drinking. When asked what would make him feel that his problems with drinking were serious enough to require immediate treatment, he replies, "If it started interfering with my work."

A follow-up appointment is scheduled in 2 weeks to monitor Alan's situation and continue discussion of treatment options. At the follow-up appointment, Alan appears more tired and fidgety and reveals that his boss had noted alcohol on his breath and suggested he take some time off. Alan accepts referral to an intensive outpatient alcoholism treatment program.

While Alan is in treatment and in the aftercare program, the NP continues to see him every 2 weeks. She prescribes trazadone 50 mg qhs for sleep and recommends regular exercise for sleep hygiene, stress relief, and weight control. She continues to monitor his GGT, which slowly returns to normal. Alan has one 3-day lapse to drinking while in the program but is able to resume abstinence. Alan is able to maintain both his marriage and his job.

Like any chronic, relapsing disorder, alcohol dependence in remission requires regular follow-up. The NP acquaints herself with Alan's recovery plan and asks him at each visit about craving for alcohol, any lapses to drinking, and the effectiveness of relapse prevention techniques learned in the treatment program. The basics of health maintenance, such as a nutritious diet, regular exercise, adequate rest, and effective coping strategies for psychosocial stressors, are emphasized as important components of a clean and sober lifestyle.

CASE STUDY 2

Mary is a 27-year-old married African-American woman who was seen at her first prenatal appointment accompanied by her husband. At that time she was confirmed to be 8 weeks' pregnant. She is employed full-time as a clerical worker for the state in which she resides. This is her first pregnancy. Her husband, aged 30, is employed full-time as a computer programmer in a large private corporation.

Mary began smoking Newports at age 20, before she was married. Both her parents are lifetime nonsmokers. She reports that she lights up her first cigarette about 20 minutes after waking, as soon as the coffee is ready. She smokes approximately 15 cigarettes each day, usually during work breaks and after dinner. Her FTND score is recorded as 6. She has seriously attempted to quit smoking one time in the past and remained abstinent for 4 days. Her husband is also a smoker and reportedly consumes about 1 pack per day of Marlboro Lights. He is interested in quitting and has attempted to do so three times in the past; his longest period of abstinence was 3 months. Neither Mary nor her husband used nicotine replacement or other pharmacotherapy with previous attempts to quit smoking.

On completion of the prenatal examination, the NP strongly advises Mary to quit smoking immediately, citing the risks of continued smoking to Mary and her fetus, and offers to assist with the cessation process. The NP recommends that Mary receive individual intensive counseling that is available on-site at the prenatal clinic. During the remainder of this visit, the NP reviews the program materials and schedules an appointment for the following week at the clinic. Mary is encouraged to rely on behavioral counseling and cognitive/behavioral skill training and to forego the use of nicotine replacement at this time. The NP also advises Mary's spouse to participate in the quitting process and encourages him to consider nicotine replacement therapy. The NP suggests that Mary's husband contact the occupational health department at his worksite for further treatment.

Mary and her husband enter treatment, as recommended. Both benefit from quitting simultaneously and serve as support for each other. A major portion of treatment includes adjusting to high-risk situations in which smoking occurs (e.g., during work-breaks and after dinner). Both develop substitute strategies for these "trigger" situations. For example, Mary goes to the indoor employee lounge during breaks and relaxes with other nonsmoking coworkers, rather than stepping outside with smokers to light up. Her husband uses a nicotine patch on a daily basis (and ad lib gum, while at work) and remains at his computer and keeps busy during periods of cravings. In the evenings, after dinner, Mary and her husband have discussed how quitting was the best gift they could give their new baby.

The NP assesses progress with cessation and reinforces the importance of remaining nonsmokers at each subsequent prenatal visit, because clinician support and interest in the couple are vital components of the cessation program. Although Mary and her spouse have been successful in quitting smoking in the short-term, the NP continues to address abstinence on the birth of their baby, because it is well known that during the postpartum period, mothers are at high risk for relapse. At this time health risks to the infant from environmental tobacco smoke exposure should be emphasized. The same principles of treatment are applicable during the postpartum period, and the NP will recommend nicotine replacement therapy if Mary relapses. However, if Mary breast-feeds her infant, the use of these drugs must be carefully weighed. Additional pharmacotherapy, such as bupropion and nicotine replacement, should be considered for her spouse if he resumes smoking.

SELECTED RESEARCH

With the initiation of the federal government's guidelines for tobacco treatment (e.g., AHRQ clinical practice guideline), emphasis has been placed on both educating providers about tobacco cessation interventions, as well as encouraging their participation in treatment. Recently Block et al[94] investigated attitudes about tobacco and practices of health care providers in the upper Midwest. A survey was sent to chiropractors, dentists, nurse practitioners/physician assistants, physicians (primary care and specialists), and public health nurses in this part of the United States. Findings (N = 614; 52% response rate) indicated that although all provider groups wanted education about tobacco treatment methods, primary care physicians, nurse practitioners/physician assistants, and public health nurses were more likely to assess, treat, encourage cessation, have the necessary skills/knowledge about treatment, perceive fewer barriers to treatment, and want further education, when compared with specialist physicians, dentists, and chiropractors.

Recently tobacco policy interventions have also been demonstrated to reduce smoking. Moskowitz, Lin, and Hudes[95] investigated the effect of local workplace smoking laws in California to determine whether these laws enhance smoking cessation. Data were analyzed from the 1990 California Tobacco Survey of adult indoor workers (N = 4680) who were current cigarette smokers or reported smoking in the 6 months before the survey. Smokers who were employed in localities that had a strong workplace ordinance were more likely to report the existence of a worksite policy (OR = 1.6, 95% CI = 1.2, 2.2) compared with those in towns with no workplace ordinance. Also, smokers in these same localities were more likely to report quitting smoking in the prior 6 months (OR = 1.5; 95% CI = 1.1, 1.7). These findings translated into an estimated 26.4% of smokers quitting in the prior 6 months in localities with strong ordinances, compared with 19.1% in towns without ordinances.

Individual coping efforts during smoking cessation were assessed by O'Connell et al,[96] who collected real-time quantitative and qualitative data using ecological momentary assessment methods. Thirty-six cigarette smokers who were attempting to quit smoking used tape recorders and palm-top computers to record 3 consecutive days during their first 10 days of cessation. Information from the sample about coping responses indicated that a total of 1047 coping responses were used during 389 coping episodes. On average, each participant experienced 3.6 coping episodes per day and reported an average of 2.7 coping responses per episode, of which 67% were behavioral and 33% cognitive in nature. The more times the smoker had quit previously, the smaller the number of coping responses they reported per episode. Women and individuals in high arousal states were more likely to use behavioral distraction as a coping strategy.

For additional reading about cigarette smoking, the recent review by Bergent and Caporas is recommended.[97]

Client motivation and readiness for change has received increased attention as a factor contributing to the success of addiction treatment. Project MATCH, the largest study of alcoholism treatment ever conducted, found that Motivational Enhancement Therapy (MET) was as effective as the other two treatment conditions (Cognitive Behavioral Coping Skills Therapy and Twelve-Step Facilitation Therapy), even though MET was delivered in four sessions and the other two therapies required twelve sessions.[98]

The purpose of a recent study by Kinstler[99] was to discover whether the stages identified by the transtheoretical model of change[100] were compatible with the phases of a military rehabilitation program for alcohol dependence. The University of Rhode Island Change Assessment Questionnaire (URICA) was administered to 203 volunteers from three phases of the program: entering intensive inpatient treatment, completing the intensive portion of the treatment, and concluding continuing care.

The study found that persons entering treatment were significantly more likely to be in the precontemplation stage (lack of acknowledgement that alcohol use is a problem), and significantly less likely to be in the action stage (implementing behavior change) or maintenance stage (consolidating behavior change). Persons completing intensive treatment were significantly more likely to be in the contemplation stage (considering the need for change). Clients in all three treatment phases were most likely to be in either the contemplation or action stages, although there was considerable variation within groups. Kinstler concluded that assessment of client stage of change and stage-specific interventions would improve treatment outcomes.

QUESTIONS FOR FUTURE STUDY

Smoking

Individual Treatment of Nicotine Addiction. The majority of smokers are interested in quitting, although most have tried and failed.[74] To address this, the federal government has created a Tobacco Use and Dependence Clinical Practice Guideline for implementation with tobacco users in a variety of settings.[85] The guideline includes intensive counseling recommendations, as well as brief interventions that can be delivered by health care providers in a range of treatment settings.

Nicotine replacement products and other forms of new medications will increase the options available for use in treatment. Further research must be conducted to determine which are the most efficacious methods, as well as how to tailor tobacco cessation interventions to specific sociocultural, biological, and psychological subgroups of smokers. Included within these populations are those at particularly high-risk, such as adolescent tobacco users, pregnant women, mentally ill individuals, and underserved groups.

Research should also be conducted to determine which settings and media offer the best opportunities for delivering treatment. Nurses have been shown to be effective interventionists and their contribution to tobacco dependence treatment, especially as it relates to health services research, should be studied.[101] The relationship between treatment costs and cessation, as well as reimbursement to providers, also deserves further investigation.

Policy Research. Tobacco-related policies that increased the price of cigarettes and restricted smoking in the workplace and other public settings have influenced the prevalence of smoking significantly.[22,102] Further research must be conducted to determine the impact of other public policy initiatives on tobacco initiation and cessation. For example, tobacco counteradvertising techniques, similar to campaigns conducted in California and Massachusetts, should be replicated nationally to determine their influence on consumption patterns among various subgroups of tobacco users. Also, policies that limit access to tobacco among youth and require regulation of tobacco products to protect the consumer should be developed and tested to determine whether these methods affect smoking behavior. Finally, research that evaluates the effect of implementing clean indoor air policies on tobacco use should be expanded, especially at local and state levels.

Biobehavioral Research. The relationship between the biology of tobacco dependence and subsequent tobacco use behavior represents a critical dimension of nicotine addiction. Genetic factors that may predispose a person to become dependent on tobacco have recently received widespread attention. Research is being conducted to identify and characterize subgroups of smokers and the genetic mechanisms that may be central to the metabolism of nicotine.[103] Other genes have been reported to be involved with the dopaminergic reward hypothesis of nicotine dependence.[104] Findings from these studies will be useful for identifying groups at high-risk for tobacco use. The results of these studies will assist researchers who are interested in developing prevention and cessation strategies for these vulnerable groups.

Drug and Alcohol Abuse

The question of how to prevent drug abuse and addiction is a key issue for nurses, because a public health approach is generally considered to be both more effective and more cost-effective than the current emphasis on law enforcement and individual treatment. Although school-based substance abuse prevention programs are widespread, the failure of such efforts to substantially reduce youth drug use indicates a need to design, implement, and study more effective approaches.[105]

Another research issue crucial to nurses is the testing of effective approaches for motivating patients to reduce substance use. In addition to widespread use of motivational and harm reduction approaches to addiction, the concept of "harm reduction" is being considered within the smoking cessation arena, with scientists and clinicians asking whether reductions in consumption will improve long-term health outcomes. Cessation and reduction of use should also be studied with regard to cost-effectiveness of treatment, especially among certain high-risk groups, such as pregnant women, whose quitting may introduce significant economic and health-related savings to society.

There is currently a large amount of research being conducted related to the basic brain mechanisms involved in addiction, with the goal of developing better medications to prevent or reverse the addictive process. For instance, animal research has identified a substance, MK-801, that interferes with the process of associative learning (sensitization) involved with alcohol addiction.[106] Understanding of the functions of this compound may lead to development of drugs that can modulate drug-related sensitization.

REFERENCES

1. American Psychiatric Association. (2000). *Diagnostic and statistical manual of mental disorders* (4th ed., text revision), Washington, D.C.: Author.
2. Allen, K.M. (1996). *Nursing care of the addicted client.* Philadelphia: Lippincott.
3. Leshner, A.I. (1997, April). Drug abuse and addiction are biomedical problems. *Hospital Practice* (Special Report), 2-5.

4. U.S. Department of Health and Human Services (1988). The health consequences of smoking. Nicotine addiction. A report of the Surgeon General. Public Health Service. Centers for Disease Control. Center for Health Promotion and Education. Office on Smoking and Health. Rockville, MD: DHHS Publication No. (CDC) 88-8406.
5. Regier, D.A., Farmer, M.E., Rae, D.S., Locke, B.Z., Keith, S.J., Judd, L.L., et al. (1990). Comorbidity of mental disorders with alcohol and other drug abuse: Results from the Epidemiologic Catchment Area (ECA) study. *Journal of the American Medical Association 264*(19), 2511-2518.
6. Kessler, R.C., McGonagle, K.A., Zhao, S., Nelson, C.B., Hughes, M., Eshleman, S., et al. (1994). Lifetime and 12-month prevalence of DSM-IIIR psychiatric disorders in the United States. *Archives of General Psychiatry 51*(1), 8-19.
7. Centers for Disease Control and Prevention. (1999). Cigarette smoking among adults—United States, 1997. *Morbidity and Mortality Weekly Report 48,* 993-996.
8. Centers for Disease Control and Prevention. (2000). Tobacco use among middle and high school students—United States 1999. *Morbidity and Mortality Weekly 49,* 49-53.
9. Pierce, J.P., Fiore, M.C., Novotny, T.E., Hatziandreu, E.J., & Davis, R.M. (1989). Trends in cigarette smoking in the United States: Educational differences are increasing. *Journal of the American Medical Association 26,* 56-60.
10. U.S. Department of Health and Human Services. (1996). National Household Survey on Drug Abuse, Main Findings 1994. (DHHS Publication No. 96-3085). Rockville, Md.: SAMHSA Office of Applied Studies.
11. Fillmore, K.M., Hartka, E., Johnstone, B.M., Leino, V., Motoyoshi, M., & Temple, M.T. (1989). Life course variation in drinking: A meta-analysis of multiple longitudinal studies from the Collaborative Alcohol-Related Longitudinal Project. Paper presented at the Alcohol Epidemiology Symposium, Maastricht, The Netherlands.
12. Center for Substance Abuse Treatment. (1999). Cultural issues in substance abuse treatment. Rockville, Md.: U.S. Department of Health and Human Services.
13. U.S. Department of Health and Human Services. (1998). Tobacco use among U.S. racial/ethnic groups—African Americans, American Indian and Alaska natives, Asian Americans and Pacific Islanders, and Hispanics: A report of the Surgeon General. Atlanta: U.S. Department of Health and Human Services, Centers for Disease Control and Prevention.
14. Comings, D.E. (1996). Genetic factors in drug abuse and dependence. In H.W. Gordon, & M.D. Glantz (eds.), Individual differences in the biobehavioral etiology of drug abuse. NIDA Research Monograph 159 (pp. 16-38). Rockville, Md.: National Institute on Drug Abuse.
15. Donovan, J.M. (1986). An etiologic model of alcoholism. *American Journal of Psychiatry 143*(1), 1-11.
16. Gordon, H.W., & Glantz, M.D. (1996). Introduction: Individual differences in the biobehavioral etiology of drug abuse. In H.W. Gordon, & M.D. Glantz (eds.), Individual differences in the biobehavioral etiology of drug abuse, NIDA Research Monograph 159 (pp. 1-15). Rockville, Md.: National Institute on Drug Abuse.
17. Westermeyer, J. (1995). Ethnic and cultural factors in dual disorders. In A.F. Lehman, & L.B. Dixon (eds.), *Double jeopardy: Chronic mental illness and substance use disorders* (pp. 27-46). Chur, Switzerland: Harwood Academic Publishers.
18. McIntyre-Kingsolver, K.O., Lichtenstein, E., & Mermelstein, R.J. (1983). Spouse training in a multicomponent smoking cessation program. *Journal of Consulting and Clinical Psychology 51,* 632-633.
19. Ockene, J.K., Benfari, R.C., Nuttall, R.L., Hurwitz, I., & Ockene, I.S. (1982). Relationship of psychosocial factors to smoking behavior change in an intervention program. *Preventive Medicine 11,* 13-28.
20. McCourt, F. (1996). *Angela's ashes.* New York: Scribner.
21. U.S. Department of Health and Human Services. (1989). Reducing the health consequences of smoking. A report of the Surgeon General. Public Health Service. Rockville, Md.
22. Chaloupka, F.J. (1999). Macro-social influences: The effects of prices and tobacco-control policies on the demand for tobacco products. *Nicotine and Tobacco Research 1,* S105-S109.
23. Centers for Disease Control and Prevention. (1998). Response to increases in cigarette prices by race/ethnicity, income, and age groups—United States, 1976-1993. *Morbidity and Mortality Weekly Report 47,* 605-609.
24. Johnson, B.D, & Muffler, J. (1997). Determinants and perpetuators of substance abuse: Sociocultural. In J.H. Lowinson, P. Ruiz, R.B. Millman, & J.G. Langrod (eds.), *Substance abuse: A comprehensive textbook* (3rd ed., pp. 107-117). Baltimore: Williams & Wilkins.
25. McGue, M., Lykken, D.T., & Iacono, W.G. (1996). Genotype-environment correlations and interactions in the etiology of substance abuse and related behaviors. In H.W. Gordon, & M.D. Glantz, (eds.), Individual differences in the biobehavioral etiology of drug abuse. *NIDA Research Monograph 159* (pp. 49-72). Rockville, Md.: National Institute on Drug Abuse.
26. Pomerleau, O.F. (1997). Co-factors for smoking and evolutionary psychobiology. *Addiction. 92,* 397-408.
27. Marlatt, G.A. (1985). Relapse prevention: Theoretical rationale and overview of the model. In G.A. Marlatt, & J.R. Gordon (eds.), *Relapse prevention: Maintenance strategies in the treatment of addictive behaviors* (pp. 3-70). New York: Guilford Press.
28. Noordsy, D.L., Drake, R.E., Teague, G.B., Osher, F.C., Hurlbut, S.C., Beaudett, M.S., et al. (1991). Subjective experiences related to alcohol use among schizophrenics. *Journal of Nervous and Mental Disease 179*(7), 410-414.
29. Khantzian, E.J. (1985). The self-medication hypothesis of addictive disorders: Focus on heroin and cocaine dependence. *American Journal of Psychiatry 142*(11), 1259-1264.
30. O'Connell, K.A., & Shiffman, S. (1988). Negative affect smoking and smoking relapse. *Journal of Substance Abuse 1,* 25-33.
31. Glassman, A.H., Helzer, J.E., Covey, L.S., Cottler, L.B., Stetner, F., Tipp, J.E., & Johnson, J. (1990). Smoking, smoking cessation and major depression. *Journal of the American Medical Association 264,* 1546-1549.
32. Ziedonis, D.M., & George, T.P. (1997). Schizophrenia and nicotine use: Report of a pilot smoking cessation program and review of neurobiological and clinical issues. *Schizophrenia Bulletin 23,* 247-254.
33. Kasten, B.P. (1996). The client with a dual diagnosis. In H.S. Wilson, & C.R. Kneisl, (eds.), *Psychiatric nursing* (5th ed.), pp. 616-631. Menlo Park, Calif.: Addison-Wesley.
34. Kendler, K.S., Karkowski, L.M., Neale, M.C., & Prescott, C.A. (2000). Illicit psychoactive substance use, heavy use, abuse, and dependence in a U.S. population-based sample of male twins. *Archives of General Psychiatry 57*(3), 261-269.

35. Prescott, C.A., & Kendler, K.S. (1999). Genetic and environmental contributions to alcohol abuse and dependence in a population-based sample of male twins. *American Journal of Psychiatry 156*(1), 34-40.
36. Kendler, K.S., Neale, M.C., Heath, A.C., Kessler, R.C., & Eaves, L.J. (1994). A twin-family study of alcoholism in women. *American Journal of Psychiatry 151,* 707-715.
37. Cotton, N.S. (1979). The familial incidence of alcoholism. *Journal of Studies on Alcohol 40,* 89-116.
38. Schuckit, M.A. (1987). Biological vulnerability to alcoholism. *Journal of Consulting Psychology 55,* 1-9
39. Anthenelli, R.M., & Schuckit, M.A. (1997). Genetics. In J.H. Lowinson, P. Ruiz, R.B. Millman, & J.G. Langrod (eds.), *Substance abuse: A comprehensive textbook* (3rd ed., pp. 41-51). Baltimore: Williams & Wilkins.
40. Cadoret, R.J., O'Gorman, T.W., Troughton, E., & Heywood, E. (1985). Alcoholism and antisocial personality: Interrelationships, genetic and environmental factors. *Archives of General Psychiatry 42,* 161-167.
41. Cloninger, C.R., Bohman, M., & Sigvardsson, S. (1981). Inheritance of alcohol abuse: Cross-fostering analysis of adopted men. *Archives of General Psychiatry 38,* 861-868.
42. Reus, V.I., & Freimer, N.B. (1997). Understanding the genetic basis of mood disorders: Where do we stand? *American Journal of Human Genetics 60,* 1283-1288.
43. Cederlof, R. (1966). The twin method in epidemiological studies on chronic disease. Doctoral dissertation, Academy of the University of Stockholm, Sweden.
44. Cederlof, R., Friberg, L., Lundman, T. (1977). The interactions of smoking, environment, and heredity and their implications for disease etiology. A report of epidemiological studies in the Swedish twin registries. *Acta Medica Scandinavica Supplement 612,* 1-128.
45. Kaprio, J., Koskenvuo, M., Sarna, S. (1981). Cigarette smoking, use of alcohol, and leisure time physical activity among same-sexed adult male twins. In L. Gedda, P. Parise, & W.E. Nance (eds). *Twin research 3. Part C, Epidemiological and clinical studies* (pp. 37-46). New York: Wiley-Liss.
46. Swan, G.E., Cardon, L.R., Carmelli, D. (1996). The consumption of tobacco, alcohol, and caffeine in Caucasian male twins: A multivariate genetic analysis. *Journal of Substance Abuse 8,* 19-31.
47. Self, D.W. (1997, April). Neurobiological adaptations to drug use. *Hospital Practice* (Special Report), 5-9.
48. Robinson, T.E., & Berridge, K.C. (1993). The neural basis of drug craving: An incentive-sensitization theory of addiction. *Brain Research Reviews 18,* 247-291.
49. Stitzer, M.L., & de Wit, H. (1998). Abuse liability of nicotine. In N. Benowitz (ed.). *Nicotine safety and toxicity* (pp. 119-132). New York: Oxford University Press.
50. Lyvers, M. (1998). Drug addiction as a physical disease: The role of physical dependence and other chronic drug-induced neurophysiological changes in compulsive drug self-administration. *Experimental and Clinical Psychopharmacology 6*(1), 107-125.
51. Koob, G.F. (1997, April). Neurochemical explanations for addiction. *Hospital Practice* (Special Report), 12-15.
52. Pomerleau, O.F., & Pomerleau, C. (1984). Neuroregulators and the reinforcement of smoking: toward a biobehavioral explanation. *Neuroscience and Biobehavioral Review 8,* 501-513.
53. Volkow, N.D. (1997, April). The role of the dopamine system in addiction. *Hospital Practice* (Special Report), 22-26.
54. Volkow, N.D., Wang, G.J., Fowler, J.S., Hitzemann, R., Angrist, B., Gatley, S.J., et al. (1999). Association of methylphenidate-induced craving with changes in right striato-orbitofrontal metabolism in cocaine abusers: Implication in addiction. *American Journal of Psychiatry 156*(1), 19-26.
55. Maltzman, I. (1994). Why alcoholism is a disease. *Journal of Psychoactive Drugs 26*(1), 13-30.
56. Childress, A.R., Mozley, D., McElgin, W., Fitzgerald, J., Reivich, M., & O'Brien, C.P. (1999). Limbic activation during cue-induced cocaine craving. *American Journal of Psychiatry 156*(1), 11-18.
57. Schuckit, M.A., Daeppen, J., Danko, G.P., Tripp, M.L., Smith, T.L., Li, T., et al. (1999). Clinical implications for four drugs of the DSM-IV distinction between substance dependence with and without a physiological component. *American Journal of Psychiatry 156*(1), 41-49.
58. Tsai, G., & Coyle, J.T. (1998). The role of glutamatergic neurotransmission in the pathophysiology of alcoholism. *Annual Review of Medicine 49,* 173-184.
59. Russell, M.A.H. (1990). Nicotine intake and its control over smoking. In S. Wonnacott, M.A.H. Russell, & I.P. Stolerman (eds.). *Nicotine psychopharmacology: Molecular, cellular and behavioural aspects* (pp. 374-418). New York: Oxford University Press.
60. Romach, M.K., & Sellers, E.M. (1991). Management of the alcohol withdrawal syndrome. *Annual Review of Medicine 42,* 323-340.
61. Shiffman, S., & Jarvik, M.E. (1976). Smoking withdrawal symptoms in two weeks of abstinence. *Psychopharmacology 50,* 35-39.
62. Schneider, N., & Jarvik, M.E. (1984). Time course of smoking withdrawal symptoms as a function of nicotine replacement. *Psychopharmacology 82,* 143-144.
63. Shiffman, S. (1979). The tobacco withdrawal syndrome. *NIDA Research Monograph Series 23,* 158-184.
64. Center for Substance Abuse Treatment. (1997). A guide to substance abuse treatment for primary care clinicians. Rockville, Md.: U.S. Department of Health and Human Services.
65. Gold, M.S. (1997). Cocaine (and crack): Clinical aspects. In J.H. Lowinson, P. Ruiz, R.B. Millman, & J.G. Langrod (eds.), Substance abuse: A comprehensive textbook (3rd ed.), (pp. 181-199). Baltimore: Williams & Wilkins.
66. Goodwin, D.W., & Gabrielli, W.F. (1997). Alcohol: Clinical aspects. In J.H. Lowinson, P. Ruiz, R.B. Millman, & J.G. Langrod (eds.), *Substance abuse: A comprehensive textbook* (3rd ed., pp. 142-148). Baltimore: Williams & Wilkins.
67. Giannini, J.A. (1997). *Drugs of abuse* (2nd ed.), Los Angeles: Practice Management Information.
68. Centers for Disease Control. (1994). Cigarette smoking among adults—United States, 1992 and changes in the definition of current cigarette smoking. *Morbidity and Mortality Weekly Report 34,* 342-346.
69. Velicer, W.F., Prochaska, J.O., Rossi, J.S., & Snow, M.G. (1992). Assessing outcome in smoking cessation studies. *Psychological Bulletin 111,* 23-41.
70. Hariharan, M., & VanNoord, T. (1991). Liquid-chromatographic determination of nicotine and cotinine in urine from passive smokers: Comparison with gas chromatography with a nitrogen-specific detector. *Clinical Chemistry 37,* 1276-1280.
71. Jarvis, M.J., Russell, M.A.H., Saloojee, Y. (1980). Expired air carbon monoxide: A simple test of tobacco smoke intake. *British Medical Journal 281,* 484-485.
72. Benowitz, N. (1983). The use of biological fluid samples in assessing tobacco smoke consumption. *NIDA Research Monograph 48,* 6-16.

73. Heatherton, T.F., Kozlowski, L.T., Frecker, R.C., & Fagerstrom, K.O. (1991). The Fagerstrom Test for Nicotine Dependence: A revision of the Fagerstrom Tolerance Questionnaire. *British Journal of Addictions 86,* 1119-1127.
74. Fiore, M.C., Bailey, W.C., Cohen, S.J., Dorfman, S.F., Goldstein, M.G., Gritz, E.R., et al. (1996). *Smoking cessation.* Clinical Practice Guideline No. 18. Rockville, Md.: U.S. Department of Health and Human Services, Public Health Service, Agency for Health Care Policy and Research. AHCPR Publication No. 96-0692.
75. Miller, W.R. (1996). Motivational Interviewing: Research, practice, and puzzles. *Addictive Behaviors 21*(6), 835-842.
76. Samet, J.H., Rollnick, S., & Barnes, H. (1996). Beyond CAGE: A brief clinical approach after detection of substance abuse. *Archives of Internal Medicine 156,* 2287-2293.
77. American Society of Addiction Medicine. *Patient placement criteria for the treatment of substance-related disorders* (2nd ed.). Washington, D.C.: Author.
78. Hurt, R.D., Dale, L.C., Offord, K.P., Bruce, B.K., McClain, F.L., Eberman, K.M. (1992). Inpatient treatment of severe nicotine dependence. *Mayo Clinic Proceedings 67,* 823-826.
79. Center for Substance Abuse Treatment. (1995). *Detoxification from alcohol and other drugs.* Rockville, Md.: U.S. Department of Health and Human Services.
80. O'Brien, C.P. (1996). Recent developments in the pharmacotherapy of substance abuse. *Journal of Consulting and Clinical Psychology 64*(4), 677-686.
81. Treatment for alcoholism. (2000). *Harvard Mental Health Letter 16*(11), 1-4.
82. O'Malley, S.S., Jaffe, A.J., Chang, G., Rode, S., Schottenfeld, R., Meyer, R.E., & Rounsaville, B. (1996). Six-month follow-up of naltrexone and psychotherapy for alcohol dependence. *Archives of General Psychiatry 53*(3), 217-222.
83. Johnson, B.A., & Ait-Daoud, N. (1999). Medications to treat alcoholism. *Alcohol Research and Health 23*(2), 99-106.
84. Gross J., & Stitzer, M. (1989). Nicotine replacement: Ten week effects on tobacco withdrawal symptoms. *Psychopharmacology 98,* 334-341.
85. Fiore, M.C., Bailey, W.C., Cohen, S.J., Dorfman, S.F., Goldstein, M.G., Gritz, E.R., et al. (2000). *Treating tobacco use and dependence: Clinical practice guideline.* Rockville, Md.: U.S. Department of Health and Human Services.
86. Schneider, M.G., Olmstead, R., Mody, F.V., Doan, K., Franzon, M., Jarvik, M.E., Steinberg, C. (1995). Efficacy of a nicotine nasal spray in smoking cessation: A placebo-controlled, double-blind trial. *Addiction 90,* 1671-1682.
87. Tonneson, P., Norregaard, J., Mikkelson, K. (1993). A double-blind trial of a nicotine inhaler for smoking cessation. *Journal of the American Medical Association 269,* 1268-1271.
88. Kornitzer, M., Boutsen, M., Dramaix, M., Thijs, J., & Gustavsson, G. (1995). Combined use of nicotine patch and gum in smoking cessation: A placebo-controlled clinical trial. *Preventive Medicine 24,* 41-47.
89. Jorenby, D.E., Leischow, S.J., Nides, M.A., Rennard, S.I., Johnston, J.A., Hughes, A.R., et al. (1999). A controlled trial of sustained-release bupropion, a nicotine patch, or both for smoking cessation. *New England Journal of Medicine 340,* 685-691.
90. Marlatt, G.A. (1996). Harm reduction: Come as you are. *Addictive Behaviors 21*(6), 779-788.
91. Miller, W.R., & Rollnick, S. (1991). *Motivational interviewing: Preparing people to change addictive behavior.* New York: Guilford Press.
92. Carroll, K.M. (1998). *A cognitive-behavioral approach: Treating cocaine addiction. National Institute on Drug Abuse therapy manuals for drug addiction.* Rockville, Md.: National Institute on Drug Abuse.
93. Alcoholics Anonymous. (1986). *If you are a professional.* New York: Alcoholics Anonymous World Services.
94. Block, D.E., Hutton, K.H., & Johnson, K.M. (2000). Differences in tobacco assessment and intervention practices: A regional snapshot. *Preventive Medicine 30,* 282-287.
95. Moskowitz, J.M., Lin, A., & Hudes, E.S. (2000). The impact of workplace smoking ordinances in California on smoking cessation. *American Journal of Public Health 90,* 757-761.
96. O'Connell, K.A., Gerkovich, M.M., Cook, M.R., Shiffman, S., Hickcox, M., & Kakolewski, K.E. (1998). Coping in real time: Using ecological momentary assessment techniques to assess coping with the urge to smoke. *Research in Nursing and Health 21,* 487-497.
97. Bergen, A.W., & Caporaso, N. (1999). Cigarette smoking. *Journal of the National Cancer Institute 91,* 1365-1374.
98. Project MATCH Research Group. (1997). Matching alcoholism treatments to client heterogeneity: Project MATCH posttreatment drinking outcomes. *Journal of Studies on Alcohol 58*(1), 7-29.
99. Kinstler, D.P. (2000). Examining the relevance of the transtheoretical model of change within an alcohol dependency treatment program. *Journal of Addictions Nursing 12*(1), 17-22.
100. Prochaska, J.O., & DiClemente, C.C. (1986). Toward a comprehensive model of change. In W.R. Miller, & N. Heather (eds.), *Treating addictive behaviors: Processes of change* (pp. 3-27). New York: Plenum Press.
101. Houston-Miller, N., Smith, P.M., DeBusk, R.F., Sobel, D., & Taylor, C.B. (1997). Smoking cessation in hospitalized patients. *Archives of Internal Medicine 157,* 409-415.
102. Farrelly, M.C., Evans, W., & Sfekas, A.E.S. (1999). The impact of workplace smoking bans: Results from a national survey. *Tobacco Control 8,* 272-277.
103. Pianezza, M.L., Sellars, E.M., & Tyndale, R.F. (1998). Nicotine metabolism defect reduces smoking. *Nature 393,* 750-751.
104. Lerman, C., Caporaso, N., Main, D., Audrain, J., Boyd, N.R., Bowman, E.D., et al. (1998). Depression and self-medication with nicotine: The modifying influence of the dopamine D4 receptor gene. *Health Psychology 17,* 56-62.
105. Brown, J.H. (2001). Youth, drugs, and resilience education. *Journal of Drug Education 31*(1), 83-122.
106. Ravven, W. (2000). Scientists find link between alcohol and drug addiction. *Newsbreak 15*(8), 3.

SECTION II

Alterations in Cognition

Cognition is a complex interaction of physiological and neuropsychological processes that allow a person to perceive and interact with his or her environment. Alterations in cognition can be defined as changes in an individual's perception and behavior that impairs his or her ability to interact with the internal and external environment and to respond to change. Examples of cognitive functions include consciousness, memory, language, perceptions, judgment, reasoning, and mood.

Alterations in cognition occur insidiously, over many months or years, or acutely, within seconds or minutes, and result in observable changes in one or more of these functions. Examples of pathophysiological phenomena related to cognition include delirium, disorientation, altered consciousness, confusion, stupor, dementia, psychosis, dissociation, and coma. These phenomena are caused by a variety of pathophysiological mechanisms, such as impaired cerebral blood flow, hypovolemia, hyperglycemia or hypoglycemia, infarction, electrolyte imbalances, fever, abnormalities in neurotransmitter systems, and neuronal degeneration.

The two chapters in this section, Chapter 8 (Dementia) and Chapter 9 (Acute Confusion), explore two important phenomena with different pathophysiological mechanisms, time patterns, risk groups, and behavioral changes. These phenomena involve complex interrelationships and processes; multiple theories of causation and the effect of moderator variables have been posited. Confusion and dementia are human responses to biological or psychosocial processes. They are repeatedly observed by nurses across a wide range of acute care and chronic care settings. As the population ages and numbers of critically ill patients increase, these phenomena will continue to be seen more frequently in both chronically and critically ill persons. Confusion and dementia associated with such illnesses as ICU psychosis and Alzheimer's disease bring about changes in behavior that create tremendous burdens on family, caregivers, health care providers, and the health care system at large.

These two phenomena must be differentiated for optimal health outcomes in chronic care and acute health care situations. Knowledge of the mechanisms and manifestations of dementia and confusion provides professional nurses with information that can be used to enhance their observations and the assessment needed to correctly diagnose and treat the phenomena. Several types of clinical therapies are presented, including biomedical and cognitive-behavioral therapies that can be used by the nurse, patient, and family to manage the illness.

Studies by nurses that have most recently begun to describe these phenomena and scientifically test various treatments are presented. The chapters in this section provide theoretical and empirical knowledge as a basis for professional nursing practice and research.

CHAPTER

8 Dementia

KATHY RICHARDS, WANDA CRUMPTON & PAO-FENG TSAI

DEFINITION

Older persons experience changes in their ability to store and recall new information as part of the normal process of aging. These subtle differences that occur with aging do not meet the criteria for dementia. *Dementia* is defined as the loss of multiple acquired cognitive and emotional abilities sufficient to interfere with activities of daily living (ADLs).[1]

Diagnostic criteria for dementia include impairment in short- and long-term memory, an impairment in abstract thinking, impaired judgment, disturbance in higher cortical function, and personality changes.[2] Memory and intellectual diminishment must be sufficient to cause social and occupational impairments. Other criteria include language and visuospatial difficulties.[3] The onset of dementia is gradual and insidious.[4]

One widely recognized category of dementia is Alzheimer's disease. Criteria presented in the *Diagnostic and Statistical Manual of Mental Disorders*[5] for Alzheimer's disease include memory impairment, aphasia, apraxia, agnosia, disturbance in executive thinking, impairment in social or occupational function, significant decline from previous level of functioning, and a gradual onset and continuing cognitive decline (Box 8-1). Other types of dementia that will be presented in this chapter include vascular dementia, frontal lobe dementia, Huntington's disease, Creutzfeldt-Jakob disease, and human immunodeficiency virus (HIV) dementia.

PREVALENCE AND POPULATIONS AT RISK

During the past 40 years, the median age of the North American population has increased from 29.8 years to 42.1 years.[6] As Baby Boomers age, this median age will continue to move upward. This increase in age will be accompanied by an increase in the number of persons with dementia.

The prevalence of dementia is 1% at age 60 and doubles for every 5 years of age. This prevalence becomes 30% to -50% by age 85.[1] The U.S. Preventative Services Task Force reported that dementia affects 0.8% to 1.6% of persons 65 to 74 years old, 7% to 8% of persons 75 to 84 years old, and 18% to 32% of persons age 85 and older.[7] Dementia is present in 50% to 66% of the 1.3 million residents of American nursing homes. Approximately 4 million Americans have been diagnosed with Alzheimer's disease, the disorder that may account for up to 70% of all cases of dementia. This number is expected to increase to 9 million by the year 2040.[3] Multiinfarct or vascular dementia accounts for 10% to 20% of dementias; other causes are rare.[1]

BOX 8-1 Diagnostic Criteria for Dementia of the Alzheimer's Type

- Memory impairment and one or more of the following: aphasia (language disturbance), apraxia (impaired ability to carry out motor activities despite intact motor function), agnosia (failure to recognize or identify objects despite intact sensory function), disturbances in executive functioning (i.e., planning, organizing, sequencing, abstracting)
- Cognitive deficits severe enough to cause impairment in social and occupational functioning
- Gradual onset with continued decline
- Deficits must not be caused by other conditions
- Deficits do not occur only during the course of delirium

Adapted from American Psychiatric Association. (2000). *Diagnostic and statistical manual of mental disorders* (4th ed.). Washington, D.C.

Up to 30% of the 1 to 1.5 million Americans infected with HIV will manifest some form of cognitive impairment. Moderate to severe immunosuppression; constitutional symptoms such as anemia, weight loss, and poor nutrition; and systemic opportunistic infections place the patient infected with HIV at a higher risk for developing dementia.[8]

RISK FACTORS

Many factors have been identified as possible causative agents of dementia. These agents may cause reversible or irreversible dementia. Reversible causes include inflammation, infection, nutrition, toxicity, mass lesions, and complex partial status epilepticus. Inflammatory causes may include sarcoidosis and central nervous system complications of systemic lupus erythematosis. Infections caused by fungi, tuberculosis, *Listeria monocytogenes,* Lyme disease, and syphilis have been implicated in dementia cases. Vitamin B_{12} deficiencies and toxic reactions from prescription medications may contribute to dementia. Subdural hematoma, communicating hydrocephalus, and meningiomas and other tumors may cause dementia.[1] Other frequent reversible causes of dementia are depression, alcohol abuse, and polypharmacy.

Irreversible causes account for the majority of dementias. These causes may be classified as degenerative, vascular, metabolic, and neoplastic. Degenerative conditions include Alzheimer's disease, Pick's disease, Huntington's disease, and Parkinson's disease. Multiinfarct dementias and disseminated intravascular coagulation are vascular causes. Metabolic conditions include storage diseases that are characterized by accumulation of abnormal material in cells of the nervous system such as neuronal ceroid lipofuscinoses. Leukodystrophies represent inborn errors of metabolism resulting from a defective gene that cause morphological changes in the white matter of the central nervous system. Neoplastic disorders causing dementia include meningeal metastases and gliomatosis cerebri.[1]

Risk of Alzheimer's disease increases with advancing age. Presence of the apolipoprotein E (ApoE) has been shown to play a role in the development of Alzheimer's disease. The ApoE e-4 allele increases the risk and the ApoE e-2 allele decreases risk. Without a family history, the lifetime risk of Alzheimer's disease increases from 9% without the ApoE e-4 allele to 29% in persons with one copy of the ApoE e-4 allele. Individuals who are homozygous for the ApoE e-4 have an 83% chance of developing Alzheimer's disease during their lifetime.[8]

Several other factors have been implicated in the development of Alzheimer's disease. Fifty percent of persons with first-degree relatives who have Alzheimer's disease will develop the condition before age 90. Previous head injury, female sex, and lower education levels have also been shown to be risk factors for developing the disease. Women have a higher risk than men of developing dementia after the age of 80. Before age 80, the risk is higher in men. Studies also indicate that a lower educational level presents a higher risk of developing Alzheimer's disease, although adjustment for education did not change the risk for women.[9] Premorbid intelligence may also play a significant role in the development of dementia. Persons with a greater cognitive reserve are able to delay the symptoms of dementia and are able to cope for a longer period of time before the dementia is apparent.[10] Breitner[11] suggested that the use of nonsteroidal antiinflammatory drugs, aspirin, and histamine H_2-receptor antagonists may delay the onset or reduce the risk of developing Alzheimer's disease. It also has been reported that estrogen replacement therapy might lower the risk of developing the disease.[12]

Persons with cerebrovascular disease have an increased risk of vascular or multiinfarct dementia. Vascular dementia occurs more often in men, especially those with hypertension or other cardiovascular risk factors. A longitudinal study by Moroney et al[13] found that high levels of low-density lipoprotein increased the risk of dementia associated with stroke. This risk factor is potentially modifiable by diet and exercise.

MECHANISMS

Patients with Alzheimer's disease exhibit characteristic morphological changes in their brains. These alterations include generalized atrophy of the cerebral cortex, cortical neuritic plaques, and neurofibrillary tangles. Neuritic plaques are formed when beta-amyloid, a normally soluble substance, becomes insoluble in the presence of Alzheimer's disease.[12] Neuritic plaques are composed of enlarged axons, synaptic terminals, and dendrites. Amyloid composes 70% of the material in the plaque core. These plaques are surrounded by proliferating astrocytes and microglial cells. Neurofibrillary tangles are filamentous inclusions that develop within the pyramidal neuronal soma and may extend into dendrites.[14a] The distribution of neurofibrillary tangles is specific to the association cortex and does not affect the sensory or motor cortex. While the number of neuritic plaques and neurofibrillary tangles have been associated with the severity of dementia, the most important correlate appears to be the loss of synapse.[8] The degenerative process of Alzheimer's disease also affects the neurotransmitter-specific subcortical nuclei that project to the cortex. Choline acetyltransferase, which is responsible for the synthesis of acetylcholine, is reduced. Reduction in the synthesis results in profound memory disturbances and irreversible impairment of cognitive function. In late stages of the disease, gamma-aminobutyric acid (GABA) and serotonin are affected. Postmortem studies indicate that changes in serotonergic neurotransmission may be linked more to behavioral disturbances rather than cognitive dysfunction. Neurons that release excitatory amino acids demonstrate chemical and pathological changes that strongly correlate with dementia.[14]

Lewy bodies are intraneuronal eosinophilic inclusion bodies that may be seen in the brainstem and cortex. Lewy bodies are composed of masses of filaments that are similar to neurofilaments. However, the precise molecular composition is unknown. A mutation in the alpha-synuclein gene has been identified in familial Parkinson's disease. This gene has been found to be a major component of Lewy bodies. The diagnostic hallmark of Parkinson's disease is the presence of Lewy bodies, along with neuron loss in the medial substantia nigra. Lewy bodies found in the limbic cortex and neocortex produce cognitive failure and psychosis.[8,15,16]

Pick's disease, also known as frontotemporal dementia, is manifested by progressive aphasia and personality changes. Although Pick bodies, round neuronal inclusions, give the disease its name, they are an uncommon finding on autopsy. Atrophy of the temporal lobes is demonstrated on neuroimaging. Frontotemporal dementia has been linked to chromosomes three and seventeen.[17]

Brains of HIV-infected individuals with cognitive impairment show cerebral atrophy. This type of dementia is considered to be subcortical in the initial presentation and more global with deterioration. Ventricular enlargement, particularly in the frontal and temporal lobes is seen, along with abnormalities of the sulci and deep cerebral white matter.[8]

PATHOLOGICAL CONSEQUENCES

The progressive decline in cognitive functioning that is seen in irreversible causes of dementia such as Alzheimer's and Pick's disease results in many changes in functioning for elders with dementia.[18] One important change is a partial or total misrepresentation of the environment. Persons with dementia have difficulty identifying incoming information and attaching meaning to it even if sensory functioning is intact. Partial understanding of incoming stimuli may confuse them. For example, elders with dementia may be less able to compensate for the decreased visual acuity common in aging because they cannot supply from memory details of the environment.[18] This difficulty in accurate perception of incoming stimuli can lead to anxiety, delusions, and problematic behaviors. Persons with Alzheimer's dementia also have difficulty perceiving contrast (separating foreground from background objects), which further impairs their visual acuity.

An additional perceptual deficit common in Alzheimer's dementia is agnosia. Agnosia is difficulty with object recognition although no visual or sensory deficit is present.[18] Visuospatial perception allows persons to recognize directions and patterns in the environment. Dysfunction in visuospatial perception may cause persons with dementia to lose their way, even in familiar surroundings.

The inability to initiate and carry out previously learned tasks in the absence of any motor weakness, sensory impairments, or decreased language comprehension is called *apraxia*. In persons with dementia, apraxia is apparent during ADLs such as dressing or preparing a meal. Apraxia of gait occurs in the later stages of Alzheimer's disease and may cause falls.[18]

Incontinence of bowel and bladder is common in persons with dementia. Contributing factors to incontinence include the fact that persons with dementia may be unable to recognize the sensation of fullness, be unable to find the bathroom, or are unable to undress themselves.

Another common consequence of dementia is anxiety.[18] Cognitively impaired persons are vulnerable to anxiety. Restlessness and agitation may signal anxiety. As they become unsure of their surroundings or what is expected of them, they react with fear and distress.[18] Anxiety and agitation may follow the inability to complete a task once regarded as simple. Depression is another frequently observed consequence of dementia.

Reduced ability to communicate verbally and in writing is another consequence of dementia. Persons with dementia may be unable to communicate their pain or discomfort, hunger, thirst, or other sensations.

Problematic behaviors, such as physical and verbal aggression, verbally nonaggressive behaviors, and wandering are common consequences of dementia. In fact, more than half (53.7%) of nursing home residents display problematic behaviors, with aggression

(34.3%) occurring the most often, according to analysis of data from the 1987 National Medical Expenditure Survey.[19] The confusion and disinhibition experienced by persons with dementia may result in a susceptibility to violent outbursts and sudden acts of physical or verbal aggression. Cursing, hitting, spitting, or kicking occur in some elders with dementia. Verbally nonaggressive behaviors, such as screaming, or loud repetition of a phrase, such as "don't do that," may also occur. In progressive dementias, declining cognitive functioning results in many physical and emotional consequences for elders with dementia and their caregivers such as inability to perform self-care activities like bathing and dressing.

Another disabling consequence of many persons with dementia is sleep disturbance. Their sleep is light and inefficient, and they awake often during the night.[20,21] While awake they may scream or wander into other residents' rooms. One study found persons in a nursing home, 60% of whom had dementia, slept only 66% of the night.[22] In addition to poor nighttime sleep, persons with dementia often sleep in the daytime. In 24-hour sleep recordings of persons with dementia in nursing homes, 10% to 20% of the total 24-hour sleep time occurred during the daytime, with frequent napping episodes of light sleep (stages 1 and 2 non–rapid eye movement [REM] sleep) and nighttime sleep involving frequent awakenings and decreased REM sleep.[23,24] In another study, daytime sleep of persons with dementia in a nursing home consisted of 22 transitions from wake to sleep, with each wake interval averaging only 33 minutes.[25] In a series of studies in a clinical research ward or hospital, napping increased as cognition deteriorated.[26,27] Because they spend 40% of the night awake and obtain light sleep during their daytime naps, persons with dementia receive little restorative sleep.[26-28]

Disturbed nighttime sleep in persons with dementia may stem from the following physiological states: (1) chronic illness,[21] (2) a higher incidence of sleep-related respiratory deterioration and periodic limb movements in persons with dementia than in nondemented elders,[21] and (3) dysregulation of the circadian and homeostatic sleep-wake processes caused by neuronal pathophysiology.[21] Other causes, which behavioral or environmental interventions can address, include (1) disruptive nighttime environmental events such as noise from staff and other persons and undimmed lighting,[29,30] (2) low levels of daytime bright light exposure,[21] and (3) inactivity and boredom leading to excessive daytime napping.[21,31]

Another pathological consequence of dementia is inactivity. Persons with dementia have lost many of the cognitive, functional, and social abilities necessary to participate in traditional social and physical activities. Inactivity results in isolation, lack of stimulation, loss of self-esteem, increased disability, and problematic behaviors.[32]

RELATED PATHOPHYSIOLOGICAL CONCEPTS AND DIFFERENTIAL DIAGNOSIS

When assessing patients with dementia, nurses must consider other phenomena that manifest in a similar manner to dementia and whose presence make an accurate diagnosis of dementia difficult. Depression, delirium, and schizophrenia share several common signs and symptoms with dementia and can occur concurrently with dementia.

Depression is defined as a morbid sadness, dejection, or melancholy. It is associated with disturbances of sleep and appetite and loss of interest in almost everything. Thinking ability and attention span are reduced.[1] Depression may be an early sign of Alzheimer's disease; it should be recognized and treated. Affective symptoms are common in persons with dementia, but are both underrecognized and undertreated. These symptoms cause significant distress to patients and their caregivers.[33] Depression is associated with wandering, aggression, constant requests for help, complaining and negativism, and impaired ability to complete ADLs and may accelerate loss of functioning.[34] Anxiety, including worrying over minor issues, disturbed sleep, and complaints of aches and pains, may be more prevalent in mild-to-moderately cognitively impaired persons who have insight into their memory problems and in persons with coexisting physical illness.[34]

Delirium is often mistaken for dementia (see Chapter 9, Acute Confusion). *Delirium* is defined as a disturbance of consciousness that is accompanied by a change in cognition that cannot be accounted for by a preexisting dementia. Delirium usually develops over a period of hours or days and tends to fluctuate during the course of the day. It is a direct physiological consequence of many medical conditions (e.g., hypoxemia, electrolyte imbalances, hyperglycemia or hypoglycemia), substance intoxication or withdrawal, use of medications (particularly benzodiazepines), or exposure to a toxin.[1] Delirium can be differentiated from dementia by its acute onset, fluctuations in cognitive impairment over the course of the day, and disruptions in attention.[35]

Although dementia and schizophrenia share some similar features, such as diminished function in all dimensions, poor judgment, and impaired abstract thinking,[36] they have some distinct features that usually make their differentiation fairly straightforward. *Schizophrenia* is a chronic, severe psychiatric condition characterized by (usually) auditory hallucinations, delusions, disorganized speech, and/or bizarre behavior having a relapsing and remitting course.[37] Schizophrenia initially manifests in adolescence or early adulthood, while the onset of dementia is usually middle to late adulthood. With schizophrenia there is no evidence of brain pathology and the person's sensorium remains intact.[3]

Not only is it important for the nurse to differentiate dementia from other similar phenomena, but to assist in differentiating the causes of dementia. The following discussion compares and contrasts the presenting signs and symptoms of a number of medical conditions that cause dementia.

Specific presentations of dementia depend on which particular abilities are compromised. Impairments may occur in memory, language, spatial perception, cognition, attention, motor control, emotion, and motivation.[8] Additional symptoms include recent memory loss, difficulty performing familiar tasks, language problems, poor judgment, disorientation of time and place, personality changes, difficulty with abstract thinking, loss of initiative, and mood or behavioral changes.[4]

The cause of dementia may be determined by the presentation of symptoms. Many times the first sign exhibited in Alzheimer's disease is declarative memory impairment, manifested by forgetfulness. Declarative memory is used to recollect information consciously and intentionally.

Vascular or multiinfarct dementia results from cerebrovascular disease and usually occurs shortly after a myocardial infarction or other cardiovascular or cerebrovascular event. Symptoms occur in a stepwise fashion with significant mental deterioration after each event. Symptoms are usually accompanied by neurological evidence of a cerebrovascular disease such as paralysis of a limb, dysphagia, or headaches.[33]

Subcortical disorders, such as Parkinson's disease and Lewy body disease, cause defects in memory, motor function, and executive function while language is left intact. However, for patients with Parkinson's disease, tremor and rigidity are present for years before cognitive symptoms are exhibited. Typical presentation of Lewy body dementia is similar to delirium, with fluctuating confusion, deficits in attention, and visual hallucinations. Other common features are rigid-akinetic parkinsonism, intermittent loss of consciousness, and falls.[16,38]

Frontal lobe dementias, such as Pick's disease, present with an early onset of behavioral changes, changes in judgment, and mild defects of memory and visuospatial orientation. Other prominent symptoms include disinhibition, compulsiveness, impatience, sexual inappropriateness, and labile-affect.

Huntington's disease presents with rapid, jerky muscle spasms that occur in the arms and legs. Other manifestations include progressive rigidity, akinesia, irritability, and antisocial or psychotic behavior.[33]

Myoclonic jerks can suggest a rare, rapidly progressing dementing illness known as Creutzfeldt-Jakob disease. This disease may be contracted by eating infected beef brain, eyes, or spinal cord tissue. It may be transmitted to clinicians through contact with contaminated human brain tissue or surgical instruments. Dementia associated with anemia or liver failure may also present with myoclonic jerks.[33]

Patients with normal-pressure hydrocephalus caused by an imbalance between the production and resorption of the cerebral spinal fluid present with gait apraxia, dementia, and urinary incontinence. They exhibit a slow, unsteady, wide-based gait with short steps and difficulty lifting their feet. Impaired attention, poor memory, and poor executive function also are prominent symptoms.[1]

Patients with HIV dementia present with mental slowness, diminished concentration, and a decline in memory. Changes in behavior may occur, such as lethargy, apathy, diminished emotional response, and psychosis. The patient may also be clumsy and demonstrate gait abnormalities, tremor, and reduced motor control.[1]

Head trauma can be a significant cause of dementia. Common in professional boxers, this dementia is known as *dementia pugilistica*. The speed at which a person is able to process information is slowed, and attention span, memory, and problem-solving skills are impaired. A factor that distinguishes head trauma–induced dementia from other dementias is the fact that some of the symptoms may lessen with time.[33]

Alcohol-related causes of dementia include niacin deficiency and thiamin deficiency. Whipple's disease causes dementia, along with ophthalmoplegia and myoclonus. This disease, caused by a rod-shaped bacillus, *Tropheryma whippelii*, occurs predominantly in middle-aged men, particularly farmers.[8]

MANIFESTATION AND SURVEILLANCE

Early dementia is often viewed by patients, family members, and health care professionals as a normal consequence of aging. Families seem to suppress the awareness that a loved one is developing cognitive changes. They tend to offer excuses and rationales for the functional losses. The diagnosis of dementia has threatening implications, including loss of autonomy, dignity, and self.[6]

Persons with dementia have symptoms of cognitive decline and an impaired ability to carry out basic and instrumental ADLs. Early forgetfulness and gradual difficulties with executive functioning (balancing checkbooks, planning vacations) occur, although social functioning is usually preserved. The ability to accomplish familiar tasks, such as driving, using the telephone, and self-care activities, is usually preserved in the early stages. An inability to perform these activities may be the first sign that family members observe. Behavioral changes, such as asking the same question repeatedly, inability to take messages, and getting lost are suggestive of dementing illness.[12] In later stages, persons with dementia may be unable to recall familiar objects or newly learned information. As the dementia progresses, behavioral symptoms, such as irritability, apathy, wandering, psychosis, and agitation occur. Eventually persons with progressive dementia become completely dependent.[12]

Nurses should assess for dementia if patients or their families are concerned about cognitive decline. Interviewing patients and their caregivers and performing a comprehensive clinical assessment will provide the information to make the diagnosis of dementia.[12]

A detailed history from the patient and family may provide many valuable clues. The history will assist the nurse with information to help determine the duration and cause of dementia. Crucial components of the history include recent onset of symptoms, progression of symptoms, duration of symptoms, comorbid medical illness, and medications (specifically, antidepressants, sedatives, antiparkinsonian drugs, anticonvulsants, antihypertensives, opioids, and antihistamines). It is also important to collect any history of alcohol use, family and psychosocial history, and data on social support networks, education, literacy, and living arrangements. The history should include questions about identified neurological and psychiatric disorders, substance abuse, and exposure to environmental toxins. The nurse should compare previous cognitive performance with current status and assess multiple dimensions of cognitive abilities (memory, abstract thinking, spatial ability, handling complex tasks, language, and behavior).[12]

The nurse should question the patient and family regarding family history of dementia. Rare families have autosomal dominant forms of the Alzheimer's disease, so called *familial Alzheimer's disease,* in which 50% of each generation, regardless of gender, succumb to Alzheimer's disease, usually by midlife.[39]

A comprehensive physical examination, including detailed neurological and mental status examinations, is necessary to diagnose dementia. Chronic cognitive impairment may result from reduced cerebral oxygen perfusion associated with advanced cardiac or pulmonary disease, while focal neurological signs suggest cerebrovascular disease.[12]

Cognitive functioning should be assessed using mental status assessment instruments, such as the Mini-Mental State Examination (MMSE)[40] or the Severe Impairment Battery.[41] Repeated administration of screening tests over time allows the clinician to gauge progression of cognitive decline. However, neither of these tests captures the full range of participants' anticipated cognitive impairments, each being limited by either ceiling or floor effects. The MMSE is a 30-item standardized cognitive screen with orientation, registration, short-term memory, attention/concentration, language, and constructional capacity items (scores 0 to 30). A score less than twenty-four is the accepted cutoff for a diagnosis of dementia,[42,43] although education and age can also influence this score.[42] Test-retest reliability (24-hour) is 0.83.[44] Researchers established validity by correlating the MMSE with the standardized psychiatric clinical diagnosis ($r = 0.82 - 0.87$), the Short Portable Mental Status Questionnaire ($r = 0.83$), and the Cognitive Capacity Screening Examination ($r = 0.88$).[42,45] Administration time is about 10 minutes. Although the MMSE is widely used, its purpose is for screening. The MMSE is not sufficiently sensitive compared with comprehensive neuropsychological evaluations, especially among patients who are well educated or severely demented.

The Severe Impairment Battery,[41] a 39-item battery, designed for the severely demented patient, includes six major subscales: attention, orientation, language, memory, visuospatial ability, and construction. It also has brief evaluations of praxis and the patient's ability to respond when someone calls his or her name. Possible scores range from 0 to 100. Scores of less than 63 on the Severe Impairment Battery indicate very severe impairment and correspond to less than 4 on the MMSE. Interrater reliability for total Severe Impairment Battery score stands at 0.99, with subscale reliabilities from 0.89

(praxis) to 1.00 (orienting to name).[46] To establish validity of the Severe Impairment Battery, developers compared patients' performance on the Severe Impairment Battery with performance on the MMSE ($r = 0.76$, $p < 0.001$, $n = 70$) and the Mattis Dementia Rating Scale ($r = 0.88$, $p < 0.001$, $n = 55$). Administration time increases with level of cognitive impairment and takes about 20 minutes with the most severe cases.

Determining the cause of cognitive impairment is the next step after dementia is diagnosed. In most cases, the medical and psychiatric evaluation is sufficient to make the diagnosis, however, further evaluation is always indicated when dementia is progressive, presents with atypical symptoms, such as aphasia, or is of uncertain etiological origin. Dementia may be caused, in some cases, by reversible disorders. Although truly reversible dementia syndromes are uncommon, diagnostic testing for coexistent disorders that may exacerbate dementia or cause delirium is required. Depression, alcohol use, and drug toxicity are among the most frequent causes of reversible dementia with symptoms of Alzheimer's disease.[12]

Laboratory testing that includes a complete blood count, metabolic profile, thyroid function tests, vitamin B_{12} testing, and serological test for syphilis is necessary. Metabolic dysfunction and reversible causes of dementia must be ruled out.[12]

Neuroimaging studies can aid in the diagnosis of patients with recent-onset dementia, focal neurological signs, atypical symptoms, or uncertain diagnosis. Computed tomography or magnetic resonance can reveal brain hematomas, tumors, abscesses, strokes, arteriovenous malformations, and hydrocephalus. The role of diagnostic imaging studies such as single-photon emission computed tomography and positron emission tomography has not been fully determined.[12]

If metastatic cancer, meningitis, tertiary syphilis, hydrocephalus, encephalitis, demyelinating disease, immunosuppression, or inflammatory disease is suspected, lumbar puncture should be done.[12] Patients with abnormal mental status test results and normal physical functioning should receive neuropsychological testing.[12] Box 8-2 summarizes the dementia assessment process.

After dementia is diagnosed and the cause for the cognitive impairment has been determined, nurses should conduct serial assessments of cognitive functioning (MMSE) to monitor disease progression. Sudden declines in cognitive status may be caused by conditions superimposed on dementia such as delirium or depression.

As dementia progresses, problematic behaviors, such as wandering, screaming, and hitting frequently develop. These behaviors cause great difficulty for home caregivers and frequently result in nursing home placement. The nurse should question caregivers about the occurrence of the behaviors, their frequency, circumstances in which they usually occur, and their immediate antecedents. This information is critical for assisting caregivers to prevent and manage problematic behaviors.

Disturbed sleep, frequently associated with nocturnal wandering and escalation of problematic behaviors ("sundowning") occurs in many persons with dementia. Caregivers and persons with dementia (if possible) should be questioned about sleep disturbance. The assessment should include questions regarding the patient's usual sleep schedule, time required to fall asleep, number and length of awakenings, loud snoring or breathing pauses during sleep, leg twitching during sleep, unusual sensations in the legs that interfere with sleep, daytime activities, and napping.

Affective symptoms are common in persons with dementia, yet they are under-recognized. While it is relatively simple to ascertain a cognitively intact person's affect through self report and interviews, it is much more difficult to determine affective symptoms in persons with dementia who may have difficulty communicating their internal states.[18] Investigators have elicited the affective state of persons with mild cognitive impairment by using self-report[47] and moderate-to-severe dementia through family and caregiver interviews.[48] Family, caregivers, and health care providers can evaluate affect from facial expression, motor behaviors, and relevant verbal cues.

Dementia Care Mapping is an observational method for evaluating the process of dementia care.[48] Its central premise is that persons with dementia retain the ability to communicate through powerful nonverbal and verbal cues. Dementia Care Mapping entails one or more observers being present in the care environment for one or more 3- to 6-hour periods. The observers attempt to blend in to the setting. They record what has been happening to each resident in successive periods of 5 minutes, such as eating, wandering, or sleeping and the concomitant state of well-being or ill-being is also recorded on a Likert-type scale. They also record episodes in which the person with dementia is subjected to personal detraction (such as a hurtful remark), whether verbal or physical. Interrater reliability of the method was 0.85. Persons with dementia can be

BOX 8-2 Dementia Assessment Process

History and Physical Examination

Symptoms: memory loss, change in ADLs, language, cognition, and emotion
Review of prescribed and over-the-counter medications
Psychosocial evaluation
Family history
Caregiver evaluation
Comprehensive physical examination
  Neurological
  Neuropsychological assessment

Interdisciplinary and Multidisciplinary Team Assessment

Physician
Geriatrician
Neurologist
Neuropsychologist or psychiatrist
Nurse
Social worker
Physical or occupational therapist
Pharmacist

Laboratory Studies

Complete blood cell count
Metabolic profile
Thyroid profile
Vitamin B_{12} level
Syphilis serology

Imaging Studies

Computed tomography (CT)
Magnetic resonance imaging (MRI)

Other Studies

Lumbar puncture
Neuropsychological testing
Electroencephalography (EEG)
Single-photon emission computed tomography (SPECT)
Positron emission tomography (PET)

Adapted from Daly, M.P.M. (1999). Diagnosis and management of Alzheimer's disease. *Journal of the American Board of Family Practice 12,* 375-385.

compared based on the units of care (or lack of care) provided. The environment can be characterized by the types of behavior and activity it encourages. Another outcome of this method is the Dementia Care Quotient of the overall efficiency and quality of care delivery.

Pain is highly prevalent in the elderly due to the frequent occurrence of painful musculoskeletal conditions such as arthritis and osteoporosis. Pain often is unrecognized and untreated in patients with dementia because it is very difficult to assess. In a study of 339 nursing home residents (mean age, 87 years) cognitively impaired residents were prescribed and administered significantly less analgesic medication than those who were more cognitively intact.[49] Untreated pain can exacerbate the behavioral disturbances in dementia. Therefore, these findings underscore the need for more effective assessment of pain in this population and education of health care providers regarding pain management in cognitively impaired persons. To date, asking persons with dementia if they have pain, observing for nonverbal cues such as difficulty walking, grimacing, or change in eating or activity patterns, and paying attention to verbal cues such as crying or repetition of words or phrases such as "Oh, oh, oh" are recommended assessment techniques for pain (see Chapter 12, Pain).[18,50]

Caring for an elder with dementia frequently takes a toll on the health of the caregiver. Many caregivers are elderly women who may be in poor health themselves. The nurse also should question the caregiver to determine how he or she is coping emotionally and physically with the caregiver role and the availability and utilization of family and community support networks.

CLINICAL MANAGEMENT

The goals of treatment in persons with dementia are to (1) improve or at least slow loss of memory and cognition, (2) maintain functional independence by allowing them to remain in the least restrictive environments possible, and (3) provide for their comfort and dignity.

Pharmacological

Cognition. Many of the larger studies of cognition-enhancing drugs have involved drugs that inhibit the enzyme acetylcholinesterase, although findings from major new studies on estrogen and selegiline have also been reported. The effect sizes of these drugs are modest.[51] Only some patients show a meaningful response, and these individual effects may be obscured in clinical trials reporting mean outcome data on cognitive functioning. The acetylcholinesterase inhibitor, Donepezil at a dosage of 5 to 10 mg/day has shown significant improvement in cognition and global functioning (as measured by the Alzheimer's Disease Assessment Scale–cognitive subscale and the Clinician's Interview-Based Impression of Change with caregiver input) in patients with Alzheimer's, and preliminary data indicate clinical benefit in patients with subcortical vascular dementia.[51] In early trials of two other acetylcholinesterase inhibitors, rivastigmine (mean dose, 3.7 mg/day) and physostigmine (12 to 15 mg 2 to 3 times daily), modest benefits occurred in cognition as measured by the Alzheimer's Disease Assessment Scale–cognitive subscale and the Clinician's Interview-Based Impression of Change with caregiver input.[51]

Epidemiological studies have suggested that hormone replacement therapy may be protective against later development of Alzheimer's disease, but recent clinical trials do not support the routine use of estrogen replacement therapy in the treatment of Alzheimer's disease.[51] Further testing is required to determine whether estrogen is useful in preventing or delaying the onset of Alzheimer's disease.

Two studies have reported that selegiline, an irreversible inhibitor of monoamine oxidase type B, is associated with apparent slowing of the progression of Alzheimer's disease, although the findings require replication in a larger sample.[52,53] At present, the published findings on selegiline are not sufficient to recommend its routine clinical use for patients with Alzheimer's disease.[51]

Other promising drugs currently undergoing testing include denbufylline, a xanthine derivative; D-cycloserine, an N-methyl-D-aspartate glutamate receptor partial agonist that is used as an antibiotic to treat tuberculosis; colostrinin, a proline-rich polypeptide complex; and nicotine transdermal patches. The association between nonsteroidal anti-inflammatory drugs (NSAIDs) and a reduced risk of Alzheimer's disease has not been confirmed, but these drugs may protect the brain from the reactive glial and microglial responses associated with A (beta) deposition.[54] Another encouraging recent finding is that antioxidants, such as vitamin E, may halt or reverse the underlying disease process.[54]

Behavioral Symptoms. In a review of the biological basis for using cholinergic therapies to treat the neuropsychiatric symptoms of Alzheimer's dementia, Levy et al[55] noted that there is evidence that tacrine, donepezil, rivastigmine and metrifonate may improve neuropsychiatric symptoms. In a clinical trial, carbamazepine 300 mg/day was significantly better than placebo at reducing agitation and aggression in nursing home patients.[56]

Antipsychotic drugs have been the mainstay of treatment for psychotic symptoms and problem behaviors in persons with dementia. However, conventional antipsychotic medications result in adverse effects including sedation, postural hypotension, and extrapyramidal effects. In addition, they are only moderately effective. A metaanalysis examining the effect of conventional antipsychotics for patients with Alzheimer's disease found that only 20% of patients responded favorably to neuroleptics.[57] However, the newer atypical antipsychotics may be more effective. Two recently reported clinical trials have shown that low doses of the atypical antipsychotic risperidone are effective in reducing both physical and verbal aggression in nursing residents with dementia.[58,59]

The management of depression or anxiety in dementia sufferers has not been extensively investigated. Medications found to be effective in treating depression in persons with dementia include paroxetine, imipramine, and citalopram.[34]

As previously stated, assessing and treating pain in elders with cognitive impairment is difficult. Studies have shown that the prevalence of pain in nursing home residents is between 71% and 83%, and that persons with dementia receive significantly less pain medication than their cognitively intact peers.[49] Health care providers should prescribe and nurses should administer analgesics for pain in elders with dementia.

Summary. Significant advances have been made in the drug treatment of cognitive impairment, behavioral symptoms, and depression in dementia. Studies on the acetylcholinesterase inhibitors, donepezil and rivastigmine, have established their role in the treatment of patient's with mild-to-moderate Alzheimer's disease. Studies on the use of resperidione for treating behavioral symptoms in institutionalized patients with dementia have clarified its potential benefits and limitations. Unfortunately, there are no drugs with clinically significant disease-modifying effects. Pharmacological interventions should be used as part of a detailed management plan.[51]

Behavioral

Behavioral interventions are a safe treatment strategy that is recommended for behavioral complications by the nursing home regulation of the American Health Care Association.[60] The origin of behavioral interventions is from psychology[61] and the use of it is based on two premises. First, environmental factors, especially behaviors of nursing staff, affect behaviors of demented elders.[62] Second, a problematic behavior can be modified and exchanged for more acceptable behaviors.[63] The goal of a behavioral intervention is to modify or change unwanted behaviors through the process of relearning.[64] Mildly demented elderly persons are able to relearn through cognitive approaches, such as reality orientation and social training techniques, whereas in severely demented elders behavioral strategies are more effective than cognitive interventions.[65]

The most commonly occurring problematic behaviors include disruptive vocalization, wandering, and physical and verbal aggression. Typical antecedents of such behaviors include overstimulation (e.g., cold and noisy), boredom, loneliness, physical discomfort (e.g., pain), mental distortion (e.g., paranoia), and conflicts with other residents.[62,66] The Need-Driven Dementia-Compromised Behavior Model posits that problematic behavior is a function of the person-environment interaction and that the antecedents of the behaviors are needs that the persons with dementia are unable to express because of their cognitive dysfunction.[66] They have grouped person factors in four categories: neurological (brain regions, neurotransmitters, and circadian circuitry), neuropsychological (intellectual and cognitive abilities, perceptual, language, and sensory skills, motor ability, and affect), physiological (physiological states such as sleep disturbance and health status), and sociodemographic (demographics, and personal history factors). They group environmental factors along two dimensions: physical (macro- and micro-level) and social (social contact, network, and caregiver).

Carefully assessing and eliminating antecedents (or needs) will prevent the occurrence of some problematic behaviors. Manipulating antecedents and/or altering consequences of problematic behaviors can effectively reduce the incidence of the undesirable behaviors even in severely demented elders.

Behavioral interventions for problematic behaviors mainly focus on altering the consequences of the behavior. Positive reinforcement, such as the attention from staff, is provided to the demented elder who either changes the inappropriate behavior or shows a desirable behavior.[18,67] Other positive reinforcements include allowing the elder to receive a special treat, such as his favorite food or television program.[64,67] Gugel[63] noted that demented elders responded better to positive rather than negative reinforcement. The modification of problematic behaviors often involves multiple strategies as well as other types of intervention. Many studies of these interventions were case reports or had small sample sizes. However, these studies suggested that even at the late stage of dementia, patients are still able to learn.[68]

Another application of behavioral interventions is improvement of dressing independence in elders with dementia. Beck et al[69] conducted a pretest/delayed posttest clinical trial of behavioral strategies to promote dressing independence in 90 nursing home residents with dementia (average MMSE = 7.35). The research team prescribed strategies specific for the resident's cognitive and physical abilities following analysis of their cognitive functioning, physical abilities, and videotapes of them as they were being dressed by the nursing home staff. The results showed significantly improved independence without a clinically relevant increase in caregiver time (less than 1 minute).

Another application of behavioral strategies in persons with dementia is prompted voiding. Schnelle et al have conducted a number of studies using prompted voiding to maintain continence and individualized incontinence care in nursing home residents, many of whom were demented.[70-73] The results of these studies indicate that prompted voiding reduces incontinence in nursing home residents and individualized nighttime incontinence care (i.e., based on each resident's risk for skin problems and mobility) does not lead to increased skin breakdown.

One technique that has been used to improve the quality of life for individuals with dementia is reality orientation. In the method of reality orientation, information is provided to the person to help them better understand their surroundings. This information may include the day, date, time, weather, or other details. Spector, Davies, Woods, and Orrell[74] conducted an evaluation of the effectiveness of reality orientation by reviewing previously completed studies which involved the use of classroom reality orientation. Interventions in these studies included 30 to 60 minutes of group therapy with a minimum of four participants. The review concluded that reality orientation exhibited benefits on both cognition and behavior of persons with dementia.

Summary. The modification of behaviors often involves multiple behavioral strategies as well as other types of interventions. Successful behavioral interventions involve extensive staff training and education in the nature of the disease process, seeking individualized cues for behaviors, and the use of self as the therapeutic tool to reduce unwanted behaviors and encourage appropriate behaviors.

Environmental

Design of the physical environment is an important aid in the care of people with dementia. More than simply decorative, design is a therapeutic resource to promote well-being, functionality, and decrease problem behaviors in persons with dementia. Day et al[75] conducted a comprehensive systematic review of the literature on therapeutic design of environments for people with dementia. Some of the recommendations for therapeutic environments include small, homelike units with separation of demented residents from cognitively intact residents, and outdoor areas such as gardens. The review did not include the sensory or social environment such as music or pets. Box 8-3 summarizes their findings.

Research on the sensory and social environment of elders with dementia is accumulating. Interpersonal engagement, social activities, and exercise have been shown to be effective in reducing problematic behaviors and improving psychological well-being of elders with dementia. For example, in a 6-month observational study, Kutner et al[76] found that friendship was associated with fewer agitated behaviors. The authors suggested that interpersonal engagement contributes to the well being of persons with moderate dementia. In another study the authors[77] found significant improvements in depression in persons with Alzheimer's disease who met criteria for minor or major depressive disorder who received pleasurable events and caregiver problem solving.

Activity interventions are most effective if they are individualized based on an assessment of each person's past interests and preferences. Activities such as stimulus items, social interaction, presentation of videotapes, music, exercise, and audiotapes engage persons with dementia and help decrease problematic behaviors. Activities absorb and divert attention, and activities based on individual interests may be most effective. For example, in 32 nursing home residents with dementia, problematic behaviors, as measured by the Cohen-Mansfield Agitation Inventory, significantly decreased after three activities: (1) social interaction (55%), (2) presentation of a videotape of a family member (46%), and (3) use of music (31%).[78] In 22 nursing home residents with dementia, agitated behaviors declined by 50% after they participated in a 40-minute exercise/movement program for 28 days.[79] In a study of relaxing music at meal time, verbal agitation decreased in 29 persons with dementia in a nursing home.[80]

Another activity intervention, Video Respite, is a series of twenty 53-minute generic videotapes using acting professionals that the investigators designed to capture the interest of persons with dementia.[81] Content in one video consisted of a friendly visitor asking questions about familiar things like parents, growing up, babies, pets, and gardens. A clinical trial of the intervention in 31 persons with dementia living in their homes showed that 84% remained seated during the entire 33-minute video, paid attention, and responded verbally. Caregivers used the videotapes an average of 14 times during a month. In Simulated Presence Therapy, persons with dementia listen to an audiotape of a "conversation" entailing cherished memories, anecdotes about family, and other experiences in the life of the person with dementia.[82] The investigators reported a statistically significant increase in happy facial expression and interest in 54 nursing home residents with dementia.

In a study of the nursing home environment, two corridors in a nursing home were enhanced.[83] One

BOX 8-3 Recommendations for the Therapeutic Design and Planning of Dementia Environments

- Incorporate small inpatient units
- Separate demented residents from cognitively intact residents
- Provide respite care as a complement to home care
- If possible, relocate residents in intact units rather than individually
- Incorporate noninstitutional design (personalized rooms, homelike furnishings) throughout the facility and in dining rooms in particular
- Decrease environmental stimulation
- Incorporate brighter light levels
- Cover panic bars and door knobs to reduce unwanted exiting
- Use therapeutic design features such as a garden in outdoor areas
- Consider making toilets more visible to reduce incontinence
- Eliminate environmental factors such as unfamiliar, fearful, or noisy equipment, high water levels, and poor lighting that increase stress in bathing

Data from Day, K., Carreon, D., & Stump, C. (2000). The therapeutic design of environments for people with dementia: A review of the empirical research. *Gerontologist 40*, 397-416.

corridor included nature scenes and the other one featured a home-and-people scene from the early 1940s and 1950s. Benches were available for persons with dementia to sit and look at the scenes. Persons with dementia spent significantly more time in the enhanced corridors compared with the baseline. Decreases in pacing and physically nonaggressive, physically aggressive, and verbally aggressive behaviors occurred, but they did not reach statistical significance. Confusion did not change with the enhanced corridors; however, a significant increase in pleasure occurred with the nature scene.

Camp et al[84] compared a Montessori-based activity program and a traditional activity program with art therapy, musical programs, exercise programs, movies, cards, and discussion groups in 19 persons with dementia who participated in an adult daycare program. The Montessori-based activity program was based on the philosophy that learning begins at the simplest level and becomes more complex. Four categories of engagement were studied: constructive (behavior demonstrated in response to the activity), passive (looking or listening to the activity), nonengagement (sleeping, staring off in space or away from activity), and self-engagement (behavior during a transition period between activities or when the persons with dementia chose not to participate). Self-engagement and nonengagement occurred in the traditional activity and never occurred during the Montessori-based activity. Throughout the 9-month study, persons in the Montessori-based program demonstrated significantly more constructive engagement and significantly less passive engagement than the control group.

Summary. The social and physical environment should be safe, with a level of stimulation that is appropriate given the person's lifelong patterns of engagement with others. Social activities, exercise, and interpersonal involvement have been shown to increase well-being in elders with dementia and reduce problematic behaviors.

CONCEPTUAL MODEL

The Need-driven Dementia-compromised Behavior (NDB) model changes the prevalent view of dementia-related behaviors as "disruptive" to a perspective that these behaviors are potentially understandable.[66,85] The model proposes behaviors such as wandering or repetitive questioning are actions or behaviors that persons with dementia engage in to pursue goals or meet perceived needs. Thus problem behaviors commonly seen in persons with dementia are called *NDB*. This model offers a useful perspective for organizing, integrating, and applying relevant research to the complex issue of behaviors commonly occurring in persons with dementia.

The NDB model holds that behaviors in persons with dementia arise partly as expressions of needs and reflect the interaction of salient background (i.e., relatively stable) and proximal (i.e., more contextual and dynamic) variables. Background variables represent the person's lifelong pattern of needs fulfillment, while proximal variables within the person or environment may trigger a dementia-compromised attempt to fulfill needs. Proximal variables induce a need state and precipitate problem behaviors, given the context of risk-producing background variables. Although disruptive, problematic, or ineffective from an observer's viewpoint, these behaviors may constitute the persons' most integrated and meaningful effort to declare needs.

The NDB model (1) defines and describes the constellation of behaviors associated with dementia and (2) outlines the processes that generate these behaviors. In addition, the model can serve as a framework for deriving interventions and describing how they produce outcomes.[66,85] One manipulates the proximal factor that precipitates the behavior by maximizing the strengths and minimizing the weaknesses of the person's background factors. Testing of the model is needed. The NDB model is shown in Figure 8-1.

CASE STUDIES

CASE STUDY 1

Mr. C is a 68-year-old white man who was admitted to the hospital for repair of an abdominal aortic aneurysm. Past medical history includes coronary artery disease and hypertension. Current medications include diltiazem 180 mg daily, hydrochlorothiazide 25 mg daily, acetaminophen 1000 mg three to four times per day as needed for pain. He is a married retired salesman who is nonsmoking and drinks wine rarely. He and his wife report no difficulty with ADLs.

The surgery was performed without incident, and Mr. C was transferred to the surgical intensive care unit. The early postoperative course was uneventful. On the evening of the second postoperative day, Mr. C became restless, attempting to get out of bed over the rails and pull out his intravenous access line. He was disoriented to time, place, and situation. His speech was slow and incoherent at times. He became agitated and combative with nurses. He was given haloperidol 2 mg IV. A dose of lorazepam 1 mg IV was also administered when the haloperidol proved

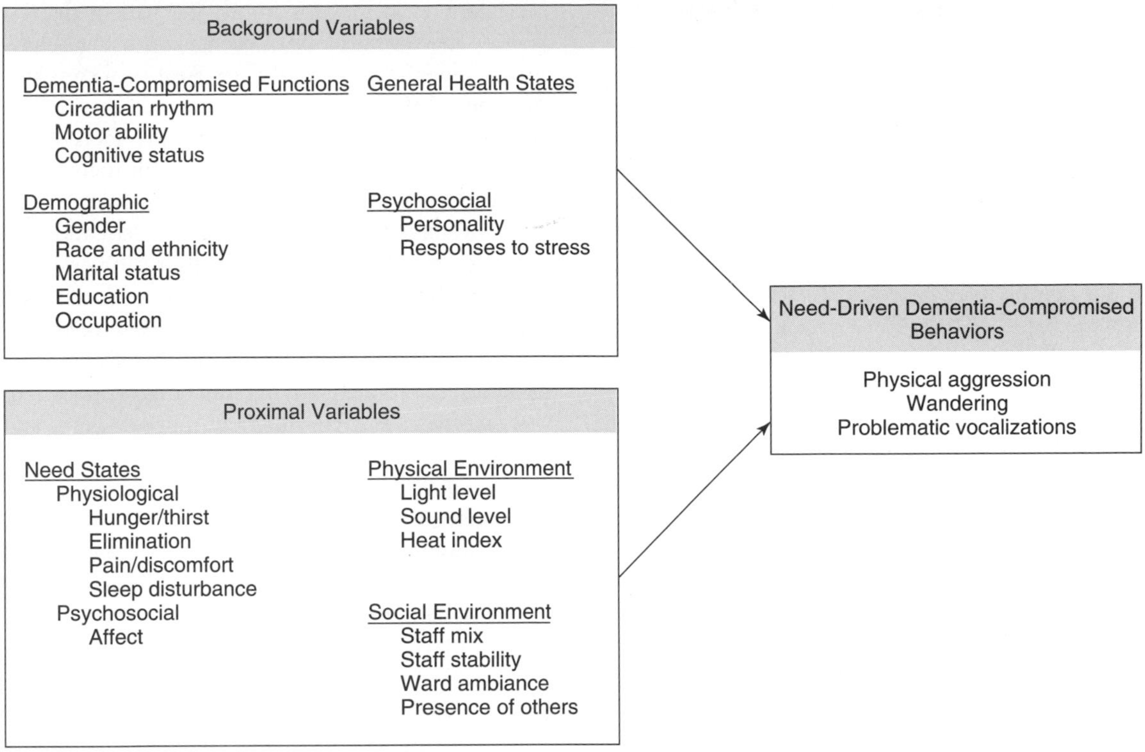

Figure 8-1 **Need-driven Dementia-compromised Behavior (NDB) model.** (Adapted from Kolanowski, A.M. [1999]. An overview of the need-driven dementia-compromised behavior model. *Journal of Gerontological Nursing 25,* 7-9.)

to be ineffective. A vest restraint was placed on the patient to prevent him from climbing out of bed.

The following morning, Mr. C was alert and oriented to person, place, time, and situation. He was unable to recall events of the previous evening. Was Mr. C demonstrating signs of dementia?

Dementia has a slow, insidious onset. Mr. C's symptoms began suddenly. The course of dementia is stable. Mr. C's course fluctuated from severe disorientation in the evening to complete lucidity the following morning. Mr. C was suffering from delirium rather than dementia.

CASE STUDY 2

Mrs. K, a 78-year-old nursing home resident with an MMSE score of 12 and probable Alzheimer's disease, suddenly began wandering up and down the hallways of the nursing home. Mrs. K has been a homemaker all of her life and has a large family who frequently come to see her in the nursing home. While wandering in the hallway she frequently goes into other resident's rooms and rummages in their drawers, lies down on their beds, and takes their things. Other residents become agitated when she comes into their rooms. During her wanderings she seems to be searching for something lost. When the nurse asks her what she is searching for, Mrs. K replies that she is looking for her room.

The nursing staff implement and evaluate the following interventions: (1) The nurses ask Mrs. K's family to bring a large wreath that contrasts with the color of the door and that will be easily visible from down the hallway. They instruct the family to attach family photos, such as pictures of Mrs. K's beloved grandchildren, to the wreath. (2) The nursing staff frequently redirect Mrs. K to her room by pointing her toward the door with the wreath and the pictures of her grandchildren. (3) The nursing staff also provide Mrs. K with a basket of clothes to fold and stack.

This case study illustrates an example of a patient who wandered and disturbed other nursing home residents. A simple environmental intervention to make the door of the patient's room unique and easily visible and an activity intervention resulted in decreased problem behaviors for Mrs. K and less disturbance for other residents.

SELECTED RESEARCH

The vast majority of nursing research related to dementia has focused on problem behaviors and caregiver burden. Research on nursing interventions for dealing with cognitive deficits of persons with dementia is less plentiful, as is research that suggests how their remaining abilities can be maximized. Much of the nursing literature is theoretical and has not been validated through research.

Horgas and Tsai[49] conducted a descriptive study on the prescription and administration of analgesic medications to treat pain in cognitively impaired nursing home residents. The sample consisted of 339 residents from four nursing homes. The mean age of the sample was 87 years, 46% were cognitively impaired, and 55% had at least one painful condition. The results indicated that persons with dementia were prescribed and administered significantly less analgesic medication, both in number and in dosage of pain drugs than cognitively intact residents. In multiple regression analysis holding the presence of painful conditions constant, more disoriented and withdrawn residents were prescribed significantly less analgesia by physicians and they were administered significantly less analgesia by nursing staff. These findings emphasize the difficulties of pain assessment in elders with dementia and need for education of health care providers about effective pain management.

Beck et al[69] conducted a clinical trial of behavioral strategies to promote dressing independence in 90 residents of eight nursing homes with dementia (average Mini Mental Status Examination score, –7.35). They used a pretest/delayed posttest design. The research team prescribed strategies specific for the resident's cognitive and physical abilities following analysis of their cognitive functioning, physical abilities, and videotapes of them as they were being dressed by the nursing home staff. A decision-making algorithm guided the prescription process. The algorithm consisted of a series of questions about cognitive abilities leading the prescriber to the strategy appropriate for the person with dementia. Standard strategies are behaviors and communication techniques that work with almost all persons with dementia. Problem-oriented strategies address particular disabilities, such as fine-motor impairment or physical limitations. The results showed significantly improved independence in dressing without a clinically relevant increase in caregiver time (less than 1 minute).

In a controlled clinical trial, Teri et al[77] compared two behavioral treatments for depression in patients with Alzheimer's disease, one emphasizing patient pleasant events and one emphasizing caregiver problem solving, to an equal-duration typical care condition and a wait list control. The focus of the pleasant events treatment was to teach caregivers behavioral strategies for improving patient depression by increasing pleasant events and using behavioral problem-solving strategies. Treatment consisted of nine 60-minute sessions, once per week, with patients and caregivers. The sessions focused on identifying, planning, and increasing pleasant events for the patient. The Pleasant Events Schedule-AD was used throughout therapy to generate ideas and help plan pleasant activities. The caregiver problem solving condition allowed caregivers more input into the content and flow of the treatment than the pleasant events intervention. Therapists used a systematic approach to problem-solving situations of concern to the caregivers and provided education, advice, and support. Seventy-two patients and their caregivers were randomly assigned to one of the four conditions and assessed preintervention, postintervention, and at a 6-month follow-up. Patients and caregivers in both behavioral treatment conditions showed significant improvement in symptoms of depression compared with the other two conditions, and these gains were maintained at follow-up. These results indicate that behavioral interventions for depression are effective strategies for treating demented patients and their caregivers.

QUESTIONS FOR FUTURE STUDY

Research is needed to determine how dementia can be prevented. Further, investigations to identify effective treatment that will prevent the devastating consequences of dementia for persons and their families are urgently needed. Another important avenue for research is experimental studies to develop and test effective interventions to improve the quality of life for persons with dementia. For example, interventions are needed to improve sleep, decrease wandering, and decrease mood disturbances in elders with dementia. Further research also is needed on methods to decrease the burden of caring for persons with dementia, such as services that would allow persons with dementia to remain at home longer. Reliable and valid instruments for pain assessment in elders with dementia are needed. Research on interventions also are needed to improve the quality of care provided in nursing home settings.

REFERENCES

1. Gabrieli, J.D., Brewer, J.B., & Vaidya, C.J. (1999). Memory. In C.G. Goetz, & E.J. Pappert (eds.), *Textbook of clinical neurology* (pp. 56-69). Philadelphia: W.B. Saunders.
2. Long, P.W. (2000). Internet mental health. [Online]. http://www.mentalhealth.com.
3. Kawas, C.H. (1999). Alzheimer's disease. In J.B. Halter, & J.G. Ouslander (eds.), *Principles of geriatric medicine*

and gerontology (4th ed., pp. 1257-1269). New York: McGraw-Hill.

4. Health, J., & Hunter, D. (2000). Neurologic health. In P.V. Meredith, & N.M. Horan (eds.), *Adult primary care* (pp. 645-691). Philadelphia: W.B. Saunders.
5. American Psychiatric Association. (2000). *Diagnostic and statistical manual of mental disorders.* (4th ed.). Washington, D.C.: Author.
6. Schultz, S. K. (2000). Dementia in the twenty-first century. *American Journal of Psychiatry 157*(5), 666-668.
7. U.S. Department of Health and Human Services. (1995). Report of the task force on aging research. Washington, D.C.: U.S. Government Printing Office.
8. Caselli, R.J., & Boeve, B.F. (1999). The degenerative dementias. In C.G. Goetz, & E.J. Pappert (eds.), *Textbook of clinical neurology* (pp. 629-653). Philadelphia: W.B. Saunders.
9. Letenneur, L., Gilleron, V., Commenges, D., Helmer, C., Orgogozo, J.M., & Dartigues, J.F. (1999). Are sex and educational level independent predictors of dementia and Alzheimer's disease? Incidence data from the PAQUID project. *Journal of Neurology, Neurosurgery, and Psychiatry 66,* 177-183.
10. Geerlings, M.I., Deeg, D.J., Penninx, B.W., Schmand, B., Jonker, C., Bouter, L.M., & van Tilburg, W. (1999). Cognitive reserve and mortality in dementia: The role of cognition, functional ability and depression. *Psychological Medicine 29,* 1219-1226.
11. Breitner, A.J. (2000). Reduced prevalence of AD in users of NSAIDs and H_2-receptor antagonists. *Neurology 54,* 2066-2071.
12. Daly, M.P.M. (1999). Diagnosis and management of Alzheimer's disease. *Journal of the American Board of Family Practice 12,* 375-384.
13. Moroney, J.T., Tang, M., Berglund, L., Small, S., Merchant, C., Bell, K., Stern, Y., & Mayeux, R. (1999). Low-density lipoprotein cholesterol and the risk of dementia with stroke. *Journal of the American Medical Association 282,* 254-260.
14. Francis, P.T., Palmer, A.M., Snape, M., & Wilcock, G.K. (1999). The cholinergic hypothesis of Alzheimer's disease: A review of progress. *Journal of Neurology, Neurosurgery, and Psychiatry 66,* 137-147.

14a. Grasby, D.C. (2001). Pathological hallmarks of Alzheimer's disease. Unpublished master's thesis, University of Tasmania, Hobart, Tasmania 7000, Australia.

15. Trojanowski, J.Q., & Lee, V.M. (1998). Aggregation of neurofilament and alpha-synuclein proteins in Lewy bodies: Implications for the pathogenesis of Parkinson's disease and Lewy body dementia. *Archives of Neurology 55,* 151-152.
16. Ballard, C., Holmes, C., McKeith, I., Neill, D., O'Brien, J., Cairns, N., et al. (1999). Psychiatric morbidity in dementia with Lewy bodies: A prospective clinical and neuropathological comparative study with Alzheimer's disease. *American Journal of Psychiatry 156,* 1039-1045.
17. Kertesz, A., & Munoz, D. (1998). Pick's disease, frontotemporal dementia, and Pick complex: Emerging concepts. *Archives of Neurology 55,* 302-304.
18. Beck, C., & Heacock, P. (1988). Nursing interventions for patients with Alzheimer's disease. *Nursing Clinics of North America 23,* 95-124.
19. Jackson, M.E., Spector, W.D., & Rabins, P.V. (1997). Risk of behavior problems among nursing home residents in the United States. *Journal of Aging and Health 9,* 451-472.
20. Dowling, G.A. (1996). Behavioral intervention strategies for sleep-activity disruption. *International Psychogeriatrics 8,* 77-86.
21. Bliwise, D.L. (2000). Dementia. In M.H. Kryger, T. Roth, & W.C. Dement (eds.), *Principles and practice of sleep medicine* (3rd ed., pp. 1058-1071). Philadelphia: W.B. Saunders.
22. Schnelle, J.F., Ouslander, J.G., Simmons, S.F., Alessi, C.A., & Gravel, M.D. (1993a). Nighttime sleep and bed mobility among incontinent nursing home residents. *Journal of the American Geriatrics Society 41,* 903-909.
23. Allen, S.R., Seiler, W.O., Stahelin, H.B., & Spiegel, R. (1987). Seventy-two hour polygraphic and behavioral recordings of wakefulness and sleep in a hospital geriatric unit: Comparison between demented and non-demented patients. *Sleep 10,* 143-159.
24. Prinz, P.N., Peskind, E.R., Vitaliano, P.P., Raskind, M.A., Eisdorfer, C., Zemcuznikov, N., et al. (1982). Changes in the sleep and waking EEGs of nondemented and demented elderly subjects. *Journal of the American Geriatrics Society 30,* 86-93.
25. Ancoli-Israel, S., Parker, L., Sinaee, R., Fell, R.L., & Kripke, D.F. (1989). Sleep fragmentation in patients from a nursing home. *Journal of Gerontology 44,* M18-M21.
26. Vitiello, M.V., & Prinz, P.N. (1989). Alzheimer's disease. Sleep and sleep/wake patterns. *Clinics in Geriatric Medicine 5,* 289-299.
27. Vitiello, M.V., Prinz, P.N., Williams, D.E., Frommlet, M.S., & Ries, R.K. (1990). Sleep disturbances in patients with mild-stage Alzheimer's disease. *Journal of Gerontology 45,* M131-M138.
28. Vitiello, M.V., Bliwise, D.L., & Prinz, P.N. (1992). Sleep in Alzheimer's disease and the sundown syndrome. *Neurology 42,* 83-93.
29. Schnelle, J.F., Cruise, P.A., Alessi, C.A., Ludlow, K., al-Samarrai, N.R., Ouslander, J.G. (1998). Sleep hygiene in physically dependent nursing home residents: Behavioral and environmental intervention implications. *Sleep 21,* 515-523.
30. Schnelle, J.F., Alassi C.A., a-Samarrai, N.R., Fricker, R.D. Jr, & Ouslander, J.G. (1999). The nursing home at night: Effects of an intervention on noise, light, and sleep. *Journal of the American Geriatrics Society 47,* 430-438.
31. Morewitz, J.H. (1988). Evaluation of excessive daytime sleepiness in the elderly. *Journal of the American Geriatrics Society 36,* 324-330.
32. Logsdon, RG., & Teri, L. (1997). The Pleasant Events Schedule-AD: Psychometric properties and relationship to depression and cognition in Alzheimer's disease patients. *Gerontologist 37,* 40-45.
33. Andresen, G. (1998). As America ages: Dx dementia: But what kind? *RN 61,* 26-30.
34. Shankar, K.K., & Orrell, M.W. (2000). Detecting and managing depression and anxiety in people with dementia. *Current Opinion in Psychiatry 13*(1), 55-59.
35. Small, G.W., Rabins, P.V., Barry, P.P., Buckholtz, N.S., DeKosky, S.T., Ferris, S.H., et al. (1997). Diagnosis and treatment of Alzheimer's disease and related disorders: Consensus statement of the American Association for Geriatric Psychiatry, the Alzheimer's Association, and the American Geriatrics Society. *Journal of the American Medical Association 278,* 1363-1371.
36. Haller, E., & Binder, R. (1994). Delirium, dementia, and amnestic disorders. In H.H. Goldman (ed.), *Review of general psychiatry.* Connecticut: Appleton & Lange.
37. Francis, A., Pincus, H.A., First, M.B., & Widiger, T.A. (1994). *A quick reference to the criteria from DSM-IV*

(4th ed., pp. 176-189). Washington, D.C., American Psychological Association.
38. McKeith, I.G., O'Brien, J.T., & Ballard, C. (1999). Diagnosing dementia with Lewy bodies. *Lancet 354,* 1227-1228.
39. Liddell, M.B., Lovestone, S., & Owen, M.J. (2001). Genetic risk of Alzheimer's disease: Advising relatives. *British Journal of Psychiatry 178,* 7-11.
40. Folstein, M.F., Folstein, S.E., & McHugh, P.R. (1975). Mini-Mental State: A practical method for grading the cognitive state of patients for the clinician. *Journal of Psychiatric Research 12,* 188-198.
41. Panisset, M., Roudier, M., Saxton, J., & Boller, F. (1993). Severe impairment battery. *Archives of Neurology 51,* 41-45.
42. Folstein, M., & McHugh, P. (1979). Psychopathology of dementia: Implications for neuropathology. In R. Katzman (ed.), *Congenital and acquired cognitive disorders.* New York: Raven Press.
43. Anthony, J.C., LeResche, L., Niaz, U., von Korff, M.R., & Folstein, M.F. (1982). Limits of the 'Mini-Mental State' as a screening test for dementia and delirium among hospital patients. *Psychological Medicine 12,* 397-408.
44. Salmon, D.P., Thomas, R.G., Pay, M.M., Booth, A., Hofstetter, C.R., Thal, L.J., et al. (2002). Alzheimer's disease can be accurately diagnosed in very mildly impaired individuals. *Neurology 59,* 1022-1028.
45. Foreman, M.D. (1987). Reliability and validity of mental status questionnaires in elderly hospitalized patients...the SPMSQ, MMSE, and CCSE. *Nursing Research 36,* 216-220.
46. Saxton, J., & McGonigle, K. (1993). *The severe impairment battery.* Suffolk, England, Thames Valley Test Co.
47. Albert, S.M., Del Castillo-Castaneda, C., Sano, M., Jacobs, D.M., Marder, K., Bell, K., et al. (1996). Quality of life in patients with Alzheimer's disease as reported by patient proxies. *Journal of the American Geriatrics Society 44,* 1342-1347.
48. Kitwood, D., & Bredin, K. (1992). A new approach to the evaluation of dementia care. *Journal of Advances in Health and Nursing Care 1,* 41-60.
49. Horgas, A.L., & Tsai, P. (1998). Analgesic drug prescription and use in cognitively impaired nursing home residents. *Nursing Research 47,* 235-242.
50. Beck, C.K. (1998). Psychosocial and behavioral interventions for Alzheimer's disease patients and their families. *American Journal of Geriatric Psychiatry 6*(2 Suppl 1), S41-S48.
51. Byrne, G.J. (2000). Drug treatment in dementia. *Current Opinion in Psychiatry 13,* 415-421.
52. Sano, M., Ernesto, C., Thomas, R.G., Klauber, M.R., Schafer, K., Grundman, M., et al. (1997). A controlled trial of selegiline, alpha-tocopherol, or both as treatment for Alzheimer's disease. *New England Journal of Medicine 336,* 1216-1222.
53. Filip, V., & Kolibas, E. (2000). Selegiline in the treatment of Alzheimer's disease: A long-term randomized placebo-controlled trial. *Journal of Psychiatry Neuroscience 24,* 234-243.
54. Emilien, G., Beyreuther, K., & Masters, C. (2000). Prospects for pharmacological intervention in Alzheimer disease. *Archives of Neurology 57,* 454-459.
55. Levy, M.L., Cummings, J.L., & Kahn-Rose, R. (1999). Neuropsychiatric symptoms and cholinergic therapy for Alzheimer's disease. *Gerontology 45,* 15-22.
56. Tariot, P.N., Erb, R., Podgorski, C.A., Cox, C., Patel, S., Jakimovich, L., et al. (1998). Efficacy and tolerability of carbamazepine for agitation and aggression in dementia. *American Journal of Psychiatry 155,* 54-61.
57. Schneider, L.S., Pollock, V.E., & Lyness, S.A. (1990). A meta-analysis of controlled trials of neuroleptic treatment in dementia. *Journal of the American Geriatrics Society 38,* 553-563.
58. De Deyn, P.P., & Rebheru, K.R.A. (1999). A randomised trial of resperidone, placebo, and haloperidol for behavioural symptoms of dementia. *Neurology 53,* 946-955.
59. Katz, I., Jeste, M.D., Mintzer, J.E., Clyde, C., Napolitano, J., Brecher, M. (1999). Comparison of risperidone and placebo for psychosis and behavioural disturbances associated with dementia: A randomised, double-blind trial. *Journal of Clinical Psychiatry 60,* 107-115.
60. American Health Care Association. (1990). The long-term care survey: Regulations, procedures, guidelines (Rep. No. Cat. No. 4697/UBP/2.5K/7/90). Washington, D.C.: Author.
61. Grasel, E. (1994). Nonpharmacological intervention strategies on aging processes: Empirical data on mental training in "normal" older people and patients with mental impairment. *Archives of Gerontology and Geriatrics 4,* 91-98.
62. Burgio, L.D., & Stevens, A.B. (1998). Behavioral interventions and motivational systems in the nursing home. In M.P. Lawton, R. Lavizzo-Morey, J.W. Rowe, V. Cristofalo, & R.W. Madsen (eds.), *Annual review of gerontology and geriatrics* (pp. 284-320). New York: Springer.
63. Gugel, R.N. (1994). Behavioral approaches for managing patients with Alzheimer's disease and related disorders. *Medical Clinics of North America 78*(4), 861-867.
64. Fares, A. (1997). Assessment and care for people with dementia. *Nursing Standard 11*(40), 49-55.
65. Carrier, L., & Brodaty, H. (1999). Mood and behaviour management. In S. Gauthier (ed.), *Clinical diagnosis and management of Alzheimer's disease* (2nd ed., pp. 229-248). London: Martin Dunitz.
66. Algase, D.L., Beck, C., Kolanowski, A., Whall, A., Berent, S., Richards, K., et al. (1996). Need-driven dementia-compromised behavior: An alternative view of disruptive behavior. *American Journal of Alzheimer's Disease 11,* 10-19.
67. Christie, M., & Ferguson, G. (1988). Can't anyone stop that screaming? *Canadian Nurse 84,* 30-32.
68. Opie, J., Rosewarne, R., & O'Connor, D.W. (1999). The efficacy of psychosocial approaches to behaviour disorders in dementia: A systematic literature review. *Australian and New Zealand Journal of Psychiatry 33,* 789-799.
69. Beck, C., Heacock, P., Mercer, S.O., Walls, R.C., Rapp, C.G., & Vogelpohl, T.S. (1997). Improving dressing behavior in cognitively impaired nursing home residents. *Nursing Research 46,* 126-132.
70. Schnelle, J.F., Cruise, P.A., Alessi, C.A., al-Samarrai, N., & Ouslander, J.G. (1998). Individualizing nighttime incontinence care in nursing home residents. *Nursing Research 47,* 197-204.
71. Schnelle, J.F., Newman, D., White, M., Abbey, J., Wallston, K.A., Fogarty, T., & Ory, M.G. (1993). Maintaining continence in nursing home residents through the application of industrial quality control. *Gerontologist 33,* 114-121.
72. Schnelle, J.F., Newman, D.R., & Fogarty, T. (1990). Management of patient continence in long-term care nursing facilities. *Gerontologist 30,* 373-376.
73. Schnelle, J.F., Ouslander, J.G., Simmons, S.F., Alessi, C.A., & Gravel, M.D. (1993b). The nighttime environment, incontinence care, and sleep disruption in nursing homes. *Journal of the American Geriatrics Society 41,* 910-914.

74. Spector, A., Davies, S., Woods, B., & Orrell, M. (2000). Reality orientation for dementia: A systematic review of the evidence of effectiveness from randomized controlled trials. *Gerontologist 40,* 206-212.
75. Day, K., Carreon, D., & Stump, C. (2000). The therapeutic design of environments for people with dementia: A review of the empirical research. *Gerontologist 40,* 397-416.
76. Kutner, N., Brown, P.J., Stavisky, R.C., Clark, W., & Green, R.C. (2000). "Friendship" interactions and expression of agitation among residents of a dementia care unit: Six-month observational data. *Research on Aging 22,* 188-205.
77. Teri, L., Logsdon, R.G., Uomoto, J., & McCurry, S.M. (1997). Behavioral treatment of depression in dementia patients: A controlled clinical trial. *Journals of Gerontology, Series B, Psychological Sciences and Social Sciences 52,* 159-166.
78. Cohen-Mansfield, J. (1995). Management of verbally disruptive behaviors in nursing home residents. *Journals of Gerontology 52A,* M369-M377.
79. Namazi, K.H., Gwinnup, P.B., & Zadorozny, C.A. (1994). A low intensity exercise/movement program for patients with Alzheimer's disease: The TEMP-AD protocol. *Journal of Aging and Physical Activity 2,* 80-92.
80. Goddaer, J., & Abraham, I.L. (1994). Effects of relaxing music on agitation during meals among nursing home residents with severe cognitive impairment. *Archives of Psychiatric Nursing 8,* 150-158.
81. Lund, D.A., Hill, R.D., Caserta, M.S., & Wright, S.D. (1995). Video respite: An innovative resource for family, professional caregivers, and persons with dementia. *Gerontologist 35,* 683-687.
82. Camberg, L., Woods, P., Ooi, W.L., Hurley, A., Volicer, L., Ashley, J., et al. (1999). Evaluation of simulated presence: A personalized approach to enhance well-being in persons with Alzheimer's disease. *Journal of the American Geriatrics Society 47,* 446-452.
83. Cohen-Mansfield, J., & Werner, P. (1998). The effects of an enhanced environment on nursing home residents who pace. *Gerontologist 38,* 199-208.
84. Camp, C.J., Judge, K.S., Bye, C.A., Fox, K.M., Bowden, J., Bell, M., et al. (1997). An intergenerational program for persons with dementia using Montessori methods. *Gerontologist 37,* 688-692.
85. Kolanowski, A. (1999). An overview of the need-driven dementia-compromised behavior model. *Journal of Gerontological Nursing 25,* 7-9.

CHAPTER

9 Acute Confusion

KENNITH CULP

DEFINITION

Acute confusion (AC) is a state of transient brain dysfunction characterized by acute onset, brief duration, and fluctuating course,[1] and frequently associated with a psychiatric disorder known as delirium.[2] AC, acute confusional state, and delirium are diagnostic terms that are often used interchangeably and are essentially synonyms for the same physiological event, best described as a broad spectrum of nonadaptive psychophysiological responses characterized by altered consciousness and disordered cognition. The terms *acute confusion* and *delirium* will be used interchangeably in this chapter.

AC is a condition of disordered cognition. It is clinically manifested in a variety of ways but may include alterations in perception, thinking, and memory; dysfunction of the reticular activating system (which influences both attention and wakefulness); and dysfunction of the autonomic nervous system (which influences both psychomotor and regulatory functions).[3] The hallmark of AC is altered attention and an acute change in mental status from baseline functioning, which may be identified clinically by a sudden onset of disorientation, decreased awareness of self or others, agitation, odd remarks or atypical verbalizations that do not fit the context of a conversation, slurred or pressured speech patterns, irritability, and/or a failure to recognize one's surroundings.[4]

The broad categorizations that describe the causes of delirium are primary cerebral diseases (e.g., encephalitis, neoplasm, trauma, epilepsy, and stroke), systemic diseases that affect the brain indirectly (e.g., metabolic imbalances, infections, fever, fluid-electrolyte problems, and cardiovascular, hepatic, and renal disease processes), exogenous substances with toxic or addictive effects (e.g., medications, illicit drugs, poisons, and occupational and environmental exposures), and environmental or psychosocial stressors (e.g., bereavement and new surroundings). This latter category is controversial; occasionally medical clinicians assert that nurses assume nonorganic causes or environmental stress too quickly and do not adequately explore pathophysiological causes. Also, it is unclear where the interaction of pain and delirium falls in the organic versus nonorganic paradigm.[5]

Although elderly persons experience acute confusion more frequently than other age groups, this phenomenon can also occur in younger adults and children.[6-8] Most commonly, the etiologies associated with AC are metabolic or systemic (Table 9-1). Frequent antecedents are fluid and electrolyte problems, drug toxicities, co-morbid disease states, pulmonary or urinary tract infections, severe pain, poor oxygenation, and endocrine disturbances.[9] Although head trauma, inflammatory processes of the brain and spinal cord, and cerebral malignancies can play a role in precipitating confusional events, in this chapter we will not place particular emphasis on these causes, because these confusional states are more readily recognized, and the etiological factors associated with them are not as "systemic" in relation to the conceptualization of delirium.

Clinical Subtypes

Some researchers argue that subtypes of delirium can be differentiated by motor activity.[10] The subtypes are (1) a quiet type: withdrawn, less attentive, and hypoactive (2) an agitated type: characterized by extensive motor activity, and (3) a mixed type: a heterogeneous manifestation of these symptoms or fluctuation between the two extremes.[11-13]

It has been hypothesized that these subtypes can be linked to etiological factors.[14] For example, patients with hepatic encephalopathy may be more likely to have somnolent delirium,[15] whereas patients with alcohol withdrawal may be more likely to have the agitated type of delirium.[16] Differences in addition to motor symptoms and attentiveness may exist as well; for example, patients with the active subtype tend to have hallucinations,

TABLE 9-1 Acute Confusion and Dementia

FEATURE	ACUTE CONFUSION	DEMENTIA
Onset and course	Develops suddenly, precise time of onset, nonprogressive, may have lucid intervals, worsens late in the day	Develops slowly over time, uncertain time of onset, gradual deterioration, generally stable over the course of the day
Consciousness	Fluctuating consciousness	Rarely altered consciousness
Thought processes	Disorganized	Impoverished
Attention	Attention altered, may be either hypoalert or hyperalert	Attention not altered until late in the disease
Perception	Illusions and hallucinations are relatively common	Illusions and hallucinations usually not present
Speech	Speech slow, incoherent	Difficulty in finding words, repetitive, near misses or invents labels
Behavior	May be agitated and restless, or sedated and withdrawn or fluctuate between hypermotor/hypomotor activity	Usually wanders about, may become agitated
Orientation	Disoriented most commonly to time, often mistaking new environment/persons for known	Orientation to person, place, and time often impaired
Age distribution	Can occur in all age groups from children through elderly, but the elderly are less resilient	Disease predominantly is of late adulthood and the elderly
Illness/medication toxicity	Medication toxicity and/or other physical illness often present	Medication toxicity and/or other physical illness rarely present
Outcome	Excellent if etiology is recognized and corrected in time	Poor, present therapeutic management focuses on slowing progression, often results in death

Adapted from Lipowski, Z.J. (1983): Transient cognitive disorders in the elderly. *American Journal of Psychiatry 140*, 1426-1436.

delusions, and illusions more often than patients with the quiet subtype. Different intervention strategies may be appropriate for each clinical subtype. These delirium subtypes may also differ in their underlying pathophysiologies, responsiveness to therapeutic interventions, and outcome. For example, some suggest that patients with cerebral hypoxia may demonstrate agitated psychomotor activity.[17]

Many researchers do not report incidence by delirium subtype, but it is described in a few studies. In one prospective study of 225 elderly patients admitted to an acute geriatric unit in a teaching hospital, 94 patients (42%) subsequently developed delirium.[18] Of these 94, 20 (21%) experienced hyperactive delirium, 27 (29%) had a hypoactive delirium, 40 (43%) had a mixed hypoactive-hyperactive psychomotor pattern, and 7 (7%) had no psychomotor disturbance. Patients with hypoactive delirium were sicker on admission, had the longest hospital stay, and were most likely to develop pressure sores. Patients with hyperactive delirium were most likely to experience a fall while in the hospital.

Part of the controversy in recognizing delirium is the moving target of diagnostic criteria. In comparing the various versions of the *Diagnostic and Statistical Manual of Mental Disorders* (DSM), one can see the evolution of these criteria over the years. For example, there is less emphasis on disorientation and memory impairment and more weight given to the presence of alterations in thought processes in DSM-IIIR than in DSM-III. The DSM-IV criteria lack an integrated neuropsychological conceptualization. The DSM-IIIR also lacks a continuum of confusional states, ranging from mild to severe. Many researchers know these limitations and, depending on the diagnostic criteria (i.e., DSM III, DSM IIIR, or DSM IV) used in any given study, there could be great variances in the frequency of cases identified.

PREVALENCE AND POPULATIONS AT RISK

AC is frequently misdiagnosed or missed altogether; thus estimates of prevalence vary widely. The precise combination of symptoms required for a firm diagnosis also remains undetermined, which has an impact on prevalence estimates.[19] In one retrospective study, the investigators reviewed hospital charts to determine whether there was documentation of delirium symptoms.[20] Researchers in this study found that 36% of the records documented symptomatology of delirium, but the diagnosis was not made. In another setting, nurses detected AC in only about one fourth of all research subjects in a long-term care facility who concurrently had been screened as positive for AC.[21] Such widespread failure to recognize this syndrome suggests a need to educate health care providers about AC and to initiate a consultation with expert clinicians when it is suspected.

The risk of developing AC is higher in severely ill patients,[22-24] persons of advanced age,[25-29] and those with limited functional abilities.[25,30,31] These major risk factors are documented not only in the case study literature, but also in at least one meta-analysis (in which male sex is also associated with greater risk).[32] Elderly postoperative patients also are at greater risk for delirium, presumably because of the use of anesthetics, anticholinergic drugs, and benzodiazepines.[33]

Delirium following surgery is very common and is a significant reason for prolonged hospitalization.[34] It is also common following severe burns in which hypoxia and hypovolemic shock are present. AC in children following admission to a burn unit has been reported.[35] Delirium in the postpartum period is relatively rare today because of the improved obstetrical care of women, but it has been reported.[36]

RISK FACTORS

Although these risk variables are not necessarily unique to delirium and may have an impact on an entire spectrum of illnesses, there is a need to classify them to identify intervention strategies.

Environmental

Environmental causes of delirium probably have underlying disturbances not only in cognition and perception, but also in disruption of neuroendocrine functioning, similar to the physiology of stress. For example, elderly residents with disruptive nocturnal behaviors in nursing homes may have experienced a room change. When residents in long-term care become isolated and do not participate in nursing home activity programs, the risk of delirium increases.[37] Other environmental factors, including the absence of windows, may increase rates of delirium in ICU patients,[38] and the appearance of costumed visitors at holiday times seems to cause confusional symptoms in some nursing home residents with dementia.[39] Diurnal fluctuations of confusional behavior suggest that time and physical environment are risk factors, specifically that late afternoon or evening increases the risk of delirium.[40,41]

Personal

Medications are the most frequent cause of delirium in older hospitalized patients, possibly because of the age-related sensitivity of the brain to the effects of drugs, as well as altered pharmacokinetics in the elderly.[42-44]

Psychotropic drugs greatly increase the risk of delirium. Opioid drugs are among the most important causes of delirium in postoperative patients. Long-acting benzodiazepines are the drugs most frequently known to cause or exacerbate confusional states in dementia patients.[45] Delirium was a major complication of treatment with tricyclic antidepressants but seems less common with newer agents.[46] Anticonvulsants can cause delirium and dementia.[47-49] Drug-induced confusion with non-psychoactive drugs is often idiosyncratic in nature, and the diagnosis is easily missed unless clinicians maintain a high index of suspicion. Histamine H_2-receptor antagonists, cardiac medications such as digoxin and beta-blockers, corticosteroids, nonsteroidal antiinflammatory agents, and antibiotics all increase the risk of AC.[50-53]

The most common physiological risk factors are hypoxia, infection, and metabolic disturbances.[27,54,55] Hypoxic events are generally associated with rapid motor behaviors, specifically a hyperattentive and hyperactive state.[3] Fever and hepatic encephalopathy are more likely to produce hypoattentive and hypomotor signs and symptoms.[43] Fluid and electrolyte imbalances, anemia, and poor nutrition are also risk factors.[56]

Developmental

Acute confusion is poorly understood in age groups other than elders. There are reports of delirium in young postpartum women,[36] adolescents with anorexia nervosa,[57] and pediatric patients,[58] but there are no large-sample epidemiological investigations in these populations. The neurophysiological thresholds in younger patients are most likely higher and thus they are less vulnerable to cerebral insult than elders are. In general, younger adults have a greater resiliency to physiological challenges than do older adults.

Children are also at risk of developing AC, especially after the delivery of anesthesia,[6,59] with fever or severe illness,[60] and with certain types of drug toxicities.[61] It is interesting to note that AC in children may vary by culture, and the content of their disorientations may be associated with childhood fantasies and beliefs.[62] Young adults can also experience delirium.[63] The risk factors for young adults are most likely similar to those already described, although some studies also point to delirium associated with alcoholism and sedative-hypnotic dependence,[64,65] postoperative pain,[5] infection,[66] and cocaine use.[67] The prevalence of AC is poorly understood in these other age groups because of a long tradition in the clinical sciences to focus delirium research on elders.[68]

Older adults have unique risk characteristics that make them more vulnerable to the onset of AC. This is because aged adults have a decreased ability to establish equilibrium when challenged with a stressful event, either physiologically[29,69,70] or environmentally.[71-74] Elders are also more likely than younger patients to develop AC as a result of taking medications because of age- and disease-associated changes in brain neurochemistry and drug metabolism. This explains why the incidence is so high in this age group and why nearly every physical illness may give rise to delirium in an elderly person.

MECHANISMS

The pathophysiology of AC is poorly understood, mostly because of the transient nature of the illness and the confounding variables introduced by coexisting physical illness and drug toxicities (even in the presence of normal dosages). It is possible that delirium is precipitated by a general reduction of cerebral metabolism. This is reflected in the concurrent presentation of cognitive impairment and the slowing of electroencephalography (EEG) background activity.

Alteration in neurotransmission has been hypothesized as a causal theory for delirium. Trzepacz[75] suggested that acetylcholine deficiency and dopamine excess, either in absolute form and/or relative to each other, may play a role in the development of delirium. These neurotransmitters work interactively, depending on the receptor subtype. The neurotransmitter acetylcholine has been suspected as a possible cause of delirium for a number of years.[76] Some medications (i.e., anticholinergics) inhibit postsynaptic muscarinic receptors, resulting in diminished function of the central neurotransmitter system.[77] Indeed, cases of drug-induced delirium have been documented in postsurgical patients and acutely ill older medical patients.[78]

Drug-Induced Delirium

Drug toxicities are more likely to occur in patients with metabolic and nutritional problems, such as hypoalbuminemia, which results in decreased protein binding of many drugs.[79] With more free drug in the blood, it is possible for more medication to cross the blood-brain barrier. Also, during illness and hospitalization, a number of new medications are introduced into the system and the sum total may exceed the ability of albumin to transport them. Hypoalbuminemia is best conceptualized as the end result of many processes—malnutrition, underfeeding combined with aggressive hydration in the hospital, losses to extravascular spaces, and decreased protein synthesis associated with hepatic disease.

Alcoholism

Alcohol withdrawal syndrome (AWS) is a unique type of delirium. The pathological mechanism in AWS is much different from the other pathologies described here and the intervention focus is on systemic detoxification.[16] Specifically, alcohol has an impact on many neurotransmitters and increases the fluidity of neuronal cell membranes, depending on the dose. The body compensates for elevated ethanol levels by increasing both hepatic and cellular pharmacokinetic tolerance.[16] Some signs and symptoms are more closely correlated with the development of AWS than other general forms of delirium: tremors; tachycardia (defined as a heart rate above 120 beats per minute in a middle-aged adult); elevated serum alcohol levels on admission to the clinic or hospital; cessation of drinking for only 6 to 8 hours; a history of epileptic seizures; and a previous history of delirious episodes associated with abrupt alcohol withdrawal.[80] The addictive nature of the etiological substance further distinguishes AWS from other types of medication-induced AC.

BOX 9-1 Organic Causes of Delirium

Intoxication

Medications: Anticholinergics, tricyclic antidepressants, lithium, sedative-hypnotics, steroids, neuroleptics, antihypertensive agents, antiarrhythmic drugs, digitalis, anticonvulsants, antiparkinsonian agents, analgesics (opiates and nonnarcotics), cimetidine

Alcohol and poisons: Heavy metals, organic solvents, methyl alcohol, ethylene glycol

Withdrawal Syndromes

Alcohol

Sedatives and hypnotics

Metabolic

Electrolyte imbalance: Elevated or decreased sodium, calcium

Hypoglycemia, hyperglycemia

Acid-base imbalance: Acidosis, alkalosis

Hypoxia

Failure of vital organs: Liver, kidney, lung

Vitamin deficiency: Thiamine (Wernicke's encephalopathy), folate, cyanocobalamin

Hyperthermia and hypothermia

Infectious

Intracranial: Encephalitis and meningitis

Systemic: Pneumonia, septicemia, influenza, urinary tract

Neurological

Space-occupying lesions: Tumor, subdural hematoma, aneurysm

Cerebrovascular diseases: Thrombosis, embolism, hemorrhage, hypertensive epilepsy

Endocrine

Thyroid: Thyrotoxicosis, myxedema

Parathyroid: Hypoparathyroidism and hyperparathyroidism

Cardiovascular

Congestive heart failure

Cardiac arrhythmia

Myocardial infarction

Multiple Etiological Factors

A number of other etiological factors associated with AC are outlined in Box 9-1. These include thyroid dysfunction and vitamin deficiencies.[31,81,82] Although there is no single explanation for explaining the increased incidence of delirium in the elderly, a delayed immune-neuroendocrine mechanism is probably the most likely culprit. As a person ages, his or her ability to adapt to stress and change in the environment is diminished when compared with that individual's younger years.

There are several physiological hypotheses on the specific endocrine tissue responsible for triggering the gradual decline in homeostatic reserve associated with the aging process,[83] but it is beyond the scope of this chapter to explore these in detail. However, this slowed response does influence neuroendocrine chemistry and does increase the likelihood of cognitive instability manifested in the signs of symptoms of AC. External environmental changes that occur suddenly might precipitate this internal, physiological imbalance and thus may explain why elders develop delirium when relocated to a new room.

There are case reports of steroid-induced AC that lend support to the neuroendocrine etiology.[51,53,84] Glucocorticoid hormones are important for coping with stress but may have deleterious effects on mood and memory when given as a medication for a prolonged period.[85] Glucocorticoids have generalized effects on brain excitability, cerebral blood flow, and oxygen consumption that can result in euphoria, psychosis, and anxiety when these medications are given in excess or abruptly discontinued. The side effects of corticosteroid withdrawal are less documented in the literature than other types of delirium. Most commonly, side effects are caused by rapid tapering or continuous use of large corticosteroid dosages.

PATHOLOGICAL CONSEQUENCES

Delirium is a disruptive, costly, and—at times—lethal condition that is associated with many adverse short-term consequences.[86] Disorientation in AC may be the result of a decreased ability to recall a recent event because of a disturbance in short-term memory.[87] Many illnesses and treatments may have a general dampening effect on memory, but for the person with AC such changes in orientation are more profound. Delirium patients may have two phases of memory alteration: general disorientation during the delirious event and a general amnesia following the period of confusion.

One of the most dire consequences of AC is increased mortality risk. Survival time was significantly shorter in those with delirium than in those without delirium in a longitudinal study of hospitalized elders.[88] Delirium appears to be an important marker of risk for death, even in older people without prior cognitive or functional impairment.[89]

AC is also associated with longer hospital length of stay (LOS), functional decline during hospitalization, falls, increased risk of developing a hospital-acquired complication, and increased admission to long-term care.[90] One prospective study compared LOS of delirious patients with controls matched by age, gender, principal diagnosis and date of admission.[91] The investigators found that hospitalized elders with delirium were statistically likely to consume more hospital resources and stayed nearly twice as long as their nondelirious cohorts. This finding has been validated by other investigators.[92,93]

Iatrogenic consequences of AC are also possible; these may occur from misdiagnosis or poor treatment resulting from failure to identify delirium or the underlying cause. The rate of "failure to detect" is pronounced. In a retrospective audit of medical records, it was suspected that 36% of the subjects had unrecognized delirium, based on physician progress notes and application of DSM-IIIR criteria for delirium.[20] Also, many nurses fail to recognize AC unless the symptoms are conspicuous. Nurses tend to recognize the hyperactive, hyperkinetic clinical subtype much more frequently than the hypoactive, hypokinetic subtype.[21]

This lack of understanding about the pathogenesis of AC leads to a number of undesirable outcomes, including increased rates of injuries.[94] Many of these are related to the inappropriate use of physical restraints,[95] which can result in asphyxiation,[96] head trauma, and bone fractures.[97] Although control of aggressive or unsafe behaviors with pharmacological or physical restraints and specific support measures may be required in special circumstances,[27] there is increasing concern that these interventions sometimes displace the primary objective of targeting the antecedent condition.[98]

RELATED PATHOPHYSIOLOGICAL CONCEPTS AND DIFFERENTIAL DIAGNOSES

A number of other phenomena and medical conditions manifest in a manner similar to acute confusion and can make the diagnosis of AC very challenging when occurring simultaneously with AC; specifically, dementia, depression, and Wernicke-Korsakoff syndrome.

Dementia

Misclassification of delirium is most common in the elderly but can occur in other age groups as well. Table 9-1 compares delirium with dementia. Dementia is the long-term loss of intellectual functioning, especially in the higher-order functions of memory, judgment, abstract thinking, reasoning, and visual-spatial relatedness, whereas delirium is a temporary state of disorganized thought.[99] (See Chapter 8, Dementia.) A hallmark difference between the two is the fact that when a person develops AC, there is a definite time point of onset, whereas in dementia, the onset of symptoms is gradual.

There is a higher rate of delirium in patients with cortical dementias (e.g., Alzheimer's disease [AD]) than in those with subcortical dementias (e.g., Parkinson's disease [PD]).[100] In one study, when PD subjects were compared with AD subjects, it was found that the PD group tended to exhibit disruptive nocturnal behavior more frequently than the AD group.[101] There are also AC risk factors specific to both types of dementia when compared with nondemented elders in nursing homes. For example, dementia patients are more likely to have a urinary tract infection, less likely to consume adequate fluids, more likely to have their medication changed, and more likely to experience an illness in which the metabolic rate is affected.[102-106]

Sundowning

There really is no clear clinical definition of sundowning, although it is easily recognized when it occurs in dementia patients. In general, sundowning is clinically identified by a circadian pattern of agitation, disruptive vocalization, occasional urinary incontinence, and confusion.[107] Possible etiological factors include disturbance in rapid eye movement (REM) sleep, episodes of sleep apnea, and a deterioration of the suprachiasmatic nucleus of the hypothalamus.[40] Management of sundowning behavior includes the treatment of any contributing physiological factors and low doses of specific neuroleptics, as well as nonpharmacological interventions, such as restriction of daytime sleep, exposure to bright lights during the day, and mild activity schedules.[108] Some researchers have also used environmental modifications to decrease the occurrence of sundowning.[109] These modifications include soft lighting, music, and elimination of stressful stimuli.[73]

Depression

Acute confusional states and the clinical symptoms of depression are often difficult to differentiate in elders. These two diagnoses are easier to delineate in younger patients. In any case, depression can occur in persons with long, chronic illnesses where there is an element of hopelessness and the person appears withdrawn.[110,111] Similar clinical manifestations can occur in AC. As stated earlier, hypokinetic delirium patients experience psychomotor slowing and their speech can be sparse.[28] Depressed elderly patients are hesitant to volunteer a verbal response, their speech is also more quiet and their behavior is more withdrawn. It is very challenging clinically to differentiate between delirium and depression; an exhaustive narrative is beyond the scope of this chapter. When depression is suspected, it is best to obtain expert geropsychiatric consultation.

Wernicke-Korsakoff Syndrome

Wernicke-Korsakoff syndrome is a type of dementia associated with chronic alcoholism and significant vitamin depletion resulting from poor nutrition and is distinctly different from delirium.[112] Wernicke-Korsakoff is characterized by a combination of motor and sensory disturbances (Wernicke's encephalopathy) and disordered memory function (Korsakoff's psychosis). This diagnosis should be a very important consideration in the treatment regimen. The pathophysiology exemplified in this syndrome is something of a cerebral "beri-beri" phenomenon that is associated with a severe deficiency of vitamin B_1 or thiamine. This severe malnutrition leads to permanent cerebral damage.

What distinguishes this syndrome from the more common types of dementia is the manifestation of ocular symptoms, mainly diplopia and horizontal nystagmus. Persons with Wernicke-Korsakoff syndrome also have a disordered gait, ataxia, and amnesia. In terms of the underlying problem, it is possible that alcohol ingestion impairs intestinal transport of thiamine.[113] Decreased thiamine intake, malabsorption of vitamins in general, and reduced storage of the small quantities ingested all play a role in the pathophysiological mechanism. The outcomes for Wernicke-Korsakoff vary according to the severity of symptoms. Ocular disturbances respond quickly to vitamin therapy,[114] but ataxia and perceptual disturbances respond much more slowly to this intervention. About one-third of those individuals with memory loss improve; however, if global amnesia is present, there is little likelihood of any major improvement in functioning.

MANIFESTATIONS AND SURVEILLANCE

The duration of AC episodes varies and has been reported to last from 1[115] to 60 days.[116] Most of the time, AC develops suddenly, within hours or days.[117] Sirois[118] documented the duration of AC in hospitalized elders in the form of incidence densities: less than 24 hours, 20%; 1 to 3 days, 30%; 3 to 5 days, 17%; 5 to 10 days, 20%; and up to 30 days, 13%. This variability is compounded by the fact that in about 10% of patients, delirium recurs during the hospitalization period. Levkoff et al[56] suggested that there is only a partial resolution of all delirium symptoms on discharge; in fact, this study reported that only 4% of patients with AC had complete resolution of all new delirium symptoms by discharge and at the 6-month follow-up only 17.7% had full resolution of symptoms.

It is difficult to identify delirium, but one significant manifestation relates to arousal and the ability to cognitively focus. Attention is altered in all of its procedural elements, including alertness and vigilance. Vigilance is the selective process in choosing which stimuli to respond to, and the ability to direct cognitive and psychomotor processes to produce a response to the stimuli. In essence, the person with AC has a diminished ability to respond selectively, as well as to mobilize, sustain, and shift attention appropriately.

There are levels of alertness and in delirium a person may be at either end of the spectrum. For example, hyperattentiveness can occur. In this state, the patient focuses on one specific stimulus and is unable to respond to all other stimuli in the environment.[18] A person with hyperattentiveness may focus on a bright, flashing light or other stimulus in the environment, shutting out all other persons and objects in the environment. Persons with decreased attention are likely to be of the somnolent type.[14] This is commonly seen in persons with hypokinetic delirium.[119] Also, a person can display both extremes over a short period. For example, alertness and attention can fluctuate even over the course of a single interview.

These changes in alertness result in altered communication. The communication change results in confabulation and *misnaming.* Misnaming refers to the use of an incorrect label or noun for an object, either related or unrelated in purpose or meaning to the actual object. It is possible that one can distinguish dementia from delirium based on the communication pattern. The speech pattern in AC can also be rambling or irrelevant, and speech is often slurred.

With delirium, it is sometimes difficult to obtain consensus from various care providers as to the validity of symptoms. This is especially true for the primary care providers who visit the patient infrequently or at set times of the day (e.g., a physician who only makes hospital rounds in the morning). Although nurses and allied health personnel are in the best position to recognize acute changes in mental status because of their constant interaction with patients at various times throughout the day, this does not mean that they always recognize AC or feel it is important to seek consultation.

There are a few physiological measures to detect delirium, but none that exclusively confirm the diagnosis. One of the more compelling physiological parameters is electroencephalograph (EEG) changes. EEG characteristics of delirium include slowing or dropout of the posterior dominant rhythm, generalized theta or delta slow-wave activity, poor organization of the background rhythm, and loss of reactivity of the EEG to eye opening and closing.[120] A less precise measure for AC related to drug-induced delirium is the serum anticholinergic activity (SAA) level.[121,122] However, some argue that SAA levels are also increased in those without delirium, such as when a fever or acute illness is present.[123]

Nursing Assessment

There are a variety of clinical assessment tools that can be used clinically to monitor and recognize AC.[124] These include the Confusion Assessment Method (CAM),[125] the Delirium Rating Scale (DRS),[126] the Mini-Mental State Examination (MMSE),[127] and the Neelon/Champagne (NEECHAM)[55] instruments. Although an extensive review of each of these is beyond the scope of this chapter, some generalized approaches are recommended.

Establishing baseline cognitive functioning is critical to monitoring patients who are vulnerable to the development of delirium. There are various ways of establishing this. Obtaining a mental status history from family, friends, and caregivers can be very useful (e.g., Does the patient recognize people familiar to him or her? Are names easily recalled?). Clinically, the MMSE is a useful assessment parameter to evaluate baseline functioning, but its use alone will not identify the presence of AC. The MMSE does aid in determining whether an acute change in a patient's mental status has occurred. Components of the MMSE are related to level of orientation, recall, and one's ability to "register" letters or numbers in sequence. When the MMSE is repeated following a suspicious change in behavior, it can document acute changes in mental status.

In general, a total score on the MMSE of 24 or higher is considered normal, but because age and education can influence "normal," the score should not have a dogmatic cut-off. In fact, it would be more accurate to consider a score relative to what is normal for the patient. If the observed MMSE is less than baseline for the patient, the nurse can proceed with screening using an instrument more sensitive to identifying AC.

As mentioned earlier, there are several instruments worth considering when screening for delirium. One of the nursing instruments that can be used is the NEECHAM Confusion Scale. This scale is divided into three categories or subscales: (1) level of responsiveness or information processing, including processing neurosensory, processing motor, and processing verbal information recognition; (2) level of behavior-appearance, motor, performance, and verbal; and (3) level of integrative physiological control, including vital function control and incontinence. It is one of the few scales that incorporates physiological data (e.g., temperature, oxygen saturation, and blood pressure) into the calculation (range 8 to 30).[128] The NEECHAM is particularly sensitive to the early onset of confusion and is highly correlated with a positive DSM-IIIR criteria rating ($r = 0.70$).[55] Information processing, the conceptual framework for developing the NEECHAM, includes assessment of the patient's ability to follow both simple and complex commands, as well as rating him or her on behavior, appearance, motor, and verbal responses. A score of 20 to 24 is considered to be mild or early AC; a score of 19 or lower is considered to be moderate to severe AC.

Ongoing surveillance is the key to determining the presence of AC. This type of surveillance is really a team effort for the nursing staff when the patient is in a health care facility. In the home setting, the family or significant other needs to be involved as well. The reason for this is that the symptoms of AC fluctuate over the course of a day, and it is entirely possible for an individual to have lucid intervals interwoven into a diurnal pattern. This means actively promoting the acquisition of assessment skills through in-service education[129] and family instruction[130] so that care providers can recognize AC.

CLINICAL MANAGEMENT

Although *delirium management* is listed in the Nursing Interventions Classification (NIC) reference, the emphasis seems to be on symptom abatement and protection from injury rather than etiologically based.[131] This is common to the medical interventions as well. These are not necessarily incorrect approaches, but should not be considered isolated from etiological evaluation and treatment. There appears to be an overwhelming notion among nurses that the behaviors of the acute confusional state are hierarchical, and that those behaviors interfering with nursing care should have priority for management (or more specifically that the behaviors need to be "contained"), so that nursing care or routines are not interfered with. Thus the "higher-order behaviors" are seen as including agitation, pulling out various tubes, and hallucinations—because they are conspicuous and increase nursing workload. Most commonly, there is an urgent call to the physician for haloperidol, chlorpromazine, or lorazepam to decrease these behaviors.

Etiologically based nursing protocols do exist for delirium. One of these focuses on identifying or suspecting drug toxicity; infection; elimination problems such as urinary tract infection and abdominal distention; new disease processes such as myocardial infarction, stroke, or changes in blood glucose; exacerbation of chronic illness; and psychosocial/environmental problems.[132] Pain management is also important, especially in elders, as this can lead to changes in cognition characteristic of AC.[50] Nurses who proceed with a systematic approach to identifying the cause, rather than focusing on the symptoms exclusively, will be able to decrease the amount of time spent in managing the patient. Also, the patient will receive better care for his or her illness.

Primary Interventions

Even before delirium occurs, primary interventions should be considered. Some have proposed a multicomponent preventive strategy focusing on cognitive impairment, sleep deprivation, immobility, visual and hearing impairment, and dehydration.[133] This protocol establishes cognitive stimulating activities (e.g., discussion of current events, structured reminiscence for dementia patients, and word games), nonpharmacological sleep interventions for patients with sleep deprivation (e.g., not awakening patients during the night for vital signs and other nursing tasks), early mobilization with minimal use of immobilizing equipment (e.g., physical restraints), ensuring that hearing and vision aids are in place, and following patients carefully for signs and symptoms of dehydration.

Dehydration, which can easily be prevented, contributes to the onset of AC through several mechanisms, including cerebral hypoperfusion, fluid and electrolyte imbalance, and poor renal excretion of drug metabolites. Volume depletion is indicated when there is an increase in the ratio of blood urea nitrogen to creatinine, and can be prevented by encouraging oral intake of fluids with non-diuretic side effects (i.e., excluding caffeine-based beverages).[134] Adequate hydration is especially important in preventing delirium in cancer patients, because this improves end of life care.[135] Nurses should also remember that resident's with dementia are sometimes unable to respond to their physiological need for water intake.

Pain management and ensuring oxygenation are also important intervention strategies. Pain treatment may consist of both pharmacological and non-pharmacological approaches (see Chapter 12, Pain). Hypoxemia is also easily identified with pulse oximetry and assessment for respiratory distress. Both of these conditions may precipitate sudden changes in cognition and complicate the clinical picture of AC because of the sometimes subtle manner in which each can present. For example, a dementia patient with pain and acute mental or behavioral change may not be able to verbalize the presence of pain. Likewise, a patient with AC, hypoxemia, and a low hemoglobin level may not have cyanosis and may have a normal pulse oximetry reading. In essence, the nurse's assessment of AC must be systematic and explore the potential etiologies of AC in order to define the correct intervention strategy.

Arthritis and other disabilities prevent some patients from consuming adequate amounts of fluids.[136,137] Improving hydration has a number of beneficial effects on other risk factors for AC, such as improving urine output, promoting the renal excretion of drug metabolites, and preventing urinary tract infection.[138] It is possible to set fluid intake goals for residents of nursing homes that are based on the patient's weight or body mass index.

Figure 9-1 proposes some intervention strategies based on the trajectory of AC. This conceptual framework also includes distinct outcomes that can be measured to evaluate the effectiveness of these interventions. Although no single intervention is likely to preclude the development of delirium, it is important to remember that if the phenomenon is promptly identified and etiologically based interventions introduced, many of the natural outcomes

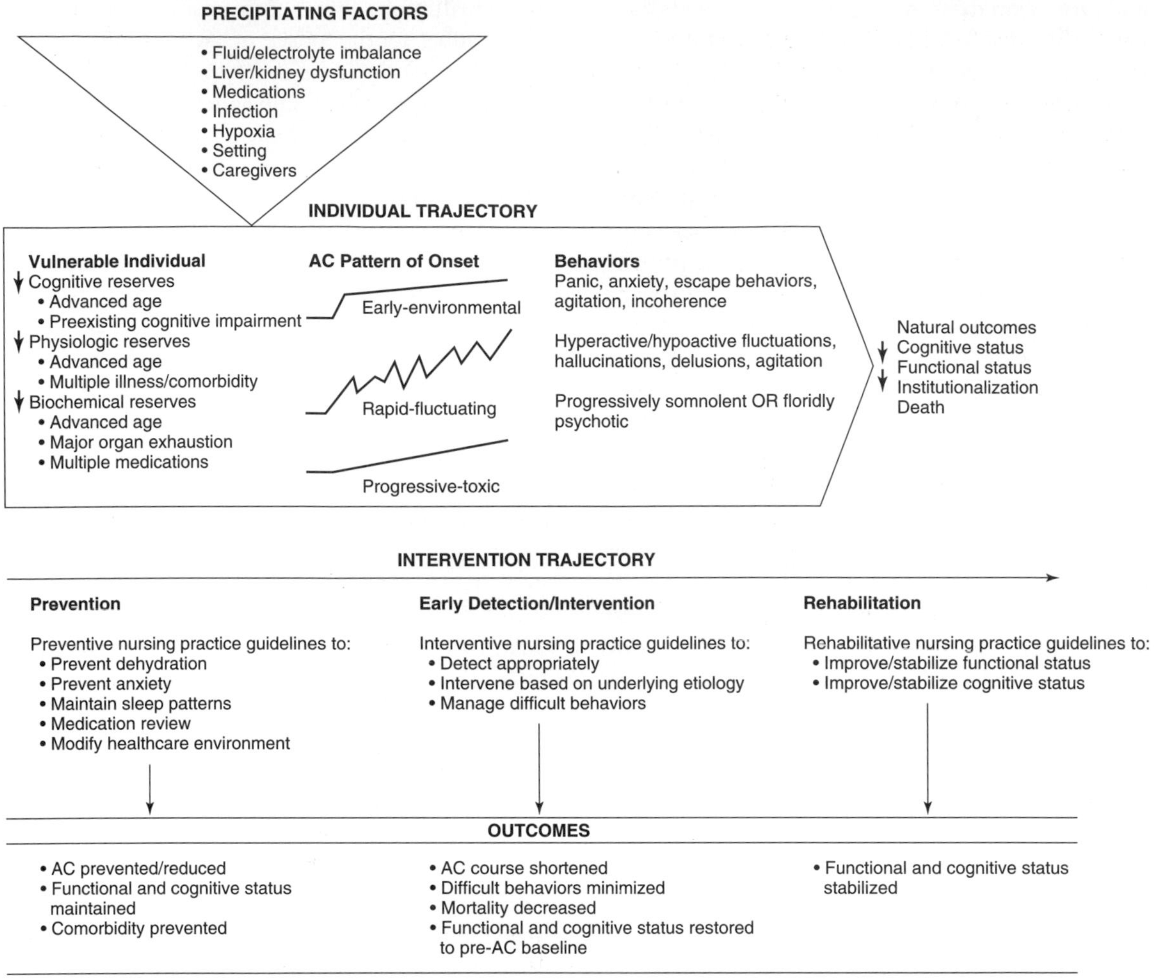

Figure 9-1 **Conceptual model for acute confusion** (AC). (From Mentes, J., Culp, K., Wakefield, B., Gaspar, P., Rapp, C.G., Mobily, P., & Tripp-Reimer, T. [1998]. Dehydration as a precipitating factor in the development of acute confusion in the frail elderly. In M.J. Arnaud, B.J. Vellas, J.L. Albarede, & P.J. Garry [eds.], *Facts, research and intervention in geriatrics: Hydration and aging* [pp. 83-100]. Paris: Springer.)

(e.g., decreased functional status and worsening cognitive status) can be avoided or at least minimized.

Staff Education

Another intervention that might be considered is not directed at the patient, but rather toward education of the staff. With the aging population and an increase in the number of individuals waiting for placement in care facilities, care providers are in substantial need of advanced education and training in the field of geropsychiatric nursing. Nurses working in long-term care facilities are frequently not prepared to manage the changing acuity levels and complex needs of their residents.[139] Continuing education workshops and in-service education programs should be developed to facilitate learning how to recognize and treat acute confusional states.

CONCEPTUAL MODEL

The degree of fluctuating symptoms observed in delirium are conceptualized from the perspective of the precipitating event leading to the onset.[134] It is important to realize that any onset and progression of symptoms is based on an individual's *neurophysiological threshold,* which is determined by age and ability to adapt to physiological, biological, and psychosocial challenge. For example, a person with dementia has a lower neurophysiological threshold than a healthy elder. A child is very resilient to fever and therefore tolerates it better than a middle-aged adult, who may develop that same temperature and later become confused.

There are also differences in the way AC is manifested in terms of the obscurity of symptoms and how rapidly those symptoms progress. Figure 9-1 illustrates a predictive model that describes the identified patterns.[3] The first type of onset is seen early in the history of the event and may be linked to environmental changes. In the elderly person with preexisting dementia this could be a new room assignment in the long-term care facility. The most common type is the rapid onset-fluctuating pattern of symptoms seen in a person where acute confusion manifests itself in the presence of illness. This could be a number of things—a change in respiratory status and hypoxemia or decreased hydration or multiple illnesses increasing in severity. The progressive-toxic pattern is seen in patients with an inability to excrete drug metabolites or in the case of multiple organ dysfunction. Most of the time the psychomotor behavior here is characteristic of the hypokinetic clinical subtype described earlier. Many times, it is this pattern that is observed in uremic and renal encephalopathies.

CASE STUDY

The following case study illustrates the challenge of diagnosing the cause of AC. A 77-year-old World War II veteran with a history of smoking, chronic obstructive pulmonary disease (COPD), and congestive heart failure (CHF) was seen in clinic for an acute exacerbation of his COPD. He had had multiple previous admissions to the hospital. He successfully quit smoking, but his shortness of breath and wheezing remained. In the past he was placed on a number of treatment regimens, including metaproterenol (Alupent) and beclomethasone metered-dose inhalers, but none of these was successful in resolving his shortness of breath. He had no history of psychiatric illness or alcohol abuse.

On admission to the VA hospital, he was treated with solumedrol 180 mg IV every 6 hours. His respiratory symptoms improved and he was changed to PO prednisone, which was tapered from 50 mg/day to 5 mg/day over a course of 1 week. He was also receiving furosemide 40 mg PO daily for his pulmonary edema. It was planned that he would go home on these maintenance doses of the prednisone and the furosemide.

However, on the morning of his discharge, a geropsychiatric nurse was called when the nurses on the general medicine unit noted an acute change in his mental status. He had become confused and disoriented, accusing the staff of trying to kick him out of the hospital when he couldn't "breathe right" and that "the nurses caused this respiratory infection." He complained of germs left behind by the nurses when they cared for him. He would stare at the red exit light by the stairwell outside his door constantly and jumped whenever someone entered the door of his room.

When the geropsychiatric nurse walked into the room, the patient was startled. He again became angry and mumbled incoherently. He had difficulty concentrating, and when the nurse started to ask him questions, his response was to look out the window. He called for his daughter loudly, peering out into the hallway. The nurse confirmed with the staff that no family members were present or had visited this morning. He claimed that there was a trail of bacteria crawling up his sheets, causing a terrible pneumonia. On his assessment, he was oriented to person, place, and year only, and did not know what month or time it was.

An arterial blood gas (ABG) was obtained that morning as it was anticipated that he might need home oxygen therapy. Hypoxia was suspected initially, but the ABG showed a pH of 7.48, $Pa{CO_2}$ 45 mm Hg, bicarbonate 32 mEq/L, a $Pa{O_2}$ 69 mm Hg, and an O_2 SAT of 89%, which was consistent with his baseline blood gases when his pulmonary problems were stable. He was afebrile, and his pulse rate was 112. His blood pressure was 100/65 and was consistent with earlier readings. An evaluation of his serum electrolytes, which were also obtained that morning, revealed a minor hyponatremia (132 mEq/L), which was assumed to be secondary to his furosemide therapy. All of his other serum electrolyte levels were within normal limits. His other medications were reviewed and, with the exception of the steroid therapy, not likely to be contributing to his confusion.

The geropsychiatric nurse consult made the following recommendations to the nursing staff: (1) initiate low-dose oxygen therapy with exertion, (2) limit the number of nurse care providers who interact with the patient, (3) reduce auditory and visual stimuli, (4) allow rest periods, adjusting the routine so sleep is not disturbed, (5) monitor the patient's attention and cognitive status hourly while awake, (6) contact the physician regarding the glucocorticoid therapy, and (7) protect the patient from injury. This last intervention did not include the application of physical restraints, but rather putting the side rails up, activating the bed alarm, and assigning a hospital volunteer to sit with and directly observe the patient.

The primary care physician was consulted immediately, and it was assumed that the delirium was a direct result of too rapidly tapering the patient's glucocorticoid therapy. Although the patient also had CHF, his blood pressure and serum digoxin levels were normal. His heart rate was elevated, and this did contribute to some decrease in his cardiac output, but it was probably the result of sympathetic nervous stimulation secondary to his delirium. The patient was promptly treated with intravenous hydrocortisone (100 mg every 6 hours). Within 24 hours his mental status improved and he was calm, attentive, and not hallucinating. A gradual taper was again initiated, and the patient was discharged 12 days later with his cognitive status intact.

SELECTED RESEARCH

Dr. Miller et al[17] studied the use of the NEECHAM (previously described) confusion scale as an assessment tool for clinicians as a part of usual nursing care. The study specifically focused on three elements of evaluating the use of the NEECHAM: After participating in an educational program on the NEECHAM, will staff nurses incorporate the assessment of AC into their usual patient care activities? Can staff nurses reliably assess acute confusion in older adults using the NEECHAM confusion scale? What impact will use of the NEECHAM confusion scale have on nurses' practice with elders?

This study involved all the RN and LPN staff on a 25-bed general medicine unit in a tertiary care teaching hospital. The NEECHAM was selected because it was an observational instrument and could be integrated into the care of patients during the course of their hospitalization. The educational program adopted by these researchers considered a number of factors related to the complexity of the assessment technique, the organizational climate of the unit, and the perceived gains by staff in adopting the assessment strategy.

After a 4- to 5-hour program of instruction on how to use the assessment scale, staff nurses assessed elderly patients for AC on admission to the unit and daily throughout their stay. The instruction included significance and clinical manifestations of AC, guided practice sessions, and how cognitive assessment can be incorporated into routine patient care activities. Research assistants (RA) collected the NEECHAM assessments daily to reduce the likelihood that the nurse would be influenced by the subject's previous day's performance on the scale. Also, the RA completed the NEECHAM on admission, the third day of hospitalization, and within 24 hours of discharge. The unit was observed for a 20-week period.

The implementation of the NEECHAM assessment technique was considered successful as indicated by a staff nurse completion rate of 81%—of a possible 185 elders admitted during the study period, 149 had admission assessments using the NEECHAM. Staff nurse scores on the NEECHAM were compared with research assistant ratings, and there were no significant differences in scores. The observed agreements were all high for the total NEECHAM score, with correlations above 0.90 for the most part, but some areas on the NEECHAM were problematic. The most variation between RA and staff ratings was on the scoring of pulse as regular or irregular—the nursing staff did not always note irregularities (kappa = 0.37). Also, there was variation in the observed rating of the subject's appearance (kappa = 0.40).

It was unclear from the research report what the sustained completion rate was on follow-up assessments, although follow-up score comparisons between staff and RA were described over time. In terms of why the NEECHAM scores were not completed all of the time, the researchers reported such unit stressors as reduced staffing, "patient crisis," implementation nursing staff being floated to other nursing units, and nurses from other units who were not familiar with the NEECHAM scale coming to work on the study unit.

For the most part, the study questions were addressed in this report. It would have been beneficial to see whether there were score variations between LPNs and RNs in the analysis or whether there were variations among RNs by educational preparation. The researchers did point out that the RA and staff nurse ratings on the NEECHAM should have been performed simultaneously, because the symptoms of AC can vary between time points in a fluctuating pattern. In general, this study did address the issues of implementing the NEECHAM confusion scale in the routine care of hospitalized elders and how successful introduction could produce fairly reliable scores.

QUESTIONS FOR FUTURE STUDY

The nature of the AC phenomenon adds complexity and methodological dilemmas to the study of delirium. The major features of delirium are that it is multidimensional, transient, potentially reversible, and variable.[140,141] However, consensus has not been reached on these characteristics, and recent research evidence is inconsistent with previously held notions about the nature of delirium.[142-144]

Relative to the multidimensional nature of delirium, it is not clear whether the multiple dimensions are cognitive and behavioral, if these two terms imply various aspects of cognition (e.g., attention, perception, and memory) or to some other unspecified dimensions.[4] Yet, the multidimensional nature of delirium has profound measurement implications. For example, the DSM-IV definition for delirium lacks an integrated neuropsychological conceptualization to aid recognition, specifically a continuum of confusional states from mild to severe.

In the current state of the science, little is known about the outcomes for mildly delirious patients. Do patients who experience mild AC have outcomes similar to those who have more advanced forms of delirium? Are outcomes similar across age groups? It is unclear whether moderate and severe forms of delirium are associated with mortality in younger age groups as is seen in the elderly.

Dementia apparently does increase the risk of delirium, but this relationship is not well-understood. Delirium is very difficult to recognize in patients with dementia. If dementia lowers the neurophysiological threshold for AC then the biobehavioral mechanism needs to be explained. This is the greatest chasm in the scheme of proper AC diagnosis in the elderly. Although much research has been performed in elderly populations, it is very frustrating that this question has not been answered and why the study population consistently appears to be limited to hospitalized elderly.

More research needs to be initiated on the epidemiology of AC in younger populations. There simply are no population-based incidence reports for toddlers, adolescents, and young adults. Some instrument development will need to be initiated to more accurately measure AC in the pediatric groups. In the elderly, more work needs to be done to know the frequency of delirium in long-term care, because many of the epidemiological studies are conducted exclusively in hospital settings. Also, little is known about the occurrence of AC in the home and community, where many dementia patients reside before admission to a nursing home.

Restricting the study of delirium to the period of acute hospitalization limits what is known about the real trajectory of AC. Sampling almost exclusively from elderly patients hospitalized for the medical and/or surgical treatment of acute physical illnesses has generated a great deal of useful information about delirium. This is especially important since these same data demonstrate that the majority of delirious patients leave the hospital while still suffering from their delirium.[145] These data, however, have failed to inform us about the incidence and prevalence of the disorder in other or the success of interventions across the continuum of care. Other cohorts may be at equal or greater risk (e.g., frail elderly persons residing in long-term care facilities because of the ravages of chronic cognitive impairment). Moreover, knowledge is just emerging about delirium in younger adult, adolescent, and pediatric populations.

REFERENCES

1. Milisen, K., Foreman, M.D., Godderis, J., Abraham, I.L., & Broos, P.L. (1998). Delirium in the hospitalized elderly: nursing assessment and management. *Nursing Clinical North American 33*(3), 417-439.
2. Carpenito, L.J. (2000). *Nursing diagnosis: Application to clinical practice*, Philadelphia: Lippincott.
3. Neelon, V., & Champagne, M. (1992). Managing cognitive impairment: The current basis for practice. In Funk, S., et al. (eds.). *Key aspects of elder care: Managing falls, incontinence, and cognitive impairment* (pp. 239-250) New York: Springer.
4. Foreman, M., Wakefield, B., Culp, K., & Milsen, K. (2001). Delirium: An overview of the state of the science. *Journal of Gerontological Nursing 27*(4), 12-20.
5. Lynch, E.P., Lazor, M.A., Gellis, J.E., Orav, J., Goldman, L., & Marcantonio, E.R. (1998). The impact of postoperative pain on the development of postoperative delirium. *Anesthesia and Analgesics 86*(4), 781-785.
6. Aono, J., Ueda, W., Mamiya, K., Takimoto, E., & Manabe, M. (1997). Greater incidence of delirium during recovery from sevoflurane anesthesia in preschool boys. *Anesthesiology 87*(6), 1298-1300.
7. Armstrong, S.C., & Schweitzer, S.M. (1997). Delirium associated with paroxetine and benztropine combination [letter]. *American Journal Psychiatry 154*(4), 581-582.
8. Bagri, S., & Reddy, G. (1998). Delirium with manic symptoms induced by diet pills [letter]. *Journal of Clinical Psychiatry 59*(2), 83.
9. Liptzin, B. (1995). Delirium. *Archives of Family Medicine 4*(5), 453-458.
10. Liptzin, B. (1999). What criteria should be used for the diagnosis of delirium? *Dementia and Geriatric Cognitive Disorders 10*(5), 364-367.
11. Camus, V., Gonthier, R., Dubos, G., Schwed, P., & Simeone, I. (2000). Etiologic and outcome profiles in hypoactive and hyperactive subtypes of delirium. *Journal of Geriatric Psychiatry and Neurology 13*(1), 38-42.
12. Meagher, D.J., & Trzepacz, P.T. (2000). Motoric subtypes of delirium. *Seminars in Clinical Neuropsychiatry 5*(2), 75-85.
13. O'Keeffe, S.T. (1999). Clinical subtypes of delirium in the elderly. *Dementia and Geriatric Cognitive Disorders 10*(5), 380-385.
14. Ross, C.A., Peyser, C.E., Shapiro, I., & Folstein, M.F. (1991). Delirium: Phenomenologic and etiologic subtypes. *International Psychogeriatrics 3*(2), 135-147.
15. Muller, N., Klages, U., & Gunther, W. (1994). Hepatic encephalopathy presenting as delirium and mania. The possible role of bilirubin. *General Hospital Psychiatry 16*(2), 138-140.
16. Volkow, N.D., Wang, G.J., Overall, J.E., Hitzemann, R., Fowler, J.S., Pappas, N., et al. (1997). Regional brain metabolic response to lorazepam in alcoholics during

early and late alcohol detoxification. *Alcohol Clinical Experimental Research 21*(7), 1278-1284.
17. Miller, J., Neelon, V., Champagne, M., Bailey, D., Ng'andu, N., Belyea, M., et al. (1997). The assessment of acute confusion as part of nursing care. *Applied Nursing Research 10*(3), 143-151.
18. O'Keeffe, S.T., & Lavan, J.N. (1999). Clinical significance of delirium subtypes in older people. *Age and Ageing 28*(2), 115-119.
19. Levkoff, S., Cleary, P., Liptzin, B., & Evans, D.A. (1991). Epidemiology of delirium: An overview of research issues and findings. *International Psychogeriatrics 3*(2), 149-167.
20. Foreman, L.J., Cavalieri, T.A., Galski, T., Dinsmore, S., Kay, P.A., & Pomerantz, S. (1995). Occurrence and impact of suspected delirium in hospitalized elderly patients. *Journal of the American Osteopathic Association 95*(10), 588-591.
21. Culp, K., Tripp-Reimer, T., Wadle, K., Wakefield, B., Akins, J., Mobily, P., & Kundradt, M. (1997). Screening for acute confusion in elderly long-term care residents. *Journal of Neuroscience Nursing 29*(2), 86-88, 95-100.
22. van der Mast, R.C. (1998). Pathophysiology of delirium. *Journal of Geriatric Psychiatry and Neurology 11*(3), 138-145.
23. Inouye, S.K., Viscoli, C.M., Horwitz, R.I., Hurst, L.D., & Tinetti, M.E. (1993). A predictive model for delirium in hospitalized elderly medical patients based on admission characteristics. *Annals of Internal Medicine 119*(6), 474-481.
24. Eden, B.M., Foreman, M.D., & Sisk, R. (1998). Delirium: Comparison of four predictive models in hospitalized critically ill elderly patients. *Applied Nursing Research 11*(1), 27-35.
25. Marcantonio, E.R., Flacker, J.M., Michaels, M., & Resnick, N.M. (2000). Delirium is independently associated with poor functional recovery after hip fracture. *Journal of the American Geriatric Society 48*(6), 618-624.
26. Ignatavicius, D. (1999). Resolving the delirium dilemma. *Nursing 29*(10), 41-46.
27. Murphy, B.A. (2000). Delirium. *Emergency Medical Clinics of North America 18*(2), 243-252.
28. Sandberg, O., Gustafson, Y., Brannstrom, B., & Bucht, G. (1999). Clinical profile of delirium in older patients [see comments]. *Journal of the American Geriatric Society 47*(11), 1300-1306.
29. Bucht, G., Gustafson, Y., & Sandberg, O. (1999). Epidemiology of delirium. *Dementia and Geriatric Cognitive Disorders 10*(5), 315-318.
30. Lawlor, P.G., Nekolaichuk, C., Gagnon, B., Mancini, I.L., Pereira, J.L., & Bruera, E.D. (2000). Clinical utility, factor analysis, and further validation of the memorial delirium assessment scale in patients with advanced cancer: Assessing delirium in advanced cancer. *Cancer 88*(12), 2859-2867.
31. Espino, D.V., Jules-Bradley, A.C., Johnston, C.L., & Mouton, C.P. (1998). Diagnostic approach to the confused elderly patient. *American Family Physician 57*(6), 1358-1366.
32. Elie, M., Cole, M.G., Primeau, F.J., & Bellavance, F. (1998). Delirium risk factors in elderly hospitalized patients. *Journal of General Internal Medicine 13*(3), 204-212.
33. Parikh, S.S., & Chung, F. (1995). Postoperative delirium in the elderly. *Anesthesia and Analgesics 80*(6), 1223-1232.
34 Franco, K., Litaker, D., Locala, J., & Bronson, D. (2001). The cost of delirium in the surgical patient. *Psychosomatics 42*(1), 68-73.
35. Adler, R. (1992). Burns are different: The child psychiatrist on the pediatric burns ward. *Journal of Burn Care and Rehabilitation 13*(1), 28-32.
36. Sieche, A., & Giedke, H. (1999). Recurring short delirium with postpartum onset in two sisters. *Psychopathology 32*(6), 325-329.
37. Rovner, B.W., German, P.S., Broadhead, J., Morriss, R.K., Brant, L.J., Blaustein, J., & Folstein, M.F. (1990). The prevalence and management of dementia and other psychiatric disorders in nursing homes. *International Psychogeriatrics 2*(1), 13-24.
38. Wilson, L.M. (1972). Intensive care delirium. The effect of outside deprivation in a windowless unit. *Archives of Internal Medicine 130*(2), 225-226.
39. Thompson, T.L.D., & Smith, T.C. (1991). Costumed figures may produce iatrogenic symptoms in delirious patients [editorial]. *Psychosomatics 32*(1), 1-4.
40. Burney-Puckett, M. (1996). Sundown syndrome: Etiology and management. *Journal of Psychosocial Nursing and Mental Health Services 34*(5), 40-43.
41. Foreman, M.D., Wootton, J.D., Pompei, P., & Rudberg, M.A. (1993). Sentences written by older adults during mental status testing. *Applied Nursing Research 6*(4), 169-171.
42. Carter, G.L., Dawson, A.H., & Lopert, R. (1996). Drug-induced delirium. Incidence, management and prevention. *Drug Safety 15*(4), 291-301.
43. Lipowski, Z.J. (1992). Update on delirium. *Psychiatric Clinics of North America 15*(2), 335-346.
44. Stewart, R.B., & Hale, W.E. (1992). Acute confusional states in older adults and the role of polypharmacy. *Annual Review of Public Health 13,* 415-430.
45. Karlsson, I. (1999). Drugs that induce delirium. *Dementia and Geriatric Cognitive Disorders 10*(5), 412-415.
46. Oxman, T.E. (1996). Antidepressants and cognitive impairment in the elderly [published erratum appears in *Journal of Clinical Psychiatry* 1996 *57*(8), 374]. *Journal of Clinical Psychiatry 57*(Suppl 5), 38-44.
47. Ellis, J.M., & Lee, S.I. (1978). Acute prolonged confusion in later life as an ictal state. *Epilepsia 19*(2), 119-128.
48. Moore, A.R., & O'Keeffe, S.T. (1999). Drug-induced cognitive impairment in the elderly. *Drugs and Aging 15*(1), 15-28.
49. Tanimu, D.Z., Obeid, T., Awada, A., Huraib, S., & Iqbal, A. (1998). Absence status: An overlooked cause of acute confusion in hemodialysis patients. *Journal of Nephrology 11*(3), 146-147.
50. Abrahm, J.L. (2000). Advances in pain management for older adult patients. *Clinical Geriatric Medical 16*(2), 269-311.
51. Galen, D.M., Beck, M., & Buchbinder, D. (1997). Steroid psychosis after orthognathic surgery: A case report. *Journal of Oral and Maxillofacial Surgery 55*(3), 294-297.
52. Leipzig, R.M. (1998). That was the year that was: An evidence-based clinical geriatrics update. *Journal of the American Geriatric Society 46*(8), 1040-1049.
53. Vincent, F.M. (1995). The neuropsychiatric complications of corticosteroid therapy. *Comprehensive Therapy 21*(9), 524-528.
54. Foreman, M.D., & Zane, D. (1996). Nursing strategies for acute confusion in elders. *American Journal of Nursing 96*(4), 44-51.
55. Neelon, V.J., Champagne, M.T., Carlson, J.R., & Funk, S.G. (1996). The NEECHAM Confusion Scale: Construction,

validation, and clinical testing. *Nursing Research 45*(6), 324-330.
56. Levkoff, S.E., Evans, D.A., Liptzin, B., Cleary, P.D., Lipsitz, L.A., Wetle, T.T., et al. (1992). Delirium. The occurrence and persistence of symptoms among elderly hospitalized patients. *Archives of Internal Medicine 152*(2), 334-340.
57. Beumont, P.J., & Large, M. (1991). Hypophosphataemia, delirium and cardiac arrhythmia in anorexia nervosa [see comments]. *Medical Journal of Australia 155*(8), 519-522.
58. Valley, R.D., Ramza, J.T., Calhoun, P., Freid, E.B., Bailey, A.G., Kopp, V.J., et al. (1999). Tracheal extubation of deeply anesthetized pediatric patients: A comparison of isoflurane and sevoflurane. *Anesthesia and Analgesics 88*(4), 742-745.
59. Aono, J., Mamiya, K., & Manabe, M. (1999). Preoperative anxiety is associated with a high incidence of problematic behavior on emergence after halothane anesthesia in boys. *Acta Anaesthesiologica Scandinavica 43*(5), 542-544.
60. Butler, T., Islam, A., Kabir, I., & Jones, P.K. (1991). Patterns of morbidity and mortality in typhoid fever dependent on age and gender: Review of 552 hospitalized patients with diarrhea. *Review of Infectious Diseases 13*(1), 85-90.
61. Garza, M.B., Osterhoudt, K.C., & Rutstein, R. (2000). Central anticholinergic syndrome from orphenadrine in a 3 year old. *Journal of Oral and Maxillofacial Surgery and Emergency Care 16*(2), 97-98.
62. Freed, R.S., & Freed, S.A. (1990). Ghost illness of children in north India. *Medical Anthropology 12*(4), 401-417.
63. Heinik, J., Avnon, M., & Hes, J.P. (1997). Length of hospitalization and disposition of elderly vs younger delirium patients in psychiatric hospitals. *Israel Journal of Psychiatry and Related Sciences 34*(2), 115-118.
64. Forster, P.L., Buckley, R., & Phelps, M.A. (1999). Phenomenology and treatment of psychotic disorders in the psychiatric emergency service. *Psychiatric Clinics of North American 22*(4), 735-754.
65. Allgulander, C., Borg, S., & Vikander, B. (1984). A 4-6-year follow-up of 50 patients with primary dependence on sedative and hypnotic drugs. *American Journal of Psychiatry 141*(12), 1580-1582.
66. Neves, A.C., Sesso, R.D.D., Ferraz, H.B., Francisco, S., & dos Reis Filho, J.B. (1998). The diagnosis of delirium in 80 emergency unit patients. *Arquivos de Neuro-Psiuiatria 56*(2), 176-183.
67. Mott, S.H., Packer, R.J., & Soldin, S.J. (1994). Neurologic manifestations of cocaine exposure in childhood. *Pediatrics 93*(4), 557-560.
68. Lindesay, J. (1999). The concept of delirium. *Dementia and Geriatric Cognitive Disorders 10*(5), 310-314.
69. Brauer, C., Morrison, R.S., Silberzweig, S.B., & Siu, A.L. (2000). The cause of delirium in patients with hip fracture. *Archives of Internal Medicine 160*(12), 1856-1860.
70. Crawley, E.J., & Miller, J. (1998). Acute confusion among hospitalized elders in a rural hospital. *Medsurg Nursing 7*(4), 199-206.
71. Inouye, S.K., Schlesinger, M.J., & Lydon, T.J. (1999). Delirium: A symptom of how hospital care is failing older persons and a window to improve quality of hospital care. *American Journal Medical 106*(5), 565-573.
72. Britton, A., & Russell, R. (2000). Multidisciplinary team interventions for delirium in patients with chronic cognitive impairment. *Cochrane Database System Review 2*, 1-12.
73. Cohen-Mansfield, J., & Werner, P. (1997). Management of verbally disruptive behaviors in nursing home residents. *Journal of the American Geriatrics Society 52*(6), M369-377.
74. Miller, J., Neelon, V., Dalton, J., Ng'andu, N., Bailey, D., Jr., Layman, E., et al. (1996). The assessment of discomfort in elderly confused patients: A preliminary study. *Journal of Neuroscience Nursing 28*(3), 175-182.
75. Trzepacz, P.T. (2000). Is there a final common neural pathway in delirium? Focus on acetylcholine and dopamine. *Seminars in Clinical Neuropsychiatry 5*(2), 132-148.
76. Itil, T., & Fink, M. (1966). Anticholinergic drug-induced delirium: Experimental modification, quantitative EEG and behavioral correlations. *Journal of Nervous and Mental System Disorders 143*(6), 492-507.
77. Tune, L.E., & Egeli, S. (1999). Acetylcholine and delirium. *Dementia and Geriatric Cognitive Disorders 10*(5), 342-344.
78. Flacker, J.M., Cummings, V., Mach, J.R., Jr., Bettin, K., Kiely, D.K., & Wei, J. (1998). The association of serum anticholinergic activity with delirium in elderly medical patients. *American Journal of Geriatric Psychiatry 6*(1), 31-41.
79. Dickson, L.R. (1991). Hypoalbuminemia in delirium. *Psychosomatics 32*(3), 317-323.
80. Palmstierna, T. (2001). A model for predicting alcohol withdrawal delirium. *Psychiatric Services 52*(6), 820-823.
81. Buchman, N., Mendelsson, E., Lerner, V., & Kotler, M. (1999). Delirium associated with vitamin B12 deficiency after pneumonia. *Clinical Neuropharmacology 22*(6), 356-358.
82. O'Keeffe, S.T., Tormey, W.P., Glasgow, R., & Lavan, J.N. (1994). Thiamine deficiency in hospitalized elderly patients. *Gerontology 40*(1), 18-24.
83. Goya, R.G., & Bolognani, F. (1999). Homeostasis, thymic hormones and aging. *Gerontology 45*(3), 174-178.
84. Travlos, A., & Hirsch, G. (1993). Steroid psychosis: A cause of confusion on the acute spinal cord injury unit. *American Journal of Physical Medicine and Rehabilitation 74*(3), 312-315.
85. Olsson, T. (1999). Activity in the hypothalamic-pituitary-adrenal axis & delirium. *Dementia and Geriatric Cognitive Disorders 10*(5), 345-349.
86. Kamholz, B. (1998). Introduction: The puzzles of delirium [editorial]. *Journal of Geriatric Psychiatry and Neurology 11*(3), 115-117.
87. Jones, C., Griffiths, R.D., & Humphris, G. (2000). Disturbed memory and amnesia related to intensive care. *Memory 8*(2), 79-94.
88. Rockwood, K., Cosway, S., Carver, D., Jarrett, P., Stadnyk, K., & Fisk, J. (1999). The risk of dementia and death after delirium. *Age and Ageing 28*(6), 551-556.
89. Cole, M.G., Primeau, F.J., & Elie, L.M. (1998). Delirium: Prevention, treatment, and outcome studies. *Journal of Geriatric Psychiatry and Neurology 11*(3), 126-137.
90. O'Keeffe, S., & Lavan, J. (1997). The prognostic significance of delirium in older hospital patients [see comments]. *Journal of the American Geriatric Society 45*(2), 174-178.
91. Stevens, L.E., de Moore, G.M., & Simpson, J.M. (1998). Delirium in hospital: Does it increase length of stay? *Australian and New Zealand Psychiatry 32*(6), 805-808.
92. Pompei, P., Foreman, M., Rudberg, M.A., Inouye, S.K., Braund, V., & Cassel, C.K. (1994). Delirium in hospitalized older persons: Outcomes and predictors. *Journal of the American Geriatric Society 42*(8), 809-815.

93. Thomas, R.I., Cameron, D.J., & Fahs, M.C. (1988). A prospective study of delirium and prolonged hospital stay. Exploratory study. *Archives General Psychiatry 45*(10), 937-940.
94. Frank, C., Hodgetts, G., & Puxty, J. (1996). Safety and efficacy of physical restraints for the elderly. Review of the evidence. *Canadian Family Physician 42,* 2402-2409.
95. Foreman, M.D., Mion, L.C., Tryostad, L., & Fletcher, K. (1999). Standard of practice protocol: Acute confusion/delirium. NICHE Faculty. *Geriatric Nursing 20*(3), 147-152.
96. Karch, S.B., & Wetli, C.V. (1995). Agitated delirium versus positional asphyxia [letter; comment]. *Annals of Emergency Medicine 26*(6), 760-761.
97. Milliken, D. (1998). Death by restraint [editorial; comment]. *Canadian Medical Journal 158*(12), 1611-1612.
98. Inouye, S.K., & Charpentier, P.A. (1996). Precipitating factors for delirium in hospitalized elderly persons. Predictive model and interrelationship with baseline vulnerability. *Journal of the American Medical Association 275*(11), 852-857.
99. Chan, D., & Brennan, N.J. (1999). Delirium: Making the diagnosis, improving the prognosis. *Geriatrics 54*(3), 28-30.
100. Lipowski, Z.J. (1983). Transient cognitive disorders (delirium, acute confusional states) in the elderly. *American Journal Psychiatry 140*(11), 1426-1436.
101. Bliwise, D.L. (1994). What is sundowning? *Journal of the American Geriatric Society 42*(9), 1009-1011.
102. Jarrett, P.G., Rockwood, K., & Mallery, L. (1995). Behavioral problems in nursing home residents. Safe ways to manage dementia [see comments]. *Postgraduate Medicine 97*(5), 189-191, 195-196.
103. Tejera, C.A., Saravay, S.M., Goldman, E., & Gluck, L. (1994). Diphenhydramine-induced delirium in elderly hospitalized patients with mild dementia. *Psychosomatics 35*(4), 399-402.
104. Meagher, D.J., O'Hanlon, D., O'Mahony, E., Casey, P.R., & Trzepacz, P.T. (1998). Relationship between etiology and phenomenologic profile in delirium [published erratum appears in *Journal of Geriatric Psychiatry and Neurology* 1999 *12*(3), following 164]. *Journal of Geriatric Psychiatry and Neurology 11*(3), 146-149.
105. Trzepacz, P.T., Mulsant, B.H., Amanda Dew, M., Pasternak, R., Sweet, R.A., & Zubenko, G.S. (1998). Is delirium different when it occurs in dementia? A study using the delirium rating scale. *Journal Neuropsychiatry Clinical Neuroscience 10*(2), 199-204.
106. Brandeis, G.H., Baumann, M.M., Hossain, M., Morris, J.N., & Resnick, N.M. (1997). The prevalence of potentially remediable urinary incontinence in frail older people: A study using the Minimum Data Set [see comments]. *Journal of the American Geriatric Society 45*(2), 179-184.
107. Evans, L.K. (1987). Sundown syndrome in institutionalized elderly. *Journal of the American Geriatric Society 35*(2), 101-108.
108. Martin, J., Marler, M., Shochat, T., & Ancoli-Israel, S. (2000). Circadian rhythms of agitation in institutionalized patients with Alzheimer's disease [in process citation]. *Chronobiology International 17*(3), 405-418.
109. Little, J.T., Satlin, A., Sunderland, T., & Volicer, L. (1995). Sundown syndrome in severely demented patients with probable Alzheimer's disease. *Journal of Geriatric Psychiatry and Neurology 8*(2), 103-106.
110. Kincaid, B.J. (1998). Delirium and depression in the elderly [letter]. *Nurse Practice 23*(2), 122-124.
111. Wattis, J. (1996). What an old age psychiatrist does. *British Medical Journal 313*(7049), 101-104.
112. Sumner, A.D., & Simons, R.J. (1994). Delirium in the hospitalized elderly. *Cleveland Clinical Journal of Medicine 61*(4), 258-262.
113. Thomson, A.D. (2000). Mechanisms of vitamin deficiency in chronic alcohol misusers and the development of the Wernicke-Korsakoff syndrome. *Alcohol and Alcoholism 35*(Suppl 1), 2-7.
114. Welch, L.W., Nimmerrichter, A., Kessler, R., King, D., Hoehn, R., Margolin, R., et al. (1996). Severe global amnesia presenting as Wernicke-Korsakoff syndrome but resulting from atypical lesions. *Psychological Medicine 26*(2), 421-425.
115. Rockwood, K. (1993). The occurrence and duration of symptoms in elderly patients with delirium. *Journal of Geronotology 48*(4), M162-166.
116. Kuroda, S., Ishizu, H., Ujike, H., Otsuki, S., Mitsunobu, K., Chuda, M., & Yamamoto, M. (1990). Senile delirium with special reference to situational factors and recurrent delirium. *Acta Medical Okayama 44*(5), 267-272.
117. Koponen, H.J. (1999). Neurochemistry and delirium. *Dementia and Geriatric Cognitive Disorders 10*(5), 339-341.
118. Sirois, F. (1988). Delirium: 100 cases. *Canadian Journal of Psychiatry 33*(5), 375-378.
119. Camus, V., Burtin, B., Simeone, I., Schwed, P., Gonthier, R., & Dubos, G. (2000). Factor analysis supports the evidence of existing hyperactive and hypoactive subtypes of delirium. *International Journal of Geriatric Psychiatry 15*(4), 313-316.
120. Jacobson, S., & Jerrier, H. (2000). EEG in delirium. *Seminars in Clinical Neuropsychiatry 5*(2), 86-92.
121. Tune, L.E. (2000). Serum anticholinergic activity levels and delirium in the elderly. *Seminars in Clinical Neuropsychiatry 5*(2), 149-153.
122. Mach, J.R., Jr., Dysken, M.W., Kuskowski, M., Richelson, E., Holden, L., & Jilk, K.M. (1995). Serum anticholinergic activity in hospitalized older persons with delirium: A preliminary study [see comments]. *Journal of the American Geriatric Society 43*(5), 491-495.
123. Flacker, J.M., & Lipsitz, L.A. (1999). Serum anticholinergic activity changes with acute illness in elderly medical patients. *Journal of the American Geriatrics Society 54*(1), M12-16.
124. Rapp, C.G., Wakefield, B., Kundrat, M., Mentes, J., Tripp-Reimer, T., Culp, K., et al. (2000). Acute confusion assessment instruments: Clinical versus research usability. *Applied Nursing Research 13*(1), 37-45.
125. Inouye, S.K., van Dyck, C.H., Alessi, C.A., Balkin, S., Siegal, A.P., & Horwitz, R.I. (1990). Clarifying confusion: The confusion assessment method. A new method for detection of delirium [see comments]. *Annals of Internal Medicine 113*(12), 941-948.
126. Trzepacz, P.T., & Dew, M.A. (1995). Further analyses of the Delirium Rating Scale. *General Hospital Psychiatry 17*(2), 75-79.
127. Folstein, M.F., Folstein, S.E., & McHugh, P.R. (1975). "Mini-mental state." A practical method for grading the cognitive state of patients for the clinician. *Journal of Psychiatric Research 12*(3), 189-198.
128. Csokasy, J. (1999). Assessment of acute confusion: Use of the NEECHAM Confusion Scale. *Applied Nursing Research 12*(1), 51-55.
129. Rapp, C., O'Nega, L., Tripp-Reimer, T., Mobily, M., Wakefield, B., Kundrat, M., et al. (2001). Training of

acute confusion resource nurses: Knowledge, perceived confidence and role. *Journal of Gerontological Nursing 27*(4), 34-40.

130. Fick, D., & Foreman, M. (2000). Consequences of not recognizing delirium superimposed on dementia in hospitalized elderly individuals. *Journal of Gerontological Nursing 26*(1), 30-40.
131. McCloskey, J.C., & Bulechek, G.M. (2000). *Nursing interventions classification (NIC)*. St. Louis: Mosby.
132. Mentes, J.C. (1995). A nursing protocol to assess causes of delirium. Identifying delirium in nursing home residents. *Journal of Gerontological Nursing 21*(2), 26-30.
133. Inouye, S.K., Bogardus, S.T., Jr., Charpentier, P.A., Leo-Summers, L., Acampora, D., Holford, T.R., et al. (1999). A multicomponent intervention to prevent delirium in hospitalized older patients [see comments]. *New England Journal Medical 340*(9), 669-676.
134. Mentes, J., Culp, K., Wakefield, B., Gaspar, P., Rapp, C.G., Mobily, P., et al. (1998). Dehydration as a precipitating factor in the development of acute confusion in the frail elderly. In Arnaud, M.J., Vellas, B., Albarede, J.L., Garry, P.J. (eds.), *Facts, research and intervention in geriatrics: Hydration and aging* (pp. 83-100). New York: Springer.
135. Lawlor, P.G., Gagnon, B., Mancini, I.L., Pereira, J.L., Hanson, J., Suarez-Almazor, M.E., et al. (2000). Occurrence, causes, and outcome of delirium in patients with advanced cancer: A prospective study. *Archives of Internal Medicine 160*(6), 786-794.
136. Mentes, J., & Buckwalter, K. (1997). Getting back to basics: Maintaining hydration to prevent acute confusion in frail elderly. *Journal of Gerontological Nursing 23*(10), 48-51.
137. Reyes-Ortiz, C.A. (1997). Dehydration, delirium, and disability in elderly patients [letter; comment]. *Journal of the American Medical Association 278*(4), 287-288.
138. Arnaud, M.J., Vellas, B.J., Albarede, J.L., & Garry, P.J. (1998). *Hydration and aging*. New York: Springer.
139. Lusk, C. (1999). Geriatric mental health education in Canada SKIPs into the 21st century. *Journal of Gerontological Nursing 25*(5), 37-42.
140. Culp, K., Mentes, J., & McConnell, E. (2001). Studying acute confusion in long-term care: Clinical investigation or secondary data analysis using the minimum data set? *Journal of Gerontological Nursing 27*(4), 41-48.
141. Lipowski, Z.J. (1991). Delirium: How its concept has developed. *International Psychogeriatrics 3*(2), 115-120.
142. Curyto, K.J., Johnson, J., TenHave, T., Mossey, J., Knott, K., & Katz, I.R. (2001). Survival of hospitalized elderly patients with delirium: A prospective study. *American Journal of Geriatric Psychiatry 9*(2), 141-147.
143. Grassi, L., Biancosino, B., Pavanati, M., Agostini, M., & Manfredini, R. (2001). Depression or hypoactive delirium? A report of ciprofloxacin-induced mental disorder in a patient with chronic obstructive pulmonary disease. *Psychotherapy and Psychosomatics 70*(1), 58-59.
144. Inouye, S.K. (2001). Delirium after hip fracture: To be or not to be? *Journal of the American Geriatric Society 49*(5), 678-679.
145. Inouye, S.K., Rushing, J.T., Foreman, M.D., Palmer, R.M., & Pompei, P. (1998). Does delirium contribute to poor hospital outcomes? A three-site epidemiologic study. *Journal of General Internal Medicine 13*(4), 234-242.

SECTION

III Alterations in Sensation

A sensation is defined as a perception and/or a feeling associated with stimulation of sensory receptors or sense organs. Sensations primarily are considered to be subjective, although some may be associated with objective phenomena, such as nausea and vomiting. Sensations are modulated by the individual's experience and perceptual processes.

Examples of sensations include taste, touch, vision, hearing, and smell. Sensations also may be synonymous with symptoms, such as dyspnea and pain; these symptoms are signs of pathological processes. All sensations may become symptoms when alterations in structure or function occur. Numerous symptoms or sensations are assessed frequently by nurses and thus fall within the domain of nursing practice and research. In fact, if nursing functions are defined as the diagnosis and treatment of human responses to actual or potential health problems, a major component of nursing practice is symptom management.

This section includes sensations that are symptoms representing pathological states, such as dyspnea, fatigue, pain, and nausea, vomiting, and retching. These altered sensations are human responses to illness that are assessed and managed frequently by nurses and are repeatedly seen across a wide range of diseases in a variety of chronic and acute clinical settings. Dyspnea (Chapter 10) reflects alterations in the sensation of breathing as a result of a variety of chemical, neural, and muscular stimuli integrated in the cortex. Fatigue (Chapter 11) occurs with many diseases, including cancer and cardiac, renal, and pulmonary disorders. Fatigue can be a distressing sensation that is experienced normally in day-to-day living or with disease and some clinical therapies. Pain may result from a variety of noxious stimuli. The kind and extent of the pain (Chapter 12) are shaped by the stimuli and the individual's perception, which is affected by personal, situational, and physiological variables. Chapter 13 discusses a sensation, nausea, which is followed by the observable behaviors of vomiting and retching.

All of these sensations involve complex interrelationships and processes. Multiple theories relating to causation and the effects of moderator variables are presented in each chapter. The scientific community has begun to appreciate the individual variation in perception and behavior and how other variables covary with these sensations. These physical sensations are influenced by numerous physiological and psychosocial processes. Adequate study of the sensations requires consideration of multiple theoretical perspectives, including information-processing theories, physiological mechanisms, psychological factors, sociocultural determinants, and developmental stages.

Pain, as a symptom, has been studied extensively, with most of the related moderator variables being well known and scientifically investigated. By contrast, dyspnea, primarily has been studied from a pathophysiological perspective, with little emphasis on relevant psychosocial variables or the meaning of the symptom to the person. Fatigue as a pervasive symptom is only recently recognized and studied in the context of health and illness. Nurse researchers have over time described and studied conceptual models and cognitive-behavioral therapies for the treatment of nausea and vomiting.

The probability that these symptoms will be reported by the individual may vary as a function of demographic variables, such as age, gender, occupation, residential status, and culture. Self-reports of sensations such as shortness of breath or fatigue differ widely, depending on the personal perception and the meaning and definition that the symptom has to the person. In addition, physical impairment does not always correlate with the reporting of frequency or severity of these sensations, indicating the importance of considering a multifactorial model that includes demographic, personal, psychosocial, and cultural variables in addition to the pathophysiological factors.

With knowledge of the mechanisms, manifestations, and clinical therapies relevant to these sensations, the professional nurse can accurately monitor the human response over time and plan appropriate interventions. The chapters in this section provide theoretical and empirical knowledge as a basis for professional nursing practice.

CHAPTER

10 Dyspnea

VIRGINIA CARRIERI-KOHLMAN & MICHAEL STULBARG

DEFINITION

Dyspnea is a clinical term for shortness of breath or breathlessness—the discomfort associated with effort in breathing or the urge to breathe. The terms *dyspnea, shortness of breath,* and *breathlessness* are used interchangeably by patients and health care providers and are considered to be synonymous in this chapter. Dyspnea is defined as the subjective sensation of difficult, uncomfortable breathing and includes both the perception of labored breathing and the reaction to the unpleasant stimuli. This definition, suggested by Comroe[1] more than four decades ago, remains one of the most descriptive and includes the most important dimensions of dyspnea: that it is subjective and therefore can be rated only by the person; that it is a feeling of discomfort; and that it includes the "reaction" to the symptom.

More recently, a consensus statement written by a multidisciplinary committee of the American Thoracic Society recommended the following definition of dyspnea: "Dyspnea is a term used to characterize a subjective experience of breathing discomfort that is comprised of qualitatively distinct sensations that vary in intensity. The experience derives from interactions among multiple physiological, psychological, social and environmental factors, and may induce secondary physiological and behavioral responses."[2] With this definition the committee acknowledged that the word dyspnea subsumes a variety of unpleasant respiratory sensations.

There is increasing evidence that dyspnea encompasses multiple sensations or clusters of qualitative respiratory sensations that may relate to underlying pathological processes.[3-10] The study of respiratory sensations began with the seminal laboratory work of Guz,[11] who described different sensations for the different laboratory stimulus of breath-holding, irritation, obstruction, and inability to obtain enough air. Janson-Bjerklie et al[3] reported that patients with obstructive, restrictive, and vascular pulmonary diseases used different words to describe their shortness of breath. Simon et al[4] found that healthy volunteers were able to distinguish between different sensations of breathlessness, depending on the stimulus, such as breath-holding, exercise, and resistive loads. These findings were extended to patients with different pulmonary conditions who completed an instrument containing 15 descriptors of respiratory sensations. These descriptors clustered into eight categories: shallow, work, suffocating, tight, air hunger, heavy, rapid, and exhalation.[5] This preliminary work has been extended by others, with descriptors related to the disease process or activity.[6-8,12,13] At present the choice of these words or clusters is not distinct enough to be used to diagnose mechanisms for dyspnea. However, as in pain, there are most certainly multiple stimuli felt by people who experience different sensations and use different words to connote those sensations.

Recent research findings also suggest that there may be important differences among ethnic groups in choices of words to describe dyspnea.[14] Failure to recognize these distinctions and understand the words an individual uses to describe dyspnea may lead to important underestimation of disease severity. It is important to distinguish dyspnea from objective changes in breathing pattern, such as tachypnea (rapid breathing), hyperpnea (increased ventilation in proportion to metabolic demands), and hyperventilation (increased ventilation in excess of metabolic demands). These changes in the pattern of ventilation may occur concurrently with dyspnea but are not synonymous with it.[1]

Similar to pain, dyspnea is thought to have an important affective component of anxiety and distress that is influenced by personal and environmental factors and health status; therefore the threshold for perception of the sensation varies widely. The stimulus intensity of "just noticeable difference" for shortness of breath may be the same among patients with similar pathological conditions of the lung, but the affective component may vary greatly and actually modulate the intensity of the symptom for the person.[2,15] Normal subjects and patients with chronic obstructive pulmonary disease (COPD) exercising in the laboratory have been able to differentiate the distress and anxiety related to dyspnea from the intensity of the sensation.[16,17] Recent neurophysiological studies have reinforced the hypothesis that there is an affective response to dyspnea with physiological stimulation of the limbic system when healthy subjects are subjected to air hunger.[18-20]

PREVALENCE AND POPULATIONS AT RISK

Dyspnea is one of the most common human responses to real or potential health problems affecting both children and adults. At one time or another, most individuals with acute or chronic pulmonary or cardiac disease will have dyspnea. The prevalence of dyspnea extends to metabolic, infectious, and neuromuscular diseases; to less pathological states, such as obesity and panic disorders[21,22]; and to nonpathological states, such as pregnancy.

For such a ubiquitous symptom, there is surprisingly little documentation on the prevalence of the symptom itself. In a recent study of 1556 seriously ill patients admitted to tertiary hospitals, 49% reported dyspnea, 51% reported pain, and 24% reported nausea.[23] Dyspnea is reported by approximately 25% of outpatients[24] and a similar proportion of the general public over 40 years of age.[25] In one study, most of the hospitalized patients who survived an acute exacerbation of COPD were short of breath for the rest of their lives.[26,27] It is estimated that 60% to 70% of pregnant women complain of dyspnea at some time during their pregnancy.[28]

The pervasiveness of dyspnea can be estimated by the prevalence of those diseases for which dyspnea is a primary symptom; pulmonary diseases, cardiac diseases and cancer of the lung. The most common chronic pulmonary diseases are obstructive, restrictive, or vascular in nature. COPD, comprising emphysema and chronic bronchitis, is the second leading cause of disability[29] and affects more than 16 million people in the United States.[30] It is estimated that COPD is responsible for more than 13.4 million physician visits and 634,000 hospitalizations each year.[29,31] Asthma affects approximately 17 million Americans, and its prevalence is growing rapidly.[32] Restrictive diseases are increasing with the prevalence of interstitial lung disease (ILD) increasing and estimated to be 80.9/100,000 in males and 67.2/100,000 in females.[33] Dyspnea occurs in pneumonias, such as *Pneumocystis carinii*, in persons infected with the human immunodeficiency virus (HIV).[34] Between 10% and 15% of patients with lung cancer have dyspnea at diagnosis, and 65% of these patients will have the symptom at some point during their illness.[35] Five multicenter national studies are consistent in showing that the commonest presenting symptom in lung cancer is breathlessness.[36] The prevalence of dyspnea increases from referral (18%) to palliative care services (79%) during the last weeks of life and is a major management problem in 25% to 78% of terminally ill patients.[37-40]

Dyspnea is most common in cardiovascular disease associated with pulmonary congestion, such as congestive heart failure (CHF), chronic cor pulmonale, valvular heart disease, and idiopathic cardiomyopathies.[41,42] Because heart disease remains the largest single cause of death in the United States, the prevalence of dyspnea may be assumed to be great in patients with CHF.

RISK FACTORS

Risk factors that adults and children have described as precipitants of their dyspnea are listed in Box 10-1.

Environmental

By far the greatest risk factor for the development of dyspnea is cigarette smoking or breathing secondhand smoke. Large prospective epidemiological studies have shown a strong association between primary and secondary cigarette smoke and the development of chronic bronchitis, emphysema, cancer of the lung, and coronary heart disease. All of these diseases result in dyspnea.[43] People with dyspnea describe increases in their dyspnea in crowded or smoke-filled rooms and in stressful or high-pressure situations. Environmental factors, such as allergens, cigarette smoke, weaning from a ventilator, and environmental conditions, such as weather and air pollution, all can trigger shortness of breath (SOB). People with allergen-sensitive or extrinsic asthma may have SOB in different seasons from exposure to grasses and molds, pollen, animal dander, dust, or air pollutants. Environmental and occupational pollution from smoke, sulfur dioxide, and ozone have been shown to trigger bronchoconstriction in asthmatic and atopic persons. Characteristics of weather, such as extreme heat or cold, wind, and fog, can also initiate dyspnea. Altitude is a known precipitant of SOB.[44]

Personal

Personal risk factors include correlates such as age, obesity, habits (including cigarette smoking and

BOX 10-1 Risk Factors Reported to Precipitate Shortness of Breath in Adults and Children

Personal Factors

Precipitating activities
- Resting
- Lying flat
- Walking level or uphill
- Housework
- Exercise
- Sexual activity
- Stooping and bending
- Hurrying
- Dressing and bathing
- Carrying heavy objects

Physical conditions
- Disease category
- Deconditioning of muscles
- Infections
- Abdominal distention
- Obesity
- Secretions
- Feeling too warm
- Fatigue
- Smoking
- Use of alcohol

Mechanical behaviors
- Talking
- Eating
- Coughing
- Laughing

Emotions or moods
- Upset
- Worry
- Anger
- Excitement
- Depression

Environmental Factors

Specific situations
- Living arrangement
- Social circumstances
- High pressure or tension
- Life events

Environmental conditions
- Altitude
- Seasonal variation
- Cigarette smoke–filled room
- Air pollution
- Weather: heat, cold, wind, fog

Allergens
- Grasses
- Molds
- Dust
- Animal dander

Adapted from Kohlman-Carrieri, V. & Janson-Bierklie, S. (1990). Coping and self-care strategies. In D.A. Mahler (ed.), Dyspnea (p. 204). Mt. Kisco, N.Y.: Futura; and Carrieri, V.K., Janson-Bjerklie, S., & Jacobs, S. (1984). The sensation of dyspnea: A review. *Heart & Lung 13,* 436-447.

alcohol use), occupation, illness, and level of fatigue. Infection, "catching a cold," abdominal distention, increased secretions, feeling too warm or too cold, and the use of alcohol or cigarettes are reported by individuals with dyspnea to be physical conditions that precipitate dyspnea. Talking, eating, coughing, or laughing can trigger dyspnea for some people. Emotional arousal of either positive or negative affect, such as being upset, worried, angry, anxious, depressed, excited, or happy may trigger breathlessness. Certain emotions, such as panic, anger, or anxiety, appear to be direct correlates of acute dyspnea.[22] The person's previous experience with the symptom, beliefs about the symptom, and illness severity affects his or her tolerance for breathlessness. Life events and stressors reported by the patient, such as "being punished" or "death of a parent," or "being excited about my trip," exacerbate breathlessness. If a person is deconditioned, physical activity will escalate dyspnea.

Developmental

To date there are no published studies that have examined the effect of aging on the symptom of dyspnea measured outside of the laboratory setting. Investigators have compared elderly with younger subjects in studies of the intensity of respiratory sensations provoked by respiratory stimuli in the laboratory. However, today it is clear that psychophysical sensitivity is not synonymous with the clinical experience of dyspnea; therefore these studies cannot be generalized to the clinical experience of dyspnea.[45,46] Tack et al[47] compared magnitude estimation of added elastic and resistive respiratory loads in a young (<30 years) and older (>60 years) sample. Sensation intensity for equal loads was significantly lower in the older group. The ventilatory response to chemical stimuli also has been found to be diminished with advancing age, and response to hypoxia and hypercapnia was reduced by nearly 50% in healthy older persons.[48,49] The findings of these few laboratory studies demonstrating that there is decreased sensitivity in elderly persons to chemical stimuli and respiratory loads, both causes of the sensation of dyspnea, suggest that the perception of dyspnea for the same pathophysiology may be diminished in the elderly. On the other hand, changes in physiological function associated with the aging process, such as declines in expiratory airflow and respiratory muscle strength, and increased ventilatory response to exercise may contribute to greater dyspnea.[50] All of these physiological changes would be expected to

BOX 10-2 Major Diseases Presenting with Dyspnea

Respiratory
- Upper airway obstruction
- Asthma
- Chronic bronchitis
- Emphysema
- Cystic fibrosis

Parenchymal lung disease
- Interstitial lung disease
- Malignancy—cancer of the lung or metastatic
- Pneumonia

Pulmonary vascular disease
- Arteriovenous malformations
- Intravascular obstruction
- Vasculitis
- Venoocclusive disease

Pleural disease
- Effusion
- Fibrosis
- Malignancy

Cardiovascular
- Decreased cardiac output
- Elevated pulmonary venous pressure
- Right to left shunt

Deconditioning

Respiratory muscle weakness/mechanical dysfunction
- Neuromuscular disorders (e.g., myasthenia gravis, amyotrophic lateral sclerosis, polio)
- Phrenic nerve dysfunction or injury
- Weakness (e.g., malnutrition thyroid disease)
- Deformities (e.g., kyphoscoliosis)
- Abdominal loading (e.g., ascites, obesity)

Miscellaneous
- Anemia
- Pregnancy
- Anxiety
- Panic disorder

Adapted from Silvestri, G.A., & Mahler, D.A. (1993). Evaluation of dyspnea in the elderly. *Patient Clinics in Chest Medicine 14*(3), 393-403.

contribute to a perception of greater dyspnea during activity in the elderly subjects.[51,52] Finally, with the decreased mobility that usually accompanies the aging process, elderly people often become deconditioned that would lead to greater dyspnea with the same activity.

Clinical States

Any disease process that involves the respiratory system can heighten the risk of the previously described pathophysiological states and therefore is a risk factor for dyspnea. Although the focus is usually on diseases of the lungs, chest wall, pleura, diaphragm, upper airway, and heart, diseases of many other organ systems, such neuromuscular, skeletal, renal, endocrine (including during pregnancy),[53] as well as rheumatological, hematological, and psychiatric factors, may affect the respiratory system and present with dyspnea.[54] Major diseases associated with increasing risk for dyspnea are listed in Box 10-2.

MECHANISMS

The knowledge of physiological and psychosocial mechanisms of dyspnea remains in the early stages of development, however, recent investigations have shed light on this complex symptom. As with other sensations, the experience results from neural activity within the part of the cerebral cortex responsible for sensory perception, and therefore, must be studied in humans. Dyspnea arises from such stimuli as exercise, breath-holding, and hypoxia that do not have a common neurophysiological pathway of peripheral receptor stimulation. It is still unclear whether there is a final common pathway for the sensation. Unlike localized sensations, such as touch or pain, which arise from peripheral stimulation, dyspnea is a visceral sensation similar to hunger or nausea, sensations that are experienced as a result of central neural activity. It is clear that dyspnea is not one sensation but many and that different types or levels of respiratory sensations relate to some extent to the type of physiological stimulus.[25] Except in patients with advanced disease who are dyspneic at rest, dyspnea usually does not occur unless there is active stimulation of breathing (e.g., by exercise, hypoxia, hypercapnia, and metabolic acidosis).[55-58] By contrast with the stimulation of breathing, voluntary increases in ventilation induce little or no dyspnea.[56,59,60] This observation led to the *key concept* in understanding the mechanisms of dyspnea: it is not only increased effort or movement of the chest wall that results in dyspnea, but rather the fact that the respiratory center must be stimulated for dyspnea to occur. Positron emission tomography (PET), used for decades to map pain pathways, has only recently been used by neurophysiologists to map the cortical activations associated with dyspnea; they have found a strong activation of the anterior insular cortex, a limbic structure, when normal volunteers experienced air hunger in the laboratory.[20,61,62] This is the first neurological evidence that emotions are activated when normal subjects have air hunger. Probable mechanisms for selected disease categories are presented in Table 10-1.

TABLE 10-1 Pathological Mechanisms for Dyspnea in Selected Diseases

DISEASE OR STATE	DISEASE	MECHANISMS
Pulmonary diseases	Emphysema, chronic bronchitis	Loss of elasticity of airways, increased secretions, altered gas exchange, hyperinflation resulting in increased EELV, causing shortening of inspiratory muscles and diaphragm, increased thoracic cage elastic recoil, respiratory muscles function at disadvantageous position on compliance curve, mechanical inefficiency of respiratory muscles leads to more effort for less volume–impedance to ventilation → increased WOB → dyspnea.
	Asthma	Inflammation of airways and increased reactivity of airways causes narrowing and constriction of airways → hyperinflation → increased resistance to ventilation → increased WOB → dyspnea.
	Cystic fibrosis	Increased secretions, increased airway hyperreactivity → increased impedance to ventilation → dyspnea.
Interstitial diseases	Idiopathic fibrosis, occupational lung diseases, ARDS, pneumonia	Lung compliance decreased–altered gas exchange → increased resistance to ventilation → more effort for same alveolar ventilation → increased WOB, increased respiratory drive from stimulation of peripheral receptors → increased minute ventilation → dyspnea.
	HIV	Pneumonitis causes decreased lung compliance → decreased alveolar ventilation → altered gas exchange and increased WOB → dyspnea.
Alterations in respiratory pump	Kyphoscoliosis	Alteration in configuration of chest wall leading to relative or absolute respiratory muscle weakness, loss of lung volume, more effort for less volume → increased WOB → dyspnea.
Neuromuscular disease	Muscular dystrophy, myasthenia gravis, amyotrophic lateral sclerosis	Weakness of respiratory muscles → inadequate ventilation, increased WOB → dyspnea. In general, degree of dyspnea is related to the respiratory muscles affected and not to the amount of ventilation achievable. Precise influence of higher cerebral centers on dyspnea in neurological diseases remains unclear.
Cardiovascular diseases	Pulmonary embolism, pulmonary hypertension	Wasted ventilation, stimulation of receptors, vagal stimulation and increased respiratory drive → increased minute ventilation → dyspnea.
Pulmonary trauma	Flail chest, fractured ribs, pneumothorax	Damage and weakness of respiratory muscles, inefficiency of respiratory pump, impedance to ventilation → increases WOB → dyspnea.
Metabolic states	Hypoxemia, hypercapnia, metabolic acidosis	Afferent signals from carotid bodies or central neuroreceptors trigger increased respiratory drive, increased minute ventilation → dyspnea.

Continued

TABLE 10-1 Pathological Mechanisms for Dyspnea in Selected Diseases—cont'd

DISEASE OR STATE	DISEASE	MECHANISMS
Lung cancer		Impedance to ventilation as a result of tumors, pleural effusions cause shortening of respiratory muscles, less length for contraction, decreased muscle strength, muscle weakness, fatigue, anxiety, altered gas exchange, decreased lung compliance, increased WOB → dyspnea.
Cardiac diseases	Mitral stenosis, LV hypertension, congestive heart failure	Pulmonary capillary hypertension and congestion cause increases in right atrial pressure, right ventricular pressure, pulmonary artery pressure and left atrial pressure. These changes in pressure are thought to activate receptors including pulmonary artery baroreceptors and left atrial mechanical receptors → increased respiratory drive → dyspnea.
Anemia		Reduction in Hgb and reduced oxygen content leads to possible tissue hypoxia. This may be responsible for an increase in respiratory drive and increased minute ventilation out of proportion to that which is usually needed → dyspnea.
Pregnancy		Dyspnea most frequently occurs for the first time in the first or second trimester before any increase in abdominal girth and may even improve as pregnancy progresses. The increased drive to breathe induced by progesterone has been suggested as one cause of dyspnea in pregnancy.
Psychological	Hyperventilation syndrome, panic disorder	Patients with panic disorder or hyperventilation syndrome may have ventilation appropriate for metabolic needs during exercise, but may hyperventilate at rest presumably because of an increased respiratory drive. Patient complains of "smothering" or inability to take a deep breath, with associated symptoms of palpitations, dizziness, light-headedness, and numbness of hands and feet and dyspnea.

ARDS, Acute respiratory distress syndrome; *EELV,* end expiratory lung volume; *WOB,* work of breathing.

Physiological Stimuli

Dyspnea is generated through a complex series of processes involving conscious awareness of the respiratory motor command to the ventilatory muscles, activation of sensory receptors, including chest wall receptors, pulmonary vagal receptors, irritant receptors and chemoreceptors; the transmission of sensory signals to the central nervous system (CNS); and the processing of those signals by higher brain centers.[2,63]

Respiratory Motor Command. It is known that factors that necessitate an increasing motor command to achieve a certain tension in the muscles, such as decreasing muscle length or increasing muscle weakness trigger a higher sense of respiratory effort.[64,65] It is believed that there is a conscious awareness of the outgoing respiratory motor command to the ventilatory muscles.[2] This separate sense of respiratory effort has been attributed to a "corolary discharge" from brainstem respiratory neurons to the sensory cortex. The sense of respiratory effort intensifies with increases in central respiratory command and is proportional to the ratio of the pressures generated by the respiratory muscles to the maximum pressure that the muscles are capable of generating.[64]

Chest Wall Receptors. Projections to the brain of afferent signals from mechanoreceptors in the joints, tendons, and muscles of the chest all shape the type of respiratory sensations. Experimental studies, including those that measured "the just noticeable difference," constraints on lung volume, and chest vibration, have demonstrated that afferents from intercostal muscles,[66] muscle,[67,68] and chest wall receptors[69] all have a preeminent role in the generation of dyspnea.

Pulmonary Vagal Receptors. Afferent information from pulmonary vagal receptors project to the brain and there is evidence that these receptors detect reductions in tidal volume and produce air hunger without feedback from chest wall receptors in studies with patients with high cervical cord transection.[70,71] In addition, vagal blockade has been shown to ameliorate dyspnea both in exercise and breath-holding.[72,73] Dyspnea associated with bronchoconstriction has been found in part to be mediated by airway receptors[74]; however, studies do not suggest that afferent activity from pulmonary receptors is a major source of the neural information that leads to exercise-induced dyspnea.

Chemoreceptors. The dyspnea associated with hypercapnia and hypoxia is primarily the result of the chemically induced increases in the output of the respiratory center. However, there is evidence that dyspnea may be directly affected by inputs from chemoreceptors with recent studies that have shown that increased P_{CO_2} produces air hunger in subjects paralyzed with neuromuscular blocking agents.[75] Additional evidence for the independent role of chemoreceptors in the generation of dyspnea are studies that have shown that the administration of oxygen reduces dyspnea out of proportion to that expected in the reduction in ventilation,[76] and the sensation of dyspnea is more intense at a given level of ventilation produced by hypercapnia than ventilation achieved by exercise or voluntary hyperventilation.[77]

Pathophysiology of Dyspnea

The most common hypothesis is that dyspnea results from a disassociation or a mismatch between central respiratory motor activity and incoming afferent information from receptors in the airways, lungs and chest wall structures.[78,79] This theory was first presented as the "length-tension" hypothesis[67] and is now referred to as *neuromechanical* or *efferent-reafferent dissociation*.[2] Dyspnea is multifactorial and results from one or more physiological and/or psychological mechanisms. Recently these have been classified in the American Thoracic Society (ATS) Statement as (1) *heightened ventilatory demand* resulting from either an increased metabolic load or increased central respiratory drive because of an excessive stimulus (e.g., hypoxemia, acidosis, and anxiety); (2) *abnormal impedance or resistance to ventilation* because of lung hyperinflation or an increased resistive load on the respiratory system (e.g., obstruction, stiff lungs, chest wall problems); (3) *respiratory muscle weakness*, presenting as either relative weakness as in hyperinflation or absolute weakness, as in myopathy, resulting in a mismatch between central respiratory motor output and achieved ventilation and subsequent dyspnea; (4) *abnormal central perception of dyspnea with an increased respiratory drive* (e.g., increasing anxiety or hyperventilation syndrome), increases the demand to breathe out of proportion for usual effort and can precipitate and enhance the sensation of dyspnea.[2] These mechanisms, with proposed treatments, are listed in Table 10-2.

PATHOLOGICAL CONSEQUENCES

Acute dyspnea associated with acute and severe hypoxemia may result in cerebral anoxia and brain injury. Dyspnea in association with hypoventilation can result in a dulling of sensory perception—the

TABLE 10-2 Treatments for Dyspnea Targeted to Pathophysiological Mechanisms

PATHOPHYSIOLOGICAL MECHANISMS	THERAPEUTIC INTERVENTION
Reduce ventilatory demand	
Reduce metabolic load	Exercise training-improve efficiency of CO_2 elimination
	Supplemental O_2 therapy
Decrease central drive	Supplemental O_2 therapy
	Pharmacological therapy
	Opiate therapy
	Anxiolytic therapy
	Alter pulmonary afferent information:
	Vibration
	Inhaled pharmacological therapy
	Fans
	Improve efficiency of CO_2 elimination:
	Alter breathing pattern
Reduce ventilatory impedance	
Reduce/counterbalance lung hyperinflation	Surgical volume reduction
	Continuous positive airway pressure
Reduce resistive load	Pharmacological therapy
Improve inspiratory muscle function	Nutrition
	Ventilatory muscle training
	Positioning
	Partial ventilatory support
	Minimizing use for steroids
Alter central perception	Cognitive behavioral approaches:
	Distraction techniques: relaxation, guided imagery, music
	Attention techniques: education, increased self-management of medications, symptom awareness, "desensitization"
	Pharmacological therapy

Adapted from American Thoracic Society (1999). Dyspnea. Mechanisms, assessment, and management: A consensus statement. *American Journal of Respiratory and Critical Care Medicine 159*, 321-340.

phenomenon of carbon dioxide narcosis. Patients with chronic lung disease, who are at risk for respiratory failure, are most likely to develop this clinical syndrome. Acute and chronic dyspnea can increase anxiety and panic that can lead to further rapid, shallow breathing that impairs ventilation and oxygenation.

Chronic dyspnea may be severe and unrelenting, or it may be present at some tolerable level but punctuated with severe exacerbations of breathlessness. Both patterns result in profound physical, psychological, emotional, and social outcomes. The pattern of the symptom becomes very important for functional consequences. People who are typically younger and experience episodic dyspnea with asthma often maintain a normal life without giving up their job or leisure activities. However, the downward spiral of increasing dyspnea, immobility, more dyspnea, deconditioning, leading to even more anxiety and dyspnea is well known for the COPD patient or those patients with interstitial diseases.[80] As these pervasive changes develop, people with chronic dyspnea often become depressed and lose hope, reinforcing physical and social isolation. Sleep disturbance, loss of appetite, and loss of physical strength, are common consequences of increasing disability in chronic lung disease, and these consequences can all be attributed to the symptom of dyspnea.[81-84]

The negative social consequences of COPD especially in terms of increasing social isolation and low levels of social support have been described.[85-88] Increased disability, loss of job, loss of friends and leisure activities, and reductions in functional status and quality of life are frequent consequences.[89,90]

Chronic dyspnea also is associated with overwhelming fatigue and physical inertia. The patient's ability and willingness to move out of the house and stay socially involved becomes seriously compromised. Many patients are unable to stay gainfully employed, as dyspnea limits their mobility. Hobbies and leisure activities need to be limited or changed to accommodate the disability, which can result in loss of friends and social support. When people are unable to carry out ADL including dressing, bathing, and caring for their homes, the need for outside resources becomes necessary and costly to the patient and his or her family.[91]

RELATED PATHOPHYSIOLOGICAL CONCEPTS

Dyspnea is a subjective perception that is modulated by a variety of physiological, cognitive, psychosocial, and behavioral factors. The severity of breathlessness varies more than might be expected with a given degree of pulmonary dysfunction. It is worse when it is unexpected, when it occurs in inappropriate situations, and when it is perceived as dangerous.[92] Physical fitness results in less dyspnea for a given exercise stimulus.[93] Studies in both normal subjects and patients with pulmonary disease have suggested that perception of the intensity of breathlessness may be influenced by prior experience of the sensation.[44,94,95] Selected physiological variables, listed in Table 10-2, reflecting pulmonary mechanics, oxygenation, and ventilation have been found to be related to some degree to dyspnea either measured by clinical measures of dyspnea or measurements during exercise.

Hypoxemia and Hypercapnia

Hypoxemia is a specific *dyspogen,* with peripheral chemoreceptors responding to a low PaO_2 and subsequent direct neural stimulation of the sensory cortex.[56] Hypoxia during exercise produces higher ratings of respiratory difficulty and breathlessness than exercise alone.[96,97] Investigators have reported that hypercapnia itself may not be a specific stimulus for breathlessness, but rather the increased ventilation that accompanies the increasing $PaCO_2$ may be the trigger for dyspnea.[98,99]

Relationships Among Dyspnea, Exercise Capacity, Lung Function, and Health-Related Quality of Life (HRQL)

Investigators have conducted factor analyses with different combinations of measures of clinical dyspnea, exercise capacity, lung function, HRQL, and demographic variables in patients with COPD. Variation in sample sizes and types of dyspnea measures make the findings difficult to compare; however, all authors found that dyspnea is a separate dimension and therefore should be measured separately from pulmonary function tests.[100,101] One group found that dyspnea at end exercise was not contained within the three separate factors of clinical measures of dyspnea, psychological variables, and HRQL.[102] Another group found that selected spirometry parameters, maximal pressures, and clinical measures of dyspnea represented three separate and independent factors.[100]

Fatigue

One of the most frequent physical correlates of dyspnea that patients describe is fatigue.[103] Patients complain of overwhelming weariness or say they are "all worn out." Indeed, some patients describe their dyspnea only in terms of fatigue. In several studies, the degree of fatigue has been related to increasing dyspnea. In a cross-sectional study of 68 COPD patients, fatigue was related ($r = 0.41$) to usual dyspnea (VAS).[3] Fatigue increased when dyspnea increased ($r = 0.47$) in a path analysis relating dyspnea, severity, functional status, and HRQL in 45 adults with COPD.[104] In nine patients receiving mechanical ventilation therapy, fatigue was related to the preweaning dyspnea score. Lung cancer patients often actually articulated dyspnea as fatigue, and patients who had the highest dyspnea had the highest fatigue.[105] In patients with asthma, fatigue was significantly elevated during high dyspnea when compared with times of lower dyspnea.[106] General fatigue correlated with depression ($r = 0.44$), and health status ($r = 0.75$) measured by the Saint George Respiratory Questionnaire, an instrument that includes an overall symptom scale as one dimension of health status, and presumably one of the most frequent symptoms COPD patients would be rating is dyspnea.[107]

Pain

Despite the high prevalence of simultaneous pain and dyspnea, only two studies to date have investigated the interaction between the perception of pain and the perception of dyspnea. One observational study conducted with seriously ill patients found that patients who have nausea and dyspnea experience more pain than patients without these symptoms, even after adjustment for depression, anxiety, disease type, disease severity, and demographics such as age and gender and psychological measures.[23] Another group of investigators studied the effects of pain (ischemic tourniquet) on dyspnea (loaded breathing) and vice versa in healthy subjects. They found that the perception of dyspnea was increased by pain; however, dyspnea did not intensify pain.[108]

Psychological States

The meaning of the symptom to the individual and his or her emotional state, personality, previous experience and cognitive function are factors likely to influence the experience and reporting of dyspnea.[109] The perception of dyspnea can be heightened in both acute and chronic anxiety states.[110] Alternative theoretical models have been proposed to explain this relationship.[110,111] Although the relationship of anxiety and dyspnea has been known clinically, this association between anxiety and dyspnea in the patient with COPD has only recently been investigated with controlled studies.[84,112-114] In patients with the hyperventilation syndrome, both dyspnea and ventilation may increase in the absence of any known physiological stimulus to breathe.[22] In such anxious patients, cognitive processes in the forebrain may stimulate respiration (and thereby dyspnea) through activation of limbic structures known to be associated with emotion.[115,116]

Most recently, PET scans of the brain have shown that the limbic system is stimulated during air hunger, providing evidence for the relationship between dyspnea and emotional responses.[117] Although it is not known whether depression or dyspnea occurs first in chronically ill patients, depression also has been associated with dyspnea in pulmonary patients.[118-120] Depressed patients often experience episodic dyspnea that fluctuates within minutes, occurs at rest, and bears little relationship to exercise.[112]

Differential Diagnosis

Acute dyspnea has limited differential diagnoses including pneumonia, pulmonary embolism, congestive heart failure, and myocardial infarction. Chronic dyspnea, however, presents more difficulty in differentiating mechanisms and causes. An initial interview to determine the "dimensions" of the symptom, including persistence or variability of the symptom, what it feels like, location, aggravating factors or triggers, individual strategies, and medications for alleviating the symptom helps the clinician to heighten the awareness of triggers and reinforce strategies the patient is using to manage his or her SOB. It is important to identify activities that provoke or relieve it. Input from family members or close acquaintances may clarify how limited a patient really is. It is worth noting that lung disease patients may report that they are more limited by "fatigue" or "leg fatigue" than by dyspnea. Key questions relate to persistence or variability of the symptom, aggravating factors (e.g., ambulation, eating, position, and exposures) and medications or activities that help relieve the symptoms. For example, intermittent dyspnea is probably caused by asthma or heart failure, whereas persistent or progressive dyspnea suggests a chronic condition, such as COPD, interstitial fibrosis, or pulmonary hypertension. Dyspnea may occur in conditions in which ventilation is stimulated by lactic acid production at relatively low levels of exercise (e.g., deconditioning, anemia, low cardiac output states). Nocturnal dyspnea is typical of asthma, CHF, gastroesophageal reflux, and nasal obstruction.[121] Dyspnea that occurs independent of physical activity suggests an allergic or a psychological problem. Dyspnea after exercise suggests exercise-induced asthma. Although emotions may affect dyspnea of any cause, psychogenic dyspnea should be suspected when dyspnea varies greatly and is unrelated to physical activity.[122] Review of factors that may affect (e.g., cigarettes, foods, and medications) or relieve (e.g., position) SOB is helpful. Obesity, cachexia, and sleep-disordered breathing may interact with other problems to increase dyspnea.

Physical Examination. Physical examination may provide vital clues to a diagnosis: respiratory rate, body habitus (e.g., cachexia and obesity), posture, use of pursed lips, use of accessory muscles, and emotional state. Abnormal chest expansion may suggest restriction or severe hyperinflation. Coughing on inspiration or expiration may suggest obstructive or interstitial lung disease, and a decrease in the intensity of the breath sounds may suggest emphysema, pneumothorax, or pleural effusion. Forced expiration may uncover focal or diffuse wheezing. The cardiac examination may suggest pulmonary hypertension (e.g., right ventricular heave and increased pulmonic sound) or right ventricular failure (e.g., jugular venous distention, hepato-jugular reflux, and pedal edema). Clubbing may be associated with many processes, notably cancer. Lower extremity edema suggests congestive failure if symmetrical and thromboembolic disease if asymmetrical.

Laboratory Evaluation. Laboratory analyses may not be helpful in the diagnosis of dyspnea. Anemia may be a clue to occult bleeding or serious systemic problems. Polycythemia may suggest chronic hypoxemia. Laboratory testing may reveal unsuspected renal disease, metabolic acidosis, or thyroid disease. Arterial blood gases may reveal unexpected hypoxemia or hypercapnia. The database should include chest x-ray evaluation, spirometry, and an electrocardiogram. (Lung function tests are discussed in the Measurement section.)

Testing of breathing reserve during exercise (fraction of maximal ventilation not used at peak exercise) is useful in distinguishing obstructive disease from cardiac disease. Exercise testing is insensitive for distinguishing cardiac disease from deconditioning.[123] Because the symptoms of panic attacks and lung disease may overlap, determination of the primary disorder may not be easy. Psychogenic dyspnea is usually a diagnosis of exclusion.

MEASUREMENT: MANIFESTATIONS AND SURVEILLANCE

Dyspnea is a subjective phenomenon that can be rated only by the person who is experiencing it; thus direct measurement is necessarily subjective. Indirect or objective measures only become important if the patient cannot communicate or if the clinician assesses that the patient is not reporting SOB that is consistent with an observed deterioration of ventilation, oxygenation, or respiratory distress. Excellent reviews and descriptions of these instruments are published elsewhere.[2,124-127] Therefore instruments that can be used in the research or clinical setting to measure dyspnea are only briefly described in Table 10-3.

Subjective Manifestations

The simplest but least sensitive measure of dyspnea is to ask the patient whether he or she is short of breath. This yes-or-no categorical measurement probably is the most frequently used method of assessing dyspnea, but gives no information about the severity or quality of the sensation.

Unidimensional Scales

Either the visual analog scale (VAS)[96] or the Modified Borg Scale for Breathlessness (Borg)[150] is currently used to measure dyspnea intensity, when the patient is confined to bed, during exercise tests, and to assess treatments.

Multidimensional Instruments: Dyspnea with Activities and Impact on Quality of Life

In an attempt to gain a more comprehensive evaluation of the impact of dyspnea on functional performance and health status, disease-specific instruments have been psychometrically tested and are being used in research and in some clinical situations. The characteristics of the instruments most widely used in research and some clinical settings are described in Table 10-3. The decision to use one or several of these instruments will depend on the research or clinical setting, the specific outcomes one wishes to measure, and the time available for administration. Because of its simplicity and its positive correlation with other measures of health status, recently it has been recommended that the British Medical Research Council (MRC) instrument be used routinely to clinically quantify the impact of dyspnea on a patient's health status.[134,151]

Measurement of the Affective Responses to Dyspnea

Studies have shown that dyspnea intensity does not change over time with worsening pulmonary status, as would be expected.[152] End-stage COPD and lung cancer patients have been reported to decrease their activity to almost immobility, while still rating their level of dyspnea at the same intensity.[105,153] Stability in dyspnea intensity may occur; however, with treatments or life events there may be changes in the anxiety or distress associated with that dyspnea. Using different instructions, the VAS or modified Borg scale can be used to measure the "anxiety" or "distress" related to dyspnea. Patients are asked to rate their response to the following questions on a Borg or VAS scale: "How anxious are you about your shortness of breath?" or "How bothersome or distressing is your shortness of breath to you?"[16,17]

Measurement of Qualitative Respiratory Sensations

As described in the Definition section, investigators continue to examine the "language of breathlessness" or the relationship between words used to describe respiratory sensations, type of disease, mechanisms, and clinical situations.[6-8,12,13,154,155] The instrument to measure qualitative respiratory sensations that has been tested and could be used to evaluate different respiratory sensations in clinical or research situations was published in 1990 by Simon et al.[5]

Objective Manifestations

Measures of respiratory distress, which include behavioral manifestations that can be observed or physiological pulmonary function parameters, can be used as indirect measures of dyspnea if the patient is unable to communicate or report the level of SOB that the health care provider believes is indicative of and detrimental to the body.

Behavioral Manifestations

Behavioral manifestations that are frequently observed when patients say they are short of breath include increased respiratory rate, restlessness,

TABLE 10-3 Unidimensional and Multidimensional Instruments to Measure Dyspnea

INSTRUMENT	DESCRIPTION	TESTING	ADVANTAGES/DISADVANTAGES
Unidimensional Scales to Measure Dyspnea During Acute Illness and Exercise			
Visual Analog Scale (VAS)	A vertical or horizontal line, most commonly 100 cm in length. Subjects indicate their dyspnea intensity by marking a line at the level of their dyspnea, either with their finger or a pencil. Anchors at the bottom and top should be "no breathlessness" and "worst imaginable" breathlessness.	The VAS is reproducible at the same level of exercise and at maximal exercise,[128,129] has high concurrent validity (r = >0.90) with the modified Borg scale, can be placed either horizontally or vertically (r = 0.97),[130] and has demonstrated sensitivity to treatment effects.[131]	VAS is more sensitive than the Borg scale.[57]
Modified Borg Scale (Borg)	10-point scale with a nonlinear scaling scheme using descriptive terms to anchor responses.	Strongly correlated with the VAS in COPD patients (r = 0.99)[132] with minute ventilation (r = 0.98) and oxygen consumption during exercise (r = 0.95).[96]	Advantages: The descriptors may help patients in selecting the sensation intensity, facilitate more absolute responses to stimuli, and allow direct comparisons between individuals. Disadvantages: The sensitivity of the scale may be blunted by "ceiling effects" triggered by the verbal descriptors and patients may tend to choose the numbers by the descriptors.
Numeric Rating Scale (NRS)	0–10 scale, no descriptors.	Correlates well with the VAS and Borg scale.[133]	Disadvantage: The lack of testing with the symptom of dyspnea and the inability to compare outcomes with others using the more standard VAS or modified Borg scale makes this scale less desirable for measuring dyspnea.
British Medical Research Council (MRC)	A five-item scale with graduated activities that would be more likely to bring on shortness of breath. The person checks the level of activity that applies to him or her. The levels range from "I only get breathless with strenuous exercise" to "I am too breathless to leave the house or I am breathless when dressing or undressing."	Extensive testing primarily as a gold standard in concurrent validity testing of other instruments.[134]	Advantages: It is simple and easy to use and can compare with others. Disadvantages: This scale requires individuals to be active, to make comparisons with others, and includes items that measure more than one level of exercise promoting dyspnea, lacking clear limits between grades.

Multidimensional Instruments: Dyspnea With Activities of Daily Living and Health Status			
Baseline Dyspnea/ Transitional Dyspnea Index (BDI/TDI)	Measures functional impairment (the degree to which activities of daily living are impaired), magnitude of effort (the overall effort exerted to perform activities), and the magnitude of task that provokes the breathing difficulty. The TDI measures the change in dyspnea from the baseline state to another point in time, typically after an intervention.[135]	Content validity was established by correlation of scores of the BDI with the Medical Research Council Scale (MRC) ($r = -0.70$, $p < 0.01$) and the Oxygen Cost Diagram (OCD) ($n = -0.54$, $p < 0.01$).[287] Interobserver agreement (interrater reliability) between physician and pulmonary technician has been evaluated and demonstrated creditable agreement of the two observers.[136] The TDI was reported to correlate with changes in the Medical Outcomes SF36 domains of physical and social function, mental health, and general health perceptions.[137]	Advantages: Extensive use, a calculated minimum clinical difference (MCID), and demonstrated sensitivity to treatments.[138-140] Disadvantage: Dyspnea is a subjective symptom, yet the health care provider, not the patient, rates the functional consequences of dyspnea with this instrument.
The Chronic Respiratory Disease Questionnaire (CRQ)	A 20-item self-report questionnaire administered by an interviewer that measures four dimensions: dyspnea, fatigue, emotional function, and mastery of breathing.[141] The patient rates the level of dyspnea he or she has with five usual individual activities.	Internal consistency for all four scales ranged from $\alpha = 0.71$ to 0.92 in authors' recent study. In both of our previous RCTs, the CRQ has been sensitive to treatment. Numerous validation studies have been published; the CRQ is a widely used and validated instrument.[142]	Advantages: Questionnaire has been used by many researchers, and outcomes from one program can be compared with others; it has demonstrated sensitivity to treatments; and a published MCID can be used to determine clinically significant changes.[140] Disadvantage: The dyspnea with ADL scale is individualized and therefore has been found to be less reliable.[143]
The Saint George Respiratory Questionnaire (SGRQ)	This is a disease specific health status 76-item questionnaire measuring three areas: symptoms, activity, and impact of disease on daily life. The symptom category elicits information about cough, sputum, wheeze, and dyspnea. Self-administered.	Test-retest reliability of the questionnaire in COPD patients is $r = 0.92$.[144] The instrument is responsive to treatments.[145]	Advantages: Thresholds of significant clinical change (MCID) are reported.[145] It is self-administered, has computerized scoring, and has extensive psychometric testing. Disadvantage: Dyspnea is not measured separate from other symptoms.

Continued

TABLE 10-3 Unidimensional and Multidimensional Instruments to Measure Dyspnea—cont'd

INSTRUMENT	DESCRIPTION	TESTING	ADVANTAGES/DISADVANTAGES
The University of California at San Diego Shortness of Breath Questionnaire (UCSDQ)	Measures SOB with daily activities before and after a rehabilitation program or therapy. Patients rate on a 6-point scale how frequently in the last week they experience SOB during 21 ADL that are associated with varying levels of exertion. Three additional questions ask about limitations caused by SOB, fear of harm from overexertion, and fear of SOB.	Early reliability and validity are reported; however, this instrument has been used in a large RCT on lung volume reduction surgery, and extensive testing will be available in the future.[146]	Advantages: Measures SOB with individual activities that could be tracked; is easy for the patient to understand; and does not take long to administer.
The Pulmonary Functional Status and Dyspnea Questionnaire (PFSDQ-M)	Self administered original instrument rating of dyspnea with164 activities in 6 categories: self care, mobility, eating, home management, social, and recreational.[147] Modified with reduction of the number of activities to 40, standardizing scaling formats, and adding a fatigue component (PFSDQ-M).[148]	Reliability of the three components was supported by internal consistency ($\alpha = 0.93$) for change experienced by the patient with activities, 0.95 for dyspnea with activities, and 0.95 for fatigue with activities. Stability of questionnaire was demonstrated on test-retest: 0.83 for dyspnea and 0.79 for fatigue with activities. The PFSDQ-M also appears to be responsive to physiological changes in lung function over time.	Advantages: The level of dyspnea for specific ADL can be monitored over time. The instrument is sensitive to small changes in dyspnea with activities.
The Pulmonary Functional Status Scale (PFSS)	Self administered questionnaire measures mental, physical, and social functioning. Dyspnea ratings are obtained in relation to several activities and reflected in a dyspnea subscale.	Reliability and validity estimates for both scales have been reported.[149]	

diaphoresis, use of accessory respiratory muscles, tremulousness, gasping breaths, pallor, interrupted or "staccato" speech, large staring eyes, frozen appearance, audible wheezing, and coughing and use of learned strategies including pursed-lips breathing. When asked, "How can other people tell when you are short of breath?" pulmonary patients named labored breathing, wheezing, rapid and open-mouth breathing, withdrawn, and a straight upright position with a frozen and immobile position.[3] Behaviors that indicate increased work of breathing (WOB) have all been shown to be related to dyspnea.

Indirect Physiological Measures of Dyspnea

In an attempt to investigate mechanisms there has been increasing study of the physiological correlates of dyspnea, especially during exercise. Physiological parameters that have been found to be related to dyspnea and can be used as indirect objective manifestations are listed in Box 10-3.

Relationship Between Clinical Measures of Dyspnea and Pulmonary Function

The relationship between pulmonary dysfunction and the severity of dyspnea may be close only within individual disease entities. This specificity to a certain disease is seen by examining the pulmonary function tests (PFT) that correlate with dyspnea in obstructive and restrictive pulmonary diseases. In obstructive disease, the following PFTs were related to dyspnea: maximal expiratory pressure (PE_{max}) ($r = 0.35$) and maximal inspiratory pressure (PI_{max}) ($r = 0.34$) were related to dyspnea measured by the baseline dyspnea index (BDI). In restrictive disease, Mahler et al[136] found that forced vital capacity (FVC) and forced expiratory volume in one second (FEV_1) was significantly correlated (0.43 to 0.49) with three different measures of dyspnea. Maximal voluntary ventilation (MVV), the largest volume in liters that can be breathed by voluntary effort per minute, had the greatest correlation ($r = 0.78$) with dyspnea in another study,[156] and peak expiratory flow rates (PEFR) was highly related ($r = 0.85$) in asthmatic patients in yet another study.[157]

A restrictive process decreases the FVC and impairs the diffusing capacity (DLCO). The resulting reduction in FVC ($r = -0.41$) and DLCO ($r = -0.50$) has been found to correlate moderately with severity of dyspnea in restrictive diseases.[158] In patients with interstitial lung disease, only PI_{max} ($r = 0.51$) and FVC ($r = 0.44$) showed significant correlations with dyspnea.[136]

BOX 10-3 Physiological Variables Related to Dyspnea in Research Studies

- Position
- Respiratory rate
- Inspiratory time
- Tidal volume
- Minute ventilation
- Accessory muscle use
- Paradoxical and dysynchronous breathing
- Hypoxia
- Hypercapnia
- Forced expiratory volume (FVC)
- Maximum inspiratory and expiratory pressures
- Dynamic hyperinflation
- End-expiratory lung volume
- End-inspiratory lung volume
- Work of breathing
- Muscle weakness

Work of Breathing

WOB is related closely to dyspnea. In fact, dyspnea has been labeled the "clinical manifestation" of the work of breathing. Manifestations of increased WOB, such as facial expressions, increased respiratory rate, the use of accessory neck and rib cage muscles of respiration, breathing, and asynchronous breathing have all been related to dyspnea.[106,159-162] A sensitive and reliable measurement of the work of breathing, the pressure time index (PTI), was related to dyspnea in a group of mechanically ventilated patients. The PTI is a measure of the work of the respiratory muscles related to the oxygen consumption of the muscles. The clinical calculation of this variable is complex and is described elsewhere.[163] If the patient is unable to rate his or her SOB, this indirect measure can be used to estimate the dyspnea felt by the patient.

Physiological Variables Related to Dyspnea During Exercise

An increase in minute ventilation (VE), an increase in respiratory rate (RR) alone and the length of inspiratory time have been related to dyspnea in normal subjects and in patients.[162,164] An early study found that 68% of the variance of breathlessness in normal subjects and those with differing respiratory diseases was explained by the following regression equation:

$$\text{Breathlessness (Y)} = 3.0\,(Ppl/pl_{max}) + 1.2\,(Vi) + 4.5\,(VT/VC) + 0.13\,(Fb) + 5.6\,(Ti/Ttot) - 6.2$$

where Ppl is the pleural pressure, Vi is the inspiratory flow rate, VT/VC is the tidal volume expressed as a percentage of the vital capacity, Fb is the respiratory rate (RR), and Ti/Ttot is the duty cycle or the inspiratory time related to the total respiratory cycle.[164] Mahler et al[131] found the strongest predictors for dyspnea in patients with asthma who were exercising were peak inspiratory flow ($P = 0.0005$), VT ($P= 0.0009$), RR ($P = 0.0001$), and peak inspiratory mouth pressure ($P = 0.0001$). These four variables explained 63% of the variance in dyspnea.

More recently there has been a growing focus on the importance of dynamic hyperinflation (DH) and the pattern of breathing and their important relationship to increasing dyspnea during exercise.[165-169] Recent studies have shown that DH during exercise is the major contributor to dyspnea. Studying the effect of inhaled beta agonist therapy on DH during exercise in COPD patients, Belman et al[165] found significant relationships between a change in dyspnea and a change in end-inspiratory lung volume/total lung capacity (EILV/TLC), a change in end expiratory lung volume/total lung capacity (EELV/TLC) and a change in neuroventilatory coupling (NVC). The best predictor of improvement in dyspnea was the reduction in the degree of DH manifested by the decrease in EILV/TLC and an improvement in neuro-ventilatory coupling (NVC). NVC was measured by peak inspiratory esophageal pressure (Pesins)/maximum capacity for pressure generation (Pcapi)/tidal volume/total lung capacity. Most recently O'Donnell et al[170]studied DH during exercise in 105 patients with COPD and found similar results. The increasing hyperinflation that restricted VT was the main contributor to dyspnea. The strongest correlate of exertional dyspnea was an index of the concurrent constraints on VT with the VT/IC (tidal volume/inspiratory capacity) accounting for 32% ($p <0.0005$) of the variance in dyspnea ratings. Less important contributing variables included VE/MVC (minute ventilation over maximal vital capacity, RR, and IRV/predicted TLC (inspiratory reserve volume/predicted total lung capacity), each accounting for 25% of the dyspnea ratings.

Surveillance

In chronically ill patients, SOB with changing activities and emotional situations can be monitored with the use of a daily log.[171-173] During an outpatient visit, a log can be used to establish a baseline and evaluate changes in the therapeutic regimen. Dyspnea with and without activity can be measured at each visit to determine patterns over time, with different seasons, varying activities, and after new treatments are initiated. Instruments that provide dimensions of the dyspnea experience (described in the Manifestations section) can be administered to track changes in the symptom and the impact on daily living. Baseline measurements recorded when patients are stable can be used to determine changes during acute exacerbations. During acute dyspnea the patient can rate his or her SOB on a VAS or modified Borg scale. Despite the individual variation and subjective nature of the symptom, the presence of perceived SOB remains a clue or prodromal indicator that the patient is not tolerating a new procedure or that the treatment is not effective. If validated instruments cannot be used, the nurse can ask the patient to rate his or her SOB on a scale of 0 to 10 in response to a certain treatment, change in position, or strategy being implemented.

CLINICAL MANAGEMENT

Therapeutic interventions for managing dyspnea are extensively reviewed elsewhere[2,27,54,127,174-177] and will only be summarized in this chapter. In the ATS Position Statement, the multidisciplinary committee recommended that whenever possible, therapeutic interventions be targeted to a specific physiological or psychological mechanism. However, the mechanism is not always known, and the committee proposed a more generic approach to treatment. These are categorized according to the mechanisms that are described in the Mechanisms section and are listed in Table 10-2. Interventions for treating dyspnea are categorized within a single targeted physiological mechanism; however, it is important to emphasize that there is considerable overlap in mechanisms addressed by a specific therapy. Many therapies, such as self-care strategies used by people with chronic SOB or comprehensive pulmonary rehabilitation programs (PR), affect several pathophysiological mechanisms.

Self-Care Strategies Reported by Patients With Dyspnea

Investigators have continued to describe self-management strategies learned and used by patients to cope with dyspnea and these have been compared across studies[105,178-181] (see Table 10-3). These strategies span every ATS category of intervention and may vary in different ethnic groups.[182] Patients should be asked to describe or list the strategies they use at home and these can be practiced and reinforced by the nurse.

Comprehensive Pulmonary Rehabilitation Programs

Comprehensive pulmonary rehabilitation programs (PR) typically target several causes dyspnea and include many or all of the therapeutic interventions listed in Table 10-2. Most PR programs include education, multiple modalities of exercise, breathing retraining, nutritional assessment, psychological support, and group interaction.[183-185] All recent RCTs have found that outpatient and home-based PR results in improvement in dyspnea during laboratory exercise and with activities of daily living (ADLs).[125,174,186-192] It remains difficult to determine the true effect of the individual components of PR programs; however, it appears that the critical treatment for improving dyspnea is exercise training.[191]

Reducing Ventilatory Demand

Exercise Training. Not all patients have access to or can afford a comprehensive PR program. Therefore it is important to recognize that exercise training alone, including upper and lower limb muscles, or weight training also improve dyspnea.[114,192-194] The number of exercise sessions necessary to achieve improvement in dyspnea is still unknown. Findings of a meta-analysis of 14 clinical trials strongly supported PR programs that include at least 4 weeks of exercise training.[195] Although some authors have suggested "high-intensity" exercise training, approximately 80% of peak $V\text{O}_2$ to promote "conditioning,"[196,197] others have found improvement in dyspnea with lower levels of intensity.[114,138,198]

Exercise "Desensitization" for Dyspnea. Repeated exercise may result in "desensitization" to the symptom (i.e., defined as less dyspnea for the same ventilatory stimulus) resulting in subjects tolerating more exercise before reaching their maximal levels of dyspnea.[94,138,189] In fact, exercise has been suggested as the strongest treatment to bring about desensitization to dyspnea.[199] Exercise training has been shown to decrease dyspnea and the affective response and increase COPD patients' self-efficacy for coping with the symptom.[114] Desensitization may be especially important, because it may occur regardless of the improvement in physical exercise performance.[114,199-201]

Energy Conservation. Ventilatory demand is also decreased by reducing the metabolic load by decreasing the respiratory effort for the patient. Energy conservation techniques result in reduction of physical effort so that less ventilatory effort is necessary, and therefore, less dyspnea.[180,184] Most of the information known about the relationship between energy conservation and dyspnea has been reported in descriptive studies of patients who use strategies that incorporate energy conservation.[105,179,180] However, teaching by the nurse has reduced dyspnea in COPD patients[202,203] and has been labeled the most important nursing function in dyspnea management.[204] Strategies that can be taught and used by patients for decreasing SOB with specific activities are published elsewhere.[127,175]

Decreasing Chemical or Neurological Central Respiratory Drive

Oxygen therapy. Subjects can walk farther and are less breathless when they are breathing oxygen.[205,206] Oxygen may also decrease dyspnea in patients who do not have a $Pa\text{O}_2$ within the existing guidelines for oxygen therapy.[207] The dose of oxygen is titrated to prevent desaturation,[208] and higher doses may be more beneficial for dyspnea during exercise.[24,98,207]

Medications. Although opiates have pharmacological effects that modulate dyspnea, including improving hypoxia and reducing ventilation during exercise,[209-211] fear of respiratory depression has discouraged their therapeutic use.[212] Opiates for stable outpatients with COPD may still be appropriate for treatment of dyspnea in carefully selected individual patients with disease that is far advanced, but not yet terminal.[27,213] Recent studies of the use of opiates in advanced cancer patients have shown promise in alleviating cancer dyspnea.[214,215] Earlier studies showed positive results for inhaled opiates[216,217]; however, later controlled studies have shown disappointing results for dyspnea in COPD.[218-221]

Although controlled studies of COPD patients have shown no benefit of anxiolytic agents,[222-224] they may still be useful in controlling dyspnea in carefully selected patients when anxiety is known to trigger their dyspnea.[225,226] It is important to determine from the patient whether anxiety is the primary symptom (i.e., which sensation they feel first or which sensation triggers the other).

There is little information on antidepressants and dyspnea. One clinical trial showed no effect of nortriptyline on dyspnea with daily activities,[227] but a recent small case series suggested that sertraline, a serotonin reuptake inhibitor, in doses of 25 to 100 mg/day may be useful in treatment of dyspnea even in patients not otherwise considered candidates for antidepressant therapy.[110]

Alter pulmonary afferent information. Treatment aimed specifically at receptors or reflex pathways has been investigated in laboratory studies. Stimulation of the nasal mucosa with oxygen cannulas,[228] in phase chest vibration,[68,69,229,230] and facial stimulation with cold air[231] have all been shown to reduce dyspnea. People with chronic dyspnea have described their use of fans or fresh air as one strategy for managing their dyspnea.[180]

Reduce Ventilatory Impedance

Reduce Resistive Load

Medications. Inhaled β_2-adrenergic agonists, inhaled anticholinergics, and sustained release theophylline have all been shown in randomized clinical trials to improve dyspnea in patients with stable COPD.[2,232] This bronchodilator therapy provides an initial minimal yet important decrease in dyspnea. Patients often report relief from dyspnea after only learning to correctly administer their medications with a metered dose inhaler and spacer.

Partial Ventilatory Support. Noninvasive continuous positive airway pressure (CPAP) and nasal pressure support ventilation (BIPAP) during exercise alleviates dyspnea provoked by exercise or by weaning from the ventilator by the addition of partial ventilatory support, which reduces the effort required to breathe.[233-235] In one study with non-intubated COPD patients, BIPAP for 2 hours for 5 consecutive days also decreased dyspnea at rest.[236]

Lung volume reduction surgery. Numerous reports have highlighted the potentially dramatic improvement in pulmonary function and dyspnea after lung volume reduction surgery.[237,238] Improvement in dyspnea may be explained by the combination of the decreased end-expiratory lung volume relative to total lung capacity, decreased respiratory rate and the ability to increase tidal volume.[169,239,240]

Improving Respiratory Muscle Function

Nutrition. Nutritional repletion can improve respiratory muscle function.[241,242] and has been found in the one study that measured dyspnea to decrease dyspnea in cachectic patients with COPD.[243,244]

Inspiratory muscle training. Although inspiratory muscle strength training is somewhat controversial,[245] a few studies have reported significant reductions in dyspnea in patients with COPD[139,246,247] and heart failure.[41]

Breathing retraining and pursed-lips breathing. Clinically, some patients report that using pursed-lips breathing (PLB) during periods of acute dyspnea or during ADL is the most important strategy they have for decreasing their SOB. The exact reason for this decrease in dyspnea during PLB is still unknown. Some have suggested that PLB provides distraction, and this enables the patient to slow his or her breathing. Investigators have found a slowing of RR; a substantial increase in VT; increased rib cage, accessory and abdominal muscle recruitment; less recruitment and resting of the diaphragm; and improved oxygen saturation; all of these changes may reduce the respiratory effort and decrease dyspnea.[248,249] To date, only physiological measures have been used in earlier studies to investigate the effect of diaphragmatic and abdominal breathing techniques on pulmonary function. The duration of treatment, type of technique, and length of measurement time varied considerably. Collectively, these studies found an increase in VT and VC and a decrease in RR, functional residual capacity (FRC), and oxygen consumption (Vo_2).[250,251] It is unclear whether these changes in lung function would result in a concomitant decrease in dyspnea.

Positioning. Patients with COPD have described the importance of "breathing stations" or places where they can rest when they are short of breath.[91] Studies have shown a decrease in dyspnea with the leaning forward position and a reduction in respiratory effort and the use of accessory muscles in the head-down position.[252,253] Patients should be allowed to assume the position in which he or she feels less shortness of breath.

Partial ventilatory support. Although it is intuitively appealing to "rest" respiratory muscles (e.g., with nasal ventilation) that are chronically "fatigued" so that they will perform better with less dyspnea,[254,255] the value of doing so has not been established.[256-258]

Medications that increase muscle strength. Medications that improve muscle contractility might also affect dyspnea.[259] Although the findings of studies are inconsistent, the value of theophylline for decreasing dyspnea is sufficient[260] to try a therapeutic trial in the persistently dyspneic COPD patient.

Alter Central Perception

Cognitive Behavioral Approaches

Education. Education focuses on symptom management versus the disease process. Teaching sessions provide patients with coping and self-care strategies that can be used in the future and enhance their feeling of control and mastery over their shortness of breath.[203,261] Principles of self-care for both acute and chronic dyspnea are described extensively elsewhere.[261,262]

Learning new strategies for managing dyspnea enhances cognitive variables, such as the perception of self-efficacy and control over the symptom.[114,263]

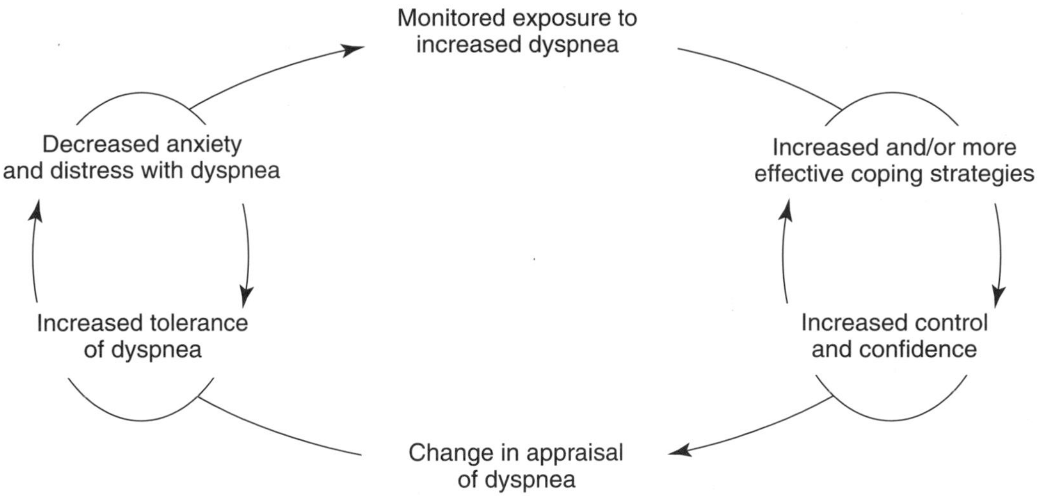

Figure 10-1 **A suggested mechanism for decreasing dyspnea and the anxiety associated with it.** (From Carrieri-Kohlman, V., Douglas, M.K., Gormley, J.M., & Stulbarg, M.S. [1993]. Desensitization and guided mastery. Treatment approaches for the management of dyspnea. *Heart & Lung* *22*[3], 226-234.)

These cognitive perceptions may have an indirect effect on the perception of dyspnea intensity or distress,[175] as shown in Figure 10-1. Patients' beliefs that they have behavioral strategies to cope with a symptom decreases the distress of the symptom in other illnesses.[264] The positive effects of education programs for patients with asthma have been established.[285] However, in patients with COPD, there is minimal study of education alone, apart from the other components of PR. Sassi-Dambron et al taught breathing strategies to be used with ADL and had the COPD patients practice these strategies, however, they found little change in multiple dyspnea measures. One earlier study using teaching and counseling by a nurse compared with three other groups (nonspecific surveillance with psychotherapy, analytic psychotherapy from experienced psychotherapists, and supportive psychotherapy from experienced psychotherapists) found that only the group treated by the nurse had a "sustained relief in breathlessness."[202] In addition, more recently, eight interactive small group education-only sessions did significantly decrease dyspnea with activity, measured by the Chronic Respiratory Disease Questionnaire (CRQ), compared with untreated controls. There were no associated changes in the 12-minute walk (MW) or pulmonary function variables.[266]

Self-Management of Medication Regimens. Clinically and during the conduct of research studies we have observed that just teaching the patient to correctly use his or her metered-dose inhaler to deliver medications may decrease reported dyspnea and increase the person's exercise performance. Education about the correct use of inhaled medications with return demonstration should be the first phase of treatment. Management of dyspnea in the face of severe episodic or continuous symptoms requires patients to learn to manipulate complex medication regimens. Patients can be taught early symptom recognition and awareness of signs and symptoms of infection so that the dose or type of medications can be altered by the patient before later contact with the physician.

Monitoring Triggers and Intensity of Shortness of Breath. Patients can discuss different factors that may make their dyspnea worse or better to individualize the experience and bring this information to their awareness.

Social Support. Clinical observations suggest that sharing with other's experiences and strategies for dealing with dyspnea may reduce the intensity of dyspnea and distress associated with it for patients with COPD[267]; however, there is also evidence that some patients need to be alone when they are experiencing extreme dyspnea.[268] In one study the level of dyspnea was related to the number of persons in the social support network. The frequency of contact with others was positively related to the intensity of dyspnea.[3]

Complementary Therapies. During acute dyspnea, distraction is often effective in the short term, because it is difficult to focus on two demands at once. Adults with asthma report using television, distancing themselves from a trigger, and other stimuli to distract themselves.[3,262] If dyspnea is increased by anxiety or panic, relaxation that is presumed to decrease anxiety would be expected to decrease dyspnea. This has been true during the actual relaxation sessions, however, the effect of relaxation treatments on subsequent dyspnea was not maintained.[269,270] Relaxation can take many forms depending on what method works for the patient.[271]

Another distraction technique is listening to music that distracts people so they do not attend to internal sensory information to the same extent.[199] During treadmill exercise, perceived "respiratory effort" (this may be dyspnea) was lower in patients with COPD while listening to music than while listening to gray noise or silence.[272] COPD patients at home decreased their dyspnea after 2 weeks with music therapy.[273] Hypnosis and biofeedback have been used in case studies with improvement in dyspnea for the individual patient.[274] Guided imagery is another method of distraction that is used clinically to increase exercise time, however, one uncontrolled study did not find changes in dyspnea with the use of guided imagery.[275] One uncontrolled study suggested that acupuncture provides short-term relief of dyspnea in cancer patients.[276] Yoga training has been shown to improve dyspnea measured by a VAS after 4 weeks with 15 subjects with chronic bronchitis[277] and "control of dyspnea attacks" in a small sample of COPD patients after 9 months.[278]

CONCEPTUAL MODELS

Physiological models relating physiological stimuli, receptors, afferent and efferent pathways, and higher centers in the brain that are thought to be involved in the genesis of dyspnea have been published.[25,63,279-282] These models provide illustrations of the complexity of the interactions among the respiratory, neurological, muscular, and chemical body systems for the perception of dyspnea to occur. Nurse researchers have been leaders in expanding this sole physiological approach to multifactorial models that emphasize both the sensory and affective dimensions of dyspnea and conceptualize dyspnea, much like pain, within a cognitive-motivational-affective framework. Models include antecedent biopsychosocial factors; cognitive-behavioral strategies to treat the symptom; and outcomes affected by the symptom, including physical performance, functional status, and quality of life.[283]

An early model for the study of dyspnea was described by Carrieri et al[284] in which antecedent personal, illness and situational factors were conceptualized as impacting on therapeutic strategies and patient coping self-care behaviors, which subsequently modulate dyspnea.[284] Several authors have published models that show the relationships among dyspnea, a subsequent decrease in activity, anxiety, and ensuing physical deconditioning.[285,286] A person-environment ecological model[287] proposed that dyspnea is a nocioceptive phenomenon and similar to pain has cognitive, motivational, and affective dimensions in addition to a sensory dimension. Perceptual sensitivity and dyspnea tolerance were major concepts addressed in the model.

Gift et al[288] proposed a middle-range "theory of unpleasant symptoms." This theory was developed by analyzing and contrasting the symptoms of fatigue and dyspnea. Dyspnea was conceptualized as having physiological and psychological dimensions similar to the distress components of pain. This theory suggests that there is a sensory component and a cognitive aspect. The important features of dyspnea were identified by comparing dyspnea in the same individual when he or she was short of breath and when he or she was not short of breath. In separate studies the psychological or distress aspects of dyspnea were found to be similar to pain and to be related to anxiety, depression, and somatization.[84,106,157] The basic structure outlined includes categories of factors (physiological, psychological, and situational) that affect one's disposition to or manifestation of the symptom, characteristics of the symptom, and the proposed performance variables affected by the symptom. Acknowledging that existing models fail to differentiate between acute and chronic dyspnea, recently a model was developed that defines chronic dyspnea as distress with varying levels of intensity, antecedents, and long-term physical, psychological, and sociocultural consequences.[283]

CASE STUDIES

The following descriptions of dyspnea are given by patients with different pulmonary disease.

CASE STUDY 1

Emphysema. GS, who is 58 years old and has emphysema, lives on disability payments he has received for the past 17 years, when his illness caused him to retire from his job as an office manager. Notably, he has a 43 pack-year history of smoking. GS is breathless dressing himself and relies on his wife for transportation, dressing, and any social activity. This severely ill man describes his dyspnea episodes as "gasping for breath," "not getting enough air," and "all closed up." His SOB, which is almost continuous, is aggravated by smoke and fumes, any physical exertion, such as walking from the bed to the bathroom in the morning, excessive humidity, or emotional arousal, such as anger and frustration. His FEV_1 is 1 L, with an FEV/FVC ratio of 46%. His grade of breathlessness on the MRC scale is 5, and he rates his usual daily dyspnea at 60 on a 100-mm VAS.

He describes behaviors that others may see him use with increasing SOB as changes in position, straining of neck muscles, especially on the left side, and sitting up straight or standing. If he is walking, he stops and does not move. GS relies primarily on medications to decrease his symptoms. He has also learned pursed-lips breathing and relaxation techniques to use when he is walking or during panic attacks. A massage by his wife to any part of his body relieves the tension and helps him to relax and breathe easier. He was taught in the past to wear loose clothes and conserve energy. He relates that when his regular medicine does not work, he is admitted to the hospital for a stay of 4 to 7 days, where he gets "more intensive treatment," such as intravenous medications and ventilatory therapy.

GS's social space is confined to his home; in fact, he has no friends in particular. Although he "still feels as good about himself as ever," he does not believe that he contributes much to the world, and this bothers him. He has given up most of his hobbies, such as golf and trips, and has trouble finding alternative activities. He prefers not to talk about his SOB because, as he emphasizes, "I don't like to burden others. I feel it brings down other people's spirits, and I don't want sympathy or pity." GS has begun to monitor his SOB with a VAS during rest and activity and feels he has "greater control" of the symptom and therefore can tolerate the symptom more.

CASE STUDY 2

Interstitial Disease. PW, 28 years old, was initially told that he had pneumonia, but after a year, a "specialist" confirmed the diagnosis of sarcoidosis. He is separated from his wife, lives alone, and continues to work as a record salesman. His dyspnea occurs "anytime, anywhere," and although he sometimes can disregard it, "it's always there." This young man describes his dyspnea as a "funny feeling, like you're going to pass out but know you're not. It's like putting salt on a sore—you know it's going to burn a little; pain down both sides of my back. I can feel fluid moving in my lungs, my heart beats fast, and I feel hot." Although physical exertion almost always brings on his SOB, strong emotions, saunas, lying down, playing with his nephew, or energy required when he's concentrating may all increase his breathing difficulty. Sitting up straight, being quiet, or taking his prescribed diazepam (Valium) are strategies he uses to diminish the "overexcited feeling" he gets when he is SOB. Others might notice his increasing SOB, because he is sweating, and "I breathe after every 10 words, compared with every 30 words for other people." PW believes that his SOB has "changed my life completely" and that he just has to deal with it: "It's a trip to change my lifestyle and know I'll be under a doctor's care for the rest of my life."

Typical of his disease pattern, remissions have allowed PW to maintain a job, perform ADL, and take trips by car or plane that do not require walking too far. His pulmonary function parameters are typical of restrictive disease, with all lung volumes decreased, a 60% of predicted vital capacity, and 70% predicted total lung capacity. Flow rates are normal. PW has little or no social support. More than decreased energy from his dyspnea, his feelings about the symptom have limited his communication and friendship with others. As he describes it: "I'm jealous of other people; they can breathe, I can't. My friends have told me I've changed; they can't help me, so why talk about it? I wouldn't depend on anyone else for anything, it's just a crutch." Typically, this patient with restrictive disease has never been taught strategies to help him cope with persistent SOB. Although he receives daily steroid treatment, he believes that "nothing can make it better; I just have to live with it."

SELECTED RESEARCH FINDINGS

The discussion of research findings will be limited to selected nursing research published since the last edition of this book. Earlier studies were reviewed in the last edition and elsewhere.[127,175,289] Research studies by nurses have continued to span all aspects of knowledge development, including perception of the symptom, validation of instruments to measure dyspnea, investigation of the correlates of dyspnea, and the study of various therapies to modulate the symptom. Meek[290] used added inspiratory airflow resistance with magnitude estimation techniques in the laboratory to examine the influence of variations in attentional focus on the judgments associated with the perception of breathlessness in normal volunteers and patients with COPD. Two conditions—the subject's typical breathing pattern and clearest memory of breathlessness—were used to alter the focus of attention and compare it with traditional techniques as a control condition (CC). There was a significant main effect for condition and an interaction effect for group by condition. There were significant differences only for the COPD group in both comparisons. It was concluded that previous exposure to sensations have an impact on judgments used to determine the intensity of a sensation given similar stimuli and, therefore, contribute to alterations in the perception of breathlessness. The findings of this study emphasize the importance of previous experience on present ratings of dyspnea.

Hardie[14] examined whether African American and white patients differed in the words they use to describe their breathlessness and/or their perception of breathlessness. Subjects with asthma (16 per group) had a provocation concentration of methacholine chloride causing a 30% fall in FEV_1. Serial PFT and measures of dyspnea were performed. Word descriptors were measured by an open-ended word descriptor questionnaire. She found significant ethnic differences in the words used to describe the sensation of breathlessness present at a 30% fall in FEV_1. African Americans used significantly more upper airway word descriptors, such as "tight throat," scared-agitated voice, "tight itchy throat," and "tough breath." Whites used significantly more lower airway or chest-wall symptom descriptors, including "deep breath," "light-headed," "out of air," "aware of breathing," and "hurts to breathe." African Americans required a 44.3% smaller mean dose of methacholine to achieve the same 30% fall in FEV_1. This study was an important advance in the study of the language of breathlessness and respiratory sensations. It reinforces the importance of being aware of ethnic differences in symptom monitoring.

Gift et al[130] continued to contribute important findings toward the measurement of clinical dyspnea. In one study, a vertical visual analog scale (VVAS) for measuring clinical dyspnea was validated. Correlation between the VVAS and horizontal VAS (HVAS) was $r = 0.97$; between the VVAS and the PEFR, correlation was $r = -0.85$, demonstrating the concurrent validity of the VVAS. Construct validity was established using the contrasted-groups approach with repeated measures. Both asthmatic patients and persons with COPD rated their dyspnea on the VVAS during times of severe and little airway obstruction. The dyspnea ratings at times of severe versus low obstruction were found to be different for both asthmatic and COPD subjects.[130] To establish the validity of a numeric rating scale as a measure of resting dyspnea, 188 patients with COPD rated their present dyspnea using the VAS and the numeric rating scale (NRS). Validity of the NRS was supported by the high correlation of its scores with scores from the VAS. Conversion of the NRS to a 0 to 100 scale and comparison with the VAS scale showed that scores were not significantly different. Scores on the NRS were obtained before and after ambulation, supporting the construct validity of the NRS scale.[133]

Nurse investigators have studied patients' memory for dyspnea and the accuracy of recall in symptom reports. Meek et al[291] examined the accuracy of self-reports of symptom intensity in patients with COPD and factors that influenced the recall of intensity. On a 0 to 10 scale subjects recalled their average greatest and least symptom intensity for the previous 14 days. No significant differences were found between recalled and actual dyspnea. The greatest contributor of the variance in the recall scores of both dyspnea and fatigue was the symptom intensity on the day of recall. Cognitive function was related to the greatest and least dyspnea scores and to the average and least recalled scores. Meek et al. suggest that there is beginning evidence that cognitive function affects symptom reporting and that current symptom intensity may impact recall of past intensity. We examined whether after an exercise session COPD patients could accurately recall the maximum ratings of dyspnea and anxiety with dyspnea they experienced during exercise training.[292] As a group, patients accurately recalled the worst dyspnea they experienced during a 30-minute exercise session. However, individual variation was substantial, limiting predictability of individual ratings. The findings supported the use of retrospective symptom ratings as a method of assessing dyspnea during exercise training.

Other investigators have studied the relationship between dyspnea and multiple psychosocial variables. Graydon et al.[293,294] studied the extent to which mood, symptoms, lung function and social support predicted the level of functioning for patients with COPD. The best predictors of patients' functioning at 30 months was their functioning at baseline, symptoms, FEV_1, and age. The most prevalent symptoms were dyspnea and fatigue, both of which were highly correlated with functioning. Another nurse researcher analyzed relationships among dyspnea and antecedent and mediator variables on quality of life. Although dyspnea was hypothesized to have a direct effect on quality of life, with a sample of 126 COPD patients, dyspnea had a direct effect on depression and only an indirect effect on quality of life.[295] Variables with direct effects on quality of life were self-esteem, depression, social support, and age. Weaver et al[296] tested an explanatory model of variables influencing functional status in 104 patients with COPD. Exercise capacity, dyspnea, and depressed mood significantly and directly influenced functional status. Dyspnea, depression, and pulmonary function indirectly influenced functional status through exercise capacity. These authors concluded that efforts to improve functional status of individuals with COPD should focus on interventions that influence exercise capacity, dyspnea, anxiety, and depressed mood. Lareau et al[152] conducted a secondary analysis to determine the direction and rate of change in the symptom of dyspnea in patients with COPD whose lung function had worsened over time. Thirty-four male subjects were followed for 5.3 ± 3.5 years. There was no significant difference in reports of dyspnea (PFSDQ) over time, despite significant reductions in lung function. Dyspnea when raising arms over the head was the only activity showing a relationship to the slope of change in FEV_1%.

In the last decade there has been an unprecedented increase in RCTs investigating the effect of PR programs on multivariate outcomes, including dyspnea.[125,174;195] One frequently cited RCT in which nurses were involved is that by Ries et al.[191] who compared the effect of a PR program with an education program similar to that offered in PR programs. Dyspnea at end exercise and with ADL decreased significantly at 2 months for the PR group but not for the education-only group. This improvement in SOB remained for 18 months; similar to the findings of other RCT over the last decade.[195] Reardon et al[138] showed that a 6-week outpatient comprehensive PR program compared with an untreated group resulted in significant improvement in exercise tolerance and dyspnea during exercise testing, as well as dyspnea with ADL (BDI/TDI).

Larson et al.[188] compared the effects of home-based inspiratory muscle training (IMT) and cycle ergometry training (CET) in patients with COPD. Patients were randomly assigned to 4 months of training in one of four groups: IMT, CET, CET + IMT, or health education (ED). Inspiratory muscle strength and endurance increased in IMT and CET + IMT groups significantly compared with CET and ED groups. Peak oxygen uptake increased and heart rate, minute ventilation, dyspnea, and leg fatigue decreased at submaximal work rates in the CET and CET + IMT groups compared with the IMT and ED groups. The combination of CET and IMT did not produce additional benefits in exercise performance and exercise-related symptoms.

We studied whether nurse coaching affected the intensity of dyspnea as well as the anxiety and distress associated with it after a 12-session exercise training program in COPD subjects.[114] Dyspnea and anxiety related to dyspnea significantly decreased relative to ventilation after the training program in both the coached and monitored-only group. Self-efficacy for walking also increased in both groups. The decrease in dyspnea was attributed in part to desensitization to the symptom, increased muscle efficiency, and comfort on the treadmill, because there was little evidence for aerobic conditioning.

The importance of exercise training for bringing about changes in dyspnea is supported by the findings of Sassi-Dambron et al in which the group who received a program of education and practice of coping strategies for dyspnea was compared with a control group who received lectures about health.[285] The education program consisted of a description of COPD; breathing strategies; progressive muscle relaxation; energy-saving techniques; panic control; and stress management. Subjects practiced coping strategies. There were no significant differences between the groups in six measures of dyspnea, with the exception that one measure of dyspnea (BDI/TDI) decreased more significantly for the group receiving the strategies and practice.

Patients with lung cancer who had completed the first line of treatment were randomized to attend a nursing clinic that offered the intervention for breathlessness or "best" supportive care.[203,297] The intervention consisted of a weekly clinic visit that included assessment of SOB, teaching effective ways of coping with SOB, exploration of the meaning of SOB, breathing control, activity pacing, relaxation techniques, and psychosocial support. The supportive care group (control) received standard management and treatment available for breathlessness and breathing assessments. Worst and best breathlessness and distress caused by the symptom was measured with a VAS. The intervention group improved their dyspnea (VAS) at rest significantly more than the control group at 8 weeks.

QUESTIONS FOR FUTURE STUDY

Dyspnea as a concept has been studied from many perspectives; however, research in all areas is needed, including perception, language, mechanisms, measurement and therapies to affect the symptom, and the study of dyspnea in other settings and across all diseases. Future research should continue to study all proposed mechanisms for dyspnea. Dynamic hyperinflation as a mechanism for exercise-induced dyspnea and the study of the limbic system response during dyspnea are exciting areas for future questions. Another important area of study are factors that affect individual differences in the discrepancy between the perception of the sensation and pathophysiology. There is beginning evidence that gender may affect the perception and rating of dyspnea as with other symptoms; these differences need to be explored.

Although in the last decade measurement of dyspnea as an outcome in the research arena has mushroomed; this knowledge has not been translated into clinical settings. Future research needs to focus on alternative methods for increasing the frequency of measurement of dyspnea in patient settings and determining whether just measuring the symptom impact treatments or outcomes. How dyspnea can be adjusted for changing activity level over time is an important future research question. Nothing is known about the individual variation in effects of differing treatments on different individuals (i.e., which strategies work with what kinds of patients). Most of the research has been with COPD patients; little is known about the types and frequency of strategies for dyspnea in other diseases including cardiac and interstitial disease.

In the future, strategies that patients have identified and that nurses have observed clinically (e.g., cold air on the face) need to be tested in patients rather than with healthy volunteers. As yet only a few nurses have studied some of the more exciting pharmacological therapies for dyspnea, such as the use of oxygen and opiates in advanced stages of illness. Because it is known that dyspnea and distress of dyspnea are modulated by psychosocial factors (e.g., self-efficacy and mood), future study of therapies may be enhanced by studying changes in related variables that may impact dyspnea. In addition, the study of dyspnea needs to be extended to acute dyspnea and advanced stages of disease. The past two decades have seen tremendous accomplishments that will form the basis for future development of knowledge related to the symptom of dyspnea.

REFERENCES

1. Comroe, J.H. (1966). Some theories of the mechanisms of dyspnea. In J.B.L. Howell & E.J.M. Campbell (eds.), *Breathlessness* (pp. 1-7). Oxford: Blackwell Scientific.
2. American Thoracic Society. (1999). Dyspnea. Mechanisms, assessment, and management: A consensus statement. *American Journal of Respiratory and Critical Care Medicine 159,* 321-340.
3. Janson-Bjerklie, S., Carrieri, V.K., & Hudes, M. (1986). The sensations of pulmonary dyspnea. *Nursing Research 35,* 154-159.
4. Simon, P.M., Schwartzstein, R.M., Weiss, J.W., Lahive, K., Fencl, V., Teghtsoonian, M., et al. (1989). Distinguishable sensations of breathlessness induced in normal volunteers. *American Review of Respiratory Disease 140,* 1021-1027.
5. Simon, P.M., Schwartzstein, R.M., Weiss, J.W., Fencl, V., Teghtsoonian, M., & Weinberger, S.E. (1990). Distinguishable types of dyspnea in patients with shortness of breath. *American Review of Respiratory Disease 142,* 1009-1014.
6. Schwartzstein, R.M. (1998). The language of dyspnea. In D.A. Mahler (ed.), *Dyspnea* (pp. 35-57). New York: Marcel Dekker.
7. Elliott, M.W., Adams, L., Cockcroft, A., MacRae, K.D., Murphy, K., & Guz, A. (1991). The language of breathlessness. Use of verbal descriptors by patients with cardiopulmonary disease. *American Review of Respiratory Disease 144,* 826-832.
8. Mahler, D.A., Harver, A., Lentine, T., Scott, J.A., Beck, K., & Schwartzstein, R.M. (1996). Descriptors of breathlessness in cardiorespiratory diseases. *American Journal of Respiratory Critical Care Medicine 154,* 1357-1363.
9. Parshall, M.B., Welsh, J.D., Brockopp, D.Y., Heiser, R.M., Schooler, M.E., & Cassidy, K.B. (2001). Reliability and validity of dyspnea sensory quality descriptors in heart failure patients treated in an emergency department. *Heart & Lung 30,* 57-65.
10. Parshall, M.B., Welsh, J.D., Brockopp, D.Y., Heiser, R.M., Schooler, M.E., & Cassidy, K.B. (2001). Dyspnea duration, distress, and intensity in emergency department visits for heart failure. *Heart & Lung 30,* 47-56.
11. Guz, A. (1977). Respiratory sensations in man. *British Medical Bulletin 33,* 175-177.
12. Moy, M.L., Lantin, M.L., Harver, A., & Schwartzstein, R.M. (1998). Language of dyspnea in assessment of patients with acute asthma treated with nebulized albuterol. *American Journal of Respiratory and Critical Care Medicine 158,* 749-753.
13. Moy, M.L., Weiss, J.W., Sparroe, D., Israel, E., & Schwartzstein, R.M. (2000). Quality of dyspnea in bronchoconstriction differs from external resistive loads. *American Journal of Respiratory and Critical Care Medicine 162,* 451-455.
14. Hardie, G.E., Janson, S., Gold, W.M., Carrieri-Kohlman, V., Boushey, H.A. (2000). Ethnic differences: word descriptors used by African-American and white asthma patients during induced bronchoconstriction. *Chest 117(4)*:935-943.
PMID: 10767221 [PubMed - indexed for MEDLINE]
15. Carrieri, K.V., Douglas, M.K., Gormley, J.M., & Stulbarg, M.S. (1993). Desensitization and guided mastery: Treatment approaches for the management of dyspnea. *Heart & Lung 22,* 226-234.
16. Carrieri-Kohlman, V., Gormley, J.M., Douglas, M.K., Paul, S.M., Stulbarg, M.S. (1996). Differentiation between dyspnea and its affective components. *Western Journal of Nursing Research 18,* 626-642.
17. Wilson, R.C., & Jones, P.W. (1991). Differentiation between the intensity of breathlessness and the distress it evokes in normal subjects during exercise. *Clinical Science 80,* 65-70.
18. Corfield, D.R., Fink, G.R., Ramsay, S.C., Murphy, K., Harty, H.R., Watson, J.D.G., et al. (1995). Evidence for

limbic system activation during CO_2-stimulated breathing in man. *Journal of Physiology 488,* 77-84.

19. Fink, G.R., Corfield, D.R., Murphy, K., Kobayashi, I., Dettmers, C., Adams, L., et al. (1996). Human cerebral activity with increasing inspiratory force: A study using positron emission tomography. *Journal of Applied Physiology 81,* 1295-1305.
20. Banzett, R.B., Mulnier, H.E., Murphy, K., Rosen, S.D., Wise, R.J., & Adams, L. (2000). Breathlessness in humans activates insular cortex. *Neuroreport 11,* 2117-2020.
21. Bass, C. (1991). Unexplained chest pain and breathlessness. *Medical Clinics of North America 75,* 1157-1173.
22. Smoller, J.W., Pollack, M.H., Otto, M.W., Rosenbaum, J.F., & Kradin, R.L. (1996). Panic anxiety, dyspnea, and respiratory disease. Theoretical and clinical considerations. *American Journal of Respiratory and Critical Care Medicine 154,* 6-17.
23. Desbiens, N.A., Mueller, R.N., Connors, A.F., & Wenger, N.S. (1997). The relationship of nausea and dyspnea to pain in seriously ill patients. *Pain 71,* 149-156.
24. Dewan, N.A., & Bell, C.W. (1994). Effect of low flow and high flow oxygen delivery on exercise tolerance and sensation of dyspnea. A study comparing the transtracheal catheter and nasal prongs. *Chest 105,* 1061-1065.
25. Stulbarg, M.S., & Adams, L. (2000). Dyspnea. In J.F. Murray & J.A. Nadel (eds.), *Textbook of respiratory medicine* (3rd ed., pp. 5441-5552). Philadelphia: W.B. Saunders.
26. Lynn, J., Ely, E.W., Zhong, Z., McNiff, K.L., Dawson, N.V., Connors, A., et al. (2000). Living and dying with chronic obstructive pulmonary diseases. *Journal of the American Geriatric Society 48,* S91-100.
27. Luce, J.M., & Luce, J.A. (2001). Management of dyspnea in patients with far-advanced lung disease. *Journal of the American Geriatric Society 285,* 1331-1337.
28. Milne, J.A., Howie, A.D., & Pack, A.I. (1978). Dyspnea during normal pregnancy. *British Journal of Obstetrics and Gynecology 85,* 260-263.
29. National Heart, Lung and Blood Institute. (2000). *Morbidity and mortality: 2000 chart book on cardiovascular, lung, and blood diseases.* Bethesda, Md.: Author.
30. Adams, P., & Hendershot, G. (1996). Current estimates from the national health interview survey. Washington, D.C.: National Center for Health Statistics. Vital and Health Statistics Series 10, No. 200.
31. Rennard, S.I. (1998). COPD: Overview of definitions, epidemiology, and factors influencing its development. *Chest 113,* 235S-241S.
32. Hartert, T.V., & Peebles, R.S. (2000). Epidemiology of asthma: The year in review. *Current Opinion in Pulmonary Medicine 6,* 4-9.
33. Coultas, D.B., Zumwalt, R.E., Black, W.C., & Sobonya, R.E. (1994). The epidemiology of interstitial lung diseases. *American Journal of Respiratory and Critical Care Medicine 150,* 967-972.
34. Janson, S., & Carrieri-Kohlman, V. (1998). Respiratory changes in HIV-related conditions. In M.R.A. Williams (ed.), *Handbook of HIV nursing* (pp. 361-386). Boston: Jones & Bartlett.
35. Twycross, R.G., & Lack, S.A. (1986). *Therapeutics I: Terminal cancer.* Edinburgh: Churchill Livingston.
36. Muers, F. (2001). Quality of life and symptom control. Lung cancer. *European Respiratory Monograph 6,* 1305-1329.
37. Roberts, D.K., Thorne, S.E., & Pearson, C. (1993). The experience of dyspnea in late-stage cancer. Patients' and nurses' perspectives. *Cancer Nursing 16,* 310-320.
38. Mercadante, S., Casucvcio, A., & Fulfaro, F. (2000). The course of symptom frequency and intensity in advanced cancer patients followed at home. *Journal of Pain and Symptom Management 20,* 104-112.
39. Edmonds, P., Higginson, I., Altmann, D., Sen-Gupta, G., & McDonnell, M. (2000). Is the presence of dyspnea a risk factor for morbidity in cancer patients? *Journal of Pain and Symptom Management 19,* 15-22.
40. Reuben, D.B., & Mor, V. (1986). Dyspnea in terminally ill cancer patients. *Chest 89,* 234-236.
41. Mancini, D.M. (1995). Pulmonary factors limiting exercise capacity in patients with heart failure. *Progress in Cardiovascular Diseases 56,* 347-370.
42. Mancini, D.M., Henson, D., LaManca, J., & Levine, S. (1992). Respiratory muscle function and dyspnea in patients with chronic congestive heart failure. *Circulation 86,* 909-918.
43. PHS Office on Smoking and Health (1984). The health consequences of smoking: A report of the Surgeon General. Rockville, Md.: Department of Health and Human Services.
44. Jones, P.W., Oldfield, W.L.G., & Wilson, R.C. (1990). Reduction in breathlessness during exercise at sea level after 4 weeks at an altitude of 4000 metres. *Journal of Physiology 422,* 105P.
45. Mahler, D.A. (1987). Dyspnea: Diagnosis and management. *Clinics of Chest Medicine 8,* 215-230.
46. Lane, R., Adams, L., & Guz, A. (1987). Is low-level respiratory resistive loading during exercise perceived as breathlessness? *Clinical Science 73,* 627-634.
47. Tack, M., Altose, M.D., & Cherniack, N.S. (1983). Effects of aging on sensation of respiratory force and displacement. *Journal of Applied Physiology 55,* 1433-1440.
48. Kronenberg, R.S., & Drage, C.W. (1973). Attentuation of the ventilatory and heart rate responses to hypoxia and hypercapnia with aging in normal men. *Journal of Clinical Investigation 52,* 1812.
49. Peterson, D.D., Pack, A.L., Silage, D.A., Fishman, A.P. et al. (1981). Effects of aging on ventilatory and occlusion pressure responses to hypoxia and hypercapnia, *American Review of Respiratory Disease 124,* 387-391.
50. Silvestri, G.A., & Mahler, D.A. (1993). Evaluation of dyspnea in the elderly patient. *Clinics in Chest Medicine 14,* 393-404.
51. Tzankoff, S.P., Robinson, S., Pyke, F.S., & Brawn, C.A. (1972). Physiological adjustments to work in older men as affected by physical training. *Journal of Applied Physiology 33,* 346.
52. Yerg, J.E.I., Seals, D.R., & Hagberg, J.M. (1985). Effect of endurance exercise training on ventilatory function in older individuals. *Journal of Applied Physiology 58,* 791.
53. Tenholder, M.F., & South, P.J. (1989). Dyspnea in pregnancy [clinical conference]. *Chest 96,* 381-388.
54. Tobin, M.J. (1990). Dyspnea. Pathophysiologic basis, clinical presentation, and management. *Archives of Internal Medicine 150,* 1604-1613.
55. Stark, R.D., Gambles, S.A., & Lewis, J.A. (1981). Methods to assess breathlessness in healthy subjects: A critical evaluation and application to analyse the acute effects of diazepam and promethazine on breathlessness induced by exercise or by exposure to raised levels of carbon dioxide. *Clinical Science 61,* 429-439.

56. Adams, L., Lane, R., Shea, S.A., Cockroft, A., & Guz, A. (1985). Breathlessness during different forms of ventilatory stimulation: A study of mechanisms in normal subjects and respiratory patients. *Clinical Science 69,* 663-672.
57. Wilson, R.C., & Jones, P.W. (1989). A comparison of the visual analogue scale and modified Borg scale for the measurement of dyspnea during exercise. *Clinical Science 76,* 277-282.
58. Lane, R., & Adams, L. (1993). Metabolic acidosis and breathlessness during exercise and hypercapnia in man. *Journal of Physiology (*Lond) *461,* 47-61.
59. Lane, R., Cockcroft, A., & Guz, A. (1987). Voluntary isocapnic hyperventilation and breathlessness during exercise in normal subjects. *Clinical Science 73,* 519-523.
60. Freedman, S., Lane, R., & Guz, A. (1987). Breathlessness and respiratory mechanics during reflex or voluntary hyperventilation in patients with chronic airflow limitation. *Clinical Science 73,* 311-318.
61. Evans, K., Banzett, R.B., McKay, L., Frackowiak, R., & Corfield, D. (2000). MRI identifies limbic cortex activation correlated with air hunger in healthy humans. *FASEB Journal 14,* A645.
62. Banzett, R.B., & Moosavi, S.H. (2001). Dyspnea and pain: Similarities and contrasts between two very unpleasant sensations. *American Pain Society Bulletin* 11.
63. Jones, N.L., & Killian, K.J. (1992). *Breathlessness: The Campbell Symposium.* McMaster University, Hamilton, Ontario, Canada.
64. Killian, K.J., Gandevia, S., Summers, E., & Campbell, E.J.M. (1984). Effect of increased lung volume on perception of breathlessness, effort and tension. *Journal of Applied Physiology 57,* 686-691.
65. Campbell, E.J.M., Gandevia, S.C., Killian, K.J., Mahutte, C.K., & Riggs, J.R.A. (1990). Changes in the perception of inspiratory resistive loads during partial curarization. *Journal of Applied Physiology 309,* 93-100.
66. Gandevia, S.C., & Macefield, G. (1989). Projection of low threshold afferents from human intercostal muscles to the cerebral cortex. *Respiratory Physiology 77,* 203-214.
67. Campbell, E.J.M., & Howell, J.B.L. (1963). The sensation of breathlessness. *British Medical Bulletin 19,* 36-40.
68. Homma, L.T., Obata, I., Sibuya, M., & Uchida, M. (1984). Gate mechanism in breathlessness caused by chest wall vibration in humans. *Journal of Applied Physiology 56,* 8-11.
69. Altose, M.D., Syed, I., & Shoos, L. (1989). *Effects of chest wall vibration on the intensity of discharge during constrained breathing. Proceedings of the International Union of Physiological Science 17,* 288.
70. Banzett, R.B., Lansing, R.W., & Brown, R. (1987). High level quadriplegics perceive lung volume change. *Journal of Applied Physiology 62,* 567-573.
71. Manning, H.L., Shea, S.A., Schwartzstein, R.M., Lansing, R.W., Brown, R., & Banzett, R.B. (1992). Reduced tidal volume increases 'air hunger' at fixed P_{CO_2} in ventilated quadriplegics. *Respiratory Physiology 90,* 19-30.
72. Davies, S.F., McQuaid, K.R., Iber, C., McArthur, C.D., Path, M.J., Beebe, D.S., et al. (1987). Extreme dyspnea from unilateral pulmonary venous obstruction. Demonstration of a vagal mechanism and relief by right vagotomy. *American Review of Respiratory Disease 136,* 184-188.
73. Guz, A., Noble, M.I.M., Eisele, J.H., & Trenchard, D. (1970). Experimental results of vagal block in cardiopulmonary disease. In R. Porter (ed.), *Breathing: Hering Breuer Centenary Symposium* (pp. 315-328). London: Churchill.
74. Taguchi, O., Kikuchi, Y., Hida, W., Iwase, N., Satoh, M., Chonan, T., et al. (1991). Effects of bronchoconstriction and external resistive loading on the sensation of dyspnea. *Journal of Applied Physiology 71,* 2183-2190.
75. Banzett, R.B., Lansing, R.W., Brown, R., Topulos, G.P., Yager, D., Steele, S.M., et al. (1990). 'Air hunger' from increased P_{CO_2} persists after complete neuromuscular block in humans. *Respiratory Physiology 81,* 1-17.
76. Lane, R., Cockcroft, A., Adams, L., & Guz, A. (1987). Arterial oxygen saturation and breathlessness in patients with chronic obstructive airways disease. *Clinical Science 72,* 693-698.
77. Chonan, T., Mulholland, M.B., Leitner, J., Altose, M.D., & Cherniack, N.S. (1990). Sensation of dyspnea during hypercapnia, exercise, and voluntary hyperventilation. *Archives of Internal Medicine 150,* 1604-1613.
78. Schwartzstein, R.M., Simon, P.M., Weiss, J.W., Fencl, V., & Weinberger, S.E. (1989). Breathlessness induced by dissociation between ventilation and chemical drive. *American Review of Respiratory Disease 139,* 1231-1237.
79. Schwartzstein, R.M., Manning, H.L., Weiss, J.W., & Weinberger, S.E. (1990). Dyspnea: A sensory experience. *Lung 168,* 185-199.
80. Casaburi, R. (1993). Exercise training in chronic obstructive lung disease. In R. Casaburi & T.L. Petty (eds.), *Principles and practice of pulmonary rehabilitation* (pp. 204-224). Philadelphia: W.B. Saunders.
81. Greenburg, G.D., Ryan, J.J., & Bourlier, P.F. (1985). Psychological and neuropsychological aspects of COPD. *Psychosomatics 26,* 29-33.
82. Agle, D.P., Baum, G.L., Chester, E.H., & Wendy, M. (1973). Multidiscipline treatment of chronic pulmonary insufficiency. 1. Psychologic aspects of rehabilitation. *Psychosomatic Medicine 35,* 41-49.
83. Heim, E., Blaser, A., & Waidelich, E. (1972). Dyspnea: Psychophysiologic relationships. *Psychosomatic Medicine 34,* 405-423.
84. Gift, A., Plaut, M., & Jacox, A. (1986). Psychologic and physiologic factors related to dyspnea in subjects with chronic obstructive pulmonary disease. *Heart & Lung 15,* 595-601.
85. Williams, S.J. (1989). Chronic respiratory illness and disability: A critical review of the psychosocial literature. *Social Science Medicine 28,* 791-803.
86. Williams, S.J., & Bury, M.R. (1989). Impairment disability and handicap in chronic respiratory illness. *Social Science Medicine 29,* 609-616.
87. Blake, R.L.J. (1991). Social stressors, social supports, and self-esteem as predictors of morbidity in adults with chronic lung disease. *Family Practice Research Journal 11,* 65-74.
88. Keele-Card, G., Foxall, M.J., & Barron, C.R. (1993). Loneliness, depression and social support of patients with COPD and their spouses. *Public Health Nursing 10,* 245-251.
89. Archibald, C.J., & Guidotti, T.L. (1987). Degree of objectively measured impairment and perceived shortness of breath with activities of daily living in patients with chronic obstructive pulmonary disease. *Canadian Journal of Rehabilitation 1,* 45-54.
90. Kennedy, S.M., Des Jardins, A., Kassam, A., Ricketts, M., & Chan-Yeung, M. (1994). Assessment of respiratory limitation in activities of daily life among retired workers. *American Journal of Respiratory Critical Care Medicine 149,* 575-583.

91. Fagerhaugh, S.Y. (1973). Getting around with emphysema. *American Journal of Nursing 73,* 94-99.
92. Dudley, D.L., Glaser, E.M., Jorgenson, B.N., & Logan, D.L. (1980). Psychosocial concomitants to rehabilitation in chronic obstructive pulmonary disease. Part 1. Psychosocial and psychological considerations. *Chest 77,* 413-420.
93. Adams, L., Chronos N., Lane, R., Guz, A. (1986). The measurement of breathlessness induced in normal subjects: Individual differences. *Clinical Science 70,* 131-140.
94. Belman, M.J., Brooks, L.R., Ross, D.J., & Mohsenifar, Z. (1991). Variability of breathlessness measurement in patients with chronic obstructive pulmonary disease. *Chest 99,* 566-571.
95. Wilson, R.C., & Jones, P.W. (1990). Influence of prior ventilatory experience on the estimation of breathlessness during exercise. *Clinical Science 78,* 149-153.
96. Adams, L., Chronos, N., Lane, R., & Guz, A. (1985). The measurement of breathlessness induced in normal subjects: Validity of two scaling techniques. *Clinical Science 69,* 7-16.
97. Ward, S.A., & Whipp, B.J. (1989). Effects of peripheral and central chemoreflex activation on the isopnoeic rating of breathing in exercising humans [published erratum appears in *Journal of Physiology* (Lond) 1990 Jan;420, 489]. *Journal of Physiology 411,* 27-43.
98. O'Donnell, D.E., Bain, D.J., & Webb, K.A. (1997). Factors contributing to relief of exertional breathlessness during hyperoxia in chronic airflow limitation. *American Journal of Respiratory and Critical Care Medicine 155,* 530-535.
99. Lane, R., Adams, L., Guz, A. (1990). The effects of hypoxia and hypercapnia on perceived breathlessness during exercise in humans. *Journal of Physiology* (Lond) *428,* 579-593.
100. Mahler, D.A., & Harver, A. (1992). A factor analysis of dyspnea ratings, respiratory muscle strength, and lung function in patients with chronic obstructive pulmonary disease. *American Review of Respiratory Disease 145,* 467-470.
101. Eakin, E., Sassi-Dambron, D., Ries, A., & Kaplan, R. (1995). Reliability and validity of dyspnea measures in patients with obstructive lung disease. *International Journal of Behavioral Medicine 2,* 118-134.
102. Hajiro, T., Nishimura, K., Tsukino, M., Ikeda, A., Koyama, H., & Izumi, T. (1998). Analysis of clinical methods used to evaluate dyspnea in patients with chronic obstructive pulmonary disease. *American Journal of Respiratory and Critical Care Medicine 158,* 1185-1189.
103. Gift, A.G., Pugh, L.C. (1993). Dyspnea and fatigue. *Nursing Clinics of North America 28,* 373-384.
104. Moody, L., McCormick, K., & Williams, A. (1990). Disease and symptom severity, functional status, and quality of life in chronic bronchitis and emphysema (CBE). *Journal of Behavioral Medicine 13,* 297-306.
105. Brown, M.L., Carrieri, V., Janson, B., & Dodd, M.J. (1986). Lung cancer and dyspnea: The patient's perception. *Oncology Nursing Forum 13,* 19-24.
106. Gift, A.G. (1991). Psychologic and physiologic aspects of acute dyspnea in asthmatics. *Nursing Research 40,* 196-199.
107. Breslin, E., van der Schans, C., Bereukink, S., Meek, P.M., Mercer, K., Volz, W., et al. (1998). Perception of fatigue and quality of life in patients with COPD. *Chest 114,* 958-964.
108. Nishino, T., & Shimoyama, N. (1999). Experimental pain augments. *Anesthesiology 91,* 1633-1638.
109. Chetta, A., Gerra, G., Foresi, A., Zaimovic, A., Del Donno, M., Chittolini, B., et al. (1998). Personality profiles and breathlessness perception in outpatients with different gradings of asthma. *American Journal of Respiratory and Critical Care Medicine 157,* 116-122.
110. Smoller, J.W., Pollack, M.H., Systrom, D., Kradin, R.L. (1998). Sertraline effects on dyspnea in patients with obstructive airways disease. *Psychosomatics 39,* 24-29.
111. Bess, C., & Gardner, W. (1985). Emotional influences on breathing and breathlessness. *Journal of Psychosomatic Research 29,* 599-609.
112. Dudley, D.L., Pitts-Poarch, A.R. (1980). Psychological aspects of respiratory control. *Clinics in Chest Medicine 1,* 131-143.
113. Burns, B.H., & Howell, J.B.L. (1969). Disproportionately severe breathlessness in chronic bronchitis. *Quarterly Journal of Medicine 38,* 277-294.
114. Carrieri-Kohlman, V., Gormley, J.M., Douglas, M.K., Paul, S.M., & Stulbarg, M.S. (1996). Exercise training decreases dyspnea and the distress and anxiety associated with it. Monitoring alone may be as effective as coaching. *Chest 110,* 1526-1535.
115. Munchauser, F., Mador, M., Ahuja, A., & Jacobs, L. (1990). Selective paralysis of voluntary but not limbically influenced automatic respiratory. *Archives of Neurology 48,* 1190-1192.
116. Heywood, P., Murphy, K., Corfield, D., Morrell, M., Howard, R., Guz, A. (1996). Control of breathing in man: Insights from the "locked in" syndrome. *Respiratory Physiology 106,* 13-20.
117. Banzett, R.B., Mulnier, H.E., Murphy, K., Rosen, S.D., Wise, R.J.S., & Adams, L. (2002). Dyspnea activates the limbic cortex.
118. Sandhu, H.S. (1986). Psychosocial issues in chronic obstructive pulmonary disease. *Clinics in Chest Medicine 7,* 629-642.
119. Janson, C., Bjornsson, E., Hetta, J., & Boman, G. (1994). Anxiety and depression in relation to respiratory symptoms and asthma. *American Journal of Respiratory and Critical Care Medicine 149,* 930-934.
120. Light, R.W., Merrill, E.J., Despars, J.A., Gordon, G.H., Mutalipassi, L.R.(1985). Prevalence of depression and anxiety in patients with COPD: Relationship to functional capacity. *Chest 87,* 35-38.
121. Togawa, K., Konno, A., Miyazaki, S., Yamakawa, K., & Okawa, M. (1988). Obstructive sleep dyspnea. Diagnosis and treatment. *Acta Otolaryngology Supplement* (Stockholm) *458,* 167-173.
122. Howell, J.B. (1990). Behavioural breathlessness. *Thorax 45,* 287-292.
123. Martinez, F.J., Stanopoulos, I., Acero, R., Becker, F.S., Pickering, R., & Beamis, J.F. (1994). Graded comprehensive cardiopulmonary exercise testing in the evaluation of dyspnea unexplained by routine evaluation. *Chest 105,* 168-174.
124. Pashkow, P., Ades, P.A., Emery, C.F., Frid, D.J., Houston-Miller, N., Peske, G., et al. (1995). Outcome measurement in cardiac and pulmonary rehabilitation. AACVPR Outcomes Committee. American Association of Cardiovascular and Pulmonary Rehabilitation. *Journal of Cardiopulmonary Rehabilitation 15,* 394-405.
125. ACCP/AACVPR P.R.G.P. (1997). Pulmonary rehabilitation: Joint ACCP/AACVPR evidence-based guidelines. ACCP/AACVPR Pulmonary Rehabilitation

Guidelines Panel. American College of Chest Physicians. American Association of Cardiovascular and Pulmonary Rehabilitation [see comments]. *Chest 112,* 1363-1396.
126. Mahler, D., Guyatt, G., & Jones, P. (1998). Clinical measurement of dyspnea. In Mahler, D. (ed.), *Dyspnea* (pp. 149-189). New York: Marcel Dekker.
127. Carrieri-Kohlman, V., Stulbarg, M.S. (2000). Dyspnea: Assessment and management. In J.E. Hodgkin, B.R. Celli & G.L. Connors (eds.), *Pulmonary rehabilitation: Guidelines to success* (pp. 57-89). New York: Lippincott Williams & Wilkins.
128. Muza, S.R., Silverman, M.T., Gilmore, G.C., Hellerstein, H.K., & Kelsen, S.G. (1990). Comparison of scales used to quantitate the sense of effort to breathe in patients with chronic obstructive pulmonary disease. *American Review of Respiratory Disease 141,* 909-913.
129. Mador, M.J., Rodis, A., & Magalang, U.J. (1995). Reproducibility of Borg scale measurements of dyspnea during exercise in patients with COPD. *Chest 107,* 1590-1597.
130. Gift, A.G. (1989). Validation of a vertical visual analogue scale as a measure of clinical dyspnea. *Rehabilitation Nursing 14,* 323-325.
131. Mahler, D.A., Faryniarz, K., Lentine, T., Ward, J., Olmstead, E.M., O'Connor, G.T. (1991). Measurement of breathlessness during exercise in asthmatics. Predictor variables, reliability, and responsiveness. *American Review of Respiratory Disease 144,* 39-44.
132. Lush, M.T., Janson, B.S., Carrieri, V.K., & Lovejoy, N. (1988). Dyspnea in the ventilator-assisted patient. *Heart & Lung 17,* 528-535.
133. Gift, A.G., & Narsavage, G. (1998). Validity of the numeric rating scale as a measure of dyspnea. *American Journal of Critical Care 7,* 200-204.
134. NHLBI/WHO-NIH National Heart, Lung and Blood Institute Global Initiative for Chronic Obstructive Lung Disease. (2001). Global strategy for the diagnosis, management and prevention of chronic obstructive pulmonary disease. Workshop Report Pub. No. 2701. Washington, D.C.: Author.
135. Mahler, D.A., Weinberg, D.H., Wells, C.K., & Feinstein, A.R. (1984). The measurement of dyspnea. Contents, interobserver agreement, and physiologic correlates of two new clinical indexes. *Chest 85,* 751-758.
136. Mahler, D.A., Rosiello, R.A., Harver, A., Lentine, T., McGovern, J.F., & Daubenspeck, J.A. (1987). Comparison of clinical dyspnea ratings and psychophysical measurements of respiratory sensation in obstructive airway disease. *American Review of Respiratory Disease 135,* 1229-1233.
137. Mahler, D.A., & Mackowiak, J.I. (1995). Evaluation of the short-form 36-item questionnaire to measure health-related quality of life in patients with COPD. *Chest 107,* 1585-1589.
138. Reardon, J., Awad, E., Normandin, E., Vale, F., Clark, B., & ZuWallack, R.L. (1994). The effect of comprehensive outpatient pulmonary rehabilitation on dyspnea. *Chest 105,* 1046-1052.
139. Harver, A., Mahler, D.A., & Daubenspeck, J.A. (1989). Targeted inspiratory muscle training improves respiratory muscle function and reduces dyspnea in patients with chronic obstructive pulmonary disease. *Annals of Internal Medicine 111,* 117-124.
140. Jaeschke, R., Singer, J., & Guyatt, G.H. (1989). Measurement of health status. Ascertaining the minimal clinically important difference. *Controlled Clinical Trials 10,* 407-415.
141. Guyatt, G.H., Berman, L.B., Townsend, M., Pugsley, S.O., & Chambers, L.W. (1987). A measure of quality of life for clinical trials in chronic lung disease. *Thorax 42,* 773-778.
142. Guyatt, G.H., King, D.R., Feeny, D.H., Stubbing, D., & Goldstein, R.S. (1999). Generic and specific measurement of health-related quality of life in a clinical trial of respiratory rehabilitation. *Journal of Clinical Epidemiology 52,* 187-192.
143. Wijkstra, P.J., TenVergert, E.M., Van Altena, R., Otten, V., Postma, D.S., Kraan, J., et al. (1994). Reliability and validity of the chronic respiratory questionnaire (CRQ). *Thorax 49,* 465-467.
144. Jones, P.W., Quirk, F.H., Baveystock, C.M., & Littlejohns, P. (1992). A self-complete measure of health status for chronic airflow limitation. The St. George's Respiratory Questionnaire. *American Review of Respiratory Disease 145,* 1321-1327.
145. Jones, P.W., & Bosh, T.K. (1997). Quality of life changes in COPD patients treated with salmeterol. *American Journal of Respiratory and Critical Care Medicine 155,* 1283-1289.
146. Eakin, E.G., Kaplan, R.M., & Ries, A.L. (1993). Measurement of dyspnea in chronic obstructive pulmonary disease. *Quality of Life Research 2,* 181-191.
147. Lareau, S.C., Carrieri-Kohlman, V., Janson-Bjerklie, S., & Roos, P.J. (1994). Development and testing of the Pulmonary Functional Status and Dyspnea Questionnaire (PFSDQ). *Heart & Lung 23,* 242-250.
148. Lareau, S.C., Meek, P.M., & Roos, P.J. (1998). Development and testing of the modified version of the pulmonary functional status and dyspnea questionnaire (PFSDQ-M). *Heart & Lung 27,* 159-168.
149. Weaver, T.E., & Narsavage, G.L. (1992). Physiological and psychological variables related to functional status in COPD. *Nursing Research 43,* 286-291.
150. Burdon, J.G.W., Juniper, E.F., Killian, K.J., Hargreave, F.E., & Campbell, E.J.M. (1982). The perception of breathlessness in asthma. *American Review of Respiratory Disease 126,* 825-828.
151. Bestall, J.C., Paul, E.A., Garrod, R., Garnham, R., Jones, P.W., & Wedzicha, J.A. (1999). Usefulness of the Medical Research Council (MRC) dyspnea scale as a measure of viability in patients with chronic obstructive pulmonary disease. *Thorax 54,* 581-586.
152. Lareau, S.C., Meek, P.M., Press, D., Anholm, J.D., & Roos, P.J. (1999). Dyspnea in patients with chronic obstructive pulmonary disease: Does dyspnea worsen longitudinally in the presence of declining lung function? *Heart & Lung 28,* 65-73.
153. Roberts, C.M., Bell, J., & Wedzicha, J.A. (1996). Comparison of the efficacy of a demand oxygen delivery system with continuous low flow oxygen in subjects with stable COPD and severe oxygen desaturation on walking. *Thorax 51,* 831-834.
154. O'Donnell, D.E., Bertley, J.C., Chau, L.K., & Webb, K.A. (1997). Qualitative aspects of exertional breathlessness in chronic airflow limitation: Pathophysiologic mechanisms. *American Journal of Respiratory and Critical Care Medicine 155,* 109-115.
155. O'Donnell, D.E., Chau, L., & Webb, K.A. (1998). Qualitative aspects of exertional dyspnea in patients with interstitial lung disease. *Journal of Applied Physiology 84,* 2000-2009.
156. Epler, G.R., Sabec, F.A., & Goensler, E.A. (1980). Determination of severe impairment (disability) in interstitial lung disease. *American Review of Respiratory Disease 121,* 647-659.

157. Gift, A.G., & Cahill, C.A. (1990). Psychophysiologic aspects of dyspnea in chronic obstructive pulmonary disease: A pilot study. *Heart & Lung 19,* 252-257.
158. Mahler, D.A., & Wells, C.K. (1988). Evaluation of clinical methods for rating dyspnea. *Chest 93,* 580-586.
159. Breslin, E.H., Garoutte, B.C., Kohlman, C.V., & Celli, B.R. (1990). Correlations between dyspnea, diaphragm and sternomastoid recruitment during inspiratory resistance breathing in normal subjects. *Chest 98,* 298-302.
160. Celli, B., Criner, G., & Rassulo, J. (1988). Ventilatory muscle recruitment during unsupported arm exercise in normal subjects. *Journal of Applied Physiology 64,* 1936-1941.
161. Delgado, H.R., Braun, S., Skatrud, J.B., Reddan, W.G., & Pegelow, D.F. (1982). Chest wall and abdominal motion during exercise in patients with chronic obstructive pulmonary disease. *American Review of Respiratory Disease 126,* 200-205.
162. Killian, K., Summers, E., Basalygo, M., Campbell, E. (1985). Effect on frequency of perceived magnitude of added resistive loads to breathing. *Journal of Applied Physiology 64,* 1936-1941.
163. Knebel, A.R., Janson-Bjerklie, S.L., Malley, J.D., Wilson, A.G., & Marini, J.J. (1994). Comparison of breathing comfort during weaning with two ventilatory modes. *American Journal of Respiratory and Critical Care Medicine 149,* 14-18.
164. Leblanc, P., Bowie, D.M., Summers, E., Jones, N.L., & Killian, K.J. (1986). Breathlessness and exercise in patients with cardiorespiratory disease. *American Review of Respiratory Disease 133,* 21-25.
165. Belman, M.J., Botnick, W.C., Shin, J.W. (1996). Inhaled bronchdilators reduce dynamic hyperinflation during exercise in patients with chronic obstructive pulmonary disease. *American Journal of Respiratory and Critical Care Medicine 153,* 967-975.
166. O'Donnell, D.E. (1994). Breathlessness in patients with chronic airflow limitation. Mechanisms and management. *Chest 106,* 904-912.
167. O'Donnell, D.E., & Webb, K.A. (1993). Exertional breathlessness in patients with chronic airflow limitation. The role of lung hyperinflation. *American Review of Respiratory Disease 148,* 1351-1357.
168. Lougheed, M.D., Lam, M., Forkert, L., Webb, K.A., & O'Donnell, D.E. (1993). Breathlessness during acute bronchoconstriction in asthma. Pathophysiologic mechanisms. *American Review of Respiratory Disease 148,* 1452-1459.
169. O'Donnell, D.E., Revill, S.M., & Webb, K.A. (2001). Dynamic hyperinflation and exercise intolerance in chronic obstructive pulmonary disease. *American Journal of Respiratory and Critical Care Medicine 164,* 770-777.
170. O'Donnell, D.E., Sanii, R., Giesbrecht, G., et al. (1988). Effect of continuous positive airway pressure on respiratory sensation in patients with chronic obstructive pulmonary disease during submaximal exercise. *American Review of Respiratory Disease 138,* 1185-1191.
171. Janson-Bjerklie, S., & Schnell, S. (1988). Effect of peak flow information on patterns of self-care in adult asthma. *Heart & Lung 17,* 543-549.
172. Verbrugge, L.M. (1980). Health diaries. *Medical Care 18,* 73-95.
173. Burman, M.E. (1995). Health diaries in nursing research and practice. *Image: Journal of Nursing Scholarship 27,* 147-152.
174. American Thoracic Society. (1999). Pulmonary rehabilitation—1999. *American Journal of Respiratory and Critical Care Medicine 159,* 1666-1682.
175. Carrieri-Kohlman, V., & Gormley, J. (1998). Coping strategies for dyspnea. In D. Mahler (ed.), *Dyspnea* (pp. 287-313). New York: Marcel Dekker.
176. Stulbarg, M., Belman, M., & Ries, A. (1998). Treatment of dyspnea: Physical modalities, oxygen and pharmacology. In D. Mahler (ed.), *Dyspnea* (pp. 321-362). New York: Marcel Dekker.
177. Trayner, E.M., & Celli, B.R. (1998). Strategies in the treatment of dyspnea: Disease specific. In D. Mahler (ed.), *Dyspnea* (pp. 261-285). New York: Marcel Dekker.
178. Kwiatkowski, M., Carrieri-Kohlman, V., Janson, S., Gormley, J.M., & Stulbarg, M.S. (1995). Patients with chronic obstructive pulmonary disease (COPD). In *International Conference on Pulmonary Rehabilitation and Home Ventilation.* Denver: National Jewish: Center for Immunology and Respiratory Medicine.
179. Janson-Bjerklie, S., Ferketich, S., Benner, P., & Becker, G. (1992). Clinical markers of asthma severity and risk: Importance of subjective as well as objective factors. *Heart & Lung 21,* 265-272.
180. Carrieri, V.J., & Janson-Bjerklie, S. (1986). Strategies patients use to manage the sensation of dyspnea. *Western Journal of Nursing Research 8,* 284-305.
181. Carrieri, V.K., Kieckhefer, G., Janson-Bjerklie, S., & Souza, J. (1991). The sensation of pulmonary dyspnea in school-age children. *Nursing Research 40,* 81-85.
182. Nield, M. (2000). Dyspnea self-management in African Americans. *Heart & Lung 29,* 50-55.
183. AACVPR. (1998). *Guidelines for Pulmonary Rehabilitation Programs* (2nd ed.), Champaign, Ill.: Human Kinetics.
184. Hodgkin, J.E., Celli, B.R., & Connors, G.L. (2000). *Pulmonary rehabilitation.* New York: Lippincott Williams & Wilkins.
185. Casaburi, R., & Petty, T.L. (eds.). (1993). *Principles and practice of pulmonary rehabilitation.* Philadelphia: W.B. Saunders.
186. Hernández, M.T., Rubio, T.M., Ruiz, F.O., Riera, H.S., Gil, R.S., & Gómez, J.C. (2000). Results of a home-based training program for patients with COPD. *Chest 118,* 106-114.
187. Puente-Maestu, L., Sanz, M.L., Sanz, P., Cubillo, J.M., Mayol, J., & Casaburi, R. (2000). Comparison of effects of supervised versus self-monitored training programmes in patients with chronic obstructive pulmonary disease. *European Respiratory Journal 15,* 517-525.
188. Larson, J.L., Covey, M.K., Wirtz, S.E., Berry, J.K., Alex, C.G., Langbein, W.E., et al. (1999). Cycle ergometer and inspiratory muscle training in chronic obstructive pulmonary disease. *American Journal of Respiratory and Critical Care Medicine 160,* 500-507.
189. O'Donnell, D.E., McGuire, M., Samis, L., & Webb, K.A. (1995). The impact of exercise reconditioning on breathlessness in severe chronic airflow limitation. *American Journal of Respiratory Critical Care Medicine* 2005-2013.
190. Goldstein, R.S., Gort, E.H., Stubbing, D., Avendano, M.A., & Guyatt, G.H. (1994). Randomised controlled trial of respiratory rehabilitation. *Lancet 344,* 1394-1397.
191. Ries, A.L., Kaplan, R.M., Limberg, T.M., & Prewitt, L.M. (1995). Effects of pulmonary rehabilitation on physiologic and psychosocial outcomes in patients with

chronic obstructive pulmonary disease. *Annals of Internal Medicine 122,* 823-832.

192. Lacasse, Y., Brosseau, L., Milne, S., Martin, S., Wong, E., Guyatt, G.H., Goldstein, R.S., Goldstein. Pulmonary rehabilitation for chronic obstructive pulmonary disease (Cochrane Review). In: *The Cochrane Library,* Issue 3, 2002. Oxford: Update Software.
193. Lake, F.R., Henderson, K., Briffa, T., Openshaw, J., & Musk, A.W. (1990). Upper-limb and lower-limb exercise training in patients with chronic airflow obstruction. *Chest 97,* 1077-1082.
194. Simpson, K., Killian, K., McCartney, N., Stubbing, D.G., & Jones, N.L. (1992). Randomised controlled trial of weightlifting exercise in patients with chronic airflow limitation. *Thorax 47,* 70-75.
195. Lacasse, Y., Wong, E., Guyatt, G.H., King, D., Cook, D.J., & Goldstein, R.S. (1996). Meta-analysis of respiratory rehabilitation in chronic obstructive pulmonary disease [see comments]. *Lancet 348,* 1115-1119.
196. Casaburi, R., Patessio, A., Ioli, F., Zanaboni, S., Donner, C.F., Wasserman, K. (1991). Reductions in exercise lactic acidosis and ventilation as a result of exercise training in patients with obstructive lung disease. *American Review of Respiratory Disease 143,* 9-18.
197. Punzal, P.A., Ries, A.L., Kaplan, R.M., & Prewitt, L.M. (1991). Maximum intensity exercise training in patients with chronic obstructive pulmonary disease. *Chest 100,* 618-623.
198. Niederman, M.S., Clemente, P.H., Fein, A.M., Feinsilver, S.H., Robinson, D.A., Ilowite, J.S., et al. (1991). Benefits of a multidisciplinary pulmonary rehabilitation program. Improvements are independent of lung function. *Chest 99,* 798-804.
199. Haas, F., Salazar-Schicchi, J., & Axen, K. (1993). Desensitization to dyspnea in chronic obstructive pulmonary disease. In R. Casaburi, T. Petty (eds.), *Principles and practice of pulmonary rehabilitation* (pp. 241-251). Philadelphia: W.B. Saunders.
200. Ramirez-Venegas, A., Ward, J.L., Olmstead, E.M., Tosteson, A.N., & Mahler, D.A. (1997). Effect of exercise training on dyspnea measures in patients with chronic obstructive pulmonary disease. *Journal of Cardiopulmonary Rehabilitation 17,* 103-109.
201. Belman, M. (1986). Exercise in chronic obstructive pulmonary disease. *Clinics in Chest Medicine 7,* 585-597.
202. Rosser, R., Denford, J., Heslop, A., Kinston, W., Macklin, D., Minty, K., et al. (1983). Breathlessness and psychiatric morbidity in chronic bronchitis and emphysema: A study of psychotherapeutic management. *Psychological Medicine 13,* 93-110.
203. Bredin, M., Corner, J., Krishnasamy, M., Plant, H., Bailey, C., & A'Hern, R. (1999). Multicentre randomised controlled trial of nursing intervention for breathlessness in patients with lung cancer. *British Medical Journal 318,* 901-904.
204. Gift, A.G. (1990). Dyspnea. *Nursing Clinics of North America 25,* 955-965.
205. Woodcock, A.A., Gross, E.R., & Geddes, D.M. (1981). Oxygen relieves breathlessness in "pink puffers." *Lancet 1,* 907-909.
206. Davidson, A.C., Leach, R., George, R.J.D., & Geddes, D.M. (1988). Supplemental oxygen and exercise ability in chronic obstructive lung disease. *Thorax 43,* 965-971.
207. Dean, N.C., Brown, J.K., Himelman, R.B., Doherty, J.J., Gold, W.M., & Stulbarg, M.S. (1992). Oxygen may improve dyspnea and endurance in patients with chronic obstructive pulmonary disease and only mild hypoxemia. *American Review of Respiratory Disease 146,* 941-945.
208. Tiep, B.L. (1990). Long-term home oxygen therapy. *Clinics in Chest Medicine 11,* 505-521.
209. Santiago, T.V., Johnson, J., Riley, D.J., & Edelman, N.H. (1979). Effects of morphine on ventilatory response to exercise. *Journal of Applied Physiology 47,* 112-118.
210. Sackner, M.A. (1984). Effects of hydrocodone bitartrate on breathing pattern of patients with chronic obstructive pulmonary disease and restrictive lung disease. *Mt. Sinai Medical Journal 51,* 222-226.
211. Kryger, M.H., Yacoub, O., Dosman, J., Macklem, P.T., & Anthonisen, N.R. (1976). Effect of meperidine on occlusion pressure response to hypercapnia and hypoxia with and without external inspiratory resistance. *American Review of Respiratory Disease 114,* 333-340.
212. Wilson, R.H., Hoseth, W., & Dempsey, M.E. (1954). Respiratory acidosis: Effects of decreasing respiratory minute volume in patients with severe chronic pulmonary emphysema, with specific reference to oxygen, morphine and barbiturates. *American Journal of Medicine 17,* 464-470.
213. Robin, E.D., & Burke, C.M. (1986). Single-patient randomized clinical trial. Opiates for intractable dyspnea. *Chest 90,* 888-892.
214. Mazzocato, C., Buclin, T., & Rapin, C.H. (1999). The effects of morphine on dyspnea and ventilatory function in elderly patients with advanced cancer: A randomized double-blind controlled trial. *Annals of Oncology 10,* 1511-1514.
215. Allard, P., Lamontagne, C., Bernard, P., & Trembblay, C. (1999). How effective are supplementary doses of opioids for dyspnea in terminally ill cancer patients? A randomized continuous sequential clinical trial. *Journal of Pain and Symptom Management 17,* 256-265.
216. Young, I.H., Daviskas, E., & Keena, V.A. (1989). Effect of low dose nebulized morphine on exercise endurance in patients with chronic lung disease. *Thorax 44,* 387-390.
217. Farncombe, M., Chater, S., & Gillin, A. (1994). The use of nebulized opioids for breathlessness: A chart review. *Palliative Medicine 8,* 306-312.
218. Noseda, A., Carpiaux, J.P., Markstein, C., Meyvaert, A., & de Maertelaer, V. (1997). Disabling dyspnea in patients with advanced disease: Lack of effect of nebulized morphine. *European Respiratory Journal 10,* 1079-1083.
219. Masood, A.R., Subhan, M.M., Reed, J.W., & Thomas, S.H. (1995). Effects of inhaled nebulized morphine on ventilation and breathlessness during exercise in healthy man. *Clinical Science 88,* 447-452.
220. Leung, R., Hill, P., & Burdon, J. (1996). Effect of inhaled morphine on the development of breathlessness during exercise in patients with chronic lung disease. *Thorax 51,* 596-600.
221. Chandler, S. (1999). Nebulized opioids to treat dyspnea [see comments]. *American Journal of Hospice and Palliative Care 16,* 418-422.
222. Woodcock, A.A., Gross, E.R., & Geddes, D.M. (1981). Drug treatment of breathlessness: Contrasting effects of diazepam and promethazine in pink puffers. *British Medical Journal 283,* 343-346.
223. Man, G.C.W., Hsu, K., & Sproule, B.J. (1986). Effect of alprazolam on exercise and dyspnea in patients with chronic obstructive pulmonary disease. *Chest 90,* 832-836.

224. Eimer, M., Cable T., Gal, P., Rothenberger, L.A., & McCue, J.D. (1985). Effects of clorazepate on breathlessness and exercise tolerance in patients with chronic airflow obstruction. *Journal of Family Practice 21,* 359-362.
225. Greene, J.G., Pucino, F., Carlson, J.D., Storsved, M., & Strommen, G.L. (1989). Effects of alprazolam on respiratory drive, anxiety, and dyspnea in chronic airflow obstruction: A case study. *Pharmacotherapy 9,* 34-38.
226. Mitchell-Heggs, P., Murphy, K., Minty, K., Guz, A., Patterson, S.C., Minty, P.S.B., et al. (1980). Diazepam in the treatment of dyspnea in the "pink puffer" syndrome. *Quarterly Journal of Medicine 49,* 9-20.
227. Borson, S., McDonald, G.J., Gayle, T., Deffebach, M., Lakshminarayan, S., & VanTuinen, C. (1992). Improvement in mood, physical symptoms, and function with nortriptyline for depression in patients with chronic obstructive pulmonary disease. *Psychosomatics 33,* 190-201.
228. Liss, H.P., & Grant, B.J. (1988). The effect of nasal flow on breathlessness in patients with chronic obstructive pulmonary disease. *American Review of Respiratory Disease 137,* 1285-1288.
229. Nakayama, H., Shibuya, M., Yamada, M., Suzuki, H., Arakawa, M., & Homma, I. (1998). In-phase chest wall vibration decreases dyspnea during arm elevation in chronic obstructive pulmonary disease patients [see comments]. *Internal Medicine 37,* 831-835.
230. Cristiano, L.M., & Schwartzstein, R.M. (1997). Effect of chest wall vibration on dyspnea during hypercapnia and exercise in chronic obstructive pulmonary disease. *American Journal of Respiratory and Critical Care Medicine 155,* 1552-1559.
231. Schwartzstein, R.M., Lahive, K., Pope, A., Weinberger, S.E., & Weiss, J.W. (1987). Cold facial stimulation reduces breathlessness induced in normal subjects. *American Review of Respiratory Disease 136,* 58-61.
232. Melani, A.S. (1997). Pharmacological treatment of exertional dyspnea in stable COPD patients. *Monaldi Archives for Chest Disease 52,* 354-362.
233. Petrof, B.J., Legare, M., Goldberg, P., Milic, E.J., & Gottfried, S.B. (1990). Continuous positive airway pressure reduces work of breathing and dyspnea during weaning from mechanical ventilation in severe chronic obstructive pulmonary disease. *American Review of Respiratory Disease 141,* 281-289.
234. Petrof, B.J., Calderini, E., & Gottfried, S.B. (1990). Effect of CPAP on respiratory effort and dyspnea during exercise in severe COPD. *Journal of Applied Physiology 69,* 179-188.
235. Maltais, F., Reissmann, H., & Gottfried, S.B. (1995). Pressure support reduces inspiratory effort and dyspnea during exercise in chronic airflow obstruction. *American Journal of Respiratory and Critical Care Medicine 151,* 1027-1033.
236. Renston, J.P., DiMarco, A.F., & Supinski, G.S. (1994). Respiratory muscle rest using nasal BiPAP ventilation in patients with stable severe COPD. *Chest 105,* 1053-1060.
237. Keller, C.A., Ruppel, G., Hibbett, A., Osterloh, J., & Naunheim, K.S. (1997). Thoracoscopic lung volume reduction surgery reduces dyspnea and improves exercise capacity in patients with emphysema. *American Journal of Respiratory and Critical Care Medicine 156,* 60-67.
238. Brenner, M., McKenna, R.J., Gelb, A.F., Fischel, R.J., Yoong, B., Huh, J., et al. (1997). Dyspnea response following bilateral thoracoscopic staple lung volume reduction surgery. *Chest 112,* 916-923.
239. O'Donnell, D.E., Webb, K.A., Bertley, J.C., Chau, L.K., & Conlan, A.A. (1996). Mechanisms of relief of exertional breathlessness following unilateral bullectomy and lung volume reduction surgery in emphysema. *Chest 110,* 18-27.
240. Martinez, F.J., de Oca, M.M., Whyte, R.I., Stetz, J., Gay, S.E., & Celli, B.R. (1997). Lung-volume reduction improves dyspnea, dynamic hyperinflation, and respiratory muscle function. *American Journal of Respiratory and Critical Care Medicine 155,* 1984-1990.
241. Arora, N.S., & Rochester, D.F. (1982). Respiratory muscle strength and maximal voluntary ventilation in undernourished patients. *American Review of Respiratory Disease 126,* 5-8.
242. Arora, N.S., & Rochester, D.F. (1982). Effect of body weight and muscularity on human diaphragm muscle mass, thickness and area. *Journal of Applied Physiology 52,* 64-70.
243. Efthimiou, J., Fleming, J., Gomes, C., Spiro, S.G. (1988). The effect of supplementary oral nutrition in poorly nourished patients with chronic obstructive pulmonary disease. *American Review of Respiratory Disease 137,* 1075-1082.
244. Goldstein, S.A., Thomashow, B., Askanazi, J. (1986). Functional changes during nutritional repletion in patients with lung disease. *Clinics in Chest Medicine 7,* 141-151.
245. Smith, K., Cook, D., Guyatt, G.H., Madhavan, J., Oxman, A.D. (1992). Respiratory muscle training in chronic airflow limitation: A meta-analysis. *American Review of Respiratory Disease 145,* 533-539.
246. Lisboa, C., Villafranca, C., Leiva, A., Cruz, E., Pertuzé, J., & Borzone, G. (1997). Inspiratory muscle training in chronic airflow limitation: Effect on exercise performance. *European Respiratory Journal 10,* 537-542.
247. Lisboa, C., Munoz, V., Beroiza, T., Leiva, A., & Cruz, E. (1994). Inspiratory muscle training in chronic airflow limitation: Comparison of two different training loads with a threshold device. *European Respiratory Journal 7,* 1266-1274.
248. Tiep, B.L., Burns, M., Kao, D., Madison, R., & Herrera, J. (1986). Pursed lips breathing training using ear oximetry. *Chest 90,* 218-221.
249. Breslin, E.H. (1992). The pattern of respiratory muscle recruitment during pursed-lip breathing. *Chest 101,* 75-78.
250. Miller, W.F. (1958). Physical therapeutic measures in the treatment of chronic bronchopulmonary disorders: Methods for breathing training. *American Journal of Medicine 24,* 929-940.
251. Campbell, E., & Friend, J. (1955). Action of breathing exercises in pulmonary emphysema. *Lancet 1,* 325-329.
252. Sharp, J.T., Drutz, W.S., Moisan, T., Foster, J., Machnach, W. (1980). Postural relief of dyspnea in severe chronic obstructive pulmonary disease. *American Review of Respiratory Disease 122,* 201-213.
253. Faling, L.J. (1986). Pulmonary rehabilitation—physical modalities. *Clinics in Chest Medicine 7,* 599-618.
254. Nava, S., Ambrosino, N., Zocchi, L., & Rampulla, C. (1990). Diaphragmatic rest during negative pressure ventilation by pneumowrap. Assessment in normal and COPD patients. *Chest 98,* 857-865.

255. Belman, M.J., Soo, H.G., Kuei, J.H., Shadmehr, R. (1990). Efficacy of positive vs negative pressure ventilation in unloading the respiratory muscles. *Chest 98,* 850-856.
256. Levine, S., Henson, D., & Levy, S. (1988). Respiratory muscle rest therapy. *Clinics in Chest Medicine 9,* 297-309.
257. Celli, B., Lee, H., Criner, G., Bermudez, M., Rassulo, J., Gilmartin, M., et al. (1989). Controlled trial of external negative pressure ventilation in patients with severe chronic airflow obstruction. *American Review of Respiratory Disease 140,* 1251-1256.
258. Strumpf, D.A., Millman, R.P., Carlisle, C.C., Grattan, L.M., Ryan, S.M., Erickson, A.D., et al. (1991). Nocturnal positive-pressure ventilation via nasal mask in patients with severe chronic obstructive pulmonary disease. *American Review of Respiratory Disease 144,* 1234-1239.
259. Murciano, D., Auclair, M.-H., Pariente, R., & Aubier, M. (1989). A randomized, controlled trial of theophylline in patients with severe chronic obstructive pulmonary disease. *New England Journal of Medicine 320,* 1521-1525.
260. Mahler, D.A., Matthay, R.A., Snyder, P.E., Wells, C.K., & Loke, J. (1985). Sustained-release theophylline reduces dyspnea in nonreversible obstructive airway disease. *American Review of Respiratory Disease 131,* 22-25.
261. Carrieri-Kohlman, V., & Janson-Bjerklie, S. (1990). Coping and self-care strategies. In D.A. Mahler (ed.), *Dyspnea* (pp. 201-230). Mount Kisco, N.Y.: Futura.
262. Canadian Lung Association Coping Strategies for SOB. Retrieved October 15, 2002 from http:/www.lung.ca/copd/management/coping/breathing.html.
263. Scherer, Y.K., Schmieder, L.E. (1997). The effect of a pulmonary rehabilitation program on self-efficacy, perception of dyspnea, and physical endurance. *Heart & Lung 26,* 15-22.
264. Thompson, S.C. (1981). Will it hurt less if I can control it? A complex answer to a simple question. *Psychological Bulletin 90,* 89-101.
265. Devine, E.C., & Pearcy, J. (1996). Meta-analysis of the effects of psychoeducational care in adults with chronic obstructive pulmonary disease. *Patient Education and Counseling 29,* 167-178.
266. Ashikaga, T., Vacek, P.M., Lewis, S.O. (1980). Evaluation of a community-based education program for individuals with chronic obstructive pulmonary disease. *Journal of Rehabilitation 46,* 23-27.
267. Levine, S., Weiser, P., & Gillen, J. (1986). Evaluation of a ventilatory muscle endurance training program in the rehabilitation of patients with chronic obstructive pulmonary disease. *American Review of Respiratory Disease 133,* 400-406.
268. DeVito, A.J. (1990). Dyspnea during hospitalizations for acute phase of illness as recalled by patients with chronic obstructive pulmonary disease. *Heart & Lung 19,* 186-191.
269. Gift, A.G., Moore, T., & Soeken, K. (1992). Relaxation to reduce dyspnea and anxiety in COPD patients. *Nursing Research 41,* 242-246.
270. Renfroe, K.L. (1988). Effect of progressive relaxation on dyspnea and state anxiety in patients with chronic obstructive pulmonary disease. *Heart & Lung 17,* 408-413.
271. Horsman, J. (1978). Using tape recordings to overcome panic during dyspnea. *Respiratory Care 23,* 767-768.
272. Thornby, M.A., Haas, F., & Axen, K. (1995). Effect of distractive auditory stimuli on exercise tolerance in patients with COPD. *Chest 107,* 1213-1217.
273. McBride, S., Graydon, J., Sidani, S., & Hall, L. (1999). The therapeutic use of music for dyspnea and anxiety in patients with COPD who live at home. *Journal of Holistic Nursing 17,* 229-250.
274. Aronoff, G.M., Aronoff, S., & Peck, L.W. (1975). Hypnotherapy in the treatment of bronchial asthma. *Annals of Allergy 34,* 356-362.
275. Moody, L.E., Fraser, M., & Yarandi, H. (1993). Effects of guided imagery in patients with chronic bronchitis and emphysema. *Clinical Nursing Research 2,* 478-486.
276. Filshie, J., Penn, K., Ashley, S., Davis, C.L. (1996). Acupuncture for the relief of cancer-related breathlessness. *Palliative Medicine 10,* 145-150.
277. Behera, D. (1998). Yoga therapy in chronic bronchitis. *Journal of the Association of Physicians of India 46,* 207-208.
278. Tandon, M.K. (1978). Adjunct treatment with yoga in chronic severe airways obstruction. *Thorax 33,* 514-517.
279. Cherniack, N.S. (1988). Dyspnea. In J.A. Murray & J.F. Nadel (eds.), *Textbook of respiratory medicine* (p. 393). Philadelphia: W.B. Saunders.
280. Manning, H.L., & Schwartzstein, R.M. (1995). Pathophysiology of dyspnea. *New England Journal of Medicine 333,* 1547-1553.
281. Adams, L., & Guz, A. (1991). Dyspnea on exertion. In B.J. Whipp & K. Wasserman (eds.), *Exercise: Pulmonary physiology and pathophysiology* (pp. 449-494). New York: Marcel Dekker.
282. Adams, L., & Guz, A. (1996). *Respiratory sensation.* New York: Marcel Dekker.
283. McCarley, C. (1999). A model of chronic dyspnea. *Image: Journal of Nursing Scholarship 31,* 231-236.
284. Carrieri, V., Janson-Bjerklie, S., & Jacobs, S. (1984). The sensation of dyspnea: A review. *Heart & Lung 13.*
285. Sassi-Dambron, D.E., Eakin, E.G., Ries, A.L., & Kaplan, R.M. (1995). Treatment of dyspnea in COPD. A controlled clinical trial of dyspnea management strategies [see comments]. *Chest 107,* 724-729.
286. Harver, A., & Mahler, D. (1998). Dyspnea: Sensation, symptom and illness. In D. Mahler (ed.), *Dyspnea* (pp. 1-34). New York: Marcel Dekker.
287. Steele, B., & Shaver, J. (1992). The dyspnea experience: Nociceptive properties and a model for research and practice. *Advances in Nursing Science 15,* 64-76.
288. Lenz, E.R., Pugh, L.C., Milligan, R.A., Gift, A., & Suppe, F. (1997). The middle-range theory of unpleasant symptoms: An update. *Advances in Nursing Science 19,* 14-27.
289. Carrieri-Kohlman, V., Janson, S. (1999). Managing dyspnea. In A.S. Hinshaw, S.L. Feetham, & J.L.F. Shaver (eds.), *Handbook of clinical nursing research* (pp. 379-393). Thousand Oaks, Calif.: Sage.
290. Meek, P.M. (2000). Influence of attention and judgment on perception of breathlessness in healthy individuals and patients with chronic obstructive pulmonary disease. *Nursing Research 49,* 11-19.
291. Meek, P.M., Lareau, S.C., & Anderson, D. (2001). Memory for symptoms in COPD patients: How accurate are their reports? *European Respiratory Journal 18,* 474-481.
292. Stulbarg, M., Carrieri-Kohlman, V., Gormley, J., Tsang, A., & Paul, S. (1999). Accuracy of recall of dyspnea after exercise training sessions. *Journal of Cardiopulmonary Rehabilitation 19,* 242-248.
293. Graydon, J.E., & Ross, E. (1995). Influence of symptoms, lung function, mood, and social support on level of functioning of patients with COPD. *Research in Nursing and Health 18,* 525-533.

294. Graydon, J.E., Ross, E., Webster, P.M., Goldstein, R.S., & Avendano, M. (1995). Predictors of functioning of patients with chronic obstructive pulmonary disease. *Heart & Lung 24,* 369-375.
295. Anderson, N., & Lobel, M. (1993). Negative affect and the report of symptoms and diseases. *Annals of Behavioral Medicine 15,* S85.
296. Weaver, T.E., Richmond, T.S., & Narsavage, G.L. (1997). An explanatory model of functional status in chronic obstructive pulmonary disease. *Nursing Research 46,* 26.
297. Corner, J., Plant, H., A'Hern, R., & Bailey, C. (1996). Non-pharmacological intervention for breathlessness in lung cancer. *Palliative Medicine 10,* 299-305.

CHAPTER 11

Fatigue

BARBARA F. PIPER

DEFINITION

Fatigue has been defined from several disciplinary perspectives, so many definitions exist. When fatigue is viewed as a subjective perception or sensation, it is defined as simply whatever the person says it is,[1,2] best measured by self-report. In this context, patients can self-rate their fatigue as mild, moderate, or severe or select a number between 0 and 10 on a numeric rating scale to indicate its intensity. Fatigue has been defined as a "feeling of lack of energy and tiredness not related to muscle weakness,"[3] and by its perceived and observed effects on performance of daily activities or physical performance.[4-6] Cancer-related fatigue is defined by a guidelines panel as a persistent subjective sense of unusual tiredness related to cancer or cancer treatment that interferes with usual functioning.[7] A multiple sclerosis (MS) panel defined fatigue in a similar fashion, stating that fatigue is a subjective lack of physical and/or mental energy perceived by individuals or caregivers that interferes with usual and desired activities.[8,9] The North American Nursing Diagnosis Association (NANDA)[10] defined fatigue as "an overwhelming sustained sense of exhaustion and decreased capacity for physical and mental work."

Fatigue has been defined by its underlying biological nature, such as diaphragmatic, motor, and neuromuscular fatigue. Diaphragmatic fatigue occurs in both acute and chronic respiratory conditions when the force and duration of muscle work exceeds muscle energy stores.[11] Diaphragmatic fatigue[12] and other forms of neuromuscular fatigue[13] have been described further by muscle response over time to electrical stimulation, such as high-frequency versus low-frequency fatigue. Schwid et al noted: "Motor fatigue [is] defined as the loss of the maximal capacity to generate force during exercise, [and is thought by some to be] the aspect most amenable to physiologic analysis."[14]

Fatigue has been defined by its origin or cause (i.e., central, peripheral, attentional,[15] pathological, physiological, or psychological), by its unknown cause, and by the exclusion of all other possible diseases (i.e., chronic fatigue syndrome or idiopathic chronic fatigue).[16,17] For example, chronic fatigue syndrome (CFS) is defined as medically unexplained persisting or relapsing fatigue lasting 6 or more consecutive months with four or more of the following symptoms present: subjective memory impairment, sore throat, tender lymph nodes, muscle pain, joint pain, headache, unrefreshing sleep, or postexertional malaise lasting more than 24 hours.[17]

Clinically, fatigue can be defined and described by its characteristic temporal patterns over time,[18] such as intermittent, curvilinear,[19] or roller coaster–like,[20] and by its duration, such as acute (less than 4 weeks[21] or 2[22] to 6 weeks[8]) or chronic (present on 50% of days for more than 6 weeks,[8] or lasting 1 to 6 months or longer).[13,17,23] Describing fatigue by temporal patterns may allow better identification and differentiation between fatigue patterns and their possible underlying mechanisms. Although not well-studied, it has been suggested that both acute and chronic forms of fatigue can coexist in some patients, similar to acute and chronic forms of pain.[23]

Despite the numerous fatigue definitions and descriptions that exist, no one definition or set of diagnostic criteria has been adopted.[24] Recently it has been proposed that fatigue should no longer be referred to as a symptom, but rather it should be called a syndrome that includes a complex of signs and symptoms that indicates an abnormal condition[25,26] or a disease state.[27] It may be premature to adopt a universal definition or set of diagnostic criteria until more testing of these definitions and criteria can be undertaken and a better understanding of underlying mechanisms is appreciated.

In the interim, there is an emerging consensus among health care professionals that fatigue in many clinical states is a subjective, multidimensional sensation similar to pain, best measured by the patient's self-report. Fatigue in these instances is viewed as a debilitating, unusual sense of tiredness that differs significantly from the transient, more easily relieved sense of tiredness that more commonly is experienced by healthy individuals.[2,9,18,28,29] Several dimensions have been identified,[2,9,18,27,30-32] suggesting that different underlying mechanisms may be operant.[16] As a consequence, management of fatigue and of chronic fatigue, in particular, will most likely require multimodal therapies used concurrently rather than monotherapies to alleviate its occurrence.[33]

PREVALENCE AND POPULATIONS AT RISK

Fatigue frequently precedes or accompanies most major illnesses and treatments.[21] It is a prevalent problem in cancer and cardiac patients.

Cancer

Fatigue is the most frequent and distressing symptom experienced by cancer patients receiving active treatment.[7,34-36] Patients consistently report that fatigue is more distressing than other symptoms, such as pain or nausea.[37,38] It is a nearly universal phenomenon, with prevalence rates ranging from 78% to 96%, depending on the form of treatment[39-41] and stage of disease.[42-45] Cancer survivors, those individuals in disease remission who no longer are receiving treatment, often continue to report unusual fatigue months or even years after treatment cessation.[46-48] Such fatigue is thought to be a possible late effect of cancer or its treatment. The incidence and prevalence rates for survivor fatigue range between 17%, when strict ICD-10 diagnostic criteria are applied[49] to 24% and 33%,[47] when other criteria, such as a score of 4 or more on a specific fatigue scale and a duration of 6 or more months are present,[50] to as high as 80% when less stringent criteria are applied. What constitutes valid prevalence rates in these survivors requires more study. Not well studied are the incidence rates of fatigue that may precede a cancer diagnosis and its treatment, or fatigue that occurs during palliative care or in terminally ill patients.[51] Advanced-cancer patients or patients who have specific forms of cancer, such as non–small cell lung cancer, are more likely to experience more severe fatigue than patients with less extensive disease or other types of cancers.[52]

Cardiac Fatigue

Fatigue is common in myocardial infarction (MI) patients.[53] In one prospective study, fatigue was the strongest predictor for a subsequent MI.[54] In another study, unusual fatigue was the most common prodromal symptom preceding an MI and was the fourth most common symptom during the acute MI period.[55] Two months after an MI, prevalence rates of mild to severe fatigue were reported to range from 45%[56] and 79%[57] to 84%.[58] When patients were followed 1 year after an MI, 69% of the original 45% who were fatigued at 2 months after an MI were still experiencing mild to severe fatigue.[56] In another study, fatigue was the most common symptom 2 months (79%) and 1 year (70%) after an MI.[57] In another study, 85.1% of chronic angina patients (who were predominantly African American) reported fatigue. Of these, 59.3% had a history of a prior MI.[59] Table 11-1 summarizes the prevalence rates reported.

TABLE 11-1 Prevalence and Populations at Risk

POPULATIONS AT RISK	DESCRIPTION AND PREVALENCE RATES
Primary care	In primary care settings, 11% to 25% of patients present with chronic fatigue as their chief complaint.[13,240,241] Of these, 20% to 45% will have a primary organic cause diagnosed for their fatigue, and 40% to 45% will have a primary psychiatric disorder diagnosed. The remaining patients will "either meet the Centers for Disease Control and Prevention (CDCP) criteria for CFS or [will] remain undiagnosed."[13]
Cancer	See description in text.
Cardiac	See description in text.
Caregivers of chronically ill persons	Family caregivers of cancer patients[242] and other chronically ill patients[8,18,71] are thought to be at risk for both acute and chronic forms of fatigue. In one cancer study, the only significant relationship documented with fatigue was the perception of caregiver burden.The more the caregiver perceived care of their family member to be a burden, the more fatigue was experienced by the caregiver.[242] In another study, tiredness was second only to back pain in frequency (72% versus 73%).[71]

TABLE 11-1 Prevalence and Populations at Risk—cont'd

POPULATIONS AT RISK	DESCRIPTION AND PREVALENCE RATES
Chronic fatigue syndrome (CFS)	The prevalence rates for patients that meet the strict CDCP criteria for CFS are extremely low, ranging from 0.5% to 10%.[16]
Chronic hepatitis C virus infection (HCV)	Fatigue is the most frequently reported symptom in HCV.[80] For women who are positive for the HCV antibody without serious liver disease, prevalence rates range from 75% to 97%. Higher rates are reported in women who are polymerase chain reaction (PCR)–positive for HCV genotype 1b.[80]
Chronic obstructive pulmonary disease (COPD)	In the few studies that have examined fatigue in COPD patients, fatigue is an extremely prevalent symptom,[68] ranking second only to dyspnea, which is the most frequent symptom reported.[95] Incidence rates range from 58%[68] to 91%.[243]
End-stage renal disease (ESRD)	Fatigue and tiredness are prevalent symptoms in ESRD.[203,244] In hemodialysis patients, fatigue and low energy are the two most important symptoms that affect quality of life.[202] A prevalence rate of 82% is reported for peritoneal dialysis patients,[245] and a prevalence rate between 87%[245] and 100% is reported in hemodialysis patients.[66]
HIV/AIDS	Fatigue can precede the diagnosis of HIV infection, central nervous system involvement, and opportunistic infections.[191] Fatigue prevalence rates of 17% to 60% are documented in HIV-infected adults before an AIDS diagnosis.[191,246,247] For AIDS patients, a prevalence rate of 43% to 70% is reported. Although fatigue is present across all stages of HIV, its prevalence rate may actually increase as the disease progresses and CD4 counts decline.[191]
Multiple sclerosis (MS)	In MS patients, fatigue is a common symptom early in the disease often preceding neurological disability[3] and other symptoms.[9] Prevalence rates range between 70%[110,237,248,249] and 95%.[8] Between 40% and 60% of patients describe it as their most troublesome symptom.[8,250] Although higher fatigue levels are reported in progressive disease, the degree of disability among the subtypes needs to be considered, as it may be responsible more for the differences reported.[84] It is one of the most common reasons for unemployment and "is listed as a cause of MS-related disability by the Social Security Administration."[9]
Parkinson's disease (PD)	Fatigue is a problem in PD but has not been well studied. A 44% prevalence rate was documented in one study.[251] In another study, PD patients with motor fluctuations had more fatigue than patients who did not have such fluctuations.[252] Two studies documented higher fatigue levels in PD patients compared with control subjects.[251,253]
Postpolio syndrome	Fatigue is one of the most frequently reported symptoms in polio survivors decades after initial diagnosis,[254,255] and significantly affects level of activity, performance status, and ability to concentrate.[254,256,257]
Pregnancy and postpartum period	Fatigue is a common problem during pregnancy, labor, and postpartum periods.[258] In one study, persistent fatigue was documented in 52% of women consistently over 18 months following delivery.[146]
Surgery	In postoperative patients, pronounced fatigue may persist for longer than 1 month after uncomplicated abdominal surgeries.[259] After major abdominal surgeries, approximately one third of patients will require 2 months to recover from fatigue.[260] Persistent and debilitating fatigue is more common than pain following a hysterectomy.[261] In one study, 74% of women experienced moderate to severe fatigue during the first few weeks after surgery.[262] Fatigue occurred more frequently and persisted twice as long as pain, and was the one symptom that most interfered with activities of daily living. Another study suggested that pain and fatigue could be used as measures for postoperative recovery in these women.[263]
Systemic lupus erythematosus (SLE)	Fatigue is one of the most common and disabling symptoms in SLE patients. A 74% to 90% prevalence rate is reported.[75,264] Eighty percent to 90% of women with SLE report experiencing "abnormal" fatigue.[75]

RISK FACTORS

Environmental

Environmental factors that may be related to fatigue have not been well studied. Because dyspnea can precede and is correlated with fatigue in COPD patients,[60,61] environmental conditions that exacerbate dyspnea, such as "tobacco smoke, strong odors and the weather,"[62] need to be assessed when managing fatigue. Heat sensitivity affects 60% to 80% of patients with MS and has been associated with worsening fatigue and neurological function with as little as a 0.5° Fahrenheit change in core body temperature.[8,9] This suggests that maintaining a controlled temperature environment may be an effective treatment to prevent fatigue in these patients.

Personal

Studies that explore relationships between fatigue and demographic or personal factors are beginning to be described. These personal risk factors include variables such as gender, race and ethnicity, and the existence of comorbidities. For some patients, sex may be a risk factor; for others it is not. Women are more likely to receive a fatigue diagnosis in cancer,[63-65] CFS,[16] and HIV/AIDS[22] than men, whereas no sex-fatigue relationships were documented in Hodgkin's disease survivors.[50] Fatigued women with HIV/AIDS are more likely to have significantly greater declines in functional abilities, psychological distress, and quality of life (QOL) than fatigued men.[22] Data are inconsistent in hemodialysis patients. In one study, no sex differences were documented[66]; in another, men were significantly more tired than women.[67] In one COPD study an interesting finding was documented. Although no sex differences were noted when a simple fatigue intensity scale was used (i.e., SF-36 vitality subscale), a more multidimensional scale revealed significant differences. Women in this study reported significantly more frequent, intense, and distressing fatigue than did men,[68] suggesting that the multidimensional measure contributed a more valid and comprehensive fatigue assessment than data based on intensity ratings alone.

Although a higher socioeconomic level is considered to be a risk factor for CFS, the data are conflicting.[16,50] Few studies have examined racial, ethnic, or cultural differences in the incidence, pattern, and expression of fatigue. Although there are a number of fatigue studies that have been conducted in different cultures, most studies have addressed samplings of English-speaking white subjects, with few published exceptions.[2,69-71]

In cancer patients, as the number of comorbidities increases, so too does fatigue.[2] The presence of comorbidities also has been linked to fatigue in MS patients.[8] In one cancer survivor study, a small proportion of patients who had preexisting coronary artery disease had 30% higher fatigue levels compared with control subjects.[72] Increases in systolic blood pressure are thought to promote fatigue and atherosclerosis by increasing arterial wall circumferential stress.[73] Although thyroid disorders, such as hypothyroidism, have been postulated to be associated with fatigue, this has not been well studied. Thyroid disorders often go undiagnosed[74,75] and untreated. In one study that examined this variable as a possible late effect of treatment, 70% of cancer survivors had subclinical or clinical hypothyroidism, compared with a 31% to 78% prevalence rate reported in other studies.[50] Surprisingly, patients who were receiving thyroid replacement therapy for their hypothyroidism were more fatigued than those diagnosed with hypothyroidism who were not being treated. Further study examining these relationships is warranted.[74] Other personal risk factors for fatigue include deconditioning, disease severity, malnutrition, symptom distress, the acute and late effects of treatment, and being a caregiver of someone who is chronically ill (see Table 11-1 for caregiver studies).

Patients who are fatigued are often counseled to get more rest. Such reliance on rest, however, may not be in their best interests, because it can lead to an ever-increasing downward spiral of inactivity, deconditioning, and increased fatigue.[9,13,75,76] There are conflicting data as to whether stage, severity, extent, and duration of illness are related to fatigue. Some studies have found a positive relationship,[2,8,77,78] whereas others have not.[8,50,79-81] In patients with HIV/AIDS, increasing fatigue is associated with more advanced disease.[24,77] Patients with lower CD4 counts experience significantly more daily fatigue and sleep more hours at night.[77] In patients with systemic lupus erythematosis (SLE), weak but significant correlations between disease activity and fatigue have been documented.[75] Fatigue scores are 33% higher in women with active versus inactive SLE disease, yet women with quiescent disease report significant fatigue, suggesting that the relationship between disease activity and fatigue may be nonlinear.[75] In another SLE study,[82] disease status was the only predictor of fatigue over time. No association has been documented between hepatitis severity and fatigue.[80,81] Although fatigue is more frequent in MS patients with progessive versus relapsing-remitting disease,[83,84] this finding may be an artifact of the degree of disability present.[84]

Although altered or depleted energy stores are thought to enhance the occurrence of fatigue,[11,18] the relationships between fatigue and abnormalities in metabolism, cachexia, type and extent of nutritional intake (i.e, anorexia), and body mass indices have not been well-studied. Patients who weigh less than 85% of predicted body weight are thought to experience fatigue from the loss of muscle strength.[11] Cachexia, the profound muscle wasting and weight loss that can occur in many cancer and AIDS patients, can affect fatigue and is thought to be caused by the endogenous production of cachectin or tumor necrosis factor alpha (TNF-alpha), a cytokine.[85] In end-stage renal disease (ESRD) patients, malnutrition, uremia and L-carnitine deficiencies have been implicated in causing fatigue but have not been well-studied.[86]

Although fatigue can occur as a primary symptom by itself, it more commonly occurs in conjunction with other symptoms such as pain,[52,87] insomnia,[76,87,88] and dyspnea.[52,60,88,89] In elderly, newly diagnosed cancer patients, pain, fatigue and insomnia are significant independent predictors of physical functioning over time.[90] As a consequence, increased attention is now being given to identifying symptoms that most frequently cluster with fatigue and under what circumstances,[91] and to test the hypothesis that effective treatments directed toward managing these other symptoms, may indirectly be beneficial in treating fatigue as well. Although pain and sleep disorders are common in MS patients, they have not been studied for their relationships to fatigue.[9]

Several studies have documented, that as the number of symptoms and distress from these symptoms other than fatigue increase, fatigue intensity levels increase.[15,92-94] In one study, symptom distress, defined as problems with nausea, vomiting and sleep, offered the best explanation for fatigue in women receiving chemotherapy for early stage breast cancer.[92] In another study, unrelieved symptom distress 2 weeks post surgery, predicted attentional fatigue in older women, three months post breast cancer surgery.[15] Patients with lung cancer, COPD, asthma, and pulmonary hypertension have difficulty distinguishing dyspnea from fatigue when they occur together[95] reinforcing the need to measure and treat symptom clusters affecting fatigue. In patients with AIDS, fatigue was significantly correlated with the number of AIDS-related physical symptoms including pain.[96] Similarly, significant correlations between fatigue and the number and severity of other symptoms are reported in ESRD patients.[66]

Most medications are associated with fatigue. These include antihistamines, anticholinergic agents, beta-blockers,[31] centrally acting alpha-blockers, and central nervous system (CNS) depressants such as narcotics and hypnotics.[7,13,36] In one SLE study, higher fatigue levels significantly were associated with the administration of hydroxychoroquine, but not with prednisolone or azathioprine.[7] In MS patients, medications used to treat MS symptoms and other comorbidities are associated with fatigue.[8] In the elderly, as the number of medications increases, so too does the level of fatigue.[97]

Interest is growing in studying fatigue not only as an acute effect of medical treatment or disease, but also as a more long term or late effect of disease and/or treatment.[64] As most studies are cross-sectional,[37] limited longitudinal data exist that examine the relationships over time between fatigue and late treatment effects. One Norwegian study of Hodgkin's disease patients in remission for more than 5 years, brought patients in for follow-up fatigue studies. Higher fatigue levels were documented in patients who had pulmonary dysfunction, defined as either a restrictive, obstructive or gas transfer impairment by testing.[50] Most of these patients had treatment-induced gas transfer impairment from interstitial pneumonitis. In these patients, the prevalence of chronic fatigue was two to three times higher than in survivors who did not have pulmonary impairment.[50] No significant correlations were found between fatigue and cardiac sequelae as measured by echocardiography, exercise testing, and chest x-ray evaluation.[50]

Developmental

Age may be a risk factor for certain types of fatigue. For example, the mean age range for CFS is 27 to 42 years.[16] In contrast, older women newly diagnosed with breast cancer may be more vulnerable to attentional fatigue following surgery than younger women.[98] In chemotherapy patients, an older age is associated with less fatigue.[65] In other studies, no association between age and fatigue is found.[50,79]

Mechanisms

Although various theories have been proposed to explain how fatigue occurs,[33] these theories have not been as well developed or tested as have pain theories. Because there are a number of similarities that may exist between these two sensations and their explanative theories, using pain as a model for the explication of fatigue mechanisms may be helpful. Both fatigue and pain are complex perceptions that may be explained in part by their underlying central and peripheral nervous system mechanisms.[23] It is well known that the nervous system plays a significant role in the transduction, transmission, perception, modulation and response to pain.[99] As a better understanding of the underlying neurophysiological mechanisms for pain have emerged, so too have improved conceptualizations and measurements of pain's multidimensions evolved.[23,99,100] The nervous system is postulated to play a significant role in the perception and modulation of fatigue,[21,101] and similar theory building for the conceptualization and measurement of fatigue's multidimensions is expected.[23]

Central nervous system (CNS) mechanisms proposed for fatigue include lack of motivation, impaired recruitment of motor neurons,[8,9] intermittent conduction blocks in partially demyelinated central motor pathways,[8,9] and inhibition of voluntary effort.[101-103] The action of sensory pathways on the reticular formation is thought to be critical to the understanding of these central fatigue mechanisms.[104] Chemoreceptors in fatigued muscles are thought to send feedback impulses to the reticular formation in the CNS. These impulses result in motor pathway inhibition anywhere from the voluntary centers in the brain to the spinal motor neurons.[104] This inhibition of voluntary effort can be overridden by feedback stimuli from nonfatigued muscles that stimulate the facilitatory portion of the reticular formation, resulting in decreased inhibition and decreased fatigue.[104]

Similar inhibition-facilitation mechanisms may be operant in attentional fatigue states,[74] because the ability to concentrate, focus, and direct attention involves the active inhibition of competing stimuli.[105] As mental effort is required to maintain this directed attention, prolonged mental effort can lead to fatigue of the underlying neural mechanisms that block competing or distracting stimuli.[105] Inability to perform cognitively,[28] to think clearly, direct attention, or concentrate are manifestations of this mental or cognitive fatiguing process.[106] Meyers[107] and Olin[108] discuss possible causes for neurocognitive changes seen in cancer patients.

In MS patients, metabolic disregulation is hypothesized to affect cognitive fatigue as fluctuations in brain glucose metabolism are reported.[109] In one study, patients' subjective fatigue scores significantly correlated with overall central lesion burden as measured by brain magnetic resonance imaging (MRI), suggesting a CNS origin in these patients.[3] Another study found no significant relationship on MRI.[79] A third MS study found that fatigue had an independent effect on cognitive function and was correlated significantly with pyramidal and cerebellar function.[110] Other possible metabolic causes of fatigue include decreased oxygen carrying capacity as a result of anemia, depletion of energy sources such as phosphocreatine, glycogen, muscle carnitine and mitochondrial myopathy,[111] and changes in amino acids.[112-114] In COPD patients, respiratory muscle fatigue and weakness can result from malnutrition, decreased oxygen supply,[115] and steroid use.[116]

Neurotransmitters have been proposed to mediate fatigue.[18,112] Decreased arousal, cognitive fatigue, and tiredness can occur from serotonin and the disruption of serotonergic pathways.[117] Fatigue is an important symptom of disturbed circadian rhythm,[118] and studies are in progress in cancer patients to explore the relationships that may exist among circadian patterns, fatigue, and melatonin secretion.[119-122]

Peripheral nervous system (PNS) mechanisms proposed for fatigue include impaired peripheral nerve function, neuromuscular junction transmission, abnormal coactivation of agonists and antagonists associated with spasticity,[8,9] and impaired fiber activation.[101] Impaired neuromuscular junction transmission has been implicated in causing fatigue in myasthenia gravis patients,[123] whereas disturbances in the neurotransmitter acetylcholine have been associated with causing fatigue in botulism patients.[124]

Both central and peripheral nervous system mechanisms may be involved in the overwhelming fatigue that patients with chronic fatigue syndrome, cancer, autoimmune disorders and MS experience.[21] It has been postulated that the central and peripheral release of endogenous cytokines by leukocytes, lymphocytes, and activated macrophages may be responsible for fatigue in these patients because of the effects these cytokines may have on the central and peripheral nervous systems, metabolism, and other bodily functions,[3,112,125] such as thyroid function.[126] Metabolic processes have been implicated in MS patients experiencing motor and muscle fatigue.[127] Cytokines are thought to interact with these systems to produce many of the common manifestations seen in fatigue.

Cytokines have been implicated in causing fatigue in cancer patients receiving radiation[128] and biotherapies,[125] and in patients exhibiting signs and symptoms of cognition disorders[125] and anemia.[129] The exogenous administration of cytokines, such as

TNF-alpha, interferon[130], and interleukin have been implicated in fatigue.[125] It is postulated that these cytokines produce fatigue, anorexia, and cognition disorders through direct effects on the frontal lobe, brain structural neurons, or neurotransmitters.[131] Peripheral neuropathies are reported with high-dose interferon therapies.[132] Similarly, the release of endogenous gamma interferon and TNF-alpha in response to interleukin-2 administration has been implicated in causing alterations in neuroendocrine secretion,[133] brain electrical activity,[134] and blood-brain barrier permeability.[135] In addition to their effects on the nervous system, TNF and interleukin-1 have been implicated in causing the progressive muscle wasting associated with cancer cachexia,[85] sleep induction, and fatigue.[136,137] Thus these particular cytokines may cause fatigue secondary to their effects on the body's metabolic functions.[85] Results have been disappointing and inconsistent when cytokine and fatigue studies have been conducted in cancer[64,128,138] and MS patients,[3] despite these posited relationships.[9]

PATHOLOGICAL CONSEQUENCES

Because fatigue mechanisms are not definitely determined, it is not possible to identify with certainty the pathological consequences of fatigue. Fatigue in some circumstances may affect morbidity and mortality. Patients who have had internal cardioverter defibrillators implanted for the treatment of arrythmias, and who have higher levels of mood disturbance, are more likely to have subsequent arrhythmias. These mood disturbances are independent predictors for subsequent arrhythmia events over time, after controlling for other variables.[139] In another study, fatigue was associated with an increased risk for sudden cardiac death 2 years after an MI.[140] In cancer patients, three retrospective studies suggest that the presence of fatigue at diagnosis, may predict a negative treatment and disease outcome for breast,[141] lung,[142] and malignant melanoma patients.[143] Two studies suggest that effective treatment of anemia with recombinant human erythropoietin (epoetin-alfa) in cancer patients not only may be linked to improvements in fatigue and QOL but also may be linked to improved survival rates in patients who respond to epoetin-alfa treatment.[144,145] In one longitudinal study that examined the effects of persistent postpartum fatigue in mothers over an 18-month period, "Infants' eye-hand coordination and performance developmental levels were higher if their mothers were not persistently fatigued."[146]

PSYCHOSOCIAL CONSEQUENCES

Many patients report that fatigue negatively affects their QOL,[22,24,25,61,151] physical well-being, ability to walk long distances, and ability to socialize and work.[38,61] More studies are needed that examine the extent to which fatigue affects patients' abilities, not only to return to work but also how long it takes them to return to work and its effects on maintaining or resuming full-time work status. Fatigue can decrease work capacity in cancer patients, as measured by symptom-limited cycle ergometry[50,147] and by a 12-minute walking test.[148,149] Two studies have documented marked declines in physical functioning in cancer patients when fatigue intensity scores are at a 7 level on a 0 to10 scale.[6,150] When compared with seronegative individuals, 50% of HIV/AIDS patients stated that fatigue interfered with their activities of daily living. These patients were also significantly more likely to be unemployed.[22]

RELATED PATHOPHYSIOLOGICAL CONCEPTS AND DIFFERENTIAL DIAGNOSES

Pathophysiological concepts that may be related to fatigue include anemia, insomnia, psychological distress (i.e., anxiety and depression), and muscle wasting or weakness.

Anemia

Among HIV/AIDS patients, anemia ranges from 20% to 70%, depending on treatment and extent of disease,[24] and was found to be significantly associated with fatigue in one large study.[22] Anemia is common in patients receiving chemotherapy[152] and in ESRD patients.[152] Almost all ESRD patients[153] and 50% to 60% of cancer patients have anemia.[154,155] It has been associated with increased fatigue, depression,[156] decreased QOL, and decreased ability to perform activities of daily living.[145] Anemia may affect cognitive function and mental fatigue[152,153] and may adversely affect cancer survival.[145] Preoperative and perioperative anemia is common in surgical patients[157,158] and may affect recovery. When patients respond to epoetin-alfa treatment,[158-160] less fatigue and fewer declines in functional status and improvements in QOL are reported, suggesting that effective treatment of anemia can be associated with the amelioration of fatigue in some circumstances.

Insomnia

Sleep disorders have not been well studied in clinical populations.[13] Additionally, insomnia and its specific relationship to fatigue and other variables,[161] such as hot flashes, nocturia, and disruption in melatonin rhythms, have not been well studied. In the general population, insomnia is associated with an increased risk of anxiety and depression,[162] decreased daytime performance,[163] and decreased functional status.[164] In one study, fatigued HIV/AIDS patients were significantly more likely to "sleep and nap more and have decreased midmorning alertness than HIV-seronegative individuals."[24] Similar findings were documented in women with HIV-related fatigue.[165] Two studies using wrist actigraphy (a noninvasive device worn on the wrist that continuously monitors body movement over time)[87] in cancer patients documented positive relationships between the number of nighttime awakenings and higher daytime fatigue levels.[166,167] Similarly, 50% of ESRD patients reported restless sleep patterns.[168] Problems with sleep in ESRD are significantly correlated not only with fatigue,[66] but also with higher fatigue levels.[67] In angioplasty patients, physical tiredness or fatigue was the most frequent consequence of fragmented sleep.[169] Poor sleep quality affects nearly two thirds of SLE patients, and moderate correlations with fatigue have been documented.[75] Sleep disruptions and anxiety about sleep were the most significant variables linked to fatigue in SLE patients,[170] suggesting that fatigue management strategies addressing these mediating factors are warranted.

Psychological Distress

Mood disturbances, such as anxiety[89] and depression, are frequently reported to be associated with fatigue, regardless of the underlying diagnosis.[13,23,66,75,158,171-173] Holland et al[174] suggested that health care professionals begin to use the term *psychological distress* when assessing and treating patients with anxiety and depression to reduce the societal stigma associated with these disorders. Considering the frequency that anxiety and depression go undiagnosed and untreated,[75] more attention needs to be given to diagnosing and treating these problems when considering fatigue treatment options. Fatigue can predict negative mood[175] and is significantly associated with greater psychological distress,[22] illustrating the strong interplay that may exist between these states.[175] In one study of MI patients, depression and fatigue scores formed a single factor, suggesting that these concepts were measuring the same construct, leading the authors to conclude that fatigue and depression were not conceptually distinct entities.[176] Many somatic symptoms of depression often overlap with the somatic symptoms of cancer and HIV/AIDS.[33] Because most depression inventories contain both somatic and cognitive/affective items to diagnose depression, false positives methodologically can result when these inventories are used to diagnose depression in medically ill persons.[33,177,178] When depression was assessed using only the nonsomatic items of the Center for Epidemiologic Survey of Depression Inventory (CES-D), Visser and Smets[178] documented, for the first time, different trajectory patterns of fatigue and depression over time in cancer patients receiving radiotherapy. Some studies have found no correlation between these states,[3] whereas other studies continue to find significant correlations,[86] even after controlling for the more somatic items on depression scales.[84] This suggests that there may be a common physiological pathway for these states under certain circumstances. Although depression may occur with fatigue, clinically it is important to differentiate between the two, because the care and therapies will differ, depending on the condition or circumstance. Evidence-based guidelines for the management of psychological distress exist that can guide practice.[174]

Muscle Wasting and Weakness

Loss of muscle strength, mass,[179] and muscle weakness are thought to increase the risk for fatigue.[9,11] Unfortunately, these signs and symptoms have not been well differentiated from each other, nor have they been well studied in relationship to fatigue. All too commonly, fatigue and weakness are equated as being part of the same symptom complex, as when the term *fatigue/weakness* is used. Related concepts, again not well differentiated from fatigue or weakness, include loss of strength and lack of endurance. It is important to differentiate these concepts, because the underlying mechanisms and treatments may vary. Weakness may precede the feeling of fatigue.[14] In polio survivors, no association between weakness and fatigue has been found.[180] One study documented that depletion of body cell mass, as measured by bioelectric impedance analysis, is associated with a significant increase in fatigue.[181] Sarcopenia, or a loss in muscle mass, which is associated with androgen ablation therapy in men with metastatic prostate cancer,[179] is thought to be caused by decreased testosterone levels resulting from therapy and may be responsible for fatigue in these patients. Similar relationships between muscle wasting and fatigue have been postulated in testosterone-deficient men treated for HIV/AIDS,[24] suggesting that for some HIV/AIDS patients, treatment with testosterone might be a beneficial indirect treatment for fatigue because of its hypothesized effects on anabolism, appetite, and depression.[24]

MANIFESTATIONS AND SURVEILLANCE/MEASUREMENT

There is an emerging consensus in the literature that fatigue is multidimensional, because its signs and symptoms can be categorized into various dimensions.[9,23,182,183] Table 11-2 describes several of these dimensions. Studies are needed to determine how these dimensions may vary across different clinical populations and treatments, and how they may be related to underlying mechanisms for fatigue.

Despite the existence of numerous valid and reliable scales to measure the intensity and perception of fatigue (i.e., sensory dimension),[23,184-189] fatigue assessments still have not been incorporated universally into health care settings, as has been the case for pain assessments.[24,33] Fatigue remains underreported, underdiagnosed, and undertreated.[7,24,36] Most likely a legal mandate will be required to effect this change, as now exists in clinical settings for the assessment of pain. For fatigue scales to be used in busy practice settings, not only must they be valid, reliable, and sensitive to measuring change over time, but also they should be easy to administer and score and not cause fatigue or unduly burden the subject in the process.[23] Busy health care professionals can ask patients three simple questions to assess the severity of fatigue:

1. Are you experiencing fatigue?
2. If yes, how severe is the fatigue on a 0 to 10 scale?
3. How is the fatigue interfering with your activities of daily living?

As with pain measurement,[190] measuring intensity alone may be insufficient.[68] Other methods must be used to capture its multidimensional properties.[2,68,184,187,191] For example, documenting the temporal patterns of fatigue may be important when planning treatment for fatigue. In patients followed daily over the first 3 weeks after an MI, five different patterns of fatigue were documented,[19] suggesting that patients should not be treated as a uniform group with the expectation that fatigue will uniformly dissipate over time. Similarly, in cancer patients who are receiving chemotherapy, different patterns of fatigue have been identified, depending on whether women with breast cancer exercise or

TABLE 11-2 Proposed Dimensions of Fatigue

DIMENSIONS	DESCRIPTION OF DIMENSION
Temporal	This dimension includes signs and symptoms that relate to the timing or circadian rhythm of fatigue (when it occurs during the day), onset and duration (weeks to months), pattern (daily, frequent, intermittent, constant, unrelenting, acute, or chronic)[62] and changes in the pattern over time.[23]
Sensory or physical	This dimension[23,28,183] includes intensity or severity of fatigue[182] and signs and symptoms that indicate to patients that they are fatigued.[23] Signs and symptoms may be localized to a specific body part such as having tired eyes,[23] chest or shoulders,[62] or may be more generalized over the whole body, such as feeling extremely tired, drained,[32] having no energy, feeling weak and exhausted,[23,54,62,265] or feeling "bone tired."[151] This dimension can include motor or muscle fatigue indices.[14,266]
Affective or emotional	This dimension includes signs and symptoms that reflect the person's degree of emotional distress or response to fatigue (i.e., increased irritability,[54] frustration, resentment,[32,62] and depression[183]) and the emotional meaning ascribed to fatigue (i.e., unpleasant[23,32]), and/or equating its presence to the perception that treatment is no longer working or the disease is becoming worse.[23]
Cognitive or mental	This dimension includes signs and symptoms that reflect fatigue's impact on the ability to concentrate, remember, think clearly, direct attention[23,32,62] and/or cognitively perform certain tasks.[28] In chemotherapy patients, this also may be referred to as *chemo-brain*[267] or neurocognitive dysfunction.[107,108]
Behavioral or functional	This dimension[9,23] includes signs and symptoms that reflect changes in physical performance status or performance of daily activities.[23,32,62]
Physiological	This dimension reflects the underlying mechanisms that may be causing fatigue, such as anatomical, biochemical, genetic, metabolic, neuromuscular, neurophysiological, and neuroendocrinological mechanisms.[18,23]

not,[192] or whether chemotherapy is given in short daily or weekly intravenous (IV) bolus infusions, continuous IV infusions, or by monthly dosing.[32]

For research purposes, a variety of methods have been developed to measure the outcomes of fatigue on performance. Cimprich[98,106,193] and colleagues[15] have evaluated a battery of tests in a series of studies that measure attentional fatigue and cognitive performance. Other investigators have used neurocognitive tests,[28] motor function,[14] and neuromuscular performance-based measures in their programs of fatigue research.[112] Unfortunately, these measures are labor intensive, require training, and are not well-suited for use in clinical settings.[112]

Not all patients may need an in-depth, multidimensional assessment of fatigue. It is critical to begin to identify those at high risk for chronic fatigue in order to tailor resources and therapies accordingly.[33] A score of 4 or higher on a 0 to 10 numeric rating scale may be a useful indicator for identifying those patients who require a more in-depth assessment and management of their fatigue.[6,7,36,187] With the focus on measuring quality of life and other symptoms in addition to fatigue, subjective fatigue can be measured by single or multiple items within specific subscales on instruments designed to measure other phenomena of interest such as mood states,[194] symptom distress,[195,] QOL,[151,196,197] and anemia.[184,196]

Identifying correlations between subjective and objective indicators of fatigue remains difficult[66,198] and has not been fruitful, possibly because of methodological issues.[14,23,138] As more valid and reliable subjective and objective measures of fatigue are incorporated into studies, more progress should be made,[28] because it is unclear whether this lack of correlation reflects imprecise measurement or a true lack of association.[14,64] For example, in one HIV/AIDS study, no significant correlations were found between fatigue and hemoglobin, hematocrit, albumin, and total protein values,[199] whereas in another study, higher fatigue levels and more hours slept at night, were associated with lower CD4+ counts and higher serum lactate dehydrogenase levels.[77] In one lung cancer study, weight loss did not correlate with fatigue over time during radiation therapy.[200] Until recently, findings were not always consistent in linking levels of anemia with fatigue. In a recent study of healthy subjects, increased fatigue correlated significantly with rapidly decreasing hemoglobin levels and improved dramatically when autologous PRBCs were adminisitered.[201] In one dialysis study, fatigue improved with epoetin-alfa treatment in a randomized clinical trial,[202] whereas no relationship was found between epoetin-alfa treatment and fatigue in descriptive studies,[67,203] suggesting that discrepancies in findings may be related to methodology. Similarly, no correlations have been documented between surrogate markers for liver disease and fatigue in HCV,[81,204] or between fatigue and biochemical markers in dialysis patients.[66] In MS patients, subjective reports of mental and physical fatigue have not correlated with objective measures of cognitive functioning[205,206] or changes in motor activity.[207]

CLINICAL MANAGEMENT

Few evidence-based practice guidelines or diagnostic criteria for fatigue exist that can be tested for their utility and validity in practice settings. In general, more is known about the assessment and measurement of fatigue, than is known about its management or treatment. Guidelines and diagnostic criteria that have been developed are emphasized in the following sections[7,8,16,17,36,49] as are findings from individual studies that have used valid fatigue measures.

Assessment

There are now several valid and reliable intensity scales that can be used to screen patients quickly for fatigue.[23,185,186,188] Because these scales, particularly the 0 to 10 verbal and numeric rating scales are easy to complete and score, there is no longer any excuse for this symptom to go unrecognized or unmonitored clinically. Eliciting perceived and observed effects of fatigue on performance is critical.[5]

The assessment, monitoring and treatment of fatigue is now an expected quality care indicator for oncology,[6,7,25] MS,[8] and CFS[17] care. As a consequence, each practice setting must immediately work toward incorporating these fatigue guidelines into practice settings, and incorporate a simple intensity rating scale for fatigue into documentation and patient-completed forms. Reports are beginning to appear in the literature that describe the establishment of fatigue clinics attempting to apply these guidelines, their referral patterns, and patient fatigue characteristics.[208]

An international study has validated the following intensity categories for fatigue in breast and prostate cancer patients receiving active therapy: none (0), mild (1 to 3), moderate (4 to 6), and severe (7 to 10).[6] Although these intensity levels constitute the best currently available data for evidence-based practice guidelines, they need to be tested in other clinical populations for their validity. In the interim, published fatigue reports need to begin to describe these severity ranges in scores, as reporting only the mean or median values may consistently underestimate the severity of fatigue in clinical populations[209] and fail to identify those at high risk (i.e., at moderate to severe levels) who might benefit from immediate intervention. Moderate to severe intensity levels can serve as "triggers" to alert health care professionals that these patients need to have the more comprehensive and more multidimensional assessment of fatigue conducted, followed by the initiation of treatments used alone or in combination. Additional studies are needed to determine what constitutes meaningful change in fatigue scores over time,[189] and response shifts.[210]

It is important to recognize that all patients need to be screened for fatigue at baseline as they undergo their initial diagnostic work up. Even before treatment has begun, patients may experience fatigue.[15] Such fatigue, when it precedes the initial diagnosis, can alert health care professionals that treatment for fatigue may need to be instituted earlier in the course of the illness and its treatment than is normally expected. When earlier treatment is instituted to combat fatigue, it may be effective in preventing fatigue from becoming more chronic in nature; although the timing and effectiveness of fatigue interventions, in general, need more study.

Screening and Detection

Screening should be performed repeatedly at treatment-related visits, including all follow-up visits when patients are no longer receiving active treatment. Patient self-report diaries, symptom inventories,[210] and telephone follow-up methods[210] can be used. In patients who present with chronic fatigue, a National Institutes of Health Panel has recommended that the following four relatively inexpensive screening tests be performed: an erythrocyte sedimentation rate, urinalysis, a thyroid-stimulating hormone level, and a general health panel blood test.[16,17] Additional radiological and laboratory tests can be ordered based on a high index of clinical suspicion.[13]

Differential Diagnosis

Because any chronic disease may cause fatigue,[13] health care providers must consider a variety of disease states and conditions when formulating a differential diagnosis for fatigue. In many cases, most diseases and psychiatric disorders can be excluded by a thorough history and physical examination.[13] Schematic evidence-based algorithms and diagnostic criteria can assist in making the differential diagnosis.[7,22,36,49] In general, in a patient who already has been diagnosed with an underlying disease process, the more common causes of fatigue need to be considered, ruled out, or treated. These frequently include anemia, infection, depression, sleep disorders, hypothyroidism,[74] and the use of specific medications. When a previously healthy individual presents, the workup becomes more complex, because the primary underlying medical diagnosis first must be made, depending on the patient's signs and symptoms. When assessing medications, one should review the number[97] and kind of prescribed and over-the-counter medications, including herbal supplements, and drug or alcohol abuse should be excluded. Dosages may need to be reevaluated or adjusted, and medications may need to be discontinued or others substituted, if they are determined to be the primary cause of the fatigue.[7,13,36,213]

Treatments

Because fatigue may be multifactorial, interventions need to be directed toward identifying and treating the underlying cause or causes of fatigue and tailoring the intervention to the individual's physical condition, treatment, and underlying disease status. Treatments may include monotherapies, such as the use of recombinant human erythropoietin (epoetin-alfa) in the treatment of anemia associated with chronic disease, such as chronic renal failure or cancer, or may include more multimodal therapies when the exact cause of fatigue is unknown, when it is multifactorial, or when it "clusters" with other symptoms.[33,91]

Pharmacological Therapies

Several studies have explored specific pharmacological therapies for the treatment of fatigue. The agent that has received the most attention in randomized clinical trials is epoetin-alfa.

Erythropoetin. Recombinant forms of human erythropoietin (epoetin-alfa), an endogenous hormone normally produced by the kidney, can be administered to patients with chronic renal failure, zidovidine-treated HIV-infections or nonmyeloid malignancies when patients are receiving chemotherapy or in patients diagnosed with anemia of chronic disease when fatigue is caused by anemia. Epoetin-alfa functions as a growth factor or cytokine, stimulating red blood cell production by causing the division, maturation, and differentiation of erythroid precursors in the bone marrow. It may take between two to six weeks after treatment is initiated before any improvement is seen in hematocrit and hemoglobin levels; an increase in reticulocyte count can be seen as early as 10 days after treatment is initiated in responders. Cancer patients most likely to respond are those with baseline endogenous serum erythropoietin levels less than 100 mU/ml or serum ferritin levels less than 400 mg/ml.[214] A rise in reticulocyte count of equal to or more than 40×10^9/L after 1 month may also be predictive of response. Iron supplementation may be needed during therapy in iron-deficient patients.[214,215] Studies in cancer patients suggest that maintaining a hemoglobin level between 11 and 12 g/dl may be a more appropriate target when the outcome is fatigue management.[145,212] Clinical trials are in progress to evaluate the effects of a longer-acting recombinant form of epoetin-alfa, Darbepoetin.[150,216,217]

Although anemia and fatigue may occur concurrently in some situations, they should not be equated with one another.[218] Other fatigue causes in addition to the anemia may be operating and will require therapy. Fifty percent of anemic patients treated with epoetin-alfa may not respond to therapy for a variety of reasons that are not well understood.[214]

Table 11-3 summarizes the pharmacological therapies that have been tested to treat fatigue.

Nonpharmacological Therapies

There are several nonpharmacological therapies that have been recommended to treat fatigue. The most well-studied include aerobic exercise and cognitive-behavioral therapies.

Aerobic Exercise. Aerobic exercise has been shown to decrease fatigue in AIDS[219] and MS patients.[220] Such programs have decreased fatigue in women with early stage breast cancer receiving chemotherapy,[147-149] and radiation therapy,[22] and similar findings are reported in peripheral stem cell transplant patients,[222] and cancer survivors.[7,36,192,223,224] Whether exercise mitigates fatigue in patients with respiratory problems has not been well studied.[209]

Counseling and Cognitive/Behavioral Therapies. In CFS patients, studies have shown that cognitive/behavioral therapy (CBT) has helped to alleviate fatigue.[225-228] CBT is a form of therapy that combines psychological modification of thoughts or beliefs about a symptom with some form of a behavioral modification such as activity or sleep.[227] In one trial, graded activity combined with cognitive restructuring was found to be more effective in reducing fatigue than relaxation therapy alone.[225] In another trial, cancer patients who received a 20-week nurse-directed cognitive/behavioral intervention reported less pain, fatigue, and other symptoms over time.[229] Similar findings were documented in progressive MS patients, non–randomly assigned to a 1-year, weekly outpatient rehabilitation program that combined physical, occupational, nutritional, and coping services, or to an MS control group. Significantly less fatigue, fewer symptoms, and a lower rate of declines in physical functioning were reported.[230]

One randomized clinical trial demonstrated that counseling and CBT equally reduced fatigue in patients who presented at 10 British primary care settings seeking treatment for fatigue. Although counseling represented a less costly and more widely available treatment, there was no overall cost advantage for either form of therapy.[231]

Table 11-4 summarizes the nonpharmacological therapies proposed for fatigue.

TABLE 11-3 Pharmacological Therapies Proposed for Fatigue

CLASSIFICATION OR NAME OF PHARMACOLOGICAL AGENT	DESCRIPTION AND POSSIBLE RATIONALES
Antidepressants	Antidepressants are hypothesized to be effective in improving fatigue as some act as central nervous system (CNS) stimulants. Thus the feeling of depression may be improved but the underlying cause of the fatigue may remain untreated.[174] In one study in cancer patients, antidepressant therapy improved depressive symptoms, but did not have any effect on fatigue.[268] Similar findings were reported in CFS patients.[269] In depressed patients, a retrospective analysis of 7 double-blind trials, indicated that energy levels and depression scores improved following 3 to 4 weeks of fluoxetine therapy.[270]
Appetite stimulants	Appetite stimulants may be effective in treating fatigue in some patients. For example, in HIV/AIDS patients, megestrol acetate and dronabinol may be useful if fatigue is related to anorexia.[271–273] More study is warranted.

TABLE 11-3 Pharmacological Therapies Proposed for Fatigue—cont'd

CLASSIFICATION OR NAME OF PHARMACOLOGICAL AGENT	DESCRIPTION AND POSSIBLE RATIONALES
Antiviral agents	Amantidine has been suggested as a treatment for fatigue in cancer[312] and HIV/AIDS patients[24] because of its previous success in treating fatigue in MS patients.[274] No randomized trials have been conducted.
Carnitine therapy	Oral carnitine supplements (L-carnitine) may improve fatigue in HIV patients with AZT-induced myopathy by facilitating the transport of long-chain fatty acids into the remaining healthy mitochondria, thereby increasing energy production within muscle fibers.[111,275] In hemodialysis patients, IV administered L-carnitine resulted in decreased subjective fatigue after three weekly, 24-weeks of treatment.[276] In women with CFS, no significant differences between patients and controls were found relative to carnitine serum levels. Authors concluded that at least in these women with CFS, serum carnitine deficiency does not contribute to fatigue.[277] Thus carnitine therapy is not indicated in women with CFS. More studies are needed.
3,4-diaminopyridine	In two MS studies, 3,4-diaminopyridine demonstrated improvement in subjective and muscle fatigue.[278,279]
Erythropoietin	See description in text.
Hyperimmune immunoglobulin	One Phase I study of porcine-derived hyperimmune immunoglobulin reports to have ameliorated fatigue significantly in HIV/AIDS patients.[280]
Melatonin	Administration of 2 to 5 mg of oral melatonin daily in the late afternoon has been used to treat fatigue, and jet lag in flight personnel[281–282] has not been tested in randomized clinical trials to treat fatigue in clinical populations. In one CFS study, the administration of melatonin made the symptoms of CFS worse,[118] and in another study it was not indicated in premenopausal women with CFS or fibromyalgia.[283]
Nicotinamide adenine dinucleotide (NADH)	In a pilot study, ENADA, a reduced and stabilized oral absorbable form of NADH was tested for fatigue efficacy in a randomized, double-blind, placebo-controlled, cross-over study in 26 CFS patients. Eight of 26 patients or 31% had a decrease in their fatigue. It is proposed that NADH may exert its fatigue-reducing effects by triggering increased energy production through ATP generation.[284] Further trials are warranted.
Prokarin™	In the first randomized, double-blind, placebo-controlled trial to evaluate the effects of Prokarin in MS patients, this histamine and caffeine-containing transdermal patch significantly improved fatigue scores without demonstrating significant side effects.[285] The responses were considered clinically significant as the experimental group improved their baseline scores by 37% and 45% elected to continue the medication. Based on serum caffeine level changes, the authors concluded that the fatigue improvements were not correlated with caffeine in the formulation. Further studies are warranted.
Psychostimulants	Psychostimulants such as pemoline (Cylert),[274] dextroamphetamine, and methylphenidate (Ritalin) have been suggested to treat fatigue in HIV/AIDS[24,199] and cancer[36,212] because of their effects on depression and cognition.[24] In the first double-blind, placebo-controlled trial in ambulatory HIV patients, pemoline and methylphenidate were compared to placebo. Fatigue was reduced significantly and equally in both treatment arms as was depression and psychological distress.[286] There have been no other randomized clinical trials reported in other clinical groups. The Rozans et al[287] article summarizes psychostimulant use in palliative cancer patients.
Transfusions (packed red blood cells [PRBCs])	PRBC transfusions are indicated for acute replacement of blood loss. Although anecdotal evidence from practice suggests that patients experience an improvement in their fatigue levels beginning 1 or 2 days following PRBC therapy, this has not been investigated. One study evaluated the acute effects of rapid hemodilution in eight healthy male subjects and found that fatigue levels dramatically increased as hemoglobin levels dropped rapidly and improved relatively immediately with autologous PRBC transfusion.[201]

TABLE 11-4 Nonpharmacological Therapies Proposed for Fatigue

CLASSIFICATION OR NAME OF NONPHARMACOLOGICAL AGENT	DISCUSSION AND POSSIBLE RATIONALE
Aerobic exercise	See description in text.
Attention-restoring therapies/distraction	Attention-restoring therapies/distraction have been shown to reduce attentional fatigue in breast cancer patients.[193] Further studies are warranted.
Continuous positive airway pressure	There is the suggestion in one study that nocturnal use of nasal CPAP may decrease the inspiratory load that COPD patients experience during sleep and that this approach may counteract the muscle fatigue that occurs during the daytime,[288] through a variety of mechanisms.[115]
Counseling and/or cognitive-behavioral therapy	See description in text.
Energy conservation	Anecdotally, employing energy conservation techniques such as pacing or delegating activities, using assistive devices, or sitting down to perform activities are thought to decrease fatigue. Trials are in progress to test this assumption in cancer patients.[289] In MS patients, a 6-session, 2-hr/week energy conservation course taught by occupational therapists resulted in significantly less fatigue in the experimental group versus the control group.[290]
Environmental measures	In heat-sensitive, fatigued MS patients, cooling therapies and controlling environmental temperatures may be beneficial but require testing.[9]
Naps	There is the suggestion at least in one study of 12 healthy young adults, that a 10-minute afternoon nap results in a more immediate and measurable improvement in subjective alertness and cognitive performance than occurs following a 30-minute nap after nocturnal sleep restriction.[291] Clearly more studies with clinical populations are warranted.
Nutrition	Nutritional approaches to prevent or treat fatigue in clinical populations have not been well studied.[292–294] There is one study that examined the effects of either a high iron-containing diet or an iron supplementation in treating fatigued, iron-deficient women of childbearing age. Both fatigue and mental health significantly improved with treatment.[295]
Patient education and preparatory sensory information	Patient information about fatigue, its expected course during treatment, its signs and symptoms and strategies to manage are thought to be helpful but as yet remain untested.[7,36,296]
Rest	Resting the diaphragm at night has been proposed to reduce muscle fatigue and enhance ventilator weaning[11] but has not been tested. Provisions of rest periods interspersed with activity have not been studied.
Sleep hygiene	In CFS patients, treatment of the underlying sleep disorder, as measured by polysomnography, did not relieve fatigue in all cases.[297] In breast cancer patients receiving multiple cycles of chemotherapy, a pilot sleep hygiene program at least maintained fatigue levels at a mild level over time.[298] Additional trials are needed.
Resistance/strength/weight training	Anaerobic exercise such as resistance or strength and weight training has not been tested in fatigued patients, particularly when fatigue may be caused by sarcopenia or muscle loss.[34,299]
Support groups	Two prospective studies suggest that, at least in early stage malignant melanoma[300] and metastatic breast cancer,[301] weekly attendance at a professionally led psychological support group for 6 weeks or longer may decrease fatigue and increase survival time.[21,302]

CONCEPTUAL MODELS

There are a variety of theoretical and conceptual models that have been used to guide fatigue studies and explain relationships between possible fatigue variables in healthy and ill populations. Table 11-5 describes a few of these models. Each of these models and theories is in various stages of development and hypothesis testing. Although the Central/Peripheral

TABLE 11-5 Conceptual Models Proposed for Fatigue

MODEL	DESCRIPTION
Central/Peripheral Nervous System Model	In this model, both central and peripheral nervous system mechanisms are proposed and described for the study of fatigue.[101]
Levine's Energy Conservation Theory	Levine[303] was the first to propose an energy conservation theory applicable to treating fatigue. Balancing energy intake with energy expenditure is an important focus of this model and provides a basis for testing energy conservation techniques to treat fatigue.[289]
Energy and Demand Model	This model proposes that fatigue is the result of an imbalance that occurs between energy and demand. Fatigue can result from diminished available energy, disruption in energy use, restoration or acquisition, and/or increased energy demand.[304] It has not been tested clinically.
Energy-Fatigue Analysis Model	This model depicts the complex interplay between energy sources, energy transformation, energy expenditure, and energy response modifiers in studying fatigue in cancer patients.[93]
Integrated Fatigue Model (IFM)	This model identifies six fatigue dimensions at its core, and around this model's core are patterns and variables hypothesized to cause and treat fatigue. The IFM has been used to guide clinical assessment, measurement, and fatigue programs of research in a variety of populations.[18,191]
Unpleasant Symptoms Theory	This theory has three major components: multidimensional symptoms (intensity, timing/duration, distress, and quality; occurring alone or in combination), influencing factors (physiological, psychological, or situational), and performance consequences (functional/role, cognitive, and physical performance/activity level).[305] It has been tested primarily in childbearing women[146,258] and in patients with dyspnea.[305,306]
Stress Response Model	This model proposes that fatigue is an outcome of prolonged stress.[307] Interactions between the source of the stressors (physiological, psychological, or situational), and the impact of the stressors is governed by the perception of the stressor, stress resistance, available coping mechanisms and the duration of the stress response. Although proposed for assessing and managing cancer fatigue, it has not been tested clinically.
Symptom Management Model	This model, developed by the University of California San Francisco School of Nursing, addresses perception of symptoms, evaluation of symptoms, and response to symptoms across clinical settings. Management strategies are depicted from patient, family, provider, and health care system perspectives. It is being tested in a variety of clinical populations.[308]
Psychobiologic-Entropy Model	This model[294] includes primary symptoms (nausea, vomiting, fever, anxiety, and fatigue), and discusses fatigue's impact on primary symptoms and its secondary impact on functional status and fatigue.
CFS and MS Models	Structural equation models were developed to explain causative variables in perpetuating fatigue in CFS and MS patients.[309] In CFS, a sense of control and focusing on bodily symptoms predicted fatigue severity and chronicity. In MS, a different model evolved. Both models revealed that cognitive and behavioral factors are involved with subjective expression of fatigue in these patients.

Nervous System[101] and Integrated Fatigue models[18,191] are arguably the most widely recognized fatigue models, model selection depends on the research questions posed and the investigator's perspective.

CASE STUDIES

CASE STUDY 1

Marsha, a 34-year-old married woman, diagnosed with multiple myeloma, has been admitted to the hospital; she is experiencing a chemotherapy-induced nadir for neutropenia, infection, and fever. At admission she had a 101.4° F (38.6° C) fever, positive blood cultures, and significantly low laboratory values (Hgb, 7.5 g/dl; Hct, 21%; ANC: 800/mm², and platelets, 24,000/mm²). She was immediately started on IV antibiotics and IV fluids. Because she was symptomatic and severely anemic, she received two units of PRBCs.

Manifestations. Marsha describes her fatigue as having started 3 to 4 days ago, coincident with her bone marrow suppression. Her fatigue is very "unusual" for her. It is constant and does not seem to fluctuate in intensity during the day. "There is no end to it; it is continuous" (temporal dimension). She rates her fatigue intensity at "more than a 10" on a 0 to 10 scale. She states that her fatigue is different from her usual tiredness: "It's extreme." Her symptoms include an overwhelming sense of whole-body fatigue (sensory dimension). "I have no strength or force. I can't go to work like this, and everything I do takes so much more effort. I become short of breath whenever I attempt to do anything" (behavioral dimension). She denies other symptoms.

Surveillance. Because Marsha has multiple myeloma, she will continue to be at high risk for periodic infections, bleeding, and anemia from her disease and its treatment. As a consequence, she will remain at high risk for fatigue. She will need to be monitored routinely for fatigue and other side effects or complications of her disease and treatment. At each office visit, her fatigue will need to be reassessed, documented, and compared with prior visits for its intensity, functional impact, and changes in pattern over time.

Management. Treatment of Marsha's fatigue is directed toward alleviating the underlying causes of her fatigue, which in this case includes her treatment-induced neutropenia, fever and infection, severe anemia, and its associated dyspnea on exertion. Marsha will need to receive education and counseling about the signs and symptoms of fatigue and methods to manage it such as energy conservation, participation in a regular mild to moderate intensity walking program to improve her endurance, and instruction about methods to manage anemia. If her hemoglobin levels remain below 12 g/dl for an extended period, consideration should be given to initiating weekly doses of epoeitin-alfa (40,000 U) subcutaneously to maintain her hemoglobin levels between 11 and 12 g/dl to prevent the need for repeated blood cell transfusions for as long as possible in her condition.

CASE STUDY 2

Frank, a 78-year-old man diagnosed with metastatic prostate cancer, lived with his 78-year-old wife, Florence, who was gradually showing increasing signs of Alzheimer's disease. Florence had had a mild stroke 2 years ago that had left her with some residual weakness and a tendency to fall. Frank currently was receiving antiandrogen therapy for his disease. His daughter requested a home consultation because of Frank's complaints about fatigue.

Manifestations. During the home visit, Frank stated that his fatigue, which he described as a new onset of "feeling tired and weak all the time," was affecting how far he could walk, and how much he could do around the home and at church. He could not put a number to its intensity on a 0 to 10 scale or rate it as mild, moderate, or severe, stating simply that it "bothered" him. Frank always had done the home vacuuming for the couple and paid all the bills. They had remained active as a couple by taking frequent drives together, visiting with friends, and being active in their church, although these activities were beginning to be affected by their medical conditions. Frank served as one of the church donation collectors during the service. He clearly prided himself on this role. He started to cry when he admitted that he no longer could perform this role at the church. He denied signs or symptoms of weight loss or anorexia but did admit to having some recent onset of back pain and difficulty sleeping. A review of Frank's medical record revealed a rising prostate-specific antigen (PSA) level and a CT scan showing progressive disease in his bones and spine.

Surveillance and Management. Because the onset of Frank's weakness and fatigue corresponded to the onset of his pain, difficulty sleeping, and disease progression, these were identified as the primary underlying causes for his fatigue. His weakness and activity status were compounded by the muscle-wasting associated with his antiandrogen therapy. His disease responded to a change in his medical therapy, because it had become refractory to his current form of therapy; his pain responded to hydrocodone-acetaminophen (Vicodin) combined with radiation therapy to the spine. Because his fatigue, pain, sleep, and activity patterns initially improved with changes made in his medical therapy, Frank was not monitored on an ongoing basis for his fatigue after the initial consultation.

Over time however, as his disease progressed, his fatigue became a much more complicated issue to manage, as the increasing care demands of his wife were not immediately apparent to others. As Florence began to deteriorate mentally, she began to wander the apartment at night; would forget who Frank was; and would not remember to take her medications. Because Frank was Florence's primary caregiver, this put an increased strain on him, in addition to the ongoing strain and depression that he was experiencing himself as a result of his own disease progression. His inability to ask for help from others was an issue. His sleep at night became worse, because he often was up with Florence because of her nighttime wanderings. He chose not to take his pain medication as prescribed, because of his continuing fears of addiction despite education, and his need to remain "on alert" to care for Florence. One night he got up to go to the bathroom, fell, and couldn't get up again because of his pain. Florence couldn't call for help or help him physically back to bed, so Frank lay on the floor, waiting until morning to call his daughter. Following hospitalization, his pain responded to IV morphine, and with his family's help, he was able to make long-term care arrangements for his wife and settle his affairs. He died shortly thereafter. In the end, this case illustrates the need for ongoing and close surveillance for such a "high-risk" couple; the complex interplay between fatigue and effective management of other symptoms such as pain, insomnia, and psychological distress; and the multiple causes and potential treatments for caregiver role strain and fatigue.

SELECTED RESEARCH

Studies in which fatigue has been examined were incorporated throughout the chapter. A few nurse- and physician-directed studies focused on the effectiveness of exercise in ameliorating fatigue.[7,36] Others have focused on developing or comparing[6,232] instruments to quantify fatigue in clinical populations.[23,233-236] More recently, investigators have been examining the clustering of symptoms occurring with fatigue.[91] Many others have contributed to the current development of the field[208] and the creation of clinical guidelines.[7,8,17,25,36]

QUESTIONS FOR FUTURE STUDY

Few studies have examined the myriad of possible underlying anatomical, molecular, biological, or biochemical mechanisms of fatigue that may occur in clinical populations. Priority must be given to this much needed area of basic fatigue research as improved diagnostic and therapeutic options can result.[30] Emphasis needs to be placed on examining the hypothesized neuromuscular (peripheral and central), neuroendocrine, cortical, genetic, neuroimmune and inflammatory mechanisms of fatigue that may mediate arousal, sleep, pain, energy balance, and metabolism in vitro (i.e., cell cultures) and in vivo (i.e., in patients), seeking always to correlate study findings with fatigue self-reports.

Studies are needed to determine whether purported dimensions of fatigue vary among[66] and between diagnostic clinical groups, provide clues to underlying fatigue mechanisms, or facilitate the targeting of effective therapies. For example, in one MS study, pyramidal tract involvement was significantly more associated with fatigability, defined as fatigue occurring during or following exercise, when compared with aesthenia, defined as fatigue occurring at rest, without exercise, where immunoactivation parameters were more significantly associated with this symptomatology.[237]

Prospective, repeated, measure-designed studies are needed to elucidate patterns of fatigue that may not only precede a diagnosis but that may occur over time as patients go through treatment and recover from the acute and long-term effects of the disease and treatment. Documenting such patterns will help to better identify those at risk, to schedule and time fatigue treatments more effectively, and to identify underlying fatigue mechanisms. Studies are needed to explore the patterns and relationships between treatment and disease-related neurocognitive side effects[107,108] and mental and physical fatigue. Such patterns need to be compared for differences that may exist as a consequence of demographic factors, such as age, gender, ethnicity, and culture[69,88,110,238]; by disease factors such as type, extent, and severity of disease[52] and the number and type of comorbidities present; and by treatment factors such as type,[41,239] number (i.e., monotherapy versus combined therapy), dose, routes,[32] duration,[32] and length of time off treatment.[47]

Fatigue intensity scores need to be reported not only as means, percentages, and median values, but also in terms of none, mild, moderate, and severe levels with relevant correlational and regression analyses performed. This will enable professionals to predict better, who is at risk for fatigue and when in the course of their disease or treatment, the trajectory of fatigue can be expected to occur. Treatment can then be initiated earlier and be targeted better to those at high risk. As a consequence, the more chronic forms of fatigue may be prevented, leading to improved benefits both for society, the individual, and the family.

Studies are needed that address morbidity, mortality, economic, and return to work outcomes as a consequence of fatigue. Populations in which fatigue needs to be studied include patients who are receiving palliative or terminal care and those individuals who are receiving preventive care because they are at high risk for disease or its recurrence. Evidence-based practice guidelines and diagnostic criteria need to be tested[7,25,36,49] in a variety of settings and be revised periodically based on new evidence. Because fatigue may "cluster" with other symptoms, studies are needed to determine whether effective treatment of symptoms other than fatigue can indirectly and positively affect fatigue as well. Fatigue intervention studies are needed for the following:

- To replicate and extend effective strategies previously tested in one sample or treatment method
- To explore the "best" timing, dose, and duration of interventions in relation to treatment and disease trajectories
- To determine the effects of interventions on underlying fatigue mechanisms
- To evaluate and compare cost effectiveness, percent of adherence, side effects, and subject or provider burden

- To evaluate fatigue outcomes in terms of disease and treatment responses and morbidity and mortality rates

In summary, although advances have been made in the assessment and measurement of fatigue and in the development of evidence-based guidelines, much remains to be done to incorporate these findings into practice settings, to identify underlying mechanisms, and to prescribe effective therapies that prevent and treat this prevalent and distressing symptom.

REFERENCES

1. Glaus, A. (1993). Assessment of fatigue in cancer and no-cancer patients. *Journal of Supportive Care in Cancer 1,* 305-315.
2. Glaus, A., Crow, R., & Hammond, S. (1996). A qualitative study to explore the concept of fatigue/tiredness in cancer patients and healthy individuals. *Journal of Supportive Care in Cancer 4,* 82-86.
3. Columbo, B., Martinelli Boneschi, F., Rossi, P., Rovaris, M., Maderna, L., Filippi, M., et al. (2000). MRI and motor evoked potential findings in nondisabled multiple sclerosis patients with and without symptoms of fatigue. *Journal of Neurology 247,* 506-509.
4. Curt, G.A. (2000). Impact of fatigue on quality of life in oncology patients. *Seminars in Hematology 37* (4 Suppl 6), 14-17.
5. Curt, G.A. (2000). The impact of fatigue on patients with cancer: Overview of fatigue 1 and 2: *Oncologist 5*(Suppl 2), 9-12.
6. Piper, B.F., Dodd, M.J., Ream, E., Richardson, A., Berger, A.M., Lynch, J., et al. (1999). Improving the clinical measurement of cancer treatment-related fatigue. Better health through nursing research: International State of the Science [Abstract. p. 99], Washington, D.C.: ANA.
7. Mock, V., Atkinson, A., Barsevick, A., Cella, D., Cimprich, B., Cleeland, C., et al. (2000). NCCN practice guidelines for cancer-related fatigue. *Oncology 14*(11A), 151-161.
8. Multiple Sclerosis Council for Clinical Practice Guidelines. (1998). Fatigue and multiple sclerosis: Evidence-based management strategies for fatigue in multiple sclerosis. Washington, D.C.
9. Sliwa, J.A. (2000). Neuromuscular rehabilitation and electrodiagnosis. 1. Central neurologic disorders. *Archives of Physical Medicine and Rehabilitation 81,* S3-S112.
10. North American Nursing Diagnosis Association (NANDA). (2001-2002). *NANDA Nursing Diagnoses: Definitions and Classification.* Philadelphia: NANDA.
11. Burns, S.M. (1991). Preventing diaphragm fatigue in the ventilated patient. *Dimensions of Critical Care Nursing 10*(1), 13-20.
12. Aubier, M., Farkas, G., De Troyer, A., Mozes, R., & Roussos, C. (1981). Detection of diaphragm fatigue in man by phrenic stimulation. *Journal of Applied Physiology 50*(3), 538-544.
13. Epstein, K.R. (1995). The chronically fatigued patient. *Medical Clinics of North America 79*(2), 315-327.
14. Schwid, S.R., Thornton, C.A., Pandya, S., Manzur, K.L., Sanjak, M., McDermott, M.P., et al. (1999). Quantitative assessment of motor strength and fatigue in MS. *Neurology 53*(1), 743-750.
15. Cimprich, B., & Ronis, D.L. (2001). Attention and symptom distress in women with and without breast cancer. *Nursing Research 50*(2), 86-94.
16. Ang, D.C., & Calabrese, L.H. (1999). A common-sense approach to chronic fatigue in primary care. *Cleveland Clinic Journal of Medicine 66*(6), 343-351.
17. Fukuda, K., Straus, S.E., Hickie, I., Sharpe, M.C., Dobbins, J.G., & Komaroff, A. (1994). The chronic fatigue syndrome: A comprehensive approach to its definition and study. International Chronic Fatigue Syndrome Study Group. *Annals of Internal Medicine 121,* 953-958.
18. Piper, B.F., Lindsey, A.M., & Dodd, M.J. (1987). Fatigue mechanisms in cancer patients: Developing nursing theory. *Oncology Nursing Forum 14*(6), 17-23.
19. Lee, H., Kohlman, G.C.V., Lee, K., & Schiller, N.B. (2000). Fatigue, mood, and hemodynamic patterns after myocardial infarction. *Applied Nursing Research 13*(2), 60-69.
20. Berger, A. (1998). Patterns of fatigue and activity and rest during adjuvant breast cancer chemotherapy. *Oncology Nursing Forum 25*(1), 1-62.
21. Piper, B.F. (1993). Fatigue. In V. Carrieri-Kohlman, A.M. Lindsey, & C.M. West (eds.), *Pathophysiological phenomena in nursing* (2nd ed., pp. 279-302). Philadelphia: W.B. Saunders.
22. Breitbart, W., McDonald, M.V., Rosenfeld, B., Monkman, N.D., & Passik, S. (1998). Fatigue in ambulatory AIDS patients. *Journal of Symptom Management 15*(3), 159-167.
23. Piper, B.F. (1997). Measuring fatigue. In M. Frank-Stromborg, & S.J. Olsen (eds.), *Instruments for clinical health-care research* (2nd ed, pp. 482-494). Sudbury, Mass.: Jones & Bartlett.
24. Groopman, J.E. (1998). Fatigue and cancer and HIV/AIDS. *Oncology 12*(3), 335-344.
25. Cella, D., Peterman, A., Passik, S., et al. (1998). Progress toward guidelines for the management of fatigue. *Oncology 12*(Suppl 11A), 369-377.
26. Winningham, M.L. (2000). The puzzle of fatigue: How do you nail pudding to the wall? In M.L. Winningham & M. Barton-Burke (eds.), *Fatigue in Cancer* (pp. 3-29). Sudbury, Mass.: Jones & Bartlett.
27. Miaskowski, C. (2002). The Lesage/Portnoy article reviewed. *Oncology 16*(3), 385-386.
28. Krupp, L.B., & Elkins, L.E. (2000). Fatigue and declines in cognitive functioning in multiple sclerosis. *Neurology 55,* 934-939.
29. Poulson, M.J. (2001). The art of oncology: When the tumor is not the target: Not just tired. *Journal of Clinical Oncology 19*(21), 4180-4181.
30. Gutstein, H.B. (2001). The biologic basis of fatigue. *Cancer 92*(6 Suppl), 1678-1683.
31. Potempa, K., Lopez, M., Reid, C., & Lawson, L. (1986). Chronic fatigue. *Image 18,* 165-169.
32. Richardson, A., Ream, E., & Wilson-Barnett, J. (1998). Fatigue in patients receiving chemotherapy: Patterns of change. *Cancer Nursing 21*(1), 17-30.
33. Piper, B.F. (1998). The Groopman article reviewed. *Oncology 12*(3), 345-346.
34. Al-Majid, S., & McCarthy, D.O. (2001). Cancer-induced fatigue and skeletal muscle wasting: The role of exercise. *Biological Research for Nursing 2*(3), 186-197.
35. Chang, V.T., Hwang, S.S., Feuerman, M., Kasimis, B. (2000). Symptom and quality of life survey of medical

oncology patients at a veteran's affairs medical center. *Cancer 88,* 1175-1183.
36. Mock, V., Atkinson, A., Barsevick, A., Cella, D., Cimprich, B., Cleeland, C., et al. (2001). NCCN Cancer-related fatigue guideline. The Complete Library of NCCN Oncology Practice Guidelines [CD-ROM], NCCN: Rockledge, PA, 2001. http://www.nccn.org.
37. Stone, P., Richardson, A., Ream, E., Smith, A.G., Kerr, D.J., & Kearney, N. (2000). Cancer-related fatigue: Inevitable, unimportant and untreatable? Results of a multi-centre patient survey. *Annals of Oncology 11,* 971-975.
38. Vogelzang, N., Brietbart, W., Cella, D., Curt, G.A., Groopman, J.E., Horning, S.J., et al. (1997). Patient, caregiver, and oncologist perceptions of cancer-related fatigue: Results of a tri-part assessment survey. *Seminars in Hematology 34*(Suppl 2), 4-12.
39. Hickok, J.T., Morrow, G.R., McDonald, S., & Bellg, A.J. (1996). Frequency and correlates of fatigue in lung cancer patients receiving radiation therapy: Implications for management. *Journal of Pain and Symptom Management 11*(6), 370-377.
40. Nail, L.M., Jones, L.S., Greene, D., & Schipper, D.L. (1991). Use and perceived efficacy of self-care activities in patients receiving chemotherapy. *Oncology Nursing Forum 18,* 883-887.
41. Woo, B., Dibble, S.L., Piper, B.F., Keating, S.B., & Weiss, M.C. (1998). Differences by treatment methods in women with breast cancer. *Oncology Nursing Forum 25*(5), 915-920.
42. Donnelly, S., & Walsh, D. (1995). The symptoms of advanced cancer. *Seminars in Oncology 22*(2 Suppl 3), 67-72.
43. Krishnasamy, M. (2000). Fatigue in advanced cancer-meaning before measurement? *International Journal of Nursing Studies 37*(5), 401-414.
44. Stone, P., Hardy, J., Broadley, K., Tookman, A.J., Kurowska, A., & A'Hern, R. (1999). Fatigue in advanced cancer. *European Journal of Cancer 34,* 1670-1676.
45. Vanio, A., & Auvinen, A. (1996). Prevalence of symptoms among patients with advanced cancer: An international collaborative study, symptom prevalence group. *Journal of Pain and Symptom Management 2*(1), 3-10.
46. Androwski, M.A., Curan, S.L., & Lightner, R. (1998). Off-treatment fatigue in breast cancer survivors: A controlled comparison. *Journal of Behavioral Medicine 21*(1), 1-18.
47. Bower, J.E., Ganz, P.A., Desmond, K.A., Rowland, J.H., Meyerwitz, B.E., & Belin, T.R. (2000). Fatigue in breast cancer survivors: Occurrence, correlates, and impact on quality of life. *Journal of Clinical Oncology 18*(4), 743-753.
48. Broekel, J.A., Jacobsen, P.B., Horton, J., Balducci, L., & Lyman, G.H. (1998). Characteristics and correlates of fatigue after adjuvant chemotherapy for breast cancer. *Journal of Clinical Oncology 16*(5), 1689-1696.
49. Cella, D., Davis, K., Breitbart, W., & Curt, G. (2001). Cancer-related fatigue: Prevalence of proposed diagnostic criteria in a United States sample of cancer survivors. *Journal of Clinical Oncology 19*(14), 3385-3391.
50. Knobel, H., Loge, J.H., Lund, M.B., Forfang, K., Nome, O., & Kaasa, S. (2001). Late medical complications and fatigue in Hodgkin's Disease survivors. *Journal of Clinical Oncology 19*(13), 3226-3233.
51. Porock, D., Kristjanson, L.J., Tinnelly, K., Duke, T., & Blight, J. (2000). An exercise intervention for advanced cancer patients experiencing fatigue: A pilot study. *Journal of Palliative Care 16*(3), 30-36.
52. Stone, P., Richards, M., A'Hern, R., & Hardy, J. (2000). A study to investigate the prevalence, severity and correlates of fatigue among patients with cancer in comparison with a control group of volunteers without cancer. *Annals of Oncology 11*(5), 561-567.
53. Havik, O.E., & Maeland, J.C. (1990). Patterns of emotional reactions after a myocardial infarction. *Journal of Psychosomatic Research 34,* 271-285.
54. Appels, A., Kop, W.J., & Schouten, E. (2000). The nature of depressive symptomatology preceding myocardial infarction. *Behavioral Medicine 26*(2), 86-89.
55. McSweeney, J.C., & Crane, P.B. (2000). Challanging the rules: Women's prodromal and acute symptoms of myocardial infarction. *Research in Nursing and Health 23*(2), 135-146.
56. Mayou, R. (1979). The course and determinants of reactions to myocardial infarction. *British Journal of Psychiatry 134,* 584-594.
57. Wiklund, I., Sanne, H., Vedin, A., & Wilhelmsson, C. (1984). Psychosocial outcome one year after a first myocardial infarction. *Journal of the American Medical Association 215,* 1292-1296.
58. Hentinin, M. (1986). Teaching and adaptation of patients with myocardial infarction. *International Journal of Nursing Study 23,* 125-138.
59. Kimble, L.P., Dunbar, S.B., McGuire, D.B., De, A., Fazio, S., & Strickland, O.L. (2001). Cardiac instrument development in a low-literacy population: The revised Chest Discomfort Diary. *Heart & Lung 30*(4), 312-320.
60. Lee, R., Graydon, J., & Ross, E. (1991). Effects of psychological well-being, physical status and social support on oxygen-dependent COPD patients' level of functioning. *Research in Nursing and Health 14,* 323-328.
61. Ream, E., & Richardson, A. (1997). Fatigue in patients with cancer and chronic obstructive airways disease: A phenomenological inquiry. *International Journal of Nursing Studies 34*(1), 44-53.
62. Small, S., & Lamb, M. (1999). Fatigue in chronic illness: The experience of individuals with chronic obstructive pulmonary disease and with asthma. *Journal of Advanced Nursing 30*(2), 469-478.
63. Heinonen, H., Volin, L., Uutela, A., Zevon, M., Barrich, C., & Ruutu, T. (2001). Gender-associated differences in the quality of life after allogeneic BMT. *Bone Marrow Transplant 28*(5), 503-509.
64. Knobel, H., Loge, J.H., Nordoy, T., Kolstad, A.L., Espevik, T., Kvalog, S., & Kaasa, S. (2000). High level of fatigue in lymphoma patients treated with high dose therapy. *Journal of Pain and Symptom Management 19*(6), 446-456.
65. Redeker, N.S., Lev, E.L., & Ruggiero, J. (2000). Insomnia, fatigue, anxiety, depression, and quality of life of cancer patients undergoing chemotherapy. *Scholarly Inquiry for Nursing Practice 14*(4), 275-298.
66. McCann, K., & Boore, J.R.P. (2000). Fatigue in persons with renal failure who require maintenance haemodialysis. *Journal of Advanced Nursing 32*(5), 1132-1142.
67. Brunier, G.M., & Graydon, J. (1993). The influence of physical activity on fatigue in patients with ESRD on hemodialysis. *ANNA Journal 20*(4), 457-531.
68. Gift, A.G., & Shepard, C.E. (1999). Fatigue and other symptoms in patients with chronic obstructive pulmonary disease: Do women and men differ? *Journal of Obstetric, Gynecologic, and Neonatal Nursing 28*(2), 201-208.

69. Chan, C.W., & Molassiotis, A. (2001). The impact of fatigue on Chinese cancer patients in Hong Kong. *Supportive Care in Cancer 9*(1), 18-24.
70. Lee, E. (2001). Fatigue and hope: Relationships to psychosocial adjustment in Korean women with breast cancer. *Applied Nursing Research 14*(2), 87-93.
71. Roca Roger, M., Ubeda Bonet, I., Fuentelsaz Gallego, C., Lopez Pisa, R., Pont Ribas, A., Garcia Vinets, L., & Pedrey Oriol, R. (2000). Impact of caregiving on the health of family caregivers. *Ater Primaira 26*(4), 217-223.
72. Loge, J.H., Ekeberg, O., & Kaasa, S. (1998). Fatigue in the general Norwegian population: Normative data and associations. *Journal of Psychosomatic Research 45*, 53-65.
73. Nichols, W.W., & Edwards, D.G. (2001). Arterial elastance and wave reflection augmentation of systolic blood pressure: Deleterious effects and implications for therapy. *Journal of Cardiovascular and Pharmacologic Therapeutics 6*(1), 5-21.
74. Carnaris, G.J., Manowitz, N.R., Mayor, G., & Ridgway, E.C. (2000). The Colorado thyroid disease prevalence study. *Archives of Internal Medicine 160*, 526-534.
75. Tench, C.M., McCurdie, I., White, P.D., & D'Cruz, D.P. (2000). The prevalence and associations of fatigue in systemic lupus erythematosus. *Rheumatology 39*, 1249-1254.
76. Winningham, M.L., Nail, L.M., Burke, M.B., Brophy, L., Cimprich, B., Jones, L., et al. (1994). Fatigue and the cancer experience: The state of the knowledge. *Oncology Nursing Forum 21*(1), 23-36.
77. Darko, D.F., McCutchan, J.A., Kripke, D.F., Gillin, J.C., & Golshan, S. (1992). Fatigue, sleep disturbances, disability and indices of progression of HIV infection. *American Journal of Psychiatry 149*, 514-520.
78. Neidig, J.L., Nickel, J., Smith, B., Brashers, D., Para, M. & Fass, R. (1996). Self-reported symptoms in HIV infection. Proceedings of the International Conference on AIDS (Vancouver), (Abstract TuB176, p. 231).
79. Bakshi, R., Miletich, R.S., Henschel, K., Shaikh, Z.A., Janardhan, V., Wasay, M., et al. (1999). Fatigue in multiple sclerosis: Cross-sectional correlation with brain MRI findings in 71 patients. *Neurology 53*, 1151-1153.
80. Goh, J., Coughlan, B., Quinn, J., O'Keane, J.C., & Crowe, J. (1999). Fatigue does not correlate with the degree of hepatitis or the presence of autoimmune disorders in chronic hepatitis C infection. *European Journal of Gastroenterology and Hepatology 11*(8), 833-838.
81. Nelles, S., Abbey, S., Stewart, D.E., Margulies, M., Wanles, I.R., & Heathcote, E.J. (1996). Fatigue assessment in patients with hepatitis C [Abstract]. *Gastroenterology 110*, A1276.
82. Tayer, W.G., Nicassio, P.M., Weisman, M.H., Schuman, C., & Daly, J. (2001). Disease status predicts fatigue in systemic lupus erythematosus. *Journal of Rheumatology 28*(9), 1999-2007.
83. Jacobs, L.W., Wende, K.E., Brownscheidle, C.M., Apatoff, B., Coyle, P.K., Goodman, A., et al. (1999). A profile of multiple sclerosis: The New York multiple sclerosis consortium, *Multiple Sclerosis 5*(5), 369-376.
84. Kroencke, D.C., Lynch, S.G., & Denney, D.R. (2000). Fatigue in multiple sclerosis: Relationship to depression, disability, and disease pattern. *Multiple Sclerosis 6*, 131-136.
85. St. Pierre, B., Kasper, C.E., & Lindsey, A.M. (1992). Fatigue mechanisms in patients with cancer: Effects of tumor necrosis factor and exercise on skeletal muscle. *Oncology Nursing Forum 19*(3), 419-425.
86. Gaston-Johansson, F., Fall-Dickson, J.M., Bakos, A.B., & Kennedy, M.J. (1999). Fatigue, pain, and depression in pre-autotransplant breast cancer patients. *Cancer Practice 7*(5), 240-247.
87. Berger, A.M., VonEssen, S., Kuhn, B.R., Piper, B.F., Farr, L., Agrawal, S., et al. (2002). Feasibility of a sleep intervention during adjuvant breast cancer chemotherapy. *Oncology Nursing Forum 29*(10), 1431-1441.
88. Okuyama, T., Akechi, T., Kugaya, A., Okamura, H., Imoto, S., Nakano, T., et al. (2000). Factors correlated with fatigue in disease-free breast cancer patients: Application of the Cancer Fatigue Scale. *Supportive Care in Cancer 8*(3), 215-222.
89. Stone, P., Richards, M., A'Hern, R., & Hardy, J. (2001). Fatigue in patients with cancers of the breast or prostate undergoing radical radiotherapy. *Journal of Pain and Symptom Management 22*(6), 1007-1015.
90. Given, B., Given, C., Azzouz, F., & Strommel, M. (2001). Physical functioning of elderly cancer patients prior to diagnosis and following initial treatment. *Nursing Research 50*(4), 222-232.
91. Dodd, M.J., Miaskowski, C., & Paul, S.M. (2001). Symptom clusters and their effect on the functional status of patients with cancer. *Oncology Nursing Forum 28*(3), 465-470.
92. Berger, A.M., & Walker, S.N. (2001). An explanatory model of fatigue in women receiving adjuvant breast cancer chemotherapy. *Nursing Research 50*(1), 43-52.
93. Irvine, D., Vincent, L., Graydon, J.E., Bubela, N., & Thompson, L. (1994). The prevalence and correlated of fatigue in patients receiving treatment with chemotherapy and radiotherapy. *Cancer Nursing 17*(5), 367-378.
94. Irvine, D.M., Vincent, L., Graydon, J.E., & Bubela, N. (1998). Fatigue in women with breast cancer receiving radiation therapy. *Cancer Nursing 21*(2), 127-135.
95. Jansen-Bjerklie, S., Carrieri, V.K., & Hudes, M. (1986). The sensations of pulmonary dyspnea. *Nursing Research 35*, 154-159.
96. Wilson, I.B., & Cleary, P.D. (1996). Clinical predictors of functioning in persons with acquired immunodeficiency syndrome. *Medical Care 34*, 610-623.
97. Liao, S., & Ferrell, B.A. (2000). Fatigue in an older population. *Journal of American Geriatrics 48*(4), 426-430.
98. Cimprich, B. (1998). Age and extent of surgery affect attention in women treated for breast cancer. *Research in Nursing and Health 21*, 229-238.
99. National Institute of Nursing Research. (1994). Symptom management: Acute pain. A report of the NINR priority expert panel on symptom management acute pain. Bethesda, Md.: U.S. Department of Health and Human Services.
100. McGuire, D.B. (1992). Comprehensive and multidimensional assessment and measurement of pain. *Journal of Pain and Symptom Management 7*(5), 312-319.
101. Gibson, H., & Edwards, R.H.T. (1985). Muscular exercise and fatigue. *Sports Medicine 2*, 120-132.
102. Maclaren, D.P.M., Gibson, H., Parry-Billings, M., & Edwards, R.H.T. (1989). A review of metabolic and physiological factors in fatigue. *Exercise and Sports Sciences Reviews 17*, 29-66.
103. Poteliakoff, A. (1981). Adrenocortical activity and some clinical findings in acute and chronic fatigue. *Journal of Psychosomatic Research 25*, 91-95.
104. Asmussen, E. (1979). Muscle fatigue. *Medicine and Science in Sports and Exercise 11*, 313-321.

105. Kaplan, S., & Kaplan, R. (1982). *Environment and cognition.* New York: Prager.
106. Cimprich, B. (1992). Attentional fatigue following breast cancer surgery. *Research in Nursing and Health 15,* 199-207.
107. Meyers, C.A. (2000). Neurocognitive dysfunction in cancer patients. *Oncology 14*(1), 75-85.
108. Olin, J.J. (2001). Cognitive function after systemic therapy for breast cancer. *Oncology 15*(5). Retrieved from www.cancernetwork.com/journals/oncology/o0105c.htm.
109. Benton, D., Parker, P., & Donohoe, R. (1996). The supply of glucose to the brain and cognitive functioning. *Journal of Biosocial Science 28*(4), 463-479.
110. Casanova, B., Coret, F., & Landate, L. (2000). A study of various scales of fatigue and impact on the quality of life among patients with multiple sclerosis. *Revista de Neurologia 30*(12), 1235-1241.
111. Dalakas, M.C., Leon-Monzon, M.E., Bernardini, I., Gahl, W.A., & Jay, C.A. (1994). Zidovodine-induced mitochondrial myopathy associated with muscle carnitine deficiency and lipid storage. *Annals of Neurology 35*(4), 482-487.
112. Elkins, L.E., Krupp, L.B., & Sherl, W. (2000). The measurement of fatigue and contributing neuropsychiatric factors. *Seminars in Clinical Neuropsychiatry 5*(1), 58-61.
113. Newsholme, E.A., & Blomstrand, E. (1996). The plasma level of some amino acids and physical and mental fatigue. *Experimentia 52,* 413-415.
114. Parry-Billings, M., Blomstrand, E., & McAndrew, N. (1990). A communicational link between skeletal muscle, brain, and cells of the immune system. *International Journal of Sports Medicine 11,* S122-S128.
115. Nardini, S. (1995). Respiratory muscle function and COPD. *Monaldi Archives of Chest Diseases 50,* 325-336.
116. Decramer, M., Laquet, L.M., Fagard, R., & Rogiers, P. (1994). Corticosteroids contribute to muscle weakness in chronic airflow obstruction. *American Journal of Respiratory Critical Care Medicine 150,* 11-16.
117. Heliman, K.M., & Watson, R.T. (1997). Fatigue. *Neurology Network Communication 1,* 283-287.
118. van de Luit, L., van der Meulen, J., Cleophas, T.J.M., & Zwinderman, A.H. (1998). Amplified amplitudes of circadian rhythms and nighttime hypotension in patients with chronic fatigue syndrome: Improvement by Inoamil but not by melatonin. *Angiology: The Journal of Vascular Diseases 49*(11), 903-908.
119. Anderson, P.R., Dean, G.E., Grant, M.M., & Kelly, H.A. (1996). A pilot test of physiologic fatigue indicators in healthy controls [Abstract 36]. *Oncology Nursing Forum 23*(2), 318.
120. Dean, G.E., Anderson, P.R., & Grant, M. (1999). Comparing fatigue in women: Breast cancer survivors with healthy controls [Abstract 66]. *Oncology Nursing Forum 26*(2), 370.
121. Mormont, M.C., Waterhouse, J., Bleuzen, P., Giacchetti, S., Jani, A., Bogdan, A., et al. (2000). Marked 24-h rest/activity rhythms are associated with better quality of life, better response, and linear survival in patients with metastatic colorectal cancer and good performance status. *Clinical Cancer Research 6*(8), 3038-3045.
122. Payne, J.K., Rabinowitz, I., & Piper, B.F. (2002). Physiological biomarkers of cancer treatment-related fatigue (Abstract 191). *Oncology Nursing Forum 29*(2), 376.
123. Vollestad, N.K., & Sejersted, O.M. (1988). Biochemical correlates of fatigue. *European Journal of Applied Physiology 57,* 336-347.
124. Cohen, F.L., & Hardin, S.B. (1989). Fatigue in patients with catastrophic illness. In S.G. Funk, E.M. Tournquist, M.T. Champagne, L.A. Copp, & R.A. Weise (eds.), *Key aspects of comfort: Management of pain, fatigue, and nausea* (pp. 208-216). New York: Springer.
125. Piper, B.F., Rieger, P.T., Brophy, L., Haeuber, D., Hood, L.E., Lyver, A., et al. (1989). Recent advances in the management of biotherapy-related side effects: Fatigue. *Oncology Nursing Forum 16*(6 Suppl), 27-34.
126. Jones, T.H., Wadler, S., & Hupart, K.H. (1998). Endocrine-mediated mechanisms of fatigue during treatment with interferon-alpha. *Seminars in Oncology 25,* 54-63.
127. Kent-Braun, J., Sharma, K., Weiner, M., & Miller, R.G. (1994). Effects of exercise on muscle activation and metabolism in multiple sclerosis. *Muscle & Nerve 17,* 1162-1169.
128. Greenberg, D.B., Gray, J.L., Mannix, C.M., Eisenthal, S., & Carey, M. (1993). Treatment-related fatigue and serum interleukin-1 levels in patients during external beam irradiation for prostate cancer. *Journal of Symptom Management 8*(4), 196-200.
129. Barlogie, B., & Beck, T. (1993). Recombinant human erythropoietin and the anemia of multiple myeloma. *Stem Cells 11,* 88-94.
130. Malik, U.R., Makower D.F., & Wadler, S. (2001). Interferon-mediated fatigue. *Cancer 92*(6 Suppl), 1664-1668.
131. Adams, F., Quesada, J.R., & Gutterman, J.U. (1984). Neuropsychiatric manifestations of human leukocyte interferon therapy in patients with cancer. *Journal of the American Medical Association 252*(1), 938-941.
132. Bernsen, P.L.J.A., Wong-Chung, R.D., & Janssen, J.T. (1985). Neurologic amyotrophy and polyradiculopathy during interferon therapy. *Lancet 1*(8419), 50.
133. Besedovsky, H.O., del Rey, A.E., & Sorkin, E. (1985). Immune-neuroendocrine interactions. *Journal of Immunology 135*(Suppl 2), 750S-754S.
134. Krueger, J.M., Walter, J., Dinnarello, C.A., Wolff, S.M., & Chedid, L. (1984). Sleep-promoting effects of endogenous pyrogen (interleukin-1). *American Journal of Physiology 246*(6, pt 2), R994-R999.
135. Denikoff, K.D., Rubinow, D.R., Papa, M.Z., Simpson, C., Seipp, C.A., Lotze, M.T., et al. (1987). The neuropsychiatric effects of treatment with interleukin and lymphokine-activated killer cells. *Annals of Internal Medicine 107*(3), 293-300.
136. Chao, C.C., DeLa Hunt, M., Hu, S., Close, K., & Peterson, P.K. (1992). Immunologically mediated fatigue: A murine model. *Clinical Immunology and Immunopathology 64,* 161-165.
137. Moldofsky, H., Lue, F.A., Eisen, J., Keystone, E., & Gorcznski, R.M. (1986). The relationship between interleukin-1 and immune functions to sleep in humans. *Psychosomatic Medicine 48,* 309-318.
138. Geinitz, H., Zimmermann, F.B., Stoll, P., Thamm, R., Kaffenberger, W., Ansorg, K., et al. (2001). Fatigue, serum cytokine levels, and blood cell counts during radiotherapy of patients with breast cancer. *International Journal of Radiation Oncology, Biology, Physics 51*(3), 691-698.
139. Dunbar, S.B., Kimble, L.P., Jenkins, L.S., Hawthorne, M., Dudley, W., Slemmons, M., et al. (1999). Association of mood disturbance and arrhythmis events in patients after cardioverter defibrillator implantation. *Depression and Anxiety 9*(4), 163-168.
140. Irvine, J., Basinki, A., Baka, B., Jandciu, S., Paquette, M., Cairns, J., et al. (1999). Depression and risk of sudden cardiac death after acute myocardial infarction: Testing

for the confounding effects of fatigue. *Psychosomatic Medicine 61*(6), 729-737.

141. Levy, S.M., Herberman, R.B., Maluish, A.M., Schlien, B., & Lippman, M. (1985). Prognostic risk assessment in primary breast cancer by behavioral and immunological parameters. *Health Psychology 4,* 99-113.
142. Kukell, W.A., McCorkle, R., & Driever, M. (1986). Symptom distress, psychosocial variables, and survival from lung cancer. *Journal of Psychosocial Oncology 4,* 91-104.
143. Temoshok, l. (1987). In consultation: Discussion of psychosocial factors related to outcome in cutaneous malignant melanoma: A matched samples design. *Oncology News Update 2,* 6-7.
144. Caro, J.J., Salas, M., Ward, A., & Goss, G. (2001). Anemia as an independent prognostic factor for survival in patients with cancer: A systematic, quantitative review. *Cancer 91,* 2214-2221.
145. Littlewood, T.J., Bajetta, E., Nortier, J.W.R., Vercammen, E., & Rapoport, B. (2001). Effects of epoetin alfa on hematologic parameters and quality of life in cancer patients receiving nonplatinum chemotherapy: Results of a randomized, double-blind, placebo-controlled trial. *Journal of Clinical Oncology 19*(11), 2865-2874.
146. Parks, P.L. Lenz, E.R., Milligan, R.A., & Han, H.R. (1999). What happens when fatigue lingers for 18 months after delivery? *Journal of Obstetric, Gynecologic, and Neonatal Nursing 28*(1), 87-93.
147. MacVicar, S.B., & Winningham, M.L. (1986). Promoting the functional capacity of cancer patients. *Cancer Bulletin 38,* 235-239.
148. Mock, V., Burke, M.B., Sheehan, P.K., Creaton, E.M., Winningham, M.L., McKenney-Tedders, S., et al. (1994). A nursing rehabilitation program for women with breast cancer receiving adjuvant chemotherapy. *Oncology Nursing Forum 21*(5), 899-908.
149. Schwartz, A.L. (2000). Daily fatigue patterns and effect of exercise in women with breast cancer. *Cancer Practice 8*(1), 16-24.
150. Wang, X.S., Giralt, S.A., Mendoza, T.R., Engstrom, M.C., Johnson, B.A., Peterson, N., et al. (2002). Clinical factors associated with cancer-related fatigue in patients being treated for leukemia and non-Hodgkin's lymphoma. *Journal of Clinical Oncology 20*(50), 1319-1328.
151. Ferrell, B.R., Grant, G.E., Dean. G.E., Funk, B., & Ly, J. (1996). "Bone tired": The experience of fatigue and its impact on quality of life. *Oncology Nursing Forum 23*(10), 1539-1547.
152. Gordon, M.S. (2002). *Impact of anemia on cognitive function in patients with cancer: The anemia disease state slide lecture kit.* Springfield, N.J.: Scientific Therapeutics Information, Inc. (http://www.stimedinfo.com).
153. Tong, E.M., & Nissenson, A.R. (2001). Erythropoeitin and anemia. *Seminars in Nephrology 21,* 190-203.
154. Bron, D., Meuleman, N., & Mascaux, C. (2001). Biological basis of anemia. *Seminars in Oncology 28*(Suppl 8), 1-6.
155. Groopman, J.E., & Itri, L.M. (1999). Chemotherapy-induced anemia in adults: Incidence and treatment. *Journal of the National Cancer Institute 91,* 1616-1634.
156. Glaus, A., & Muller, S. (2000). Hemoglobin and fatigue in cancer patients: Inseparable twins? *Schwizerische Medizinische Wochenschrift 130*(13), 471-477.
157. Bachmann, G.A. (2001). Epoetin alfa use in gynecology: Past, present and future. *Journal of Reproductive Medicine 46*(5 Suppl), 539-544.
158. Stovall, T.G. (2001). Clinical experiences with epoetin alfa in the management of hemoglobin levels in orthopedic surgery and cancer: Implications for use in gynecologic surgery. *Journal of Reproductive Medicine 46*(5 Suppl), 531-538.
159. Gabrilove, J.L., Cleeland, C.S., Livingston, R.B., Sarokhan, B., Winer, E., & Einhorn, L.H. (2001). Clinical evaluation of once-weekly dosing of epoeitin alfa in chemotherapy patients: Improvements in hemoglobin and quality of life are similar to three-times-weekly dosing. *Journal of Clinical Oncology 19*(11), 2875-2882.
160. Glaspy, J., Bukowski, R., Steinberg, D., Taylor, C., Tchekmedyian, S., & Vadhan-Raj, S., for the Procrit Study Group (1997). Impact of therapy with epoetin alfa on clinical outcomes in patients with nonmyeloid malignancies during cancer chemotherapy in community oncology practice. *Journal of Clinical Oncology 15,* 1218-1234.
161. Lee, K. (2001). Sleep and fatigue. *Annual Review of Nursing Research 19,* 249-273.
162. Ford, D.E., & Kamerow, D.B. (1989). Epidemiologic study of sleep disturbances and psychiatric disorders. *Journal of the American Medical Association 262,* 1479-1484.
163. Morin, C.M. (1993). *Insomnia: Psychological assessment and management.* New York: Guilford Press.
164. Winningham, M. (1992). How exercise mitigates fatigue: Implications for people receiving cancer therapy (pp. 16-21). In J. Johnson (ed.), *The biotherapy of cancer—V: Symposium proceedings presented at the 16th annual Oncology Nursing Society Congress, San Antonio, Texas.* Pittsburgh: Oncology Nursing Press/Roche Laboratories.
165. Lee, K.A., Portillo, C.J., & Miramontes, H. (2001). The influence of sleep and activity patterns on fatigue in women with HIV/AIDS. *Journal of the Association of Nurses in AIDS Care 12*(Suppl), 19-27.
166. Berger, A.M., & Farr, L. (1999). The influence of daytime inactivity and nighttime restlessness on cancer-related fatigue. *Oncology Nursing Forum 26*(10), 1663-1671.
167. Berger, A.M., & Higginbotham, P. (2000). Correlates of fatigue during and following adjuvant breast cancer chemotherapy, *Oncology Nursing Forum 27*(90), 1443-1448.
168. Devins, G.M., Edworthy, S.M., Paul, L.C., Mandin, H., Seland, T.P., Klein, G., et al. (1993). Restless sleep, illness intrusiveness, and depressive symptoms in three chronic illness conditions: Rheumatoid arthritis, end-stage renal disease, and multiple sclerosis. *Journal of Psychosomatic Medicine 37*(2), 163-170.
169. Edell-Gustafsson, U.M., & Hetta, J.E. (2001). Fragmented sleep and tiredness in males and females one year after percutaneous transluminal coronary angioplasty (PTCA). *Journal of Advanced Nursing 34*(2), 203-211.
170. McKinley, P., Ouellette, S.C., & Winkel, G.H. (1995). The contributions of disease activity, sleep patterns, and depression to fatigue in systemic lupus erythematosus. *Arthritis and Rheumatism 38*(6), 826-834.
171. Loge, J.H., Abrahamsen, A.F., Ekeberg, O., & Kaasa, S. (2000). Fatigue and psychiatric morbidity in Hodgkins disease survivors. *Journal of Pain and Symptom Management 19,* 91-99.
172. Moody, L., McCormick, K., & Williams, A.R. (1991). Psychophysiologic correlates of quality of life in chronic bronchitis and emphysema. *Western Journal of Nursing Research 13*(3), 336-352.
173. Schwartz, C.E., Coulthard-Morris, L., & Zeng, Q. (1996). Psychosocial correlates of fatigue in multiple sclerosis. *Archives of Physical Medicine and Rehabilitation 77,* 165-170.

174. Holland, J.C., Benedetti, C., Breitbart, W.S., Dudley, M.M., Fleishman, S., Fobair, P., et al. NCCN distress management guideline. The Complete Library of NCCN Oncology Practice Guidelines [CD-ROM], Rockledge, PA: NCCN, 2001 (http://www.nccn.org).
175. Small, S.P., & Graydon, J.E. (1992). Perceived uncertainty, physical symptoms, and negative mood in hospitalized patients with chronic obstructive pulmonary disease. *Heart & Lung 21*(6), 568-574.
176. Wojciechowski, F.L., Strik, J.J., Falger, P., Lousberg, R., & Honig, A. (2000). The relationship between depression and vital exhaustion symptomatology post-myocardial infarction. *Acta Psychiatrica Scandanavica 102*(5), 359-365.
177. Kalichman, S.C., Sikkema, K.J., & Somlai, A. (1995). Assessing persons with human immunodeficiency virus (HIV) infection using the Beck Depression Inventory: Disease processes and other confounds. *Journal of Personality Assessment 64,* 86-100.
178. Visser, M.R.M., & Smets, E.M.A. (1998). Fatigue, depression, and quality of life in cancer patients: How are they related? *Journal of Supportive Care in Cancer 6*(2), 101-108.
179. Stone, P., Hardy, J., Huddart, R., A'Hern, R., & Richards, M. (2000). Fatigue in patients with prostate cancer receiving hormone therapy. *European Journal of Cancer 36*(9), 1134-1141.
180. Farbu, E., Rekard, T., Aarli, J.A., & Gilhus, N.E. (2001). Polio survivors-well educated and hard working. *Journal of Neurology 248*(6), 500-505.
181. Wagner, G.J., Fernando, S.J., & Rabkin, G. (2000). Psychological and physical health correlates of body cell mass depletion among HIV+ men. *Journal of Psychosomatic Research 49*(1), 55-57.
182. Potempa, K.M. (1993). Chronic fatigue. *Annual Review of Nursing Research 11,* 57-76.
183. Ream, E., & Richardson, A. (1996). Fatigue: A concept analysis. *International Journal of Nursing Studies 33*(5), 519-529.
184. Cella, D. (1997). The Functional Assessment of Cancer Therapy-Anemia (FACT-AN) Scale: A new tool for the assessment of outcomes on cancer anemia and fatigue. *Seminars in Hematology 34*(Suppl 2), 13-19.
185. Meek, P.M., Nail, L.M., Barsevick, A., Schwartz, A.L., Stephen, S., Whitmer, K., et al. (2000). Psychometric testing of fatigue instruments for use with cancer patients. *Nursing Research 49*(4), 181-190.
186. Mendoza, T.R., Wang, X.S., Cleeland, C.S., Morrissey, M., Johnson, B.A., Wendt, J.R., et al. (1999). The rapid assessment of fatigue severity in cancer patients: Use of the Brief Fatigue Inventory. *Cancer 85*(5), 1186-1196.
187. Piper, B.F., Dibble, S.L., Dodd, M.J., Weiss, M.C., Slaughter, R.E., & Paul, S.M. (1998). The revised Piper Fatigue Scale: Psychometric evaluation in women with breast cancer. *Oncology Nursing Forum 25*(4), 677-684.
188. Schwartz, A. (1999). Additional construct validity of the Schwartz Cancer Fatigue Scale, *Journal of Nursing Measurement 7*(1), 35-45.
189. Schwartz, A.L., Meek, P.M., Nail, L.M., Fargo, J., Lundquist, M., Donofrio, M., et al. (2002). Measurement of fatigue: Determining minimally important clinical differences. *Journal of Clinical Epidemiology 55*(3), 239-244.
190. Wang, X.S., Mendoza, T.R., Gao, S.Z., & Cleeland, C.S. (2000). The Chinese version of the Brief Pain Inventory (BPI-C): Its development and use in a study of cancer pain. *Pain 67*(2-3), 407-416.
191. Piper, B.F. (1998). Fatigue. In M.E. Ropka & A. Williams (eds.), *Handbook of HIV nursing and symptom management* (pp. 449-470). Boston: Jones & Bartlett.
192. Schwartz, A.L. (1998). Patterns of exercise and fatigue in physically active cancer survivors. *Oncology Nursing Forum 25*(3), 485-491.
193. Cimprich, B. (1993). Development of an intervention to restore attention in cancer patients. *Cancer Nursing 16*(2), 83-92.
194. McNair, D.M., Lorr, M., & Droppleman, L.F. (1992). *EdITS manual for the Profile of Mood States.* San Diego: EdITS/Educational and Industrial Testing Service.
195. McCorkle, R., & Young, K. (1978). Development of a symptom distress scale. *Cancer Nursing 1,* 373-378.
196. Cella, D. (1998). Factors influencing quality of life in cancer patients: Anemia and fatigue. *Seminars in Oncology 25*(3 Suppl 7), 43-46.
197. Ferrell, B.R., Grant, M.M., Funk, B.M., Otis-Green, S.A., & Garcia, N.J. (1998). Quality of life in breast cancer survivors: Implications for developing support services. *Oncology Nursing Forum 25*(5), 887-895.
198. Giovannoni, G., Thompson, A.J., Miller, D.H., & Thompson, E.J. (2001). Fatigue is not associated with raised inflammatory markers in multiple sclerosis. *Neurology 57*(4), 676-681.
199. O'Dell, M.W., Meighen, M., & Riggs, R.V. (1996). Correlates of fatigue in HIV infection prior to AIDS: A pilot study. *Disability and Rehabilitation 18*(5), 249-254.
200. Beach, P., Siebeneck, B., Buderer, N.F., & Ferner, T. (2001). Relationship between fatigue and nutritional status in patients receiving radiation therapy to treat lung cancer. *Oncology Nursing Forum 28*(6), 1027-1031.
201. Toy, P., Feiner, J., Viele, M.K., Watson, J., Yeap, H., & Weiskopf, R.B. (2000). Fatigue during acute isovolemic anemia in healthy resting humans. *Transfusion 40*(4), 457-460.
202. Laupacis, A., Muirhead, N., Keown, P., & Wong, C. (1992). A disease-specific questionnaire for assessing quality of life in patients on hemodialysis. *Nephron 60,* 302-306.
203. Cardenas, D., & Kutner, N. (1982). The problem of fatigue in dialysis patients. *Nephron 30,* 336-340.
204. Mahls, T.C., Daniels, K., Dahhan, W., & Donnelly, K. (1996). Fatigue in patients with chronic hepatitis C [Abstract]. *Gastroenterology 110,* A1254.
205. Krupp, L.B., Masur, D., Schwartz, J., Coyle, P.K., Langenbach, L.J., Fernquist, S.R., et al. (1991). Cognitive functioning in late Lyme borreliosis. *Archives of Neurology 48,* 1125-1129.
206. Paul, R., Beatty, W., Schneider, R., Blanco, C., & Hames, K. (1998). Cognitive and physical fatigue in multiple sclerosis: Relations between self-report and objective performance. *Applied Neuropsychology 5,* 143-148.
207. Sheean, G.L., Murray, N.M.F., Rothwell, J.C., Miller, D.H., & Thompson, A.J. (1998). An open-labelled clinical and electrophysiological study of 3,4-diaminopyridine in the treatment of fatigue in multiple sclerosis. *Brain 121,* 967-975.
208. Escalante, C.P., Grover, T., Johnson, B.A., Harle, M., Guo, H., Mendoza, T.R., et al. (2001). A fatigue clinic in a comprehensive cancer center: Design and experiences. *Cancer 92*(6 Suppl), 1708-1713.
209. Small, S.P., & Lamb, M. (2000). Measurement of fatigue in chronic obstructive pulmonary disease and in asthma. *International Journal of Nursing Studies 37,* 127-133.

210. Sprangers, M.A., Van Dam, F.S., Broersen, J., Lodder, L., Wever, L., Visser, M.R., et al. (1999). Revealing response shift in longitudinal research on fatigue—the use of the thentest approach. *Acta Oncologica 38*(6), 709-718.
211. Cleeland, C.S. (2000). Cancer-related symptoms. *Seminars in Radiation Oncology 10*(3), 175-190.
212. Lesage, P., & Portenoy, R.K. (2002). Management of fatigue in the cancer patient. *Oncology 16*(3), 373-378, 381.
213. Hlatky, M.A., Boothroyd, D., Villinghoff, E., Sharp, P., Whooly, M.A. (2002). Quality of life and depressive symptoms in postmenopausal women after receiving hormone therapy: Results from the Heart and Estrogen/Progestin Replacement Study (HERS) trial. *Journal of the American Medical Association 287*(5), 591-597.
214. Glaspy, J., & Cavill, I. (1999). Role of iron optimizing response of anemic cancer patients to erythropoetin. *Oncology 13*(4). Retrieved from www.cancernetwork.com/journals/oncology/o9904a.htm.
215. Sabbatini, P., Cella, D., Chanan-Khan, A., Cleeland, C., Coccia, P.F., Demetri, G.D., et al. (2001). NCCN cancer and treatment-related anemia guideline. The complete library of NCCN oncology practice guidelines [CD-ROM]. Rockledge, Pa.: NCCN (http://www.nccn.org).
216. Demetri, G.D. (2001). Anaemia and its functional consequences in cancer patients: Current challenges in management and prospects for improving therapy. *British Journal of Cancer 84*(Suppl 1), 31-37.
217. Glaspy, J., Jadeja, J., Justice, G., Kessler, J., Richards, D., Schwartzberg, L., et al. (2001). Darbepoetin alfa administered every 1 or 2 weeks (with no loss of dose efficiency) alleviates anemia in patients with solid tumors. Presented at the 43rd American Society of Hematology annual meeting, December 10, 2001, Orlando, Fla.
218. Hrushesky, W.J.M., & Wood, P.A. (1999). The Galspy/Cavill article reviewed. *Oncology 13*(4). Retrieved from www.cancernetwork.com/journals/oncology/o9904a.htm.
219. Smith, B.A., Neidig, J.L., Mitchell, G.L., Para, M.F., & Fass, R.J. (2001). Aerobic exercise: Effects on parameters related to fatigue, dyspnea, weight and body composition in HIV-infected adults. *AIDS 15*(6), 693-701.
220. Ponichtera-Mulcare, J.A. (1993). Exercise and multiple sclerosis. *Medicine and Science in Sports and Exercise 25*, 451-465.
221. Mock, V., Dow, K.H., Meares, C., et al. (1997). Effects of exercise on fatigue, physical functioning, and emotional distress during radiation therapy. *Oncology Nursing Forum 24*(6), 991-1000.
222. Dimeo, F.C., Stieglitz, R.D., Novelli-Fischer, U., Fetscher, S., & Keul, J. (1999). Effects of physical activity on the fatigue and psychologic status of cancer patients during chemotherapy. *Cancer 85*(10), 2273-2277.
223. Dimeo, F., Fetscher, S., Lange, W., Mertelsmann, R., & Keul, J. (1997). Effects of aerobic exercise on the physical performance and incidence or treatment-related complications after high-dose chemotherapy. *Blood 90*(9), 3390-3394.
224. Dimeo, F., Rumberger, B.G., & Keul, J. (1998). Aerobic exercise as therapy for cancer fatigue. *Medicine and Science in Sports and Exercise 39*(4), 475-478.
225. Deale, A., Chalder, T., Marks, I., & Wessely, S. (1997). Cognitive behavior therapy for chronic fatigue syndrome: A randomized clinical trial. *American Journal of Psychiatry 154*(3), 408-414.
226. Friedberg, F., & Krupp, L.B. (1994). A comparison of cognitive behavioral treatment for chronic fatigue syndrome and primary depression. *Clinical Infectious Diseases 18*, S105-S110.
227. Price, J.R., & Couper, J. (2001). Cognitive behaviour therapy for chronic fatigue syndrome in adults (Cochrane Review). *The Cochrane Library*, Issue 4. Oxford, England: Update Software.
228. Sharpe, M., Hawton, K., Simkin, S., Surawy, C., Hackmann, A., Klimes, I., et al. (1996). Cognitive behavior therapy for the chronic fatigue syndrome: A randomized controlled trial. *British Medical Journal 312*, 22-26.
229. Given, B., McCorkle, R., Cimprich, B., & Given, C. (2002). Pain and fatigue management: Results of a nursing randomized clinical trial [Abstract 34]. *Oncology Nursing Forum 29*(2), 340.
230. DiFabio, R.P., Soderberg, J., Choi, T., Hansen, C.R., & Schapiro, R.T. (1998). Extended outpatient rehabilitation: Its influence on symptom frequency, fatigue, and functional status for persons with progressive multiple sclerosis. *Archives of Physical Medicine and Rehabilitation 79*, 141-146.
231. Chisholm, D., Godfrey, E., Ridsdale, L., Chalder, T., King, M., Seed, P., et al. (2001). Chronic fatigue in general practice: Economic evaluation of counseling versus cognitive behaviour therapy. *British Journal of General Practice 51*(462), 15-18.
232. Taylor, R.R., Jason, L.A., & Torres, A. (2000). Fatigue rating scales: An empirical comparison. *Psychological Medicine 30*(4), 849-856.
233. Barroso, J., & Lynn, M.R. (2002). Psychometric properties of the HIV-related fatigue scale. *Journal of the Association of Nurses in AIDS Care 13*(1), 66-75.
234. Bormann, J., Shively, M., Smith, T.L., & Gifford, A.L. (2001). Measurement of fatigue in HIV-positive adults. Reliability and validity of the Global Fatigue Index. *Journal of the Association of Nurses in AIDS Care 12*(3), 75-83.
235. Hann, D.M., Deniston, M.M., & Baker, F. (2000). Measurement of fatigue in cancer patients: Further validation of the Fatigue Symptom Inventory. *Quality of Life Research 9*(7), 847-854.
236. Kleinman, L., Zodet, M.W., Hakim, Z., Aledort, J., Barker, C., Chan, K., Krupp, L., & Reviche, D. (2000). Psychometric evaluation of the fatigue severity scale for use in chronic hepatitis C. *Quality of Life Research 9*(5), 499-508.
237. Iriate, J., Subira, M.L., & de Castro, P. (2000). Modalities of fatigue in multiple sclerosis: Correlation with clinical and biological factors. *Multiple Sclerosis 6*, 124-130.
238. Servaes, P., van der Werf, S., Prins, J., Verhagen, S., & Bleijenberg, G. (2001). Fatigue in disease-free cancer patients compared with fatigue in patients with chronic fatigue syndrome. *Supportive Care in Cancer 9*(1), 11-17.
239. Schwartz, A.L., Nail, L.M., Chen, S., Meek, P., Barsevick, A.M., King, M.E., & Jones, L.S. (2000). Fatigue patterns observed in patients receiving chemotherapy and radiotherapy. *Cancer Investigator 18*(1), 11-19.
240. Kroenke, K., Wood, D.R., Mangelstorff, D., Meier, N.J., & Powell, J.B. (1988). Chronic fatigue in primary care. *Journal of the American Medical Association 260*, 929-934.
241. Mcdonald, E., David, A.S., Pelosi, A.J., & Mann, A.H. (1993). Chronic fatigue in primary care attenders. *Psychological Medicine 23*, 987-998.

242. Jensen, S., & Given, B. (1991). Fatigue affecting family care givers of cancer patients, *Cancer Nursing 14,* 181-187.
243 Kinsman, R.A., Yaroush, R.A., Fernandez, E., Dirks, J.F., Schocket, M., & Fukuhara, J. (1983). Symptoms and the experience in chronic bronchitis and emphysema. *Chest 83,* 755-761.
244. Srivastava, R. (1989). Fatigue in end stage renal disease patients. In S. Funk, E. Tornquist, M. Champagne, A. Copp, & R. Wiese (eds.), *Management of pain, fatigue, and nausea.* New York: Springer.
245. Merkus, M.P., Jager, K.J., Dekker, F.W., deHaan, R.J., Boeschoten, E.W., & Krediet, R.T. (1999). Physical symptoms and quality of life in patients in chronic dialysis: Results of the Netherlands Cooperative Study on Adequacy of Dialysis (NECOSAD). *Nephrology, Dialysis, and Transplant 14*(5), 1163-1170.
246. Adinolfi, A. (2001). Assessment and treatment of HIV-related fatigue. *Journal of the Association of Nurses in AIDS Care 12*(Suppl), 29-38.
247. Miramontes, H. (2001). Treatment fatigue. *Journal of the Association of Nurses in AIDS Care 12*(Suppl), 90-92.
248. Freal, J.E., Kraft, G.H., & Coryell, J.K. (1984). Symptomatic fatigue in multiple sclerosis. *Archives of Physical Medicine and Rehabilitation 65,* 135-138.
249. Krupp, L.B., Alvarez, L.A., LaRocca, N.G., & Scheinberg, L.C. (1988). Fatigue in multiple sclerosis. *Archives of Neurology 45,* 435-437.
250. Murray, T.J. (1985). Amantidine therapy for fatigue in multipe sclerosis. *Canadian Journal of Neurological Science 12,* 251-254.
251. Karlsen, K., Larsen, J.P., Tandberg, E., & Jorgensen, K. (1999). Fatigue in Parkinson's disease. *Movement Disorders 14*(2), 237-241.
252. Larsen, J.P., Karlsen, K., & Tandberg, E. (2000). Clinical problems in non-fluctuating patients with Parkinson's disease: A community-based study. *Movement Disorders 15*(5), 826-829.
253. Lou, J.S., Kearns, G., Oken, B., Sexton, G., & Nutt, J. (2001). Exacerbated physical fatigue and mental fatigue in Parkinson's disease. *Movement Disorders 16*(2), 190-196.
254. Halstead, L.S., Wiechers, D.O., & Rossi, C.D. (1985). Late effects of poliomyelitis: A national survey. In L.S. Halstead, & D.O. Wiechers (eds.), *Late effects of poliomyelitis* (pp. 11-31). Miami: Symposia Foundation.
255. Rankmore, D., & Oake, W. (1985). Ontario March of Dimes Survey: Late effects of poliomyelitis. Toronto: March of Dimes Provincial Office, 60 Overlea Blvd, M4 H1 B6.
256. Berlly, M.H., Strauser, W.W., & Hall, K.M. (1991). Fatigue in postpolio syndrome. *Archives of Physical Medicine and Rehabilitation 72,* 115-118.
257. Bruno, R.L., Frick, N.M., & Cohen, J. (1991). Polioencephalitis, stress, and the etiology of post-polio sequelae. *Orthopedics 14,* 1269-1276.
258. Pugh, L.C., Milligan, R., Parks, P.L., Lenz, E.R., & Kitzman, H. (1999). Clinical approaches in the assessment of childbearing fatigue. *Journal of Obstetric, Gynecologic, and Neonatal Nursing 28*(1), 74-80.
259. Petersson, B., Wernerman, J., Waller, S.O., von der Decken, A., & Vinnars, E. (1990). Elective abdominal surgery depresses muscle protein synthesis and increases subjective fatigue: Effects lasting more than 30 days. *British Journal of Surgery 77,* 796-800.
260. Kehlet, H. (1988). Anesthetic technique and surgical convalescence. *Acta Chirurgica Scandinavica 550* (Suppl), 182-191.
261. Rock, J.A. (2001). Quality-of-life assessment in gynecologic surgery. *Journal of Reproductive Medicine 46*(5 Suppl), 515-519.
262. DeCherney, A.H., Bachmann, G., Isaacson, K., & Gall, S. (2002). Postoperative fatigue negatively impacts the daily lives of patients recovering from hysterectomy. *Obstetrics & Gynecology 99*(1), 51-57.
263. Rorarius, M.G., Kujansuu, E., Baer, G.A., Suominen, P., Teisala, R., Miettinen, A., et al. (2001). Laparoscopically assisted vaginal and abdominal hysterectomy: Comparison of postoperative pain fatigue and systemic response: A case-control study. *European Journal of Anesthesiology 18*(8), 530-539.
264. Robb-Nicholson, L.C., Daltroy, L., Eaton, H., Gall, V., Wright, E., Hartley, L.H., et al. (1989). Effects of aerobic conditioning in lupus fatigue: A pilot study. *British Journal of Rheumatology 28,* 500-505.
265. Dean, G.E., & Stahl, C. (2002). Increasing the visibility of patient fatigue. *Seminars in Oncology Nursing 18*(1), 20-27.
266. Djaldetti, R., Ziv, I., Achiron, A., & Melamed, E. (1996). Fatigue in multiple sclerosis compared with chronic fatigue syndrome: A quantitative assessment. *Neurology 46,* 632-635.
267. Chemobrain: Chemotherapy side effect? (1996). *Patient Perspectives,* April, 1-2.
268. Morrow, G.R., Hickok, J.T., Raubertas, R.F., Flynn, P.J., Hynes, H.E., Banerjee, T.K., et al. (2001). Effect of an SSRI antidepressant on fatigue and depression in 738 cancer patients treated with chemotherapy: A URCC CCOP study [Abstract 1531]. *Proceedings of the American Society of Clinical Oncology 20,* 384A.
269. Vercoulen, J.H.M.M., Swanink, C.M.A., Zitman, F.G., Vreden, S.G.S., Hoofs, M.P.E., Fennis, J.F.M., et al. (1996). A randomized, double-blind, placebo-controlled study of fluoxetine in chronic fatigue syndrome. *Lancet 347,* 858-861.
270. Judge, R., Plewes, J.M., Kumar, V., Kohe, S.C., & Kopp, J.B. (2000). Changes in energy during treatment of depression: An analysis of fluoxetine in double-blind, placebo-controlled trials. *Journal of Clinical Psychopharmacology 20*(6), 666-672.
271. Gorbach, S.L., Knox, T.A., Roubenoff, R. (1993). Nutrition grand rounds: Interactions between nutrition and infection with human immunodeficiency virus. *Nutrition Reviews 51*(8), 226-234.
272. Oster, M.H., Enders, S.R., Samuels, S.J. Cone, L.A., Hooton, T.M., Browder, H.P., et al. (1994). Megestrol acetate in patients with AIDS and cachexia. *Annals of Internal Medicine 121,* 400-408.
273. Ungarvarski, P.J., & Hurley, P.M. (1995). Nursing research in HIV/AIDS home care: Part 2. *Home Healthcare Nurse 13*(4), 9-13.
274. Krupp, L.B., Coyle, P.K., Doscher, N.P., Miller, A., Cross, A.H., Jandorf, M.A., et al. (1995). Fatigue therapy in MS: Results of a double-blind, randomized, parallel trial of amantidine, pemoline and placebo. *Neurology 45,* 1956-1961.
275. DeSimone, C., Tzantzoglou, S., Famularo, G., Moreeti, S., Paoletti, F., Vullo, V., & Delia, S. (1993). High dose L-carnitine improves immunologic and metabolic parameters in AIDS patients. *Immunopharmacology and Immunotoxicology 15*(1), 1-12.

276. Brass, E.P., Adler, S., Sietsema, K.E., Hiatt, W.R., Orlando, A.M., & Amoto, A. (2001). Intravenous L-carnitine increases plasma carnitine, reduces fatigue, and may preserve exercise capacity in hemodialysis patients. *American Journal of Kidney Diseases 37*(5), 1018-1028.
277. Soetekouw, P.M., Wevers, R.N., Vreken, P., Elving, L.D., Janssen, A.J., van der Veen, Y., et al. (2000). Normal carnitine levels in patients with chronic fatigue syndrome. *Netherlands Journal of Medicine 57*(1), 20-24.
278. Bever, C.T., Jr., Andersen, P.A., Leslie, J., Panitch, H.S., Dhib-Jalbut, S., Khan, O.A., et al. (1996). Treatment with oral 3,4-diaminopyridine improves leg strength in multiple sclerosis patients: Results of a randomized, double-blind, placebo-controlled, crossover trial. *Neurology 47,* 1457-1462.
279. Polman, C.H., Bertelsmann, F.W., de Waal, R., van Diemen, H.A., Uitdehaag, B.M., van Loenen, A.C., et al. (1994). 4-aminopyridine in the treatment of patients with multiple sclerosis: Long-term efficacy and safety. *Archives of Neurology 51,* 292-296.
280. Osther, K., Wiik, A., Black, F.F., Skinhoj, P., Kellermann, G., Ugen, K.E., et al. (1992). PASSHIV-1 treatment of patients with HIV-1 infection: A preliminary report of a phase I trial of hyperimmune porcine immunoglobulin to HIV-1. *AIDS 6,* 1457-1464.
281. Arendt, J., Borbely, A.A., Franey, C., & Wright, J. (1984). The effects of chronic, small doses of melatonin given in the late afternoon on fatigue in man: A preliminary study. *Neuroscience Letters 45*(30), 317-321.
282. Arendt, J., Bojkowski, C., Folkard, S., Franey, C., Marks, V., Minors, D., et al. (1985). Some effects of melatonin and the control of its secretion in humans. *Ciba Foundation Symposium 117,* 266-283.
283. Korszun, A., Sackett-Lundeen, L., Papadopoulos, E., Brucksch, C., Masterson, L., Engelberg, N.C., et al. (1999). Melatonin levels in women with fibromyalgia and chronic fatigue syndrome. *Journal of Rheumatology 26,* 2675-2680.
284. Forsyth, L.M., Preuss, H.G., MacDowell, A.L., Chiazze, L., Jr., Birkmayer, D., & Bellanti, D. (1999). Therapeutic effects of oral NADH on the symptoms of patients with chronic fatigue syndrome. *Annals of Allergy, Asthma, & Immunology 82*(2), 185-191.
285. Gillson, G., Richards, T.L., Smith, R.B., & Wright, J.V. (2002). A double-blind pilot study of the effect of Prokarin on fatigue in multiple sclerosis. *Multiple Sclerosis 8*(1), 30-35.
286. Breitbart, W., Rosenfeld, B., Kaim, M., & Funesti-Esch, J. (2001). A randomized double-blind placebo-controlled trial of psychostimulants for the treatment of fatigue in ambulatory patient with human immunodeficiency virus. *Archives of Internal Medicine 161*(3), 411-420.
287. Rozans, M., Dreisbach, A., Lertora, J.J.L., & Kahn, M.J. (2002). Palliative uses of Methylphenidate in patients with cancer: A review. *Journal of Clinical Oncology 20*(1), 335-339.
288. Mezzanotte, W.S., Tangel, D.J., Fox, A.M., Ballard, R.D., & White, D.P. (1994). Nocturnal nasal continuous positive airway pressure in patients with chronic obstructive pulmonary disease. *Thorax 50,* 1569-1574.
289. Barsevick, A.M., Sweeney, C., Beck, S., Dudley, W., Whitmer, K., & Nail, L. (2002). A randomized trial of energy conservation training versus attentional control during cancer treatment [Poster Abstract 195]. *Oncology Nursing Forum 29*(2), 377.
290. Mathiowetz, V., Matuska, K.M., & Murphy, M.E. (2001). Efficacy of an energy conservation course for persons with multiple sclerosis. *Archives of Physical Medicine and Rehabilitation 82*(4), 449-456.
291. Tietzel, A.J., & Lack, L.C. (2001). The short-term benefits of brief and long naps following nocturnal sleep restriction. *Sleep 24*(3), 293-300.
292. Kalman, D., & Villani, L.J. (1997). Nutritional aspects of cancer-related fatigue. *Journal of the American Dietetic Association 97,* 650-654.
293. Winningham, M.L. (2001). Strategies for managing cancer-related fatigue: A rebailitation approach. *Cancer 92*(4 Suppl), 988-997.
294. Winningham, M.L. (2000). The foundations of energetics: Fatigue, fuel, and functioning. In M.L. Winningham & M. Barton-Burke (eds.), *Fatigue in cancer: A multidimensional approach* (pp. 31-53). Sudbury, Mass.: Jones & Bartlett.
295. Patterson, A.J., Brown, W.J., Roberts, D.C., & Seldon, M.R. (2001). Dietary treament of iron deficiency in women of childbearing age. *American Journal of Clinical Nutrition 74*(5), 650-656.
296. Troy, N.W., & Dalgas-Pelish, P. (1995). Development of a self-care guide for post-partum fatigue. *Applied Nursing Research 8*(2), 92-101.
297. Krupp, L.B., Jandorf, L., Coyle, P.K., & Mendelson, W.B. (1993). Sleep in chronic fatigue syndrome. *Journal of Psychosomatic Research 37,* 325-331.
298. Berger, A.M., Higgenbotham, P., VonEssen, S., Kuhn, B., Piper, B., & Agrawal, S. (2002). Outcomes of a sleep intervention following adjuvant chemotherapy [Abstract 8]. *Oncology Nursing Forum 29*(2), 333.
299. Cella, D. (2002). The Lesage/Portenoy article reviewed. *Oncology 16*(30), 381-382, 385.
300. Fawzy, F.I., Cousins, N., Fawzy, N.W., & Kemeny, M.E. (1990). A structured psychiatric intervention for cancer patients. *Archives of General Psychiatry 47,* 720-725.
301. Spiegel, D., Bloom, J.R., & Yalom, I.D. (1981). Group support for metastatic cancer patients: A randomized prospective outcome study. *Archives of General Psychiatry 38,* 527-533.
302. Spiegel, D., Bloom, J.R., Kraemer, H.C., & Gottheil, E. (1989). Effect of psychosocial treatment on survival of patients with metastatic breast cancer. *Lancet 2,* 888-891.
303. Levine, M. (1973). *Introduction to clinical nursing* (2nd ed.). Philadelphia: F.A. Davis.
304. Cahill, C.A. (1999). Differential diagnosis of fatigue in women. *Journal of Obstetric, Gynecologic, and Neonatal Nursing 28*(1), 81-86.
305. Lenz, E.R., Pugh, L.C., Milligan, R.A., Gift, A., & Suppe, F. (1997). The middle-range theory of unpleasant symptoms: An update. *Advances in Nursing Science 19*(3), 14-27.
306. Lenz, E.E., Suppe, F., Gift, A.G., & Milligan, R.A. (1995). Collaborative development of middle-range nursing theories: Toward a theory of unpleasant symptoms. *Advances in Nursing Science 17*(3), 1-13.
307. Aistars, J. (1987). Fatigue in the cancer patient: A conceptual approach to a clinical problem. *Oncology Nursing Forum 14,* 25-30.
308. Dodd, M.J., Jansen, S., Facione, N., Faucett, J., Froelicher, E.S., Humphreys, J., et al. (2001). Advancing the science of symptom management. *Journal of Advanced Nursing 33*(5), 668-676.
309. Vercoulen, J.H.M.M., Swanink, C.M.A., Galama, J.M.D., Fennis, J.F.M., Jongen, P.J.H., Hommes, O.R., et al. (1998). The persistence of fatigue in chronic fatigue syndrome and multiple sclerosis: Development of a model. *Journal of Psychosomatic Research 45*(6), 507-517.

CHAPTER 12 Pain

KATHLEEN A. PUNTILLO, CHRISTINE MIASKOWSKI, & GRETCHEN SUMMER

DEFINITION

Pain is a complex experience with sensory, affective, behavioral, and cognitive characteristics. Although pain is ubiquitous, an individual's unique integration of pain characteristics makes it a very personal experience. Definitions of pain are intended to provide meaning to the phenomenon, to attempt to explain its characteristics and mechanisms, and to provide direction to clinicians and researchers. Because of its unique personal nature, pain has been defined as "whatever the experiencing person says it is, existing whenever he says it does."[1] Another well-established definition of pain is that it is "an unpleasant sensory and emotional experience associated with actual or potential tissue damage, or described in terms of such damage."[2] In fact, pain is described in many ways; for example, in anatomical terms (back pain) or according to its duration (acute, recurrent, or chronic). A more current recommendation is to classify pain into the following categories: transient pain (i.e., a brief response to a noxious stimulus without negative sequelae); tissue injury pain; and nervous system pain.[3] This approach promotes our understanding of pain mechanisms, concentrates on symptoms regardless of disease process, and focuses on interventions that are optimal treatment modalities. The focus of this chapter is on the pathophysiological phenomenon of pain in adults.

PREVALENCE AND POPULATIONS AT RISK

Transient pain seldom requires professional interventions. On the other hand, tissue injury pain and nervous system pain are associated with many clinical conditions. Tissue injury pain is derived from surgical and trauma-related injuries, among other conditions, or it may be iatrogenically induced. Nervous system pain is associated with many chronic pain conditions. Cancer pain can occur from both tissue injury and nervous system alterations. An understanding of the prevalence of some of these conditions reinforces the need for attention and effective interventions.

Tissue Injury Pain

Surgical Pain. Almost 24 million surgeries were performed in the United States in 1994,[4] and pain accompanies most of these procedures. Surveys of surgical patients demonstrated that almost half of all hospitalized postoperative patients did not receive adequate pain relief.[5,6] In other studies, less than half of the pain medication prescribed for patients with moderate to severe levels of pain had been administered.[7,8] In a small group of cardiac surgery patients (n = 9), the average amount of opioid (expressed in morphine equivalents) administered during the first three postoperative days was only 14 mg/day.[9] In a larger follow-up study that included 74 cardiac and abdominal surgery patients, the average dose of opioid analgesic for the first 3 postoperative days was even less (i.e., 10.9 mg/day).[10] When postoperative opioid administration patterns were compared between cardiac surgery patients younger than (n = 39) versus older than (n = 41) 65 years of age, those older than 65 fared less well.[11] The older group received less opioid analgesics, although this finding only approached significance on days 2 and 3. Regardless of age, all patients received significantly less opioids than they were prescribed across all study days, with the average amount ranging from 8.8 mg to 15.9 mg/day. These studies emphasize the risk of inadequate pain relief for patients undergoing surgery.

This risk of inadequate postoperative pain relief can have physiological consequences. All surgical patients commonly have changes in biological cascade systems that may lead to organ dysfunction and morbidity. This dysfunction and morbidity can be exaggerated in patients with unrelieved pain.[12] Documented negative patient outcomes have included decreased pulmonary function,[13] as well as decreased mobility, increased incidence of complications, and increased length of hospital stay.[14] Effective treatment of postoperative pain may modify negative biological responses to surgery.[12]

Trauma-Related Pain. It is estimated that almost 4 million individuals per year are admitted to hospitals in the United States with a primary diagnosis of traumatic injury.[15] Injuries to soft tissues and bones following trauma account for a large proportion of the medical workload in the United States.[16] Pain can become both a short- and long-term problem for injured patients, even though some patients may not feel pain at the time of an injury.[17] Patients with blunt trauma often have serious injuries, such as multiple rib fractures, pulmonary contusions, abdominal injuries, axial spine injuries, and/or lower extremity fractures.[18] All of them can be potential sources of substantial pain. Pain can, and often does, persist beyond the acute phase of hospital recovery. Posttrauma patients have reported chronic pain and severe psychological stress. Geisser et al[19] examined differences in pain and affective disturbances (e.g., posttraumatic stress disorder [PTSD]) in a sample of 241 patients with chronic pain. Chronic pain in 150 of the patients without PTSD had not originated from a traumatic accident; chronic pain in 46 of the patients with low PTSD resulted from a traumatic accident; chronic pain in 45 of the patients with high PTSD resulted from a traumatic accident. Although actual pain scores derived from the pain rating index of the McGill Pain Questionnaire were not reported, patients in the accident/high PTSD group were reported to have significantly higher levels of pain compared with the other two groups. In another sample of 121 patients with current and chronic pain resulting from injury and referred to a tertiary-care rehabilitation program, there was a considerable proportion (more than 50%) who displayed symptoms of PTSD.[20] Immediate and consistent attention to trauma-related pain may help prevent the development of persistent, intractable pain, as well as help to eliminate a cause of PTSD.

Burn Pain. Burns are among the most painful of all traumatic injuries.[21-23] In the United States, it is estimated that between 1.4 and 2 million people seek medical treatment annually for a burn injury, with up to 75,000 of those requiring hospitalization because of the extent of the burn, associated injury, or comorbid conditions.[24-26] Economic status[26] and geographic location[27,28] contribute to the risk of being burned, whereas the cause of the burn is more closely related to age,[29] occupation, and participation in recreational activities.[30]

In a recent survey, 100% of adult burn patients surveyed ($n = 65$) reported they suffered from pain, with 35% describing their overall pain experience as severe.[31] The depth of a burn is an indicator of how painful the burn is likely to be. Contrary to popular belief, full thickness burns are often painful.[32] In addition, deeper burns are more commonly associated with chronic sensory problems such as chronic pain, dysesthesias (also known as deafferentation pain or neuropathic pain), and/or paresthesias long after healing has occurred.[33-35] Three components characterize the pain that occurs following a burn:[36]

1. Background pain: Constant pain, always in the "background," that occurs at rest in burned areas and skin graft donor sites
2. Breakthrough pain: Intermittent pain that "breaks through" the analgesia provided for the background pain (e.g., during simple activities, such as changing position, turning in bed, and walking)
3. Procedural pain: The most intense pain that occurs in response to manipulations of the wound that are necessary during wound debridement and dressing changes, which must be performed daily or even several times a day to accomplish healing.

Each component requires a separate management plan with special attention being given to providing an adequate dosage range to address the extreme variability of burn pain. Opioids continue to be the first line of treatment for these three components of burn pain. Oftentimes, however, prescribed doses well within the recommended dosage range are woefully inadequate to control the intense pain associated with burns.

Tissue Pain that is Iatrogenically Induced. Iatrogenic pain is pain induced as a result of a health care intervention. It often accompanies diagnostic or treatment-related procedures, such as the treatments for cancer discussed later. Indeed, thousands of painful procedures are performed every day in numerous settings. That fact, in and of itself, may serve as a barrier to adequate pain control since the procedure and its accompanying pain becomes so commonplace for health care providers that it is ignored. Many commonly performed procedures are very painful. In fact, the common procedure of turning a patient was rated by patients to be the most painful of six common procedures performed on more than 6000 hospitalized patients.[37] Health care professionals may infer that the pain associated with procedures such as turning is rapid and benign, something that the individual "needs to put up with." Despite that inference, procedural pain can be both a physiological and psychological stressor to patients.

Nervous System Pain

Chronic Neuropathic Pain. Although not all chronic pain is categorized as neuropathic, pain that occurs as a result of injury to or dysfunction of the nervous system (i.e., nervous system pain) is associated with many chronic pain conditions. The time frame for when an acute painful condition becomes a chronic condition lacks a clear definition. The International Association for the Study of Pain (IASP) Subcommittee on Taxonomy identified three categories of chronic pain: less than 1 month, 1 to 6 months, and more than 6 months, depending on the painful condition.[38] For clinical purposes, many clinicians consider pain of greater than 3 months' duration to be chronic. This type of pain is now frequently referred to as persistent pain. In a recent review of the epidemiological studies of chronic nonmalignant pain,[39] prevalence rates varied from 2% to 40% of the population. The types of pain included in the category of chronic pain are numerous and can include low-back pain, headache, pain associated with degenerative joint diseases, pain associated with fibromyalgia, central pain syndromes, abdominal pain syndromes, musculoskeletal pain syndromes, and facial pain. More specific neuropathic chronic pain syndromes include diabetic neuropathy, postherpetic neuralgia, poststroke pain, trigeminal neuralgia, and complex regional pain syndrome.

Neuropathic pain can occur with numerous medical conditions such as AIDS, MS, arterial and venous insufficiency, and cerebrovascular accident, most of which have a substantial neuropathic component. The prevalence of pain associated with AIDS has been best categorized, with prevalence ranging from 28% to 97%. The prevalence of pain increases as the disease progresses.[40-49] The most common pain problems in patients with HIV disease include peripheral neuropathies, headache, pharyngeal pain, abdominal pain, arthralgias, myalgias, and painful dermatological conditions.[40,43,49]

Tissue and Nervous System Pain

Cancer. Patients with cancer can experience tissue pain, nervous system pain, or a combination of both. Approximately 50% of patients receiving active treatment for cancer experience pain, and more than 70% of patients in the advanced stages of the disease experience pain. Of cancer patients who experience pain, 40% to 50% reported that their pain was of moderate to severe intensity, and another 25% to 30% described their pain as severe.[50]

In a recent international study,[51] the mechanisms underlying a variety of chronic pain problems were categorized as somatic (71.6%), visceral (34.7%), and neuropathic (39.7%) in origin. The major pain syndromes comprised joint and bone lesions (41.7% of patients), visceral lesions (28.1%), soft tissue infiltration (28.3%), and peripheral nerve injuries (27.8%). A large majority of cancer patients (92.5%) had one or more pains caused by the cancer, and 20.8% of the patients had one or more pains caused by cancer therapy.

Secondary pain may result from certain cancer treatments. For example, mucositis pain can occur with the administration of chemotherapy or radiation therapy. Chemotherapy-induced mucositis usually occurs 2 to 10 days after the initiation of therapy. The drugs most commonly associated with severe mucositis include amsacrine, bleomycin, dactinomycin, daunorubicin, doxorubicin, epirubicin, floxuridine, 5-fluorouracil, and methotrexate.[52] Pain is usually associated with erythema and inflammation of the oral mucosa. The inflammation may progress to areas of ulceration. In addition, the development of infections may exacerbate the pain. Radiation treatments produce oral mucositis at doses of 2000 to 2500 cGys. Pain associated with radiation-induced mucositis is variable. However, pain may be severe enough to interfere with nutritional intake.

MECHANISMS

The gate control theory, reported by Melzack and Wall in 1965,[53] revolutionized the understanding of pain transmission and modulation mechanisms (Figure 12-1). This theory hypothesized that both nociceptive and nonnociceptive peripheral sensory transmission fibers synapse on the same spinal cord cells that transmit pain sensations to the brain. Inhibitory interneurons in the spinal cord can influence these central transmission cells by interrupting the balance between small diameter (pain) fibers and large diameter (nonpain) fibers. When large-diameter nonpain fibers are less active, compared with pain fibers, pain transmission cells are stimulated. By contrast, when large-diameter nonpain fibers are stimulated, inhibitory interneurons block pain transmission to higher centers. Higher control processes within the CNS can influence pain transmission in the spinal cord by delivering descending inhibitory messages to the spinal cord.

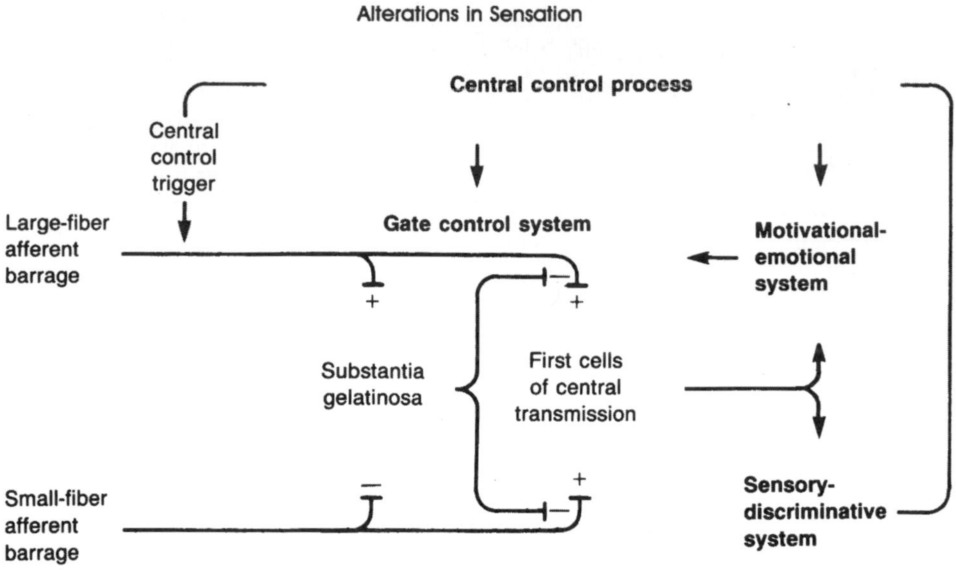

Figure 12-1 **The gate control model, which proposes a balance of activity between large afferent nonpain fibers and small pain fibers that synapse on transmission cells in the spinal cord. Peripheral fiber activity is modulated by substantia gelatinosa cells. Sensory-discriminative and motivational-emotional systems transmit impulses from spinal cord to brain. Central control processes influence the gate control system. + = excitation, − = inhibition** (From Chapman, C.R., & Bonica, J.J. [1983]. *Current concepts: Acute pain* [p. 11]. Pharmacia, Peapack NJ.)

The concept of neuroplasticity, developed in the late 1970s, revolutionized fundamental thinking about pain processing. This concept suggests that the nervous system is not a hard-wired system, but a dynamic system that can interact with other physiological systems and change over time. This idea led Melzack[54] to revise the gate control theory of pain. His revised theory was designed to help clinicians and researchers better understand and study the human experience of pain. He called this revised theory the *neuromatrix theory of pain* (Figure 12-2). This theory proposes that the neurosignature for the pain experience (i.e., the signal that the nervous system recognizes as acute or chronic pain) is determined by the synaptic architecture of the neuromatrix. According to Melzack, the neuromatrix is a genetically built-in matrix of neurons whose spacial distribution and synaptic links are initially determined genetically and are later influenced and modified by sensory inputs. Loops between the thalamus, cortex, and limbic systems (i.e., some of the structures that compose the neuromatrix) diverge to permit parallel processing in different components of the neuromatrix and converge to permit interactions between the output products of the processing. The cyclical processing and synthesis of nerve impulses in the neuromatrix imposes a characteristic output pattern, or *neurosignature*.[54] This theory conceptualizes pain as a multidimensional experience that is produced by multiple influences, including physical and psychological factors.

Pain processing occurs in large part through a series of interactions within the peripheral and central nervous systems. The major neurophysiological mechanisms involved in pain processing are transduction, transmission, modulation, and perception. Transduction is the process by which noxious stimuli lead to electrical activity in appropriate sensory nerve endings.[55] Primary afferent nociceptors (i.e., A-delta and C-fibers) are the nerve fibers involved in transduction. Activation of A-delta and C-fibers generate impulses that are carried to the dorsal horn of the spinal cord.

Primary afferent nociceptors can respond to mechanical, thermal, and chemical stimuli that are painful. Activation of primary afferent nociceptors usually begins with some type of tissue injury or damage that sets in motion an inflammatory process. The process of inflammation involves a variety of inflammatory mediators (e.g., cytokines and neuropeptides) that activate and sensitize primary afferent nociceptors.[56] These mediators are released from circulating leukocytes, platelets, vascular endothelial cells, immune cells, as well as from

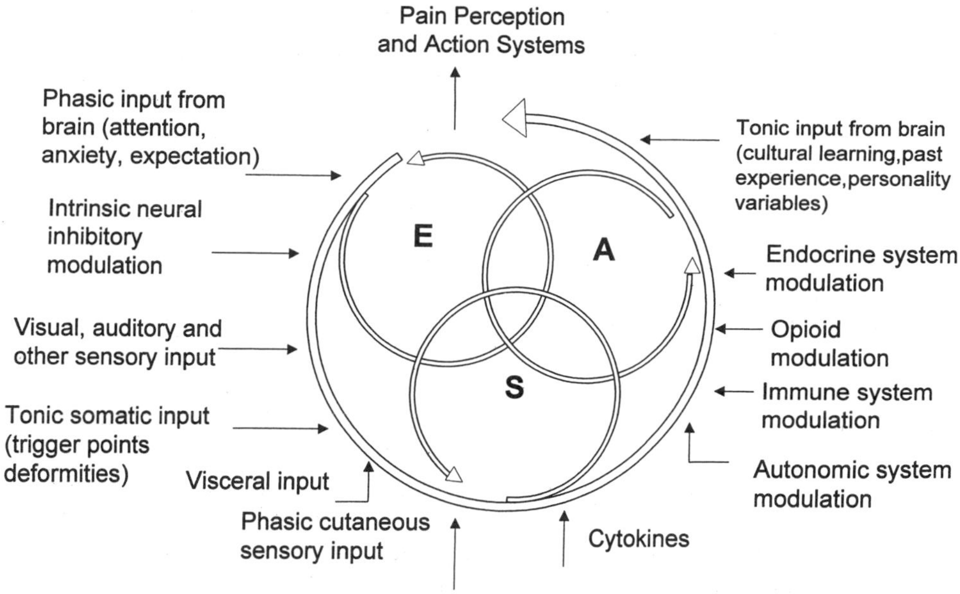

Figure 12-2 **The body-self neuromatrix. The neuromatrix comprises a widely distributed neural network that includes somatosensory, limbic, and thalamocortical components. The synaptic architecture of the neuromatrix is determined by genetic and sensory influences. Multiple inputs act on the neuromatrix, contributing to output. (*A,* Affective-motivational; *E,* evaluative-cognitive dimensions of the pain experience; *S,* sensory-discriminative.)** (From Melzack, R. [1999]. From the gate to the neuromatrix. *Pain 6,* S125.)

cells within the peripheral nervous system (PNS). The result of the inflammatory process on primary afferent nociceptors is twofold: (1) direct excitation of C-fibers that leads to activation of C-fiber terminals and pain and (2) sensitization of C-fibers (i.e., a noxious stimulus produces intense pain; also called hyperalgesia). These inflammatory mediators interact to form a complex series of events that change the function of primary afferent neurons in the short term. They also can alter gene transcription that results in long-term alterations in the biochemistry of sensory neurons.[57]

Transmission refers to the process whereby the electrochemical nerve impulse is relayed to structures in the central nervous system (CNS) whose activity produces the sensation of pain.[55] The first stage of transmission involves the conduction of impulses in primary afferents to the spinal cord. At the spinal cord, spinal cord neurons are activated that relay the pain signal to the brain. The receipt of the pain signal in the brain elicits the subjective sensation of pain.

The biochemistry of the synapse in the dorsal horn of the spinal cord is extremely complex. The neurotransmitters present in the dorsal horn of the spinal cord are released in response to activity in either afferent fibers, local intrinsic spinal neurons, or from the endings of neurons descending from the brain. These transmitters are concentrated in the dorsal horn of the spinal cord in an area called the substantia gelatinosa, one of the densest neuronal areas in the CNS and crucial for pain transmission and modulation.[58] Specific neurotransmitters increase or decrease pain transmission. In addition, different neurotransmitters and different receptors appear to be involved in the transmission of acute and chronic pain.

It is suspected that transmission from C-fibers after very brief or acute mechanical or thermal stimulation involves glutamate and aspartate, which act on the alpha-amino-3-hydroxyl-5-methyl-4-isoxazole-propionic acid (AMPA) receptor to produce long-lasting excitations. If the stimulus is maintained and/or its frequency or intensity is increased, the subsequent release of neurotransmitters contributes to pain transmission and allows N-methyl-D-aspartate (NMDA) receptors to become activated. The activation of NMDA receptors results in the release of a series of neurotransmitters that amplifies the pain signal and may underlie many forms of central hyperalgesia and lead to the development of chronic pain.[59-61] A more detailed discussion of persistent pain is presented later in the chapter.

The output neurons from the dorsal horn of the spinal cord cross in the anterior white commissure and ascend the spinal cord in the anterolateral quadrant (ALQ). The ALQ has two ascending pathways: the spinothalamic tract (STT) and the spinorecticular tract (SRT). The STT ascends through the lateral edge of the medulla, lateral pons, and midbrain to the thalamus. From the thalamus, neurons project to the somatosensory cortex. The STT transmits aspects of acute pain (e.g., location, intensity, and quality) and alerts an individual to a potentially threatening event.[62] The neurons in the SRT ascend from the ALQ to the recticular formation, the pontine and medullary areas, and the medial thalamic nuclei. The SRT contributes to the affective processing of pain by connecting ascending information about pain from the brainstem to limbic structures through noradrenergic bundles.[63]

The modulation of pain is extremely complex. Pain modulation can occur through segmental modulation (e.g., at the level of the spinal cord) and through descending modulation. These modulating systems contain the body's own endogenous neurotransmitters (e.g., endorphin, enkephalin, and serotonin) that are involved in the processing of painful stimuli. In addition, these systems can be modulated by pharmacological and nonpharmacological approaches. For example, the use of relaxation techniques or guided imagery may activate the release of endogenous neurotransmitters that modulate an individual's response to acute or chronic pain.

The final pain process is perception. The anatomical and neurochemical correlates involved in this process are poorly understood. Newer techniques, such as positron emission tomography (PET) are providing insights into pain perception. For example, changes in neural activity in the thalamus were found in patients with neuropathic pain who underwent a PET scan.[64,65]

A CONCEPTUAL MODEL OF PAIN

In 1965, the gate control model of pain proposed by Melzack and Wall[53] remarkably altered the approach to pain research and treatment. The model placed emphasis on CNS mechanisms of pain rather than the previous concentration on peripheral factors. It also highlighted the importance of the brain as an active system that filters, selects, and modulates inputs.[54] That is, higher CNS control processes can influence the spinal gate control system by delivering descending inhibitory messages (see Figure 12-1). Although the gate control model is not considered complete, it provides one of the most important conceptual approaches to understanding pain mechanisms and to explaining the effectiveness of certain interventions. The neuromatrix theory,[54] discussed in the previous section on mechanisms, augmented the gate control model to further our understanding of pain.

PATHOLOGICAL CONSEQUENCES OF PAIN

Over the past decade, a focus on reducing adverse outcomes in patients with pain has highlighted the potential effects of pain on homeostasis. The stress response stimulated by pain has profound pathological consequences.[66-68] (See Chapter 14 for an in-depth discussion of the stress response.) Stress evokes autonomic responses that markedly increase adrenergic neural activity and plasma catecholamine concentrations.[69] Increased circulating catecholamines can cause arteriolar vasoconstriction, impair tissue perfusion, and reduce tissue-oxygen partial pressure.[70] Pain-induced reflex responses may adversely influence respiratory function, increase cardiac demands, decrease intestinal motility, and initiate skeletal muscle spasms.[71] Other responses triggered by pain induce catabolic hypermetabolism such as hyperglycemia, lipolysis, and breakdown of muscle to provide protein substrate.[72] Catabolic stimulation and hypoxemia impair wound healing[73-80] and increase the risk of wound infection (see Wound Healing, Chapter 17). All may contribute to fatigue and prolonged convalescence.[81]

A considerable amount of effort has been focused on evaluating the effects of pain on immune function. Altered immune function has been attributed to direct CNS innervation of the immune system, to stress-elicited changes in circulating levels of hormones, and to stress-elicited coping behaviors (e.g., smoking, poor diet, and alcohol use) that can further diminish immune response. (For reviews of this topic, see references 82, 83, and 84.) Findings from a number of studies suggest that stressful experiences are associated with quantitative and functional changes in immune parameters such as decreases in the number of cytotoxic T cells (CD8 lymphocytes) and a reduction in neutrophil phagocytic activity.[85] These important cellular components of the immune system are responsible for destroying viral and bacterial invaders.

Pain has been shown to suppress natural killer cell activity,[86,87] which performs a critical function in the immune system by destroying cancer cells before they have a chance to proliferate. Studies with rats found that the tumor-enhancing effects of pain were significantly reduced in animals who received morphine following a surgical procedure compared with the animals who did not receive morphine.[88] The exact mechanisms by which pain effects the immune system are not completely understood. Further research is needed to elucidate the mechanisms involved and their implications for health and illness.

Acute pain is the greatest risk factor for the development of debilitating pathophysiological chronic pain. Rather than tissue damage, nerve damage is the most common underlying cause of persistent chronic pain syndromes.[89] Pain of this nature is also called neuropathic pain. Persistent pain can have an inflammatory cause as well, resulting from peripheral tissue damage and inflammation that lead to changes in neural afferent activity, neuromediator release, and structural alterations.[90-92] Two kinds of pathophysiological modifications in the responsiveness of the nervous system result in persistent pain: peripheral sensitization (i.e., a reduction in the threshold of nociceptor afferent peripheral terminals in the area of the injury) and central sensitization (i.e., an activity-dependent increase in the excitability of spinal neurons).[93] Together, these changes contribute to a postinjury hypersensitivity state that manifests itself as an increase in the neural responses to noxious stimuli and as a decrease in pain threshold.

Persistent pain syndromes are also associated with injuries that result in an absence of nociceptive input from the periphery or the spinal cord. Examples include phantom pain, pain experienced by paraplegics below the level of a total spinal cord transection, and pain that results from normally nonnoxious stimuli, such as touch.[94]

Another example of pain experienced as a result of the loss of sensory input into the CNS is deafferentation pain. Deafferentation pain can occur as a result of avulsion of a peripheral or central nerve, such as when dorsal roots are traumatically severed from the cord. Even though nociceptive signals are unable to be conducted directly with the cord and travel to the brain, the patient often feels excruciating pain.[95]

Chronic, intractable pain can also result from spontaneous lesions in nociceptive pathways in the CNS. For example, thalamic syndrome is the term used to describe pain caused by lesions in the thalamus. The thalamus functions as a "central relay station" that directs and modulates neural signal transmissions to and from other parts of the brain. Thalamic lesions are the source of severe, poorly localized pain as well as other noxious sensations that are completely independent of where the sensation is actually felt in the body.[95] Although thalamic syndrome is the most frequently observed central pain syndrome,[96] lesions can occur in other ascending nociceptive pathways as well.

Persistent pain results in major changes in neural synaptic and neurotransmitter profiles that expand or contract based on sensory input. These changes result in a change in the biochemistry as well as the function of affected sensory neurons, resulting in a very different nervous system than existed before the original painful stimulus.

RELATED PATHOPHYSIOLOGICAL CONCEPTS

Unrelieved pain results not only in the development and maintenance of persistent pain, but also in a range of comorbid pathophysiological responses.[97] Short-term pathophysiological consequences may include fatigue and sleep disturbances as well as acute anxiety disorders, while long-term consequences may include depression and PTSD.

Fatigue and Sleep Disturbance

Fatigue and sleep disturbances can occur with both acute and chronic pain and can disrupt the patient's ability to function physically and cognitively. Clinical studies have supported a relationship between pain, fatigue, and sleeplessness. For example, fatigue accompanied and followed episodes of pain in patients with chronic back pain and was related to pain intensity.[98] Both fatigue and sleep disturbances can have a negative impact on the patient's mood and quality of life.[99] Treatments for pain, fatigue, and sleep disturbances may include the use of analgesics, tricyclic antidepressants, and aerobic fitness programs.[100]

Fear and Anxiety

The function of acute pain is to warn the body of impending danger. Therefore the natural responses to the system are fear and anxiety. However, there are clear differences between these two responses. Fear is an alarm reaction to an immediate threat that typically results in sympathetic nervous system (SNS) arousal and the desire to escape.[101] Anxiety is an emotion associated with negative affect and apprehensive anticipation of potential threats. The anxious individual is hypervigilant and has increased muscle tension. There is a clear relationship between anxiety and pain report.[102] However, fear and anxiety have different effects on human pain thresholds. Anxiety appeared to induce hyperalgesia, while fear increased pain thresholds and induced analgesia.[103] These findings have clinical implications. That is, patients who are fearful when exposed to a threatening event may have less pain than patients who are anxious because of anticipation of an unpredictable, threatening event.

Depression

"If pain persists and treatment fails, it is not surprising that depression sets in."[104] As obvious as this statement may appear, depression has a close relationship with chronic pain, and this relationship remains a source of controversy within the medical community. What is not in dispute, however, is that depression is extremely common in patients suffering from chronic pain disorders.[105-113] In fact, the preponderance of evidence linking depression and chronic pain has led some researchers to postulate there is a causal relationship between the two symptoms.[105,114] For example, Nesse[115] theorized that depression and chronic pain share common biochemical pathways that have evolved as a result of dysregulation of adaptive responses over time.

Traditionally, speculation as to the comorbidity between depression and chronic nonmalignant pain disorders (CNPDs) fell into two distinct theoretical camps: psychological or biological. For example, Eisendrath[116] viewed chronic pain as a psychiatric problem because of its frequent association with psychiatric disorders such as somatization, hypochondriasis, factitious physical illnesses, and pain related to psychosocial problems. In contrast, Ruolf[117] suggested a physiological basis for the comorbidity of depression and pain. He claimed that 50% of chronic pain sufferers also suffer from depression because depression and chronic pain share common biological pathways. Recently, it was proposed that different hypotheses may apply to different types of CNPDs and different types of depression.[107] To date, no hypotheses have earned widespread support for any specific causal relationship.

Posttraumatic Stress Disorder

As noted earlier, chronic pain was found to be a risk factor for posttraumatic stress disorder (PTSD).[118] Estimates are high for patients referred for psychological treatment of chronic pain, with 50% reported to have PTSD.[119] In one of the few studies that compared PTSD and chronic pain in injured workers (n = 139), 95.2% were found to be in pain and 34.7% were diagnosed with PTSD.[20] These findings suggest that PTSD is a significant aspect of the clinical presentation of injured workers in chronic pain.[20]

MANIFESTATIONS AND SURVEILLANCE

Verbal Manifestations

The most valid and reliable indicator of pain is the patient's self-report of the pain experience. To determine the cause of the pain, patients should be asked to provide the following information about the pain problem: description of the pain, location and radiation of the pain, severity of the pain, aggravating and relieving factors, and previous treatment modalities and their effectiveness. In most instances, ongoing assessments of the patient's pain can be accomplished by asking the patient to rate the intensity/severity of the pain using a 0 to 10 numeric rating scale. The following question can be asked "On a scale of 0 to 10, with 0 being 'no pain' and 10 being 'the worst pain you can imagine,' how much do you hurt right now (on average, at its worst)? Published pain guidelines[14,120] include many examples of self-report pain instruments. The important point is to choose age-, language-, and situation-appropriate pain rating scales to assure accurate and consistent evaluations. (Table12-1 lists examples of pain self-report instruments.)

Behavioral Responses to Pain

Behaviors associated with pain are both conscious and unconscious, including characteristic facial expressions and varying degrees of movement or immobilization of torso and limbs. Several sophisticated observational techniques and rating scales have been developed to assess objective behaviors that accompany a pain experience.[124,125] Concordance between patients' ratings of their pain and evaluations by health care professionals who observed patients' behaviors were shown to be modestly low.[126,127] One cause for this discrepancy is that patients do not always exhibit painful behaviors, because there are individual variations in responses to pain.[128]

Conversely, patient behaviors may be exaggerated, leading health care professionals to disregard their validity as pain indicators. Concordance between patients and health professionals can be improved when health professionals use a structured, systematic method of pain assessment that includes observation of behavioral signs of

TABLE 12-1 Valid and Reliable Pain Measurement Tools*

AGE GROUP	APPROPRIATE PAIN ASSESSMENT TOOL	ASSESSMENT INFORMATION
Adults	Numerical rating scales (most frequently used—may also be used to measure emotional dimension; e.g., level of distress in response to pain) Visual analogue scales (Huskisson, 1974)† Word descriptor scales	Subjective, quantitative measure of pain severity
	McGill Pain Questionnaire (Melzack, 1983)‡	Multidimensional—includes sensory, emotional and cognitive dimensions of pain, as well as location
Elderly adults	Numerical rating scales	Unidimensional
	Faces pain rating scale (Herr, Mobily, Kohout, & Wagenaar, 1998)§	(sensory dimension)—subjective, quantitative measure of pain severity

*Broken lines indicate a potential overlap (i.e., the same information may or may not be applicable, depending on age and/or use of instrument).
†Adapted from Huskisson, E.C. (1974). Measurement of pain. *Lancet ii, 1127-1131.*
‡Melzack, R. (1983). The McGill Pain Questionnaire. In Melzack, R. (ed.), *Pain Measurement and Assessment* (pp. 41-47). New York: Raven Press.
§Herr, K.A., Mobily, P.R., Kohout, F.J., & Wagner, D. (1998). Evaluation of the Faces Pain Scale for use with the elderly. *The Clinical Journal of Pain 14,* 29-38.

pain.[129,130] Moderate to strong correlations were found between ICU nurses' ratings of patients' pain and the patients' own pain intensity ratings after a structured pain assessment tool was used to assess the patients' pain. This assessment tool included behavioral and physiological signs of pain.[129] Using multiple measures of pain can provide a more complete picture of the total pain experience.

Physiological Responses to Pain

Acute pain often activates a sudden SNS response that includes elevation of heart and respiratory rates and blood pressure, pallor, perspiration, flushing, pupil dilation, and drops in levels of transcutaneous oxygen saturation lasting a few minutes to an hour. Very intense and brief pain can be followed by a rebound parasympathetic nervous system response. SNS and PNS responses to pain can become dampened over time and, thus, not present even though pain persists.[131] Physiological responses are influenced by attention, habituation, distraction, or predictability.[132,133] Because the physiological responses are not unique to pain, they should be evaluated within the context of other pain measures such as the patient's own report or behavioral signs of pain as well as the patient's clinical situation.[128] For example, it is reasonable to assume that increased heart rate and blood pressure during a painful procedure are correlates of the patient's pain and should be assumed to be pain indicators.

Differential Diagnosis

Pain is a multidimensional experience, and it is essential to evaluate each of the dimensions during a comprehensive pain assessment. This would include, whenever possible, the patient's self-report of pain intensity and its location; its onset and duration; and its associated distress. Recent recommendations regarding categorizing pain according to possible mechanisms, such as tissue pain or nervous system pain,[3] provide the clinician a classification system to aid in differential diagnosis. For example, patients' descriptions can lead the clinician to differentiate the mechanism according to tissue injury pain or nervous system injury pain. The language used by patients to describe their pain also helps to differentiate among pain causes and sequelae. For example, peripheral nerve injury is often characterized as having a burning quality, while visceral pain is frequently described as stabbing or cramping.[128] Even in the same patients, pain quality words can differ according to the type of pain being experienced. Patients undergoing procedures most frequently described their procedure-related pain as sharp, stinging, stabbing, shooting, and awful, while they described their baseline (i.e., preprocedural) pain most often as aching, tender, and dull.[37] These examples emphasize the importance of conducting a comprehensive pain assessment to make the differential diagnosis of the etiology of the pain.

Age and Cultural-Related Issues

The elderly and patients for whom English is not their primary language[131] are less able to advocate for themselves because they cannot, or do not, communicate their pain treatment needs. Therefore age and cultural-related issues increase the vulnerability of certain patients to suffer needless pain. This communication problem is of particular concern because the very young and the very old are most at risk for increased morbidity and mortality as a result of the pathophysiological consequences of pain.[66,68] Recognition of the special needs of these patients can help nurses to provide effective pain management.

Elderly patients present unique challenges to obtaining an accurate pain assessment upon which to base analgesic treatment. For example, elderly patients often minimize their complaints of pain because they confuse the pain of interest with pain associated with aging and/or other health problems. In addition, elderly patients are reluctant to report symptoms of pain because they believe their complaints are bothersome to nurses.[135] Moreover, visual, hearing, and psychomotor impairment that is common in the elderly frequently interfere with comprehension and effective use of a pain scale.[14,136] Vision difficulties may be reduced by providing additional lighting, a magnifying glass, and/or by using an enlarged version of a pain assessment tool. Creating a quiet environment with as few distractions as possible will result in a more accurate pain assessment at any age. In addition, using a tool that is compatible with the patient's physical capabilities will reduce problems related to psychomotor impairment. Because of problems with memory and abstraction,[137] elderly patients often require more time to master a new skill. Careful and gentle repetitive explanations when introducing a pain assessment method should result in increased comprehension and thus more accurate findings on which to base a pain management plan.

Effective analgesia in this vulnerable patient population is particularly challenging but also particularly important in order to decrease suffering and prevent pathophysiological consequences of pain. Determining the most effective course of analgesia requires reliable assessment which can and must be obtained despite the challenges posed by patients at the extreme ends of the age spectrum.

It is well established that cultural attitudes toward pain vary widely from one cultural group to another.[138] What is less understood, however, is that greater individual differences exist *within* ethnic communities than *between* them.[139-141] Therefore assessing a patient's pain based on cultural bias (e.g., stereotyping) is harmful at worst and inaccurate at best. As shown in Box 12-1, the single most reliable method of determining the existence, and severity, of the patient's pain is self-report.[142] All pain tools, however, are to a certain degree language dependent. Thus establishing an effective method of pain assessment is essential to provide quality nursing care. Most importantly, recognizing and respecting different cultural attitudes toward pain and establishing

BOX 12-1 Hierarchy of Reliability and Validity of Basic Measures of Pain Intensity

1. Patient's self-report using a pain rating scale, such as the Numerical Rating Scale (NRS), Visual Analogue Scale (VAS), McGill Pain Questionnaire (Melzack, 1983).
2. Pathological conditions or procedures that usually cause pain.
3. Behaviors (e.g., facial expressions, body movements, crying).
4. Report of pain from parent, family, or others close to patient. These individuals may be asked to give proxy pain ratings—guesses about the intensity of the patient's pain.
5. Physiological measures. These are the least sensitive indicators of pain.

Adapted from McCaffrey, M., & Pasero, C. (1999). *Pain: Clinical manual* (p. 95). St. Louis: Mosby.
Information from Acute Pain Management Guideline Panel. (1992). *Acute pain management in adults: Operative procedures*. Quick reference guide for clinicians, AHCPR Pub. No. 92-0019, Rockville, Md.: Agency for Health Care Policy and Research, Public Health Service, U.S. Department of Health and Human Services; Acute Pain Management Guideline Panel. (1992). *Acute pain management in infants, children and adolescents*: Operative and medical procedures. Quick reference guide for clinicians, AHCPR Pub. No. 92-0020, Rockville, Md.: Agency for Health Care Policy and Research, Public Health Service, U.S. Department of Health and Human Services; and McGrath, P.J., Beyer, J., Cleeland, C., Eland, J., McGrath, P.A., & Portenoy, R. (1990). American Academy of Pediatrics Report of the Subcommittee on Assessment and Methodological Issues in the Management of Pain in Childhood Cancer. *Pediatrics 86*(Suppl 5), 814-817.

treatment goals consistent with those attitudes will help address pain more effectively, diminish pathophysiological consequences of the pain, and improve outcomes[147] (see Box 12-1).

CLINICAL MANAGEMENT

In 1992, postoperative pain management guidelines disseminated throughout the United States stressed the importance of aggressive attention to pain management after surgery.[14] They outlined recommendations for proper pain assessment, use of specific analgesics as well as nonpharmacological interventions, and patient preparation as active participants in pain management plans. While there is evidence of certain benefits derived from use of these guidelines,[148] improvement in short-term and long-term outcomes of postoperative pain still falls short of being optimal.

Pharmacological

The effective management of acute and chronic pain often requires the use of analgesic medications. The number of pain medications and the types of formulations for pain medications has grown exponentially in the past several years. Traditionally, pain medications were divided into nonopioid, opioid, and adjuvant analgesics. Current approaches group analgesics based on their pharmacological class or their mechanism of action (e.g., acetaminophen, aspirin, nonsteroidal antiinflammatory drugs [NSAIDs], opioids, antidepressants, anticonvulsants, and oral local anesthetics).

Acetaminophen, aspirin, and the NSAIDs are a diverse group of compounds that share certain pharmacological and therapeutic properties. They exert their analgesic effect primarily through actions in the peripheral nervous system. Aspirin and the nonselective NSAIDs produce their analgesic effects by inhibiting the action of the enzyme cyclooxygenase and decreasing the production of prostaglandins. Prostaglandins are the chemical mediators produced during tissue injury that activate primary afferent nociceptors.[149]

One of the recent developments in the pharmacological management of pain is the discovery that two forms of cyclooxygenase exist, namely cyclooxygenase-1 (COX-1) and cyclooxygenase-2 (COX-2). The COX-1 enzyme is constitutive and produces prostaglandins with physiologically protective functions (e.g., thromboxane for platelets, PGI_2 for the gastrointestinal mucosa, and PGE_2 for renal function).[150,151] During inflammation, the inducible form of the enzyme (i.e., COX-2) is produced in macrophages by cytokines and also by nitric oxide. Nonselective NSAIDs inhibit both of these isoenzymes. Inhibition of the COX-1 enzyme with nonselective NSAIDs is associated with an increased incidence of gastric and renal side effects. However, inhibition of the COX-2 enzyme with either nonselective NSAIDs or selective COX-2 antagonists produces analgesic effects. The new selective COX-2 antagonists have the same analgesic potency as the nonselective NSAIDs already in use, but they have a reduced side effect profile.[150,151]

Opioid analgesics exert their analgesic effects by binding to opioid receptors located in supraspinal, spinal, and peripheral sites. They hyperpolarize the neural membrane by potassium current activation or through suppression of calcium currents. These actions block neurotransmitter release and pain transmission.[152]

A large number of opioid analgesics are available for the management of acute and chronic pain (e.g., morphine, fentanyl, hydromorphone, methadone, and oxycodone). The management of acute pain is best accomplished with the use of short-acting opioid analgesics (e.g., codeine, fentanyl, hydromorphone, and morphine). By contrast, the management of chronic pain that requires opioid analgesics is best accomplished with the use of long-acting formulations (e.g., sustained-release morphine or oxycodone preparations, methadone, levorphanol, or transdermal fentanyl). The effective management of acute or chronic pain with an opioid analgesic requires that opioids be titrated to achieve the optimal analgesic effect with minimal side effects. One must remember that the optimal dose of an opioid analgesic varies widely among individuals. Therefore clinicians must pay careful attention to the titration of opioid analgesics.

For the management of acute pain problems, opioid analgesics should be administered on a regular schedule for the first 36 hours following a surgical procedure that is anticipated to require opioid analgesia for at least 48 hours. This approach will avoid the long delays that are associated with "as needed" administration of opioids.

A mainstay approach to the management of chronic pain, particularly chronic pain caused by cancer or other chronic medical conditions, is to administer opioid analgesics on a regular schedule. This approach maintains an adequate level of the analgesic in the patient's bloodstream. Patients who are placed on an around-the-clock dosing schedule should have orders for supplemental doses of opioids (i.e., short-acting opioid preparations) as a backup for their regularly scheduled analgesics. In addition, patients on an around-the-clock dosing schedule should be monitored for the development of tolerance. One of the first signs that a patient is developing tolerance is that he or she will report that the duration of analgesia has shortened.

Opioid analgesics produce a fairly consistent profile of side effects, including constipation, sedation, nausea and vomiting, pruritus, urinary retention, and respiratory depression. Tolerance develops to all of the side effects of opioid analgesics except constipation. Clinicians should anticipate the development of opioid-induced side effects and treat them prophylactically.

A complete discussion of the other types of analgesic medications (e.g., antidepressants, anticonvulsants, and oral local anesthetics) is beyond the scope of this chapter. Many of these drugs are used to manage neuropathic pain. In addition, many of these drugs are added to an analgesic regimen to enhance the effectiveness of other types of analgesics.

Nonpharmacological Management

The gate control theory of pain[53] provides a theoretical basis for some nonpharmacological interventions for pain. These interventions are proposed to either inhibit or modulate the ascending transmission of a noxious stimulus from the periphery or stimulate descending inhibitory control from the brain. For example, cognitive-behavioral interventions can influence the pain experience through activation of the descending neural pathways from higher brain centers that are responsible for cognition and affect, which will block pain transmission from the spinal cord area.[153] Such therapies include those that address pain coping, self-efficacy, and fear-avoidance belief.

Physical interventions, such as cutaneous stimulation through rubbing, massage, or electrical nerve stimulation, are proposed to block transmission of noxious stimuli along peripheral-to–spinal cord fibers. Peripherally applied heat causes local vasodilation that promotes circulatory removal of biomediators of pain from the site of injury, whereas cold application decreases release of pain-inducing chemicals.[154]

A review of nonpharmacological intervention studies is useful for making informed practice decisions. Keefe[153] provided an overview of studies that tested the effectiveness of cognitive-behavioral therapies (CBT) for chronic pain. Patients in these studies had received psychological interventions, such as training in pain coping, imagery, distraction, relaxation training, and communication skills. While this review did not provide extensive detail of each study, Keefe noted that outcomes for patients having received CBT were statistically and clinically superior to those of control group patients who did not receive CBT interventions.

Although nurses often use nonpharmacological interventions for the management of pain, evidence from research studies is limited. Sindhu[155] conducted a metaanalysis of nursing studies that examined nonpharmacological interventions for acute pain. She selected 49 studies from a total of 3166 abstracts reviewed, although reasons for selection were not reported. Most selected studies examined the effects of relaxation, patient teaching, and visual imagery on pain intensity. There was some evidence of a reduction in pain intensity scores in patients who received relaxation therapy or patient teaching compared with patients in the control groups. Although a pooled effect size of 0.06 was determined, there was strong heterogeneity among the effect sizes of the individual studies. The heterogeneity of samples and statistical analysis procedures limited interpretation of the findings.

A metaanalysis of 98 intervention studies tested the effects of psychoeducational care provided to adults with cancer on seven outcomes, one of which was pain.[156] Very specific study inclusion and exclusion criteria were reported. Experimental treatment groups received education, nonbehavioral/noncognitive counseling, behavioral/cognitive counseling, or a combination of these interventions. A positive treatment effect was demonstrated in 92% of the studies in which pain was measured (n = 13). A relaxation intervention had the largest and most homogeneous effect on pain, as opposed to education only or multiple behavioral strategies with or without education.

In another metaanalysis of the effect of interventions on symptom management in cancer patients, 28 randomized experimental and control group studies were analyzed.[157] Of these 28 studies, four evaluated the effects of nonpharmacological interventions on pain. One of the studies tested the effects of relaxation on pain but showed no improvement in pain scores. The other three studies showed 77% and 80% improvement rates for music and an 87% improvement rate for massage.

Relaxation strategies are often a part of multimodal chronic pain management. The effectiveness of these strategies was evaluated by a systematic review of nine studies involving 414 patients who met predefined inclusion criteria. These criteria included the use of a randomized controlled trial methodology and the use of relaxation only as the intervention.[158] There was a heterogeneity of chronic pain states that included rheumatoid arthritis, ulcerative colitis, and cancer. Only three of the nine studies showed statistically significant differences in pain scores in favor of relaxation compared with the control groups. Based on these findings, there is insufficient evidence to confirm that relaxation can reduce chronic pain.

The variability in research findings reported here demonstrates the lack of sufficient evidence at this time for the universal effectiveness of nonpharmacological interventions for pain. However, until more definitive research is forthcoming, the use of nonpharmacological interventions, either alone or as analgesic adjuncts, should be encouraged if they are appropriate for and acceptable to the patient. Table 12-2 gives examples of nonpharmacological interventions recommended for managing postoperative pain.[14] Published guidelines for cancer pain management[120] include the following recommendations concerning some interventions that have the strongest scientific evidence:

- Psychosocial interventions should be introduced early in the course of a cancer-related illness but should not be a substitute for analgesic therapy
- Patients with cancer pain should be encouraged to remain active and to participate in self-care when possible
- Prolonged immobilization should be avoided whenever possible to prevent untoward effects, such as deconditioning and joint contractures
- Education about pain, its treatments, and the ability to control it effectively should be part of every patient's treatment plan

Although not all of these recommendations have a strong research basis, the acute and cancer pain guidelines[14,120] represent the current state of knowledge regarding effective and appropriate care. The advantages of nonpharmacological interventions for pain are that they are noninvasive, usually uncomplicated in their administration, and often economical. Patients may be taught to use many of them independent of caregivers' assistance. Although nurses have for some time integrated nonpharmacological therapies into the care of patients with pain, now the use of such therapies is more acceptable to the medical community, and these are considered part of informed, responsible practice. Of a group of 362 pain specialists who responded to a survey, 80% reported using or referring patients for counseling/psychotherapy. More than 65% did the same for use of electromagnetic applications, such as transcutaneous electrical nerve stimulation (TENS), exercise interventions, and acupuncture. More than 80% of those practitioners considered use of those therapies to be a legitimate part of medical practice.[159]

Management by Family Caregivers

Family caregivers are involved in all aspects of pain management. Family caregivers have similar fears and concerns as patients about the use of pain medication (e.g., fears of addiction, fears about the development of tolerance, and fears about the side effects of pain management), particularly opioid analgesics. These fears and concerns can pose significant barriers to effective pain management. Research has shown that family caregivers tend to overestimate the amount of pain that their family member is experiencing.[160] This finding should be considered when clinicians need to rely on the family member's report of pain when the patient is not able to provide a self-report of pain intensity.

Clinicians need to include family members in all teaching sessions regarding pain management. Family members should be taught how to assess the

TABLE 12-2 Examples of Nonpharmacological Interventions for Postoperative Pain Recommended for Use by the Acute Pain Management Guideline Panel

COGNITIVE-BEHAVIORAL	PHYSICAL AGENTS
Education/instruction	Applications of heat or cold
Relaxation	Massage, exercise, and immobilization
Imagery	Transcutaneous electrical nerve stimulation
Biofeedback	

From Acute Pain Management Guideline Panel. (1992). *Acute pain management: Operative or medical procedures and trauma.* Clinical Practice Guidelines (AHCPR Pub. No. 92-0032). Rockville, Md.: Agency for Health Care Policy and Research, Public Health Service, U.S. Department of Health and Human Services.

patient's pain and how to help the patient keep a pain management diary. In addition, family caregivers should be taught about the mechanism of action of the pain medication, the dosing schedule, and how to treat side effects of pain medications. Clinicians need to discuss with patients and their family caregivers the meanings of tolerance, physical dependence, and psychological addiction. Fears and barriers should be discussed and a plan developed to optimize the management of the patient's pain.

CASE STUDY

Pain Problem. TP, a 39-year-old white man was admitted to the hospital with a pneumothorax and fractured pelvis after a motor vehicle crash. He had a history of HIV and used 120 mg of oral slow-release morphine daily over the past 6 months for associated pain. He appeared calm, but his pupils were dilated, he was diaphoretic, slightly tachycardic, and picked nervously at the sheets as he reported his pain to be a 12/10 on the 0 to 10 numerical rating scale (NRS). After evaluation in the emergency department (ED), a bolus of 5 mg of morphine was given IV. Morphine patient-controlled analgesia (PCA) was initiated at a dose of 1 mg per dose, with an 8-minute lockout and a 4-hour limit of 30 mg per standard protocol. A chest tube was placed, and he was scheduled to have the fracture surgically reduced with placement of an external fixation device later that day. Before surgery, he made multiple attempts on the PCA. The patient's partner was present, and both he and the patient were voicing concerns about the postoperative pain management plan.

Pain Management. A pain management planning conference was held before surgery involving the surgeon, anesthesiologist, the nurse and physician on the acute pain service acute pain service, the patient care nurse, the patient, and his partner. Three problems were identified: (1) opiate tolerance and withdrawal risk; (2) risk of postoperative atelectasis and pneumonia caused by discomfort on coughing, deep breathing, and turning; and (3) postoperative pain from surgical reduction of the fracture and incisional site. The patient and his partner were assured that all three problems were recognized and would be treated.

It was decided to address the first two problems immediately by initiating a continuous IV infusion of midazolam 2 mg/ml and morphine 10 mg/ml. The rate of each was titrated to produce a relaxed, alert state with an absence of withdrawal symptoms (e.g., dilated pupils, nervous behavior, diaphoresis, and tachycardia). The patient and his partner were reassured that these medications would be provided continuously, not dependent on a report of pain.

After surgery, the midazolam and morphine infusions were restarted at the preoperative levels and the patient was extubated and transferred to the critical care unit for observation before being transferred to the surgical acute care unit the following day. Once he was alert, the patient reported his pain to be a 10/10, but he appeared to be relaxed, remained alert while awake, and was able to turn, cough, and deep breathe easily with assistance. On the fifth postoperative day, the morphine and midazolam infusions were replaced with equivalent doses of oral methadone and lorazepam. A plan was made to taper their use. The opioid equivalency dose was decreased by no more than 20% every 3 days until he could safely resume taking his preoperative analgesic medication, and the lorazepam was discontinued. He was discharged and followed in the clinic until his preoperative analgesic plan of 120 mg of continuous-release oral morphine could be resumed, at which time he was referred back to his regular physician for follow-up.

Analysis. This patient with a traumatic injury requiring surgical intervention had chronic pain because of his HIV and tolerance to opioids and thus presented a challenging pain problem. High subjective reports of pain were difficult to assess. Yet it was clear to the staff that the patient was in need of maintenance analgesia while in the hospital. Having this insight helped the team to resist labeling the patient as a "drug-seeker" and enabled them to focus on his medical problems in a holistic and supportive manner. Also, the additional acute pain resulting from trauma and subsequent surgical intervention represented a legitimate need for effective pain relief. The amount of opioids administered to the patient in the ED were subtherapeutic, given his history and injuries. However, the team's approach became more aggressive as they planned preoperative and postoperative analgesic coverage. Initiating an anxiolytic agent in combination with the PCA helped to not only decrease the patient's anxiety but to decrease his perception of pain. Using a PCA device afforded the patient increased control in an environment in which he had little control and made delivery of his analgesic independent of self-reports of pain. With continuous IV analgesic delivery for immediate preoperative and postoperative pain management, the patient was able to focus on tasks related to his recovery and sleep without worrying that he would wake up in severe pain. These practical, effective solutions to each of his pain problems signaled that the team took his complaint of pain seriously. Having demonstrated that his pain was a high priority helped to increase the patient's and his partner's satisfaction with his plan of care. With a coordinated multidisciplinary team effort, identification of individual problems, and a sound plan to treat them, this patient received the support he needed from a group of health care professionals dedicated to the relief of his pain.

SELECTED RESEARCH

Genetic research will dominate basic science pain research in the coming decade. The cloning of familiar as well as new opioid receptors[161] will further facilitate this task. In addition, future research will add to the knowledge of specific "neurochemical signatures" for each type of acute and persistent pain.[162-165] Identifying similar neurochemical signatures in the future will provide insight into novel therapeutic targets for the prevention of both acute and chronic pain.

Recent research by Gear et al[166-169] documented sex differences in responses to analgesic medications. In a series of studies, the responses of men and women who had undergone surgery for removal of impacted third molars were evaluated following the administration of opioid analgesics that have activity at the kappa opioid receptor. The analgesics that were tested in these experiments included pentazocine, nalbuphine, and butorphanol. In all of these studies, women reported significantly greater analgesic effects with these opioids compared with men. In fact, when nalbuphine was administered to men in a dose of 5 mg, it actually produced antianalgesic effects (i.e., the men who received the nalbuphine experienced more pain when compared with men who had received a placebo). This research on sex differences in analgesic responses has opened up an entire field of research in this area. Undoubtedly, these findings and the findings from future studies will result in the development of sex-specific strategies for pain management.

Diagnostic- or treatment-related procedural pain is ubiquitous in clinical practice and deserves nursing attention. Puntillo et al conducted a comprehensive examination of procedural pain in the American Association of Critical Care Nurses (AACN)–sponsored Thunder Project II.[37,170] Data were obtained from 6201 patients in 164 national and five international sites. Patients had undergone one of six procedures: wound care, wound drain removal, tracheal suctioning, turning, central venous catheter insertion, and femoral sheath removal. They documented that the most painful and distressing procedure was turning and the least painful procedure was femoral sheath removal, and the least distressful was central venous catheter insertion.[37] Less than 20% of patients received opiates before procedures. In an extensive analysis of analgesic practices associated with these procedures, the researchers reported that the likelihood of receiving opioids was a factor of preprocedure pain intensity, having a femoral sheath removed, being white, and procedure duration. Those less likely to receive opioids had a medical diagnosis or were patients being tracheally suctioned.[163] Findings from the Thunder Project II provide an extensive foundation for future intervention studies for procedural pain.

QUESTIONS FOR FUTURE STUDY

Nursing research will continue to identify practical interventions employing the skillful and humanistic application of scientific knowledge to affect desired results in caring for patients.[171] Questions to be answered in the future include how best to expand on the growing body of knowledge related to the assessment of pain in patients with communication barriers. These include patients who are critically ill, elderly persons, those with dementia, and those who do not speak the same language as their health care providers. Work will continue to refine the combination of opioid and nonopioid balanced modes of treatment with complementary nonpharmacological analgesic nursing interventions.

Nursing research is needed to identify optimal patient and family education regarding how best to prepare patients to communicate their pain and how to administer treatment interventions accurately. Research is also needed to determine the best use of treatment modalities to optimize therapeutic benefits while minimizing untoward effects. Research will continue to explore the different gender and ethnic responses to analgesic interventions. Nurses will contribute to the comfort of patients at end-of-life by examining "best practices" regarding pain assessment and treatment across patient populations and clinical settings. These types of research endeavors will highlight nursing's unique ability to help the person in pain.

REFERENCES

1. McCaffery, M. (1979). *Nursing management of the patient with pain* (p. 11). Philadelphia: J.B. Lippincott.
2. International Association for Study of Pain. (1979). Pain terms: A list with definitions and notes on usage. *Pain 6,* 249-252.
3. Woolf, C.J., Bennett, G.J., Doherty, M., Dubner, R., Kidd, B., Koltzenburg, M., et al. (1998). Towards a mechanism-based classification of pain? *Pain 77,* 227-229.
4. American Hospital Association. (1994). *Guide to the health care field.* Chicago: Author.
5. Jacox, A., Ferrell, B., Heidrich, G., Hester, N, & Miaskowski, C. (1992). A guideline for the nation: Managing acute pain. *American Journal of Nursing 1992,* 49-55.
6. Jurf, J.B., & Nirschl, A. (1993). Acute postoperative pain management: A comprehensive review and update. *Critical Care Nursing Quarterly 16,* 8-25.
7. Kitson, A. (1994). Post-operative pain management: A literature review. *Journal of Clinical Nursing 3,* 7-18.

8. Tittle, M.B., & McMillan, S.C. (1994). Pain and pain-related side effects in an ICU and on a surgical unit: Nurses' management. *American Journal of Critical Care 3,* 25-30.
9. Puntillo, K.A. (1990). The pain experiences of intensive care unit patients. *Heart & Lung 19*(5), 526-533.
10. Puntillo, K.A., & Weiss, S.J. (1994). Pain: Its mediators and associated morbidity in critically ill cardiovascular surgical patients. *Nursing Research 43*(1), 31-36.
11. Lay, T.D., Puntillo, K.A., Miaskowski, C., & Wallhagen, M. (1996). Analgesics prescribed and administered to intensive care cardiac surgery patients: Does patient age make a difference? *Progress in Cardiovascular Nursing 11*(4), 17-24.
12. Kehlet, H. (1999). Acute pain control and accelerated postoperative surgical recovery. *Surgical Clinics of North America 79*(2), 431-443.
13. Brooks-Brunn, J.A. (1995). Postoperative atelectasis and pneumonia: Risk factors. *American Journal of Critical Care 4,* 340-349.
14. Acute Pain Management Guideline Panel. (1992). Acute pain management: Operative or medical procedures and trauma. Clinical Practice Guideline No. 1, AHCPR Publication No. 92-0032. Rockville, Md.: Department of Health and Human Services, Public Health Services.
15. Department of Health and Human Services. (1991). Vital and health statistics: Detailed diagnoses and procedures, National discharge summary 1988. Hyattsville, Md.: U.S. Department of Health and Human Services; Series 13, No. 107.
16. Yates, D.A., & Smith, M.A. (1994). Orthopaedic pain after trauma. In P.D. Wall & R. Melzack (eds.), *Textbook of pain* (3rd ed., pp. 409-421). Edinburgh: Churchill Livingstone.
17. Melzack, R., Wall, P.D., & Ty, T.C. (1982). Acute pain in an emergency clinic: Latency of onset and descriptor patterns related to different injuries. *Pain 14,* 33-43.
18. Mackersie, R.C., & Karagianes, T.G. (1990). Pain management following trauma and burns. *Critical Care Clinics 6,* 433-449.
19. Geisser, M.E., Roth, R.S., Bachman, J.E., & Eckert, T.A. (1996). The relationship between symptoms of post-traumatic stress disorder and pain, affective disturbance and disability among patients with accident and non-accident related pain. *Pain 66,* 207-214.
20. Asmundson, G.J.G., Norton, G.R., Allerdings, M.D., Norton, P.J., & Larsen, D.K. (1998). Posttraumatic stress disorder and work-related injury. *Journal of Anxiety Disorders 12*(1), 57-69.
21. Perry, S. (1984). Pain and anxiety in the burned child. *Journal of Trauma 24,* 191-195.
22. Gilboa, D., Friedman, M., & Tsur, H. (1994). The burn as a continuous traumatic stress: Implications for emotional treatment during hospitalization. *Journal of Burn Care and Rehabilitation 15,* 86-91.
23. Ashburn, M.A. (1995). Burn pain: The management of procedure-related pain. *Journal of Burn Care and Rehabilitation 16*(3), Part 2, 365-371.
24. Baker, S.P., O'Neill, B., Ginsberg, N.J., & Li, G. (1992). *Fire, burns and lightning. The injury fact book* (2nd ed., pp. 161-173). New York: Oxford University Press.
25. Brigham, P.A., & McLoughlin, E. (1996). Burn incidence and medical care use in the United States: Estimates, trends, and data sources. *Journal of Burn Care and Rehabilitation 17*(2), 95-107.
26. Pruitt, B.A., Mason, A.D., & Goodwin, C.W. (1990). Epidemiology of burn injury and demography of burn care facilities. In D.S. Gann (ed.), *Problems in general surgery* (pp. 235-251). Philadelphia: J.B. Lippincott.
27. Hedson, D.A., Rode, H., & Bloch, C.E. (1988). Primus stove burns in Cape Town: A costly but preventable injury. *Burns 20,* 251-252.
28. Rioja, L.F., Alonso, P.E., & Soria, M.D., Redondo, A., de la Cruz, J., & de Haro, J. (1993). Incidence of ember burns in Andalusia (Spain). *Burns 19,* 220-222.
29. Iregbulem, L.M., & Nnabuko, B.E. (1993). Epidemiology of childhood thermal burns in Enugu, Nigeria. *Burns 19,* 223-226.
30. Shergill, G., Scerri, G.V., Regan, P.J., & Roberts, A.H. (1993). Burn injuries in boating accidents. *Burns 19,* 229-231.
31. Washington State Health Care Authority. (1997, unpublished). Consumer assessment of health plans, Adult survey: The Picker Institute and the University of Massachusetts Center for Survey Research. Olympia, Washington.
32. Silbert, B.S., Osgood, P.F., & Carr, D.B. (1998). Burn pain. In T.L. Yaksh, M. Maze, C.L. Lynch, J.F. Biebuyck, et al. (eds.), *Anesthesia: Biologic foundations* (pp. 759-773). Philadelphia: Lippincott-Raven.
33. Latarjet, J., & Choinère, M. (1995). Pain in burn patients. *Burns 21,* 344-348.
34. Malenfant, A., Forget, R., Papillon, J., Amsel, R., Frigon, J.Y., & Choinère, M. (1996). Prevalence and characteristics of chronic sensory problems in burn patients. *Pain 67*(2-3), 493-500.
35. Taal, L., & Faber, A.W. (1998). Posttraumatic stress and maladjustment among adult burn survivors 1 to 2 years postburn. Part II. The interview data. *Burns 24*(5), 399-405.
36. Choinière, M. (2001). Burn pain: A unique challenge. *Pain Clinical Updates IX*(1), 1-4.
37. Puntillo, K.A., White, C., Morris, A., Perdue, S., Stanik-Hutt, J., Thompson, C., et al. (2001). Patients' perceptions and responses to procedural pain: Results from Thunder II Project. *American Journal of Critical Care 10*(4), 238-251.
38. Crombie, I.K., & Davies, H.T. (1999). Requirements for epidemiological studies. In I.K. Crombie, P.R. Croft, S.J. Linton, L. LeResche, & M. Von Korff (eds.), *Epidemiology of pain.* Seattle: IASP Press.
39. Verhaak, P.F., Kerssens, J.J., Dekker, J., Sorbi, M.J., & Bensing, J.M. (1998). Prevalence of chronic pain disorder among adults: A review of the literature. *Pain 77,* 231-239.
40. Breitbart, W., Passik, S., Bronaugh, T., Zale, C., Bluestine, S., Gomez, M., et al. (1991). Pain in the ambulatory AIDS patient: Prevalence and psychosocial correlates. Poster session presented at the 38th Annual Meeting, Academy of Psychosomatic Medicine, Atlanta.
41. Dixon, P., & Higginson, I. (1991). AIDS and cancer pain treated with slow release morphine. *Postgraduate Medicine Journal 67,* S92-S94.
42. Larue, F., Fontaine, A., & Colleau, S.M. (1997). Underestimation and undertreatment of pain in HIV disease: A multicentre study. *British Medical Journal 314*(7073), 23-28.
43. Lebovits, A.H., Lefkowitz, M., McCarthy, D., Simon, R., Wilpon, H., Jung, R., & Fried, E. (1989). The prevalence and management of pain in AIDS: A review of 134 cases. *Clinical Journal of Pain 5,* 245-248.
44. McCormack, J.P., Li, R., Zarowny, D., & Singer, J. (1993). Inadequate treatment of pain in ambulatory HIV patients. *Clinical Journal of Pain 9,* 279-283.

45. Moss, V. (1990). Palliative care in advanced HIV disease: Presentation, problems, and palliation. *AIDS 4,* S235-S242.
46. Moss, V. (1991). Patient characteristics, presentation, and problems encountered in advanced AIDS in a hospice setting—a review. *Palliative Medicine 5,* 112-116.
47. Newshan, G.T., & Wainapel, S.F. (1993). Pain characteristics and their management in persons with AIDS. *Journal of the Association of Nurses in AIDS Care* *4*(2), 53-59.
48. Schofferman, J., & Brody, R. (1990). Pain in far advanced AIDS. In C.R. Chapman, & K.M. Foley (eds.), Advances in pain research and therapy (Vol. 16, pp. 379-386). New York: Raven Press.
49. Singer, E.J., Zorilla, C., Fahy-Chandon, B., Chi, S., Syndulko, K., & Tourtellotte, W.W. (1993). Painful symptoms reported by ambulatory HIV-infected men in a longitudinal study. *Pain 54,* 15-19.
50. Bonica, J.J. (1985). Treatment of cancer pain: Current status and future need. In H.L. Fields, R. Dubner, & R. Cervero (eds.), *Advances in pain research and therapy* (Vol. 9, pp. 589-616). New York: Raven Press.
51. Caraceni, A., Portenoy, R.K., a working group of the IASP Task Force on Cancer Pain. (1999). An international survey of cancer pain characteristics and syndromes. *Pain 82,* 263-274.
52. Beck, S.L. (1999). Mucositis. In C.H. Yarbro, M.H. Frogge, & M. Goodman (eds.), *Cancer symptom management* (pp. 328-343). Boston: Jones & Bartlett.
53. Melzack, R., & Wall, P. (1965). Pain mechanisms: A new theory. *Science 150*(3699), 971-978.
54. Melzack, R. (1999). From the gate to the neuromatrix. *Pain* (Suppl 6), S121-S126.
55. Fields, H.L. (1987). *Pain.* New York: McGraw-Hill.
56. Levine, J.D., & Taiwo, Y. (1994). Inflammatory pain. In P.D. Wall, & R. Melzack (eds.), *Textbook of pain* (3rd ed., pp. 45-56). London: Churchill Livingstone.
57. Neumann, S., Doubell, T.P., Leslie, T., & Woolf, C.J. (1996). Inflammatory pain hypersensitivity mediated by phenotypic switch in myelinated primary sensory neurons. *Nature 384*(6607), 360-364.
58. Besson, J.M., & Chaouch, A. (1987). Peripheral and spinal mechanisms of nociception. *Physiological Reviews* *67*(1), 67-186.
59. Dickenson, A.H. (1994). NMDA receptor antagonists as analgesics. In H.L. Fields, & J.C. Liebeskind (eds.), *Pharmacologic approaches to the treatment of chronic pain: New concepts and critical issues. Progress in pain research and management* (Vol. 1, pp. 173-187). Seattle: IASP Press.
60. Dray, A., Urban, L., & Dickenson, A. (1994). Pharmacology of chronic pain. *Trends in Pharmacologic Sciences* *15*(6), 190-197.
61. Price, D.D., Mao, J., & Meyer, D.J. (1994). Central neural mechanisms of normal and abnormal pain states. In H.L. Fields, & J.C. Liebeskind (eds.), *Pharmacologic approaches to the treatment of chronic pain: New concepts and critical issues. Progress in pain research and management* (Vol. 1, pp. 61-84). Seattle: IASP Press.
62. Markenson, J.A. (1996). Mechanisms of chronic pain. *American Journal of Medicine 101*(Suppl 1A), 65-185.
63. Chapman, C.R. (1992). Psychological aspects of postoperative pain. *Acta Anesthesiology Belgium 43,* 41-52.
64. DiPiero, V., Jones, A.K.P., Iannotti, F, et al. (1991). Chronic pain: A PET study of the central effects of percutaneous high cervical cordotomy. *Pain 46,* 9-12.
65. Iadarola, M.J., Max, M.B., Berman, K.F., Byas-Smith, M.G., Coghill, R.C., Gracely, R.H., & Bennett, G.J. (1995). Unilateral decrease in thalamic activity observed with positron emission tomography in patients with chronic neuropathic pain. *Pain 63,* 55-64.
66. Anand, K., Phil, D., & Hickely, P. (1987). Does halothane anesthesia decrease the metabolic and endocrine stress responses of newborn infants undergoing operation? *British Medical Journal 296,* 668-672.
67. Epstein, J., & Breslow, M.J. (1999). The stress response of critical illness. *Critical Care Clinics 15*(1), 17-33.
68. Yeager, M.P., Glass, D.D., Neff, R.K., & Brinck-Johnsen, T. (1987). Epidural anesthesia and analgesia in high-risk surgical patients. *Anesthesiology 66,* 729-736.
69. Halter, J.B., Pflug, A.E., & Porte, D., Jr. (1977). Mechanism of plasma catecholamine increases during surgical stress in man. *Journal of Clinical Endocrinology and Metabolism 45*(5), 936-944.
70. Akca, O., Melischek, M., Scheck, T., Hellwagner, K., Arkilic, C.F., Kurz, A., et al. (1999). Postoperative pain and subcutaneous oxygen tension. *Lancet 354*(9172), 41-42.
71. Kehlet, H. (1995). Does analgesia benefit outcome? In M.M. Parker, M.J. Shapiro, & D.T. Porembka (eds.), *Critical care, state of the art* (pp. 213-228). Anaheim, Calif.: Society of Critical Care Medicine.
72. Hedderich, R., & Ness, T.J. (1999). Analgesia for trauma and burns. *Critical Care Clinics 15*(1), 167-184.
73. Anand, K.J. (1986). The stress response to surgical trauma: From physiological basis to therapeutic implications. *Progress in Food and Nutrition Science 10*(1-2), 67-132.
74. Cousins, M., & Power, I. (1999). Acute and postoperative pain. In Wall, P.D., & Melzack, R. (eds.), *Textbook of Pain* (4th ed., pp. 447-491). Edinburgh: Churchill Livingstone.
75. Jonsson, K., Jensen, J.A., Goodson,W.H., Scheuenstuhl, H., West, J., Hopf, H.W., & Hunt, T.K. (1991). Tissue oxygenation, anaemia and perfusion in relation to wound healing in surgical patients. *Annals of Surgery 214,* 605-613.
76. Kehlet, H. (1993). General vs. regional anesthesia. In M.C. Rogers, J.H. Tinker, & B.G. Covino, (eds.), *Principals and practice of anesthesiology* (pp. 1218-1234). St Louis: Mosby.
77. Lewis, K.S., Whipple, J.K., & Michael, K.A. (1994). Effect of analgesic treatment on the physiological consequences of acute pain. *American Journal of Hospital Pharmacy 51*(12), 1539-1554.
78. Kiecolt-Glaser, J.K., Marucha, P.T., Malarkey, W.B., Mercado, A.M., & Glaser, R. (1995). Slowing of wound healing by psychological stress. *Lancet 346*(8984), 1194-1196.
79. Rosenberg, J., & Kehlet, H. (1993). Postoperative mental confusion: Association with postoperative hypoxemia. *Surgery 114,* 76.
80. Whitney, J.D., & Heitkemper, M.M. (1999). Modifying perfusion, nutrition, and stress to promote wound healing in patients with acute wounds. *Heart & Lung 28*(2), 123-133.
81. Christensen, T., & Kehlet, H. (1993). Postoperative fatigue. *World Journal of Surgery 17,* 220.
82. Herbert, T.B., & Cohen, S. (1993). Stress and immunity in humans: A meta-analytic review. *Psychosomatic Medicine 55*(4), 364-379.
83. Kiecolt-Glaser, J.K., Glaser, R. (1995). Psychoneuroimmunology and health consequences: Data and

shared mechanisms. *Psychosomatic Medicine 57*(3), 269-274.
84. Rabin, B.S. (1999). *Stress, immune function, and health: The connection.* New York: Wiley-Liss.
85. Peterson, P.K., Chao, C.C., Molitor, T., Murtaugh, M., Strgar, F., & Sharp, R.M. (1991). Stress and pathogenesis of infectious disease. *Reviews of Infectious Diseases 13,* 710-720.
86. Beilin, B., Shavit, Y., Hart, J., Mordashov, B., Cohn, S., Notti, I., & Bessler, H. (1996). Effects of anesthesia based on large versus small doses of fentanyl on natural killer cell cytotoxicity in the perioperative period. *Anesthesia and Analgesia 82,* 492-497.
87. Pollock, R.E., Lotzova, E., & Stanford, S.D. (1991). Mechanism of surgical stress impairment of human perioperative natural killer cell cytotoxicity. *Archives of Surgery 126,* 338-342.
88. Page, G.G., & Ben-Eliyahu, S. (1997). The immune-suppressive nature of pain. *Seminars in Oncology Nursing 13*(1), 10-15.
89. Ashburn, M.A., & Staats, P.S. (1999). Management of chronic pain. *Lancet 353*(9167), 1865-1869.
90. Dubner, R., & Ruda, M.A. (1992). Activity dependent neuronal plasticity following tissue injury and inflammation. *Trends in Neurosciences 15,* 96-103.
91. Puig, S., & Sorkin, L.S. (1996). Formalin-evoked activity in identified primary afferent fibers: Systemic lidocaine suppresses phase-2 activity. *Pain 64,* 345-355.
92. Woolf, C.J., Shortland, P., & Coggeshall, R.F. (1992). Peripheral nerve injury triggers central sprouting of myelinated afferents. *Nature 355*(6355), 75-78.
93. Woolf, C.J., & Chong, M.S. (1993). Preemptive analgesia—treating postoperative pain by preventing the establishment of central sensitization. *Anesthesia and Analgesia 77*(2), 362-379.
94. Loeser, J.D., & Melzack, R. (1999). Pain: An overview. *Lancet 353,* 1607-1609.
95. Brodal, P. (1998). The somatosensory system. In P. Brodal (ed.), *The central nervous system: Structure & function* (2nd ed., pp. 185-244). New York: Oxford University Press.
96. Jessell, T.M., & Kelly, D.D. (1991). Pain and analgesia. In E.R. Kandel, J.H. Schwartz, & T.M. Jessell (eds.), *Principles of neural science* (pp. 385-399). Norwalk, Conn.: Appleton & Lange.
97. Coderre, T.J., & Katz, J. (1997). What exactly is central to the role of central neuroplasticity in persistent pain? *Behavioral and Brain Sciences 20*(3), 483-486.
98. Feuerstein, M., Carter, R.L., & Papciak, A.S. (1987). A prospective analysis of stress and fatigue in recurrent low back pain. *Pain 31,* 333-344.
99. Miaskowski, C., & Lee, K.A. (1999). Pain, fatigue, and sleep disturbances in oncology outpatients receiving radiation therapy for bone metastasis: A pilot study. *Journal of Pain and Symptom Management 17*(5), 320-332.
100. Moldofsky, H. (1989). Sleep influences on regional and diffuse pain syndromes associated with osteoarthritis. *Seminars in Arthritis and Rheumatism 18* (Suppl 2), 18-21.
101. Barlowe, D.H., Chorpita, B.F., & Turovsky, J. (1996). Fear, panic, anxiety, and disorders of emotion. In D.A. Hope (ed.). *Nebraska Symposium on Motivation, 1995: Perspectives on anxiety, panic, and fear. Current theory and research in motivation, 43* (pp. 251-328). Lincoln, Neb.: University of Nebraska Press.
102. Madland, G., Feinmann, C., & Newman, S. (2000). Factors associated with anxiety and depression in facial arthromyalgia. *Pain 84*(2-3), 225-232.
103. Rhudy, J.L., & Meagher, M.W. (2000). Fear and anxiety: Divergent effects on human pain thresholds. *Pain 84*(1), 65-75.
104. Wall, P. (1999). *Pain: The science of suffering.* London: Weidenfeld & Nicolson.
105. Banks, S., & Kerns, R. (1996). Explaining the high rates of depression in chronic pain: A diathesis—stress framework. *Psychological Bulletin 119,* 95-110.
106. Dworkin, R.H., & Gitlin, M.J. (1991). Clinical aspects of depression in chronic pain patients. *Clinical Journal of Pain 7*(2), 79-94.
107. Fishbain, D.A., Cutler, R., Rosomoff, H.L., & Rosomoff, R.S. (1997). Chronic pain-associated depression: Antecedent or consequence of chronic pain? A review. *Clinical Journal of Pain 13*(2), 116-137.
108. Gupta, M.A. (1986). Is chronic pain a variant of depressive illness? A critical review. *Canadian Journal of Psychiatry 31*(3), 241-248.
109. Kinney, R.K., Gatchel, R.J., Ellis, E., & Holt, C. (1992). Major psychological disorders in chronic TMD patients: Implications for successful management. *Journal of the American Dental Association 123*(10), 49-54.
110. Magni, G. (1987). On the relationship between chronic pain and depression when there is no organic lesion *Pain 31*(1), 1-21.
111. Marbach, J.J., & Lund, P. (1981). Depression, anhedonia, and anxiety in tempomandibular joint and other facial pain syndromes. *Pain 11*(1), 73-84.
112. Romano, J., & Turner, J. (1985). Chronic pain and depression: Does the evidence support a relationship. *Psychology Bulletin 97,* 18-34.
113. Roy, R., Thomas, M., & Matas, M. (1984). Chronic pain and clinical depression: A review. *Comprehensive Psychiatry 25,* 96-105.
114. Zelman, D.C., Howland, E.W., Nichols, S.N., & Cleeland, C.S. (1991). The effects of induced mood on laboratory pain. *Pain 46*(1), 105-111.
115. Nesse, R.M. (1999). Proximate and evolutionary studies of anxiety, stress and depression: Synergy at the interface. *Neuroscience and Biobehavioral Reviews 23,* 895-903.
116. Eisendrath, S. (1995). Psychiatric aspects of chronic pain. *Neurology 45*(Suppl 9), S26-S34.
117. Ruolf, G. (1996). Depression in the patient with chronic pain. *Texas Personnel and Guidance Association Journal 43,* S25-S43.
118. Stein, M.B., Walker, J.B., Hazen, A.L., & Forde, D.R. (1997). Full and partial posttraumatic stress disorder: Findings from a community survey. *American Journal of Psychiatry 154*(8), 1114-1119.
119. Hickling, E.J., Blanchard, E.B., Silverman, D.J., & Schwarz, S.P. (1992). Motor vehicle accidents, headaches and post-traumatic stress disorder: Assessment findings in a consecutive series. *Headache 32*(3), 147-151.
120. Cancer Pain Management Guideline Panel. (1994). Management of cancer pain. Clinical Practice Guideline No. 9. AHCPR Publications No. 94-0592. Rockville, MD.: Agency for Health Care Policy and Research, U.S. Department of Health and Human Services, Public Health Services.
121. Huskisson, E.C. (1974). Measurement of pain. *Lancet ii,* 1127-1131.
122. Melzack, R. (1983). The McGill Pain Questionnaire. In Melzack, R. (ed.), *Pain measurement and assessment* (pp. 41-47). New York: Raven Press.
123. Herr, K.A., Mobily, P.R., Kohout, F.J., & Wagner, D. (1998). Evaluation of the Faces Pain Scale for use with the elderly. *The Clinical Journal of Pain 14,* 29-38.

124. Keefe, F. (1989). Behavioral measurement of pain. In Chapman, C.R., & Loeser, J.D. (eds.), *Issues in pain management: Advances in pain research and therapy* (Vol. 12, pp. 405-424). New York, Raven Press.
125. Turk, D.C., & Melzack, R. (1992). *Handbook of pain assessment.* New York: Guilford Press.
126. Camp, L.D., & O'Sullivan, P.S. (1987). Comparison of medical, surgical and oncology patients' descriptions of pain and nurses' documentation of pain assessments. *Journal of Advanced Nursing 12,* 593-598.
127. Teyske, K., Daut, R.L., & Cleeland, C.S. (1983). Relationships between nurses' observations and patients' self-reports of pain. *Pain 16,* 289-296.
128. Katz, J., & Melzack, R. (1999). Measurement of pain. *Surgical Clinics of North America 79*(2), 231-252.
129. Puntillo, K.A., Miaskowski, C., Kehrle, K., Stannard, D., Gleeson, S., & Nye, P. (1997). Relationship between behavioral and physiological indicators of pain, critical care patients' self-reports of pain, and opioid administration. *Critical Care Medicine 25,* 1159-1166.
130. Stannard, D., Puntillo, K., Miaskowski, C., Gleeson, S., Kehrle, K., & Nye, P. (1996). Clinical judgment and management of postoperative pain in critical care patients. *American Journal of Critical Care 5,* 267-270.
131. Gracely, R.H. (1989). Pain psychophysics. In Chapman, C.R., & Loeser, J.D. (eds.), *Issues in pain measurement: Advances in pain research and therapy* (Vol. 12, pp. 211-229). New York: Raven Press.
132. Barr, R.G. (1983). Variations on the theme of pain: Pain tolerance and development changes in pain perception. In M.D. Levine, W.B. Carey, A.C. Crocker, & R.T. Gross (eds.), *Development-behavioral pediatrics* (pp. 505-512). Philadelphia: W.B. Saunders.
133. McCaffery, M., & Beebe, A. (1989). *Pain: Clinical manual for nursing practice.* St Louis: Mosby.
134. Todd, K.H., Samaroo, N., & Hoffman, J.R. (1993). Ethnicity as a risk factor for inadequate emergency department analgesia. *Journal of the American Medical Association 269,* 1537-1539.
135. Jensen, M.P., Karoly, P., & Braver, S. (1986). The measurement of clinical pain intensity: A comparison of methods. *Pain 27,* 117-126.
136. Herr, K.A., & Mobily, P.R. (1993). Comparison of selected pain assessment tools for use with the elderly. *Applied Nursing Research 6,* 39-46.
137. McCormack, H.M., Horne, D.J., & Sheather, S. (1988). Clinical applications of visual analog scales: A critical review. *Psychological Medicine 18,* 1007-1019.
138. Zborowski, M. (1969). *People in pain.* San Francisco: Josey-Bass.
139. Encandela, J.A. (1993). Social science and the study of pain since Zborowski: A need for a new agenda. *Social Science Medicine 36,* 783-791.
140. Martinelli, A.M. (1987). Pain and ethnicity: How people of different cultures experience pain. *Association of Operating Room Nurses Journal 46,* 273-278.
141. Wolff, B.B. (1985). Ethnocultural factors influencing pain and illness behavior. *Clinical Journal of Pain 1,* 23-30.
142. National Institutes of Health. (1987). The integrated approach to the management of pain. *Journal of Pain and Symptom Management 2,* 35-44.
143. McCaffery, M., & Pasero, C. (1999). *Clinical Manual.* St Louis: Mosby.
144. Acute Pain Management Guideline Panel. (1992). *Acute pain management in adults: Operative procedures. Quick reference guide for clinicians,* AHCPR Pub. No. 92-0019, Rockville, Md.: Agency for Health care policy and Research, Public Heatlh Service, U.S. Department of Health and Human Services.
145. Acute Pain Management Guideline Panel. (1992). *Acute pain management in infants, children, and adolescents: Operative and medical procedures. Quick referenced guide for clinicians,* AHCPR Pub. No. 92-0020, Rockville, Md.: Agency for Health Care Policy and Research, Public Health Service, U.S. Department of Helath and Human Services.
146. McGrath, P.J., Beyer, J., Cleeland, C., Eland, J., McGrath, P.A., & Portenoy, R. (1990). American Academy of Pediatrics Report of the Subcommittee on Assessment and Methodologic Issues in the Management of Pain in Childhood Cancer. *Pediatrics, 86* (5 Pt 2), 814-817.
147. Clark, M.M. (1983). Cultural context of medical practice. *Western Journal of Medicine 139*(6), 2-6.
148. Devine, E.C, Bevsek, S.A., Brubakken, K., Johnson, B.P., Ryan, P., Sliefert, M.K., & Rodgers, B. (1999). AHCPR clinical practice guideline on surgical pain management: Adoption and outcomes. *Research in Nursing and Health 22,* 119-130.
149. Boynton, C.S., Dick, C.F., & Mayor, G.H. (1988). NSAIDs: An overview. *Journal of Clinical Pharmacology 28,* 512-517.
150. Coleman, R.A., Smith, W.L., & Narumiya, S. (1994). Classification of prostanoid receptors: Properties, distribution, and structure of the receptors and their subtypes. *Pharmacologic Reviews 46,* 205-229.
151. Mitchell, J.A., Akarasereenont, P., Thiemermann, C., Flower, R.J., & Vane, J.R. (1993). Selectivity of nonsteroidal anti-inflammatory drugs as inhibitors of constitutive and inducible cyclooxygenase. *Proceedings of the National Academy of Sciences 90,* 11693-11697.
152. Duggan, A.W., & North, R.A. (1983). Electrophysiology of opioids. *Pharmacologic Reviews 35,* 219-282.
153. Keefe, F. (2000). Can cognitive-behavioral therapies succeed where medical treatments fail? In M. Devor, M.C. Rowbotham, & Wiesenfeld-Hallin (eds.), *Proceedings of the 9th World Congress on Pain, Progress in Pain Research and Management* (Vol. 16, pp. 1069-1084). Seattle: IASP Press.
154. Mobily, P.R. (1994). Nonpharmacologic interventions for the management of chronic pain in older women. *Journal of Women and Aging 6*(4), 89-109.
155. Sindhu, F. (1996). Are non-pharmacological nursing interventions for the management of pain effective? A meta-analysis. *Journal of Advanced Nursing 24,* 1152-1159.
156. Devine, E.C., & Westlake, S.K. (1995). The effects of psychoeducational care provided to adults with cancer: Meta-analysis of 116 studies. *Oncology Nursing Forum 22*(9), 1369-1380.
157. Smith, M.C., Holcombe, J.K., & Stullenbarger, E. (1994). A meta-analysis of intervention effectiveness for symptom management in oncology nursing research. *Oncology Nursing Forum 21*(7), 1201-1210.
158. Carroll, D., & Seers, K. (1998). Relaxation for the relief of chronic pain: A systematic review. *Journal of Advanced Nursing 27,* 476-487.
159. Berman, B.M., & Bausell, R.B. (2000). The use of nonpharmacological therapies by pain specialists. *Pain 85*(3), 313-315.
160. Yeager, K.A., Miaskowski, C., Dibble, S.L., & Wallhagen, M. (1995). Differences in pain knowledge and perception of the pain experience between outpatients with cancer and their family caregivers. *Oncology Nursing Forum 22*(8), 1235-1241.

161. Wang, J.B., Johnson, P.S., Imai, Y., Persico, A.M., Ozenberger, B.A., Eppler, C.M., et al. (1994). CDNA cloning of an orphan opiate receptor gene family member and its splice variant. *February Letters 348*(1), 75-79.
162. Boehmer, C.G., Norman, J., Catton, M., Fine, L.G., & Mantyh, P.W. (1989). High levels of mRNA coding for substance P, somatostatin and α-tubulin are expressed by rat and rabbit dorsal root ganglia neurons. *Peptides 10,* 1179-1194.
163. Dalsagaad, C.J., Ygge, J., Vincent, S.R., Ohrling, M., Dockray, G.J., & Elde, R. (1984). Peripheral projections and neuropeptide coexistence in a subpopulation of fluoride-resistant acid phosphatase reactive spinal primary sensory neurons. *Neuroscience Letters 51,* 139-144.
164. Hokfelt, T., Kellerth, J.O., Nilsson, G., & Pernow, B. (1975). Experimental immunohistochemical studies on the localization and distribution of substance P in cat primary sensory neurons. *Brain Research 100,* 235-252.
165. Levine, J.D., Fields, H.L., & Basbaum, A.I. (1993). Peptides and the primary afferent nociceptor. *Journal of Neuroscience 13,* 2273-2286.
166. Gear, R.W., Miaskowski, C., Gordon, N.C., Paul, S.M., Heller, P.H., & Levine, J.D. (1999). The kappa opioid nalbuphine produces gender- and dose-dependent analgesia and antianalgesia in patients with postoperative pain. *Pain 83*(2), 339-345.
167. Gear, R.W., Miaskowski, C., Heller, P.H., Paul, S.M., Gordon, N.C., & Levine, J.D. (1997). Benzodiazepine mediated antagonism of opioid analgesia. *Pain 71*(1), 25-29.
168. Gear, R.W., Miaskowski, C., Gordon, N.C., Paul, S.M., Heller, P.H., & Levine, J.D. (1996a). Kappa-opioids produce significantly greater analgesia in women than in men. *Nature Medicine 2*(11), 1248-1250.
169. Gear, R.W., Gordon, N.C., Heller, P.H., Paul, S., Miaskowski, C., & Levine, J.D. (1996b). Gender difference in analgesic response to the kappa-opioid pentazocine. *Neuroscience Letters 205*(3), 207-209.
170. Puntillo, K.A., Wild, L.R., Morris, A.B., Stanik-Hutt, J., Thompson, C., & White, C. (2002) Practices and predictors of analgesic interventions for adults undergoing painful procedures. *American Journal of Critical Care 11*(5), 415-429.
171. Johnson, J.L. (1994). A dialectical examination of nursing art. *Advances in Nursing Science 17*(1), 1-14.

CHAPTER

13 Nausea, Vomiting, and Retching

VERNA A. RHODES & ROXANNE W. McDANIEL

Nausea, vomiting, and retching (NVR) are three separate phenomena; they affect people with varying frequency, intensity, duration, and clinical conditions. They can be extremely distressing and even contribute to economic loss. These related phenomena may occur in isolation or in combination and have a significant impact on acceptance, continuation, and outcomes of clinical therapies. These phenomena affect populations with varying conditions, such as pregnancy, gastrointestinal (GI) upsets, and renal disease. Before the pronounced side effects of antineoplastic chemotherapy (ANCT) and radiotherapy for neoplastic conditions, limited attention was given to the study and treatment of NVR.[1-6]

DEFINITIONS

Nausea is a subjective, unobservable phenomenon of an unpleasant sensation experienced in the back of the throat and the epigastrium that may or may not culminate in vomiting.[7] The term *nausea* is best understood by most nonprofessionals as "sick to the stomach." This individual experience has been described as an unpleasant wavelike sensation at the back of the throat, in the epigastric area, or throughout the abdomen.[8] It is usually known through self-report; however, it may have some objective elements because of its intensity.[9,10] Expressions used to characterize nausea are "distressing," "overwhelming," "may cause a desire to vomit," and "all-consuming."[11,12]

Vomiting is the forceful expulsion of the contents of the stomach through the oral or nasal cavity. Both the occurrence and the frequency of vomiting can be objectively measured.[12] However, the amount of distress (physical or mental anguish, suffering, or discomfort) from vomiting is subjective. Although frequently confused with nausea, vomiting is an observable phenomenon. Most individuals have less difficulty reporting the occurrence of vomiting, the act (such as sudden or projectile), and the distress that accompanies it. Vomiting is objective and the occurrence can be assessed by another, but the distress can only be reported by the individual. Vomiting is best described as "throwing up." Other terms for this phenomenon are "upchucking," "hurling," "pitching," "barfing," and "spitting up." The latter phrase is most often associated with infants. "Driving the white porcelain bus" is a more recent descriptor by some younger individuals (referring to a toilet).[13]

Retching is an attempt to vomit without output; a rhythmic movement of the muscles of vomiting without expulsion of gastric contents.[14] Reference terms commonly used are "gagging," "dry heaves," or "attempting to vomit without results."[12] Patients are able to differentiate the frequency of occurrence and the actual distress experienced from the sensation of retching. Although vomiting and retching may occur concurrently or independently, a scientific database for each symptom is needed for symptom management and to determine the patterns of each.

PREVALENCE AND POPULATIONS AT RISK

The symptoms of NVR have plagued people over time and continue to be distressing symptoms that may interfere with an individual's quality of life (QOL). Written references to these unique symptoms have been found dating to Biblical times.[11] The first description of pregnancy nausea and vomiting (NV), written on papyrus, was dated 2000 BC.[15]

NVR are associated with a variety of life events and medical conditions. Excitement, anxiety or fear, dizziness, motion sickness, and overindulgence in food and drink can suddenly induce the symptoms of NVR. NVR symptom experiences are second only to the common cold in the cause of absenteeism.[16] NV have been the most frequently reported adverse effects of ANCT and have had a significant impact on treatment acceptance, continuation, and outcome. NVR, fatigue, and pain have been identified as the most distressing and discomforting symptoms affecting persons with both acute and chronic conditions as well as terminally ill patients.[13,15-18]

NVR are common in the first trimester of pregnancy.[19] These symptoms have a pervasive, detrimental impact on a pregnant woman's family, social, and professional life.[20] Early studies reported a high incidence of NV, 80% and 50%, respectively.[21-23] A review of studies of NV of pregnancy found that up to 90% of pregnant women experience NVR at some time during their pregnancy.[24,25] A prospective study of the frequency, duration, and severity of NV in 160 pregnant women revealed that 80% had nausea lasting all day.[26] A recent review revealed that 70% to 85% of pregnant women experienced nausea and approximately 50% experienced vomiting.[27]

Diseases of the GI system are common and place the patient at great risk for NVR. Intraabdominal disorders, such as distention and decreased motility, predispose to these symptoms. The symptoms of NVR frequently are associated or occur concomitantly with other medical conditions, including myocardial infarction and chronic renal disease.[28] The postoperative symptoms of NVR continue to be a concern with pediatric and adult surgical patients and have been shown to significantly delay discharge from the recovery area following ambulatory surgery.[29-32] The challenges of managing postoperative NVR are increasing as complex surgeries, such as laparoscopic cholecystectomy, laminectomy, hysterectomy, and knee and shoulder reconstruction, are being performed on an outpatient basis. One investigation revealed that all types of surgery lasting 2 hours or greater were twice as likely as shorter surgeries to cause patients to experience nausea.[33] Excluding ear or gastrointestinal surgical procedures, there was a 39% incidence of postoperative NV in a convenience sample of 300 patients, 18 years and older, who had general anesthesia. The investigators recommended that women and patients with surgery lasting greater than 2 hours be assessed more frequently for postoperative NV.[33] Despite advances in anesthetic practice and surgical techniques, the incidence of postoperative vomiting ranges from 20% to 30% during the first 24 hours after surgery.[34]

RISK FACTORS

Age and Development

Although the developmental stages reflecting the natural history of NVR are unknown, Norris proposed a developmental typology of the emotional origin of NVR. The first evidence of these symptoms is the "spitting up" of infancy; however, the cause is not clearly understood. A study by Cohen et al[35] found that the occurrence of postoperative NVR is low in infants and in children under 3 years of age, thus lending support to the theory that neural development of the vomiting center is a factor in the occurrence of NVR. Psychological or emotional needs of children may influence the occurrence of the symptoms. An early observation study of the emetic symptoms of 1713 postoperative patients in different age groups was coupled with a survey of other authors' work.[36] This pioneer effort concluded that children and adolescents had a higher incidence of NVR as compared with adults when they received a light halothane anesthetic rather than the emetogenic ether anesthetic. The incidence of vomiting is similar in children of all ages up to 11 years of age, when the incidence of vomiting is higher in females than in males.[36,37] Postoperative vomiting increases after puberty but tends to decrease with increasing age.[36,37] There is evidence that older patients tolerate ANCT better than younger patients. This was first explained as resulting from less aggressive ANCT in older patients; however, older patients frequently receive aggressive therapy, yet still have less NVR than younger patients.[38,39]

Craig and Powell[38] found that with only one exception, in two groups of patients (those older than 65 and those younger than 65 years of age) with breast cancer who were receiving similar ANCT protocols, younger patients consistently reported greater problems with NVR. Because women 50 years of age or younger are more likely to experience NVR, they are more prone to anticipatory NVR.[25]

Sex

Women are two to three times more likely to experience NVR and have distressing symptom experiences postoperatively and with ANCT than are men.[30,33] Studies have shown that the gender difference in the symptom occurrence may be related to female hormones, because the incidence of postoperative NVR is similar in males and females during childhood and increases in girls as menarche is approached,[37] descending after menopause to levels similar to that of males.[40,41]

Recent studies found that the phase of the menstrual cycle influences the intensity of NVR symptoms.[34] The incidence of postoperative NV varies from 50% to 75% after gynecological surgery when general anaesthesia is administered.[42] In

94 women 18 to 42 years of age who were undergoing unilateral elective thyroid surgery in Croatia, the highest occurrence of NVR was noted in the periovulatory and premenstrual periods, leading the investigators to conclude that elective surgery in young and middle-aged women is best avoided premenstrually and in the middle of their cycle,[34,43] thus suggesting that the optimal scheduling of surgical procedures should be between days 1 and 12 or days 16 and 24 of the menstrual cycle.

Pathological States

Tumor enlargement impinging on adjacent anatomical structures and limiting physiological functioning may cause severe NVR by activating mechanoreceptors in the bowel wall.[13] Some common conditions are delayed gastric emptying, gastric outlet or bowel obstruction, gastritis, hepatic or renal failure, hypercalcemia, hyponatremia, and increased intracranial pressure. Delayed gastric emptying may occur from physiological problems, such as anticholinergic effects of drugs, including opioids, or mechanical resistance (partial or complete) to emptying. Ascites, hepatomegaly, duodenal tumor, and pancreatic cancer are some of the causes of mechanical resistance.

Personal

Anxiety, stress, and patients' expectations of the occurrence of NVR symptoms are additional risk factors. Previous experience with NVR may influence individuals' concerns and behavior. Discrepancies found between the expectation of NV and the actual occurrence of these symptoms (amount, frequency, severity, and times) suggest that patients do not have accurate pretreatment expectations of the occurrence or distress of post-ANCT NVR.[44,45] Several studies have demonstrated that preparatory information and realistic expectations reduce negative mood states and improve coping behaviors used to deal with NVR.[45-47] Therefore preparatory information and early management of these dreaded symptoms enable patients to develop effective coping mechanisms and lead to improved QOL.

Patients are active participants in their treatment. Their goals and behaviors are largely determined by their perceptions of the illness.[48] In a study to investigate chemotherapy-naive patients' NVR associated with ANCT, a statistically significant relationship was found between the 329 patients' expectations of NVR symptom experience and their expectations of symptom distress. No significant relationship was reported between the expectation of the symptom and the actual symptom experience, as measured on the Index of Nausea and Vomiting.[45] These discrepancies suggest that patients did not have accurate pretreatment schema or cognitive expectations of the most commonly distressing post-ANCT experience. Previous history of NVR during pregnancy, ability to remember smells, and reported distress when blood samples were being taken predicted anticipatory NVR.[49]

Environmental

Binge eating or drinking and vomiting behaviors have been attributed to environmental influences such as sociocultural and family environmental indices (family-personal relationships). The findings of a recent study to clarify the relationship of the behaviors of binging—unrestrained indulgence—and vomiting suggested that genetic influences may be of particular relevance to the cause.[50] This study of the lifetime history of binging and vomiting of 1897 female twins found a strong association between having ever binged and having ever induced vomiting. Modeling estimates indicated that lifetime binging and vomiting were both inherited (46% and 72%) and influenced by individual-specific environmental factors (54% and 28%). A substantial overlap was noted between the genetic and individual-specific environmental factors. These data are consistent with the identification of binging and vomiting as complex traits resulting from the interplay of multiple genes and individual-specific environmental influences.

Individuals who develop motion sickness are also more prone to NVR with health care–related procedures.[36,45,46] In a report by Howarth and Finch,[51] two different strategies for exploring virtual environments provided support for maintaining a quiet position and atmosphere. Although nausea increased steadily both when the head was kept still and when head movement was encouraged while exploring the virtual world, head movement appeared to accentuate the symptoms. Other contributing factors to NVR include the emetogenic qualities of the ANCT drug agent or combination, dosage, route, time of day, and length of administration. The emetic potential of ANCT for acute NVR is noted in Table 13-1.

MECHANISMS

Neuropathophysiology of Nausea and Vomiting

The mechanisms leading to vomiting have been elucidated; however, there is limited information

TABLE 13-1 Emetogenic Potential of Antineoplastic Agents (Acute NVR)

AGENT	PERCENTAGE OF TIME AGENT INDUCES EMESIS	ONSET OF EMESIS (HR)	DURATION OF EMESIS (HR)
Cisplatin*	>90	1–6	24–120
Dacarbazine	>90	1–3	1–12
Mechlorethamine	>90	0.5–2	8–24
Streptozocin	>90	1–4	>24
Carboplatin	60–90	1–6	4–24
Carmustine*	60–90	2–4	4–24
Cyelophosphamide*	60–90	4–12	4–24
Cytarabine*	60–90	6–12	3–12
Dactinomycin	60–90	2–6	12–24
Doxorubicin	60–90	4–6	6–24
Procarbazine	60–90	24–27	Varies
Daunorubicin	30–60	2–6	6–24
Epirubicin ≤90 mg/m^2	30–60	0.25–0.5	6–24
Fluorouracil	30–60	3–6	2–24
Hexamethylmelamine/ Methenamine (oral)†	30–60	2–6	†
Idarubicin*	30–60		
Ifosfamide	30–60	2–6	4–24
Mitomycin	30–60	1–4	48–72
Mitoxantrone	30–60	2–6	6–24
Bleomycin Cytarabine* Docetaxel Etoposide Fluorouracil <1000 mg/m^2 Gemcitabine Methotrexate* Mitomycin Paclitaxel Vinblastine	10–30	3–12	1–12

Data from Hesketh, P.J., Kris, M.G., Grunberg, S.M., Beck, T., Hainsworth, J.D., Harker, G., et al. (1997). Proposal for classifying the acute emetogenicity of cancer chemotherapy. *Journal of Clinical Oncology 15,* 103-109; American Hospital Formulary Service (2001). *Drug information.* Bethesda, Md.: American Society of Health-System Pharmacists; Andrews, P.R.L., & Davis, C.J. (1993). The mechanism of emesis induced by anticancer therapies. In P.R.L. Andrews, & G.J. Sanger (eds.), *Emesis in anticancer therapy: Mechanisms and treatment* (pp. 113-161). New York: Chapman & Hall Medical; and Grunberg, S.M. (2001). Nausea and vomiting. In C.M. Haskell (ed.), *Cancer treatment* (ed. 5, pp. 327-331). Philadelphia: W.B. Saunders.
*Dose-related; potential for emesis increases with higher doses.
†Limited information on emesis onset and duration.

on the mechanism that triggers vomiting. Vomiting results from an intricate succession of physiological events mediated by afferent enervation, humoral factors, and somatic visceral musculature that are ultimately coordinated by the emetic or vomiting center in the medulla (Figure 13-1). Afferent input to the emetic center is received primarily from four sources: (1) the cerebral cortex pathway, which is stimulated by learned associations; (2) the chemoreceptor trigger zone (CTZ), located in the area postrema, which is sensitive to chemical stimuli from the cerebrospinal fluid and blood; (3) the vestibular apparatus or pathway, which activates the emetic center via body positional changes; and (4) the peripheral pathway, which is activated by neurotransmitter receptors found in the GI tract, where the vagus nerve communicates with the emetic center. The CTZ, the GI tract, and the cerebral cortex have been identified as sources of afferent input to the emetic center.[55-57] Vomiting occurs when efferent impulses are sent from the vomiting center to the salivation center, abdominal muscles, respiratory center, and cranial nerves. The area postrema does not appear to receive input from the cerebral cortex, thus not stimulating acute ANCT vomiting; however, it may stimulate the emetic

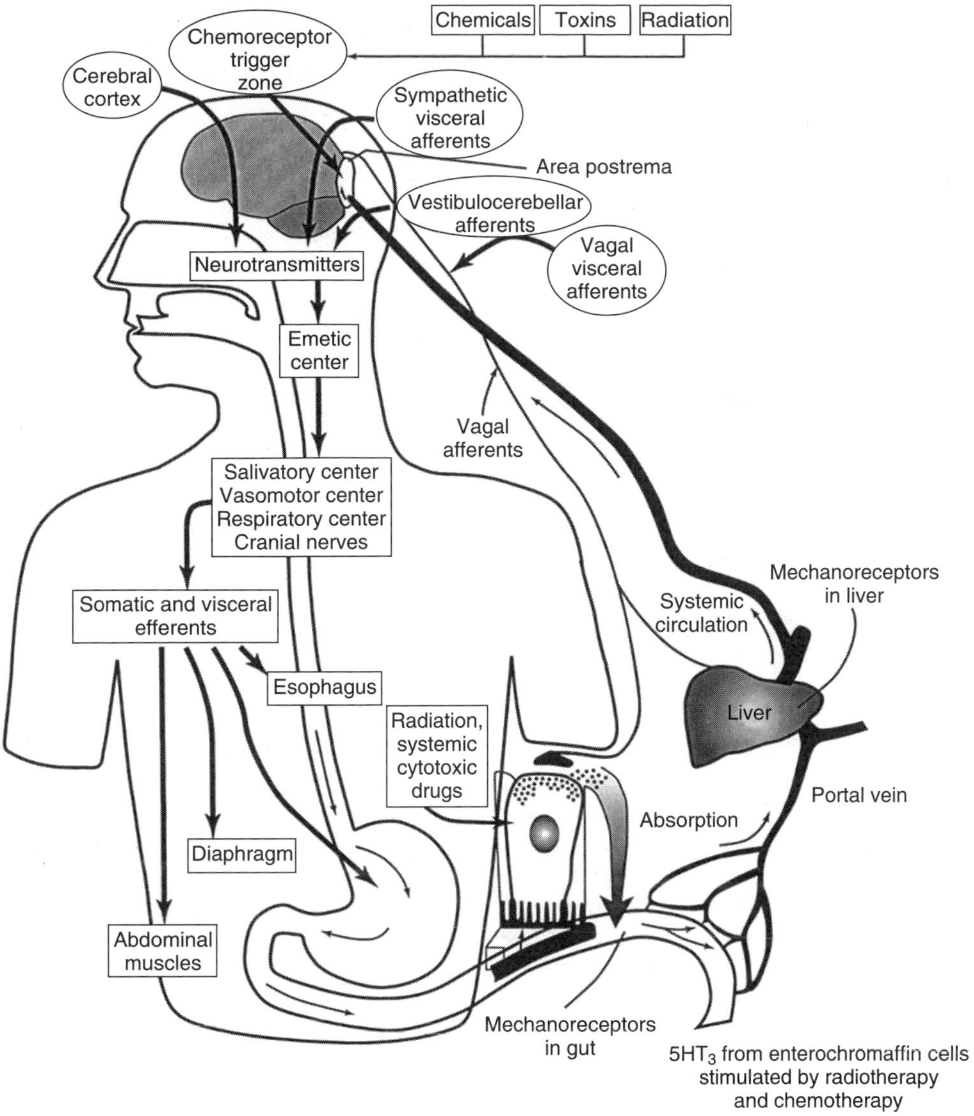

Figure 13-1 Neuropathophysiology of vomiting. (Data from Andrews, P.R.L., & Davis, C.J. [1993]. The mechanism of emesis induced by anticancer therapies. In P.R.L. Andrews, & G.J. Sanger [eds.], *Emesis in anticancer therapy: Mechanisms and treatment* [pp. 113-161]. New York: Chapman & Hall Medical; and Grunberg, S.M. (2001). Nausea and vomiting. In C.M. Haskell [ed.], *Cancer treatment* [ed. 5, pp. 327-331]. Philadelphia: W.B. Saunders.)

center in anticipatory vomiting. The mechanoreceptors in the bowel wall may be stimulated by the stretch, distortion, or direct invasion of the GI tract as a result of a tumor mass or constipation.[13,58] Similar receptors are located in visceral capsules and in parietal serosal surfaces and provide afferent input to the emetic center via the vagus and splanchnic nerves.

Dopamine, acetylcholine, histamine, and serotonin are neurotransmitters involved in the emetogenic pathways stimulated by chemotherapy and radiation.[57] The GI tract, the CTZ, and the emetic center have abundant receptors for these neurotransmitters. Serotonin or 5-hydroxytryptamine (5-HT3) is stored and released from platelets, neurons, and from high concentrations of enterochromaffin cells in the gut. The serotonin or 5-HT3 receptors are in peripheral tissues, the nucleus of the solitary tract, and the CTZ, where the majority of vagal afferents enter the brain. Peripherally, the release of serotonin from enterochromaffin cells in the gut is caused by ANCT and radiation therapy.[57] The CTZ is located within the area postrema and is exposed to both cerebrospinal fluid and the systemic circulation; therefore, substances circulating in both of these fluids can stimulate the area postrema to release neurotransmitters. Because the largest concentration of 5-HT3 receptors in the central nervous system (CNS) is in the nucleus of the solitary tract and the area postrema where the CTZ is located and where vagal afferents enter the brain, it is postulated that 5-HT3 antagonists may mediate NV by interaction with these central receptors.[56,57]

Another group of ligand-receptor pairs, molecules coordinated to a central atom in a complex synthetase, appears to play an important role in NVR.[51,56,59] Recently three tachykinin (small or medium-sized peptides) receptor genes have been cloned. They are classified as neurokinin$_1$ (NK$_1$), neurokinin$_2$, and neurokinin$_3$ receptors. Their preferred ligands, known as *neurokinins,* or with other family tachykinins, are 11-amino acid peptides that include substance P, neurokinin A, and neurokinin B.[56,59] Of these, only the NK$_1$ receptor, activated by substance P, is involved with emesis.[59,60] Interestingly, these antagonists are active against emetogenic stimuli (e.g., apomorphine and motion) that are unaffected by 5-HT3 antagonists.[57]

The neuropathophysiology of vomiting is complex. The pathogenesis of NVR in pregnancy remains poorly understood with multifactorial theories proposed combining both biologic and psychological factors.[25,61] Although the above receptors and transmitters are involved, as may be adrenergic and opioid receptors, additional research is needed to determine possible interactions and/or the specific role of different receptors.[59]

PATHOLOGICAL CONSEQUENCES

Depending on the condition or illness that precipitates NVR, the consequences may differ. For example, NVR are rarely viewed favorably by a pregnant woman. Yet morning sickness of the first trimester is associated with decreased risk of spontaneous abortion during the first 20 weeks of gestation and with increased birthweight. The association of these symptoms with a positive outcome of pregnancy may be because placental development is stimulated, energy expenditure is reduced, or nutrient intake is actually increased.[62] There may be a possible advantage for these discomforting symptoms. Findings indicate that pregnancy hormones and factors may be important for normal fetal heart development.[63] Although NVR in pregnancy affect the pregnant woman's well-being and lifestyle, the causes are not known.[24,26,62] The findings of a study of the relationship of certain demographic factors (parity, age, smoking, and employment status) and pregnancy outcomes (birth weight and sex of the infant) and the severity of NVR during pregnancy indicated that it may be possible to identify women at risk for third-trimester NVR.[64]

The stimulation of the trigeminovagal reflex arc is thought to be the primary explanation for the high rate of vomiting after strabismus surgery. Exploration of this potentially serious complication of ophthalmic surgery found a significant association between a positive intraoperative oculocardiac reflex and postoperative vomiting; children with a positive intraoperative oculocardiac reflex were 2.6 times more likely to vomit than those without the reflex.[65]

Anticipatory NVR are conditioned responses that start before the administration of ANCT regimen and exacerbate posttreatment NVR.[66,67] Approximately 30% of ANCT-naive patients who have posttreatment-induced NVR experience anticipatory symptoms by the fourth ANCT.[66,67] Despite recent pharmacological advances in the management of posttreatment ANCT, further research related to alternative treatments is critical to prevent these anticipatory symptoms and to enhance the patient's QOL throughout the illness trajectory.

Women who had experience with illnesses associated with NVR, such as stomach flu, motion sickness, surgical procedures, and pregnancies, reported higher levels of NVR when they underwent chemotherapy.[45] It is still difficult to manage postoperative NVR despite the introduction of new antiemetic drugs, in part because of previous experiences with NVR.[67,68] These appear to be examples of the influence of pretreatment schema on posttreatment NVR and have specific implications for the preparatory information and early symptom management to promote QOL for women.

Alcohol Effect

Although it is common for patients treated with cisplatin ANCT to have NVR, patients with a history of chronic, heavy alcohol intake experience less NVR from cisplatin than do those who are not heavy drinkers.[69-71] A prospective study of 37 patients with lung cancer found that 93% of patients with a history of chronic high alcohol intake had no emesis ($p = 0.013$), and the remaining 7% had fewer episodes (0 to 2) of vomiting and significantly less nausea ($p = 0.05$).[69,72] Sullivan, Leyden, and Bell[71] postulated that long-term alcohol exposure destroys the CTZ. By contrast, a comparison of the frequency and severity of GI symptoms of 48 male alcoholics and 48 nonalcoholic control subjects revealed increased GI symptoms in chronic alcoholics.[73] Both withdrawing and actively drinking alcoholics had more frequent NV, heartburn, diarrhea, and flatulence, and more severe chest pain, milk intolerance, and postprandial fullness. They concluded that alcoholics have more frequent and more severe GI symptoms that resolve quickly during abstinence and that predominantly occur while the individual is actively drinking rather than during withdrawal.[73]

RELATED PATHOPHYSIOLOGICAL CONCEPTS AND DIFFERENTIAL DIAGNOSIS

Related Symptoms

The symptom experience (symptom occurrence and symptom distress) of patients with chronic disease, such as cancer and renal disease, may vary at different phases throughout their illness. The disease itself, its treatment, concurrent disorders, or nonspecific factors may contribute to the additional symptoms of NVR. Seriously ill patients with cancer have a high symptom burden. The findings of a recent study that included 1556 patients with chronic obstructive pulmonary disease, congestive heart failure, liver failure, acute respiratory failure, and other serious illnesses concluded that patients with nausea and dyspnea have more pain than patients without these symptoms.[74] The relationship among nausea and dyspnea and pain is unknown. Although pain may cause or increase dyspnea and nausea, it is possible that improved management of dyspnea and nausea may relieve pain. Although NVR, dyspnea, and pain are symptoms that may significantly affect patients' QOL, patients receiving end-stage palliative care frequently have a variety of additional severe physical and psychosocial concomitant symptoms, including asthenia, anorexia, constipation, confusion, and mood changes.[1] Constipation (resultant colonic stretch) or increased intraabdominal pressure may stimulate the mechanoreceptor pathways to the emetic center and trigger vomiting.[75]

Tumor Burden

Limited data are available concerning the impact of tumor burden on NVR. In one study, the impact of tumor burden on NVR in 101 patients with ovarian cancer who were receiving their initial ANCT revealed that in patients with a large tumor burden (greater than 2 cm), emesis was more delayed (days 2 to 7) and their nausea more acute. The persistent delayed NV was more evident in patients 55 or older with a large residual tumor burden.[76] Although these findings were from ANCT-naive subjects with known tumor burdens, the findings stimulate questions concerning the role of tumor burden on the NVR symptom experience of subjects in the palliative care phase.

Pain or Medication Induced

Inadequate pain control may be a contributing factor for the symptoms of NVR. Some of the medications used to manage pain may also contribute to NVR. Opioids, nonsteroidal antiinflammatory drugs (NSAIDs), digoxin, anticoagulants, and anticholinergics are examples of medications that may induce NVR by chemical action at the CTZ, by serotonin release in the GI tract, through GI irritation or stasis, or a combination of these.[75] Opioids activate the CTZ and may cause NVR with gastric stasis. The area postrema has one of the highest densities of opioid receptors.[76] NVR may be caused by GI irritation from NSAIDs. Accumulation of plasma morphine, morphine-3-glucuronide, and morphine-6-glucuronide concentrations may be a causal or aggravating factor in the NV and cognitive function profile of palliative care patients with significantly impaired renal function.[75]

MANIFESTATIONS, SURVEILLANCE, AND MEASUREMENT

Vasomotor physiological responses such as hot or cold feelings, diaphoresis, increased salivation, pallor, and tachycardia may accompany NVR. Young children who are unable to articulate or describe their discomfort may manifest varied behaviors; they may rub the abdominal area, salivate, and refuse food and drink.[11,12] Nausea can be measured only subjectively. Both subjective and objective measurements of vomiting and retching are possible and useful.[12]

Often these symptom experiences, although unpleasant, are fleeting. However, if the symptom experience interferes with life routines or events or requires health care, it becomes problematic and may affect the human response of future NVR experiences decreasing the QOL.

Management of NVR includes accurate and thorough assessment of the effectiveness of both pharmacological and nonpharmacological therapies. A conceptual framework for the management of the NVR experience is illustrated in Figure 13-2. Clinical management necessitates a precise patient and family assessment. Assessment is an ongoing process that begins with the initial patient contact and continues through the pregnancy[64] or the illness trajectory. The history and physical examination

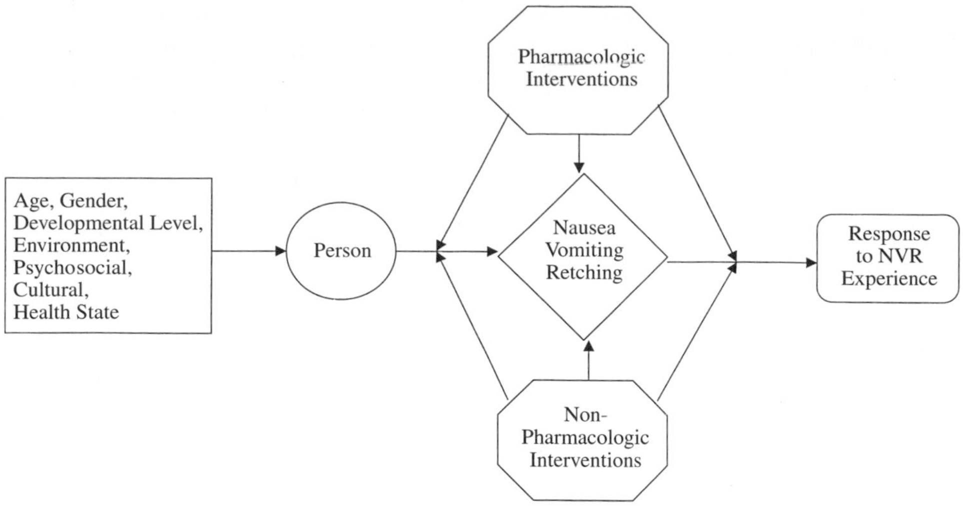

Figure 13-2 Conceptual framework for management of the nausea, vomiting, and retching experience.

should be used to differentiate separate symptoms, rather than take a global or synonymous approach when assessing NVR. Information obtained by interviews, questionnaires, or self-report instruments should use words that have the same meaning to patients, family members, and caregivers. A balance between obtaining accurate data about the specific symptom and patient or family burden must be maintained. Assessment tools that can be completed quickly and reviewed can mean less expenditure of patient energy and nursing time. These are important criteria to consider when choosing an instrument to measure the individual symptoms, determining symptom patterns, and making comparisons.

Many patients with prospective surgical malignant and nonmalignant conditions and most palliative care patients have experienced NVR during earlier therapies; therefore the clinician or researcher must avoid directing suggestive attention to the symptom. During the initial contact, the patient's prior symptomatology, methods of management, and anticipated expectations need to be assessed. Family members' and/or significant others' suggestions, evaluations, and possible assistance in recording observations and patient-stated symptomatology in a daily diary or journal may be helpful.

Patient journals, logs, or daily diaries completed by the patient or caregiver provide useful assessment information. As a result of these reflective self-report tools, family caregivers and patients frequently have developed increased experience in problem-solving, a greater sense of control, and improved self-care management.[13] Health care providers may often note patterns of symptom occurrence; self-care management strategies, including individualized pharmacological and nonpharmacological interventions; and situational or concomitant happenings. Figure 13-3 is an example of a journal.

Several comprehensive instruments include one or more of the components of NVR and are available to help assess concomitant symptomatology.[12,72,77-83] An example of this type of instrument is the Adapted Symptom Distress Scale (ASDS), a 31-item, 5-point self-report instrument that measures patients' perception of the occurrence and distress of 14 symptoms.[78] This instrument yields a total score for symptom experience, scores for symptom occurrence and distress, and subscale scores for six symptom categories. The ASDS is a highly reliable instrument with an internal consistency of 0.91 for the total occurrence and reliability for the subscales, ranging from 0.38 for the appearance subscale to 0.84 for the concentration subscale.[78] Others, such as the Symptom Distress Scale (SDS)[84] and the Memorial Symptom Assessment Scale,[85] either measure a single component or provide global measures of the concepts. The SDS is a 13-item instrument with an internal consistency alpha of 0.84. Internal consistency for physical symptoms on the Memorial Assessment Scale is 0.88.

There are instruments that specifically measure one or more of these components, such as the Index of Nausea, Vomiting, and Retching (INVR), which has eight statements that measure the three symptoms over a 12-hour time frame. The INVR has strong reliability as evidenced by an internal consistency alpha of 0.98. Another instrument is Morrow's Assessment of Nausea and Emesis

Self-Care Journal Instructions

Please keep daily records in this journal, beginning on the day of your outpatient visit. Carry the journal and a pencil with you at all times so that you can record activities and results as they occur. The more detailed your journal is, the more valuable it will be in assessing your progress. In addition, your careful records will assist us in planning your care and in serving other patients. Your help is greatly appreciated.

The directions below will help you determine what information to put in each column of the journal. In addition, please refer to the sample entries on the next page.

Date, time	Record the date and time of each entry.
How I felt before self-care activity	Record entries as often as desired and upon awakening, at noon, midafternoon or early evening, and before going to bed at night.
Self-care activity	Record the names of the medications taken and describe any action you took to improve how you were feeling.
Result	Describe how you felt an hour after completing the activity; you may use the following code: **1 = I felt better** **2 = no change** **3 = I felt worse**

Self-Care Journal Example

Sample journal entries are shown below. Remember that details are important; if in doubt, include it.

Date/Time	How I Felt Before Self-Care Activity	Self-Care Activity	Result
5/18/00 7 AM	Awakened by alarm, tired, no appetite	Showered. Tried to eat cereal and juice	**3**
8:15	Stomach feeling queasy	Took Kytril. Sat in patio recliner listening to birds	**1**
8:50	Lack of stamina	Husband drove to work. Ate 2 saltines	**2**
10:30	Hungry	Sipped coke and ate 2 pieces dry toast while sitting in recliner	**1**
12:00	Looking forward to seeing friends	Enjoyed lunch with two friends. Ate a cup of chicken soup	**1**
1:45	Feeling sick to stomach	Practiced relaxation exercises, listening to soft music. Took compazine, went home	**1**
5:30	Nauseated by smell of cooking food	Resting quietly and napped on patio for 1-2 hours	**1**
7:30	Eating cottage cheese and fruit salad	Watching an entertaining video with husband and children	**1**

Figure 13-3 Self-care journal, developed by R.A. Rhodes and P.M. Watson.

(MANE), a 17-item instrument that measures the onset, frequency, intensity, severity, and duration of chemotherapy-related NV.[86,87]

CLINICAL MANAGEMENT

Optimal clinical management of NVR includes the prevention of the symptoms and the minimization of medication side effects. Proactive nursing interventions are needed. Although accurate ongoing assessments are always essential for the recognition and monitoring the progress of the problem, it is essential that the patient's expectations about NVR be included in the initial assessment, thus permitting appropriate patient teaching to correct false assumptions and to help the patient identify symptom control measures.

Conditions such as tumor enlargement or bowel obstruction require pain control; hence careful assessment is critical to determine whether the NVR result from pharmacological agents. A recent retrospective assessment of a metoclopramide-based antiemetic regimen for chronic nausea in 100 patients with advanced cancer revealed that 32% of the patients presented with "nausea" on admission, and during the average admission, 98% developed "nausea."[4] The report suggests that nausea can be controlled in the majority of patients with the use of safe, simple, standardized antiemetic regimens. In a study of 55 pregnant women, more than 70% managed their morning sickness by adjustments in resting, eating, cooking, and increased emotional support. The particular actions identified in this study are not generally found in the literature.[16]

Pharmacological Interventions

The symptoms of NV are frequently managed with antiemetic drug therapy. Antiemetics are selected on the basis of the causes of the nausea, the pharmacological action, receptor and site, appropriate route of administration, and appropriate dose. Adequate management may require combination drug therapy. The cost-benefit of various drug combinations also needs to be considered. The variety of antiemetics and other drugs available to manage and even prevent NVR allows individualized symptom management; however, currently available pharmacological agents are still unable to provide complete protection for every patient.[44,88] Several classes of antiemetics are used in the management of NVR. The serotonin 5-HT3 antagonists represent a major improvement in the management of ANCT-induced NVR. Although 5-HT3 antagonists plus dexamethasone are considered to be the most effective antiemetic combination, their antiemetic efficacy is not maintained over multiple cycles of highly emetogenic chemotherapy and is not effective for delayed emesis.[89-93] In those cases, other antiemetic combinations are administered. Morrow et al[6] differentiated between the efficacy of these drugs on the symptoms of vomiting and nausea. Findings from two patient samples, with 300 patients treated before 5-HT3 availability and 300 patients treated with 5-HT3, showed a significant reduction in the frequency of posttreatment vomiting. It did not reduce the frequency of posttreatment nausea or in anticipatory symptoms.[6] In a study of the outcomes of antiemetic therapy following the administration of high-dose ANCT, NV continued to be significant problems through the delayed phase.[94] Thirty-two (54%) of the patients were unable to maintain oral intake, and 29 patients (49%) had two to five episodes of vomiting in 24 hours. A number of patients given serotonin type 3 receptor antagonists before high-dose ANCT developed NV that required the addition of other antiemetic medications.

The 5-HT3 drugs are very effective with elderly and young patients, can be administered every 12 hours, and have increased effectiveness in combination with dexamethasone.[68] The use of 5-HT3 receptor antagonists to relieve the NVR associated with radiation therapy and acute emetogenic chemotherapy is well documented. Tropisetron-containing combinations or tropisetron alone were more effective in the management of NV of terminal cancer patients than the conventional antiemetic combination of chlorpromazine plus dexamethasone.[95] Their use in the management of chronic nausea is less well documented. Pereira and Bruera[91] reported the successful management of intractable nausea with ondansetron in a case study of a 66-year-old woman in a palliative care unit. Currow et al[92] also found ondansetron to be effective in palliative care: 80% of patients with nausea and 71% of patients with vomiting had improvement of their symptoms. Symptom control was achieved in 80% of patients admitted with either nausea and/or vomiting.

Until recently, researchers and clinicians have underestimated the NVR of pregnancy and thus these symptoms have been undertreated. Limited use of reliable and valid NVR measurement of the patterns during pregnancy has hampered safe, scientific, pharmacological interventions.[26,61,96] Antiemetics are rarely prescribed for NVR in pregnancy. In a study of hyperemesis gravidarum, a 2-week course of methylprednisolone was more effective than promethazine.[97] Prophylactic vitamin K replacement is suggested in conditions in which hyperemesis occurs and is protracted to avoid vitamin K deficiency and coagulopathy. The adminstration of thiamine supplements to all women with prolonged vomiting during pregnancy is encouraged as prophylaxis of neurological symptoms, such as confusion, diplopia, unsteadiness, and seizures caused by Wernicke's encephalopathy.[98]

There is a general perception that medications are not safe in pregnancy, despite the fact that fewer than 30 drugs have been shown to cause major malformations in humans. A large number of women need medications in pregnancy to treat pregnancy-induced conditions, acute illnesses, and chronic diseases. Investigators in a recent study of 240 participants concluded that the perception of the risk of developmental malformations is strong, even for safe drugs, and this perception is difficult to change even when evidence is presented.[99] Many individuals consider herbal compounds useful and effective for relieving the severity of NV of pregnancy.[61] A survey of the medical literature did not find any reports of the safety of herbs used during pregnancy.[100] Of 300 nonmedical sources reviewed, 75 cited the use of herbs in pregnancy; the most commonly cited are ginger, chamomile, peppermint, and raspberry leaf for morning sickness. Although herbal remedies are often seen as safe, "drug-free" treatments for morning sickness, the contradictory information and dearth of original research related to safety indicates that these compounds should be used with caution.[100] A prospective study to evaluate the safety of echinacea in pregnancy when used for upper respiratory tract conditions suggests that gestational use of echinacea during organogenesis is not associated with an increased risk for major malformations.[101] Additional research is needed to determine the safety of herbal remedies, particularly in pregnancy.

Only a few studies have been reported on the prevention of NVR in children receiving ANCT. Older antiemetic medications, such as metoclopramide and phenothiazines, had moderate efficacy; however, they induced sedation and extrapyramidal reactions. A 5-HT3 receptor antagonist in combination with dexamethasone is recommended as standard antiemetic prophylaxis in pediatric patients receiving highly or moderately emetogenic ANCT.[102,103] Further studies are needed that investigate optimal dose and scheduling of antiemetic medications as well as their efficacy in preventing chemotherapy-induced delayed NVR and anticipatory NV in children. In a study with 80 pediatric patients undergoing major orthopedic surgeries, prophylactic administration of ondansetron (100 μg/kg) was more effective than droperidol and ondansetron (50 μg/kg) and superior to saline solution for the prevention of emesis before epidural opioids and general anesthesia were administered.[31] Granisetron 40 μg/kg was the minimum effective dose for the prevention of postoperative NV in a pediatric sample; increasing the dose to 100 μg/kg provided no demonstrable benefit.[103]

Prophylactic treatments for postoperative NVR after a variety of surgical procedures continue to be explored.[105-106] In Finland, a prophylactic combination treatment of ondansetron 8 mg with a small dose of droperidol was effective for the prevention of postoperative NV after laparoscopic surgery in patients with a high probability of NV.[105] RS-25259, a long-acting selective 5-HT3 receptor antagonist, reduced postoperative vomiting but not nausea in hysterectomy patients.[107] A single intravenous administration of tropisetron, a newer 5-HT3 receptor antagonist, has shown promise by significantly reducing postoperative NVR after elective surgery with general anesthesia.[108]

Phenothiazines have been used over time for the prevention and control of severe NV from various causes. The phenothiazines contain several different medications that may be administered rectally, which is advantageous for patients with severe NVR. The dosing schedule, which can vary from every 4 to 6 hours to every 10 to 12 hours, depends on the route of administration and preparation. They are particularly effective for delayed nausea when used in combination antiemetic regimen.[59,90] However, this category of medications may cause side effects, including drowsiness, hypotension, and extrapyramidal symptoms, especially in older patients. Change in cognitive function was strongly associated with increased use of prochlorperazine in a study of 535 patients receiving ANCT.[109] Cognitive function, global QOL, fatigue, anorexia, insomnia, and dyspnea were significantly worse in those who vomited.

Substituted benzamides, such as metoclopramide, are effective with low to moderate NV.[101] Bruera et al[4] found that a metoclopramide-based treatment regimen was effective in controlling the frequency and intensity of chronic nausea in 100 patients admitted to a palliative care unit.

Other medications that have antiemetic effects include butyrophenones, antihistamines, antiemetics, corticosteroids, and cannabinoids. Butyrophenones are major tranquilizers and are particularly effective when anxiety is associated with NV. Antihistamines, such as cyclizine and promethazine, and anticholinergics, particularly hyoscine, also exhibit an antiemetic effect. An advantage of these medications is that some can be administered with a transdermal patch, orally, or parenterally.[74] Corticosteroids are useful in heightening the effects of other antiemetics.[59,93] The use of cannabinoids for the management of NVR has been limited, although some studies have shown reduced NVR with the use of cannabinoids.[110-113] A study of the antiemetic medication preferences of practicing oncologists revealed that cannabinoids (either as marijuana smoke or oral tetrahydrocannabinol) were ranked ninth in order of preference for the treatment of mild to moderate NV, and sixth for more severe symptoms associated with chemotherapy.[111] Gonzales-Rosales and Walsh[113] found dronabinol in combination with prochlorperazine was effective in treating unresponsive NV in a patient with widespread metastatic disease.

Nonpharmacological Interventions

Nonpharmacological interventions can be used alone, in combination, or as adjuvant therapy with pharmaceutical agents to manage NVR. Although research is limited, there are studies that support the effectiveness of a variety of interventions. These interventions may be effective in controlling NVR by relaxing the patient which, when used in conjunction with antiemetics, may result in a reduction of the dose and frequency required.

Diet and Environment. Before antiemetics are prescribed, the stimuli for nausea in the environment should be reduced or eliminated. This may include minimizing sights, sounds, or smells that can initiate nausea. Unpleasant odors and smells from cooking should be eliminated. Attractively prepared food should be presented in small amounts. Cool, carbonated beverages are generally more desirable. Room-temperature and bland foods seem to be better tolerated than hot foods. Foods may taste differently due to taste changes and need to be selected accordingly. Sweet, fatty, highly salted, and spicy foods should be avoided. Experimenting with sour foods such as lemons, sour pickles, or sour hard candy is also helpful. The patient's preference or desire not to eat must be recognized since ingestion of food may cause NVR with concomitant abdominal symptoms such as pain, abdominal distention, constipation, or diarrhea.

Acupuncture/Acupressure. The use of acupuncture and acupressure to relieve NV has been found to be effective in several populations. Acupressure at the P6 (Nei-Guan) point was an effective prophylaxis for postoperative NV in a study of 200 surgical patients.[114] Stein et al[115] found that acupressure was an effective, nonpharmacological method to reduce intraoperative nausea during elective cesarean section in the awake patient. Alkaissi, Stalnert, and Kalman[116] reported that the placebo effect of acupressure decreased nausea after 24 hours, but vomiting and need of rescue antiemetics was reduced only by acupressure with the correct P6 point stimulation. However, Dibble[117] reported significant differences between two groups of women receiving chemotherapy for breast cancer in nausea and nausea intensity with the finger acupressure group reporting less intensity and experience of nausea. A review of 10 randomized trials studying the effects of acupressure, ginger, and pyridoxine on the NV of pregnancy found they were beneficial, although the data on acupressure were equivocal.[118] In a randomized, single-blind, crossover study, manual acpuncture reduced hyperemesis gravidaruim. Findings suggested that active P6 acupuncture, in combination with standard treatment, could relieve hyperemesis gravidarum more quickly than placebo.[119] Dundee et al[120,121] found that P6 acupuncture is an effective adjuvant to conventional antiemetic therapy for patients having cytotoxic medications and that it was effective when used with a large number of patients receiving chemotherapy.[120]

There has been very limited research using acupressure with terminally ill patients. Acupressure wrist bands in a small sample of hospice patients were not effective in reducing NV.[121] The causative factors of NV, such as constipation, in this population may require a different kind of management.

Music Therapy. Relaxation or hypnotic techniques serve as adjuncts to medication and other comfort measures. Frank[122] investigated the effects of music therapy and guided visual imagery on anxiety and the degree and length of NV in patients with a history of chemotherapy nausea and vomiting. Patients' perceived degree of vomiting was significantly reduced, and there was a suggestion of a decrease in the length of vomiting.

Progressive Muscle Relaxation (PMR). According to Bayuk,[123] relaxation techniques, including PMR training, guided imagery, and hypnosis, have been shown to be helpful in alleviating the NV as well as the anxiety experienced by cancer patients receiving chemotherapy. This is supported by several research studies. Cotanch and Strum[124] found that PMR may be effective in reducing side effects of nausea, vomiting, anorexia, and emotional distress that frequently accompany chemotherapy. Morrow and Hickok[125] found PMR training was effective in preventing as well as decreasing the frequency of postchemotherapy NV. A study of 60 Japanese patients receiving chemotherapy verified the effectiveness of PMR in reducing NVR.[126] There is no published research using PMR in palliative care. However, the positive results found with chemotherapy patients indicate it may be a useful strategy in palliative care.

Guided Imagery. Guided imagery has been found to be effective in decreasing NV. In one study, patients who received guided imagery had significantly less perceived degree of vomiting and a decrease in the length of vomiting with the intervention.[122] A clinical relaxation program that included guided imagery was compared to a standard antiemetic protocol for chemotherapy in another study.[127] The antiemetic protocol was more effective in preventing periods of NV; however, the total period of NV was four hours shorter with the relaxation program. The effectiveness of guided imagery when added to a standard antiemetic regimen in patients receiving chemotherapy showed that the guided imagery group experienced symptoms later than the control group, although the differences were not significantly different.[128] The guided imagery group did feel significantly more prepared, relaxed, and in control than the control group.

The research findings related to the effectiveness of nonpharmacological measures to manage NVR are limited. There is support for their use either alone or as a supplement to pharmacological agents. Nonpharmacological measures are noninvasive, can frequently be done by the patient alone, and enhance feelings of control.

CASE STUDY

The following case study illustrates the symptom experiences of nausea, vomiting, and retching associated with ANCT for breast cancer.

Mrs. H, a 48-year-old woman, was diagnosed with stage II breast cancer. She is married and has four children; the youngest is 16. With her pregnancies she had moderate nausea and vomiting, particularly during the first trimester. Just before her diagnosis of breast cancer, Mrs. H received a promotion at work to a position she has been working toward for several years. It was important for her to be able to continue to work if at all possible.

Mrs. H underwent a left modified radical mastectomy, followed by six cycles of cyclophosphamide (Cytoxan), doxorubicin (Adriamycin), and 5-fluorouracil (5FU) (CAF) chemotherapy. The chemotherapy protocol consisted of: Adriamycin 50 mg/m^2, day 1; Cytoxan 500 mg/m^2, day 1; and 5FU 500 mg/m^2, days 1 and 8. This cycle was repeated every 21 days for six cycles. Management of side effects was of the utmost importance in order to enable Mrs. H to continue working. She also was concerned about possibly feeling too drowsy, because it would interfere with work and her responsibilities at home.

The following antiemetic regimen was used for the first cycle of chemotherapy. Before beginning chemotherapy, Mrs. H was given dexamethasone (Decadron) 20 mg orally and granisetron (Kytril) 2 mg. According to her self-care journal, the evening following her first chemotherapy, she took Decadron 10 mg orally. The day after chemotherapy, she took Decadron 8 mg twice a day; the second day she took Decadron 4 mg, twice a day; and the third day she took Decadron 2 mg twice a day. In addition to Decadron, she took ondansetron (Zofran) 8 mg orally for 3 days. Prochlorperazine (Compazine) 10 mg every 6 hours, and lorazepam (Ativan) 1 mg every 4 hours were available as needed for nausea and vomiting. Mrs. H reported that she had seven episodes of vomiting, and she reported persistent nausea the first 2 days following chemotherapy. The nausea continued for 1 week. She was able to work following chemotherapy but felt the nausea interfered with her ability to do her usual quality of work.

During the second cycle of chemotherapy, the premedications were changed to control nausea and vomiting immediately after chemotherapy. Mrs. H received Decadron 20 mg, along with Zofran 32 mg via intravenous piggyback (IVPB) before her chemotherapy. Following chemotherapy she took Decadron 10 mg every 8 hours for four doses, then Decadron 8 mg, twice a day for 1 day; then 4 mg, twice a day for 1 day; then 2 mg, twice a day for 1 day; along with Zofran 8 mg orally for 3 days. Compazine and Ativan were ordered to be taken as needed for nausea and vomiting. Following this cycle, Mrs. H reported moderate nausea and two or three episodes of vomiting after chemotherapy. Although the nausea was not as severe as it was following the first cycle, she found it to be more distressful. She had persistent nausea again for 1 week after chemotherapy and found this more difficult to deal with than after the first cycle.

Although she had NV after the second cycle, Mrs. H did not want to change the medications she received to manage it. Therefore the same antiemetic regimen was followed for the third cycle of chemotherapy. The nurse instructed Mrs. H in using guided imagery and relaxation to control these symptoms. Mrs. H's NV were controlled after chemotherapy, but she again had persistent nausea for the week following chemotherapy. She tried using imagery and relaxation techniques but found it was too difficult for her to concentrate, and these alternative therapies were not effective for her.

For the fourth cycle, the premedications were the same as the previous two cycles, because vomiting that occurred immediately after chemotherapy vomiting had been controlled. Following chemotherapy, Compazine 10 mg every 6 hours around the clock for 72 hours was added to the postchemotherapy medications to control nausea. Mrs. H returned for evaluation after 2 days of taking Compazine, because she felt so groggy and weak that she felt something else was wrong. Her nausea was controlled, but Mrs. H reported that she felt too drugged and could not function as she wanted. She reported being unable to manage usual activities at home and unable to concentrate at work.

For the fifth cycle of chemotherapy, Mrs. H received the same premedications she had received the previous three cycles. After chemotherapy, the Compazine was eliminated from the antiemetic regimen because of the adverse effects she had reported. An accupressure Relief Band was prescribed and was used for 72 hours. She was instructed to apply the Relief Band when she began to feel nauseated and to wear it until she was nausea free. With the Relief Band, she reported that she experienced some nausea, but felt it was tolerable. She was able to function both at work and at home. Although she felt her energy level was decreased somewhat, she felt alert and was able to concentrate at work.

Mrs. H reported satisfaction with the management of her nausea and vomiting during the previous cycle, so the same regimen was followed for the last cycle of chemotherapy. Following chemotherapy she used the relief band and one dose of Compazine 10 mg, which prevented any NV, and did not make her feel drowsy or interfere with her activities of daily living. Following completion of this protocol, she received tamoxifen.

SELECTED RESEARCH

Much of the research on cancer patients has focused on pharmacological measures to manage NVR. The following selected research studies present some alternative methods for managing NVR in various populations.

The effectiveness of acupressure as a complement to the usual pharmacological methods to prevent and/or relieve NV was examined in 157 NV-prone postoperative patients.[129] This quasi-experimental study used acupressure wristbands (Sea-Bands) on one or both wrists of the treatment group. Subjects were placed into 5 groups: group 1 had Sea-Bands on both wrists; group 2 had Sea-Bands on one wrist; group 3 had wristbands without acupressure on both wrists; group 4 had a wristband without acupressure on one wrist; and group 5 had no wristband. Although acupressure on one or both wrists did not significantly decrease postoperative NV, these findings must be considered with caution because of the small sample size.

The effect of a preoperative fluid bolus on postoperative NV was examined with 90 female patients undergoing laparoscopic surgery.[130] The 45 women in the experimental group received a 1-L normal saline solution bolus preoperatively, whereas the 45 women in the control group received the standard fluids preoperatively. Both groups received usual care postoperatively. The two groups were similar in age, but the control group was significantly heavier. Fifty-one percent of the control group had an episode of NV, compared with 17% of the experimental group. These findings indicate that a liter of saline fluid bolus given preoperatively may decrease the incidence of postoperative NV following laparoscopic surgery.

Grealish, Lomasney, and Whiteman[131] tested the effectiveness of foot massage in relieving NV in 87 patients hospitalized with cancer. A 10-minute foot massage (5 minutes per foot) was found to have a significant immediate effect on patients' perceptions of pain, nausea, and relaxation.

QUESTIONS FOR FUTURE STUDY

Future research on NVR needs to encompass diverse populations, including those grouped by age, sex, health state, cultural background, and medical conditions. The following are suggested questions for future research:

- What instruments are appropriate, reliable, and valid to use with diverse groups?
- How can preparatory information interventions be used with various populations?
- What are the different patterns of anticipatory, acute, and delayed NVR?
- What is the relationship of concurrent symptoms that occur over time with NVR?
- How do gender differences or predisposing factors influence emetic sensitivity?
- How can clinical trials be designed to separately measure the symptoms of nausea, vomiting, and retching; and their components, occurrence, and distress?
- Are there different pharmacological interventions that will reduce the symptoms of NVR in various populations?
- Which nonpharmacological interventions are effective in reducing the symptoms of NVR in various populations?

- What interventions are effective in preventing anticipatory symptoms and enhancing the patient's quality of life?
- What are the patterns of NVR during pregnancy?

REFERENCES

1. Fainsinger, R., Miller, M.J., & Bruera, E. (1991). Symptom control during the last week of life. *Journal of Palliative Care 7,* 5-11.
2. Addington-Hall, J., & McCarthy, M. (1995). Dying from cancer: Results of a national population-based investigation. *Palliative Medicine 29,* 295-305.
3. Osoba, D., Warr, D.G., Fitch, M.I., Nakashima, L., & Warren, B. (1995). Guidelines for the optimal management of chemotherapy-induced NV: A consensus. *Canadian Journal of Oncology 5,* 381-400.
4. Bruera, E., Seifert, L., Watanabe, S., Babul, N., Darke, A., Harsanyi, Z., et al. (1996). Chronic nausea in advanced cancer patients: A retrospective assessment of a metoclopramide-based anti-emetic regimen. *Journal of Pain Symptom Management 11,* 1147-1153.
5. Kurtz, M.E., Kurtz, J.C., Given, C.C., & Given, B. (1996). Concordance of patient and caregiver symptom reports. *Cancer Practice 4,* 185-190.
6. Morrow, G.R., Roscoe, J.A., Hynes, H.E., Flynn, P.J., Pierce, H.I., & Burish, T. (1998). Progress in reducing anticipatory nausea and vomiting: A study of community practice. *Supportive Cancer Care 6*(1), 46-50.
7. Rhodes, V.A. (1997). Criteria for assessment of nausea, vomiting, and retching. *Oncology Nursing Forum Supplement 24*(7), 13-19.
8. Grant, M. (1997). Introduction: Nausea and vomiting, quality of life, and the oncology nurse. *Oncology Nursing Forum Supplement 24*(7), 5-7.
9. Guyton, A. (1980). *Textbook of medical physiology* (6th ed.). Philadelphia: W.B. Saunders.
10. Dodd, M.J., Onishi, K., Dibble, S., & Larson, P.J. (1996). Differences in nausea, vomiting, and retching between younger and older outpatients receiving cancer chemotherapy. *Cancer Nursing 19,* 155-161.
11. Norris, C.A. (1982). Nausea and vomiting. In C.A. Norris (ed.), *Concept clarification in nursing: A sampler* (pp. 81-110). Wakefield, Mass.: Nursing Resources.
12. Rhodes, V.A., Watson, P.M., Johnson, M.H., Madsen, R.W., & Beck, N.C. (1987). Patterns of nausea, vomiting, and distress in patients receiving antineoplastic drug protocols. *Oncology Nursing Forum 14*(4), 3544.
13. Rhodes, V.A., & McDaniel, R.W. (2001). Nausea, vomiting, and retching: Complex problems in palliative care. *CA: A Cancer Journal for Clinicians 51,* 232-248.
14. National Comprehensive Cancer Network. (2001). *Nausea and vomiting: Treatment guidelines for patients with cancer* (Version 1, pp. 5-36). Atlanta: American Cancer Society.
15. Andrews, P., & Whitehead, S. (1990). Pregnancy sickness. *News in Physiological Sciences (NIPS) 5,* 5-10.
16. Jenkins, M.L., & Shelton, B.J. (1989). The effectiveness of self-care actions in reducing morning sickness. In S.F. Funk, E.M. Tornquist, M.T. Champagne, L.A. Copp, & R.A. Wiese (eds.), *Key aspects of comfort: Management of pain, fatigue, and nausea* (pp. 267-272). New York: Springer.
17. Rousseau, P. (1995). Antiemetic therapy in adults with terminal disease: A brief review. *American Journal of Hospice and Palliative Care 12*(1), 13-18.
18. Sarna, L. (1998). Effectiveness of structured nursing assessment of symptom distress in advanced lung cancer. *Oncology Nursing Forum 25*(6), 1041-1048.
19. Murphy, P.A. (1998). Alternative therapies for nausea and vomiting of pregnancy. *Obstetrics & Gynecology 91,* 149-155.
20. O'Brien, B., Naber, S. (1992). Nausea and vomiting during pregnanacy: Effects on the quality of women's lives. *Birth 19,* 138-143.
21. Jarnfelt-Samsioe, A. (1987). Nausea and vomiting in pregnancy: A review. *Obstetrical and Gynecological Survey 41,* 422-427.
22. Dilorio, C.K., & van Lier, D.J. (1989). Nausea and vomiting in pregnancy. In S.F. Funk, E.M. Tornquist, M.T. Champagne, L.A. Copp, & R.A.Wiese (eds.), *Key aspects of comfort: Management of pain, fatigue, and nausea* (pp. 259-267). New York: Springer.
23. Whitehead, S.A., Andrews, P.L.R., & Chamberlanin, G.V.P. (1992). Characterization of nausea and vomiting in early pregnancy: A survey of 1000 women. *Journal of Obstetrics and Gynecology 12,* 364-369.
24. Whitehead, S.A., Holden, W.A., & Andrews, P.L.R. (1992). Pregnancy sickness. In A.L. Bianchi, L. Grelot, A.D. Miller, & G.L. King (eds.), *Mechanisms and control of emesis. Libbey: Eurotest* (pp. 297-306). (Colloque INSERM, Vol. 223). Paris: Institut National de la Santé et de la Recherche Médicale.
25. Broussard, C.N., & Richter, J.E. (1998). Nausea and vomiting of pregnancy. *Gastroenterology Clinics of North America 27,* 123-151.
26. Lacroix, R., Eason, E., & Melzack, R. (2000). Nausea and vomiting during pregnancy: A prospective study of its frequency, intensity, and patterns of change. *Obstetrics & Gynecology 182,* 931-937.
27. Jewell, D., & Young, G. (2001). Interventions for nausea and vomiting in early pregnancy. The Cochrane Library (Oxford), Issue 2 (9P). (Update Software, online or CD-ROM, updated quarterly).
28. Hawthorn, J. (1995). *Understanding and management of nausea and vomiting.* London: Blackwell.
29. Mann, A. (1998). A continuing postoperative complication: Nausea and vomiting—who is affected, why, and what are the contributing factors. *CRNA—the Clinical Forum for Nurse Anesthetists 9*(1), L19-L29.
30. Munro, H. (2000). Postoperative nausea and vomiting in children. *Journal of Perianesthesia Nursing 15*(6), 401-407.
31. Goodarzi, M. (1998). A double blind comparison of droperidol and ondansetron for prevention of emesis in children undergoing orthopaedic surgery. *Paediatric Anaesthesia 8,* 325-329.
32. Alon, E., Buchser, E., Herrera, E., Christiaens, F., De Pauw, C., Ritter, L., et al. (1998). Tropisetron for treating established postoperative nausea and vomiting: a randomized, double-blind, placebo-controlled study. *Anesthesia and Analgesia 86*(3), 617-623.
33. Gunta, K., Lewis, C., & Nuccio, S. (2000). Prevention and management of postoperative nausea and vomiting. *Orthopedic Nursing 19*(2), 39-48.
34. Konvalinka, P.A. (1999). Relationship of the menstrual cycle to postoperative incidence of emesis after laparoscopic cholecystectomy. *Clinical Excellence for Nurse Practitioners 3*(6), 353-358.

35. Cohen, M.M., Cameron, C.B., & Duncan, P.G. (1990). Pediatric anesthesia morbidity and mortality in the postoperative period. *Anesthesia and Analgesia 70,* 160-167.
36. Purkis, I.E. (1964). Postoperative Vomiting. *Canadian Anaesthetists Society Journal 11*(4), 335-352.
37. Rita, L., Goodarzi, M., & Seleny, F. (1981). Effect of low dose droperidol on postoperative vomiting in children. *Canadian Anaesthetists Society Journal 28,* 259-262.
38. Craig, J.G., & Powell, B.L. (1987). The management of nausea and vomiting in clinical oncology. *American Journal of Medical Science 293,* 34-44.
39. Jacobson, P.B., & Redd, W.H. (1988). The development and management of chemotherapy related anticipatory nausea and vomiting. *Cancer Investigations 6,* 329-336.
40. Vance, J.P., Neill, R.S., & Norris, W. (1973). The incidence and etiology of postoperative nausea and vomiting in a plastic surgical unit. *British Journal of Plastic Surgery 26,* 226-339.
41. Forrest, J.B., Cahalan, M.K., Rehder, K., Goldsmith, C.H., Levy, W.J., Strunin, L., Bota, W., Boucek, C.D., Cucchiara, R.F., & Dhamee, S. et al. (1990). Multicenter study of general anaesthesia. II: Results. *Anesthesiology 72,* 262-268.
42. Warriner, C.B., Knox, D., Belo, S., Cole, C., Finegan, B.A., & Perreault, L. (1997). Prophylactic oral dolasetron mesylate reduces nausea and vomiting after abdominal hysterectomy. The Canadian Dolasetron Study Group. *Canadian Journal of Anaesthesia 44*(11), 1167-1173.
43. Bacic, A., Rumboldt, Z., Gluncic, I., & Buklijas, J. (1998). The impact of the menstrual cycle and ondansetron on postoperative nausea and vomiting. *International Journal of Clinical Pharmacology Research 18*(4), 153-158.
44. Jacobson, O.B., Borbjerg, D.H., & Redd, W.H. (1993). Anticipatory anxiety in women receiving chemotherapy for breast cancer. *Health Psychology 12,* 469-475.
45. Rhodes, V.A., Watson, P.M., McDaniel, R.W., Hanson, B.M., & Johnson, M.H. (1995). Expectation and occurrence of postchemotherapy side effects. *Cancer Practice 3*(4), 247-253.
46. Rhodes, V.A., McDaniel, R.W., Hanson, B., Markway, E., & Johnson, M. (1994). Sensory perceptions of patients on selected antineoplastic chemotherapy protocols. *Cancer Nursing 17*(1), 45-51.
47. Johnson, J., Lauver, D., & Nail, L. (1989). Process of coping with radiation. *Journal of Counseling and Clinical Psychology 57,* 358-364.
48. Orem, D.E. (2001). Health, self-care, and deliberate action. In D.E. Orem, *Nursing: Concepts of practice* (6th ed.). St Louis: Mosby.
49. Hursti, T.J. (1995). Individual factors modifying chemotherapy related nausea and vomiting. *Karolinska Institutet Dissertation Abstracts International 56*(1), 304.
50. Sullivan, P.F., Bulik, C.M., & Kendler, K.S. (1998). Genetic epidemiology of binging and vomiting. *British Journal of Psychiatry 173,* 75-79.
51. Howarth, P.A., & Finch, M. (1999). The nauseogenicity of two methods of navigating within a virtual environment. *Applied Ergonomics 30*(1), 39-45.
52. Hesketh, P.J., Kris, M.G., Grunberg, S.M., Beck, T., Hainsworth, J.D., Harker, G., et al. (1997). Proposal for classifying the acute emetogenicity of cancer chemotherapy. *Journal of Clinical Oncology 15,* 103-109.
53. American Hospital Formulary Service. (2001). *Drug information.* Bethesda, Md.: American Society of Health-System Pharmacists.
54. Andrews, P.R.L., & Davis, C.J. (1993). The mechanism of emesis induced by anticancer therapies. In P.R.L. Andrews, & G.J. Sanger (eds.), *Emesis in anticancer therapy: Mechanisms and treatment* (pp. 113-161). New York: Chapman & Hall.
55. Grunberg, S.M. (2001). Nausea and vomiting. In C.M. Haskell (ed.), *Cancer treatment* (ed. 5, pp. 327-331). Philadelphia: W.B. Saunders.
56. Veyrat-Follet, C., Farinottik, R., & Raimer, J.L. (1997). Physiology of chemotherapy-induced emesis and antiemetic therapy: Predictive models for evaluation of new compounds. *Drugs 53,* 206-234.
57. Fozard, J.R. (1987). 5-HT3 receptors and cytotoxic drug-induced vomiting. *Trends in Pharm Sci 8,* 444-445.
58. Baines, M., Oliver, D.J., & Carter, R.L. (1995). Medical management of intestinal obstruction in patients with advanced malignant disease. *Lancet 2,* 990-993.
59. Herrstedt, J. (1998). Antiemetic research: A look to the future. *Supportive Care in Cancer 6,* 8-12.
60. Gralla, R.J. (2000). Antiemetic therapy. In R.C. Bast, D.W. Kufe, R.E. Pollock, R.R. Weichselbaum, J.F. Holland, & E. Frei (eds.), *Cancer medicine* (ed. 5, pp. 2243-2250). Lewiston, N.Y.: B.C. Decker.
61. Vutyavanich, T., Kraisarin, T., & Ruangsri, R. (2001). Ginger for nausea and vomiting in pregnancy: Randomized, double-masked, placebo-controlled trial. *Obstetrics & Gynecology 97*(4), 577-582.
62. Coad, J., Al-Rasasi, B., & Morgan, J. (2000). New insights into nausea and vomiting in pregnancy. *Midirs Midwifery Digest 10*(4), 451-454.
63. Boneva, R.S., Moore, C.A., & Botto, L., Wong, L.Y., & Erickson, J.D. (1999). Nausea during pregnancy and congenital heart defects: A population-based case-control study. *American Journal of Epidemiology 149*(8), 717-725.
64. Zhou, Q., O'Brien, B., & Relyea, J. (1999). Severity of nausea and vomiting during pregnancy: What does it predict? *Birth 26*(2), 108-114.
65. Allen, L.R., Sudesh, S., Sandramouli, S., Cooper, G., McFarlane, D., & Willshaw, H.E. (1998). The association between the oculocardiac reflex and post-operative vomiting in children undergoing strabismus surgery. *Eye 12*(Pt 2), L193-L196.
66. Fredrikson, M., Hurtsti, T., & Salmi, P., Borjeson, S., Furst, C.J., Peterson, C., et al. (1993). Conditioned nausea after cancer chemotherapy and autonomic nervous system condition ability. *Scandinavian Journal of Psychology 34,* 318-329.
67. Andrykowski, M.A. (1990). The role of anxiety in the development of anticipatory nausea in cancer chemotherapy: A review and synthesis. *Psychiatry in Medicine 52,* 957-960.
68. Fujii, Y., Toyooka, H., & Tanaka, H. (1997). Prevention of PONV with granisetron, droperidol and metoclopramide in female patients with history of motion sickness. *Cancer Anesth 44,* 820-824.
69. D'Acquisto, R., Tyson, L.B., Gralla, R.H., et al. (1986). The influence of a chronic high alcohol intake on chemotherapy-induced nausea and vomiting. *Proceedings of the American Society of Clinical Oncology,* 257.
70. Spiess, J.L., Adelstein, D.J., & Hines, J.D. (1987). Evaluation of ethanol as an antiemetic in patients receiving cisplatin. *Clinical Therapeutics 9,* 400-404.
71. Sullivan, J.R., Leyden, M.J., & Bell, R. (1983). Decreased cisplatin-induced nausea and vomiting with chronic

alcohol ingestion. *New England Journal of Medicine 309,* 796.
72. Del Favero, A., Tonato, M., & Roila, F. (1992). Issues in the measurement of nausea. *British Journal of Cancer 661,* S69-S71.
73. Fields, J.Z., Turk, A., Durkin, M., Ravi, N.V., & Keshavarzian, A. (1994). Increased gastrointestinal symptoms in chronic alcoholics. *American Journal of Gastroenterology 89,* 382-386.
74. Desbiens, N.A., Mueller-Rizner, N., & Connors, A.F., Wenger, N.S. (1997). The relationship of nausea and dyspnea to pain in seriously ill patients. *Pain 71,* 149-156.
75. Mannix, K.A. (1998). Palliation of nausea and vomiting. In D. Doyle, G.W.C. Hanks, & N. MacDonald (eds.), *Oxford textbook of palliative medicine* (2nd ed.). Oxford, England: Oxford University Press.
76. Hursti, T.J., Avall-Lundqvist, E., & Borjeson, S., Fredrikson, M., Furst, C.J., Steineck, G., et al. (1996). Impact of tumour burden on chemotherapy induced nausea and vomiting. *British Journal of Cancer 74,* 1114-1119.
77. McDaniel, R.W., & Rhodes, V.A. (1995). Symptom experience: The management of symptom occurrence and symptom distress. *Seminars in Oncology Nursing 11*(4), 232-234.
78. Rhodes, V.A., McDaniel, R.W., Homan, S.S., Johnson, M., & Madsen, R. (2000). An instrument to measure symptom experience: Symptom occurrence and symptom distress. *Cancer Nursing 23,* 49-54.
79. Cotanch, P. (1983). Relaxation training for control of nausea and vomiting in patients receiving chemotherapy. *Cancer Nursing 6,* 277-283.
80. Simms, S.G., Rhodes, V.A., & Madsen, R.W. (1993). Comparison of prochlorperazine and lorazepam antiemetic regimens in the control of postchemotherapy symptoms. *Nursing Research 42*(4), 234-239.
81. Rhodes, V.A., McDaniel, R.W., & Matthews, C.A. (1998). Hospice patient and nurses perceptions of self-care deficits based on symptom experience. *Cancer Nursing 21*(5), 312-319.
82. DeKeyser, F.G., Wainstock, J.M., Rose, L., Converse, P.J., & Dooley, W. (1998). Distress, symptom distress, and immune function in women with suspected breast cancer. *Oncology Nursing Forum 25*(8), 1415-1422.
83. Rhodes, V.A., Watson, P.M., & Johnson, M.H. (1984). Development of reliable and valid measures of nausea and vomiting. *Cancer Nursing 7*(1), 33-41.
84. McCorkle, R., & Young, K. (1978). Development of a sympton distress scale. *Cancer Nursing 1,* 373-378.
85. Portenoy, R.K., Thaler, H.T., Kornblith, A.B., Lepore, J.M., Friedlander-Klar, H., Kiyasu, E., Sobel, K., Coyle, N., Kemeny, N., & Norton, L., et al. (1994). The memorial symptom assessment scale: An instrument for the evaluation of symptom prevalence, characteristics and distress. *E J Cancer 30A*(9), 1326-1336.
86. Rhodes, V.A., & McDaniel, R.W. (1997). Measuring nausea, vomiting, and retching. In M. Frank-Stromborg, & S. Olsen (eds.), *Instruments for clinical health-care research* (2nd ed., pp. 509-517). Sudbury, Mass.: Jones & Bartlett.
87. Rhodes, V. A., & McDaniel, R.W. (1999). The Index of Nausea, Vomiting, and Retching: A new format of the Index of Nausea and Vomiting. *Oncology Nursing Forum 26,* 889-894.
88. Morrow, G.R., Ballatori, E., Groshen, S., & Olver, I. (1998). Statistical considerations in the design, conduct and analyses of antiemetic clinical trials: An emerging consensus. *Supportive Care in Cancer 6*(3), 261-265.
89. Andrykowski, M.A., Jacobsen, P.B., Marks, E., Gorfinkle, K., Hakes, T.B., Kaufman, R.J., Currie, V.E., Holland, J.C., & Redd, W.H. (1988). Prevalence, predictors, and course of anticipatory nausea in women receiving chemotherapy for breast cancer. *Cancer 62,* 2607-2613.
90. Gandara, D.R., Harvey, W.H., Monaghan, G.G., Perez, E.A., Stokes, C., Bryson, J.C., Finn, A.L., Hesketh, P.J. (1992). The delayed emesis syndrome from cisplatin: Phase III evaluation of ondansetron versus placebo. *Seminars in Oncology 19,* 67-71.
91. Pereira, J., & Bruera, E. (1996). Successful management of intractable nausea with ondansetron: A case study. *Journal of Palliative Care 12*(2), 47-50.
92. Currow, D.C., Coughlan, M., Fardell, B., & Cooney, N.J. (1997). Use of ondansetron in palliative medicine. *Journal of Pain Symptom Management 13*(5), 302-307.
93. Brown, S., North, D., Marvel, M.K., & Fons, R. (1992). Acupressure wrist bands to relieve nausea and vomiting in hospice patients: Do they work? *American Journal of Hospital Palliative Care 9,* 26-29.
94. Trovato, J.A., Stull, D.M., & Finley, R.S. (1998). Outcomes of antiemetic therapy after the administration of high-dose antineoplastic agents. *American Journal of Health-System Pharmacists 55*(12), 1269-1274.
95. Mystakidou, K., Befon, S., Liossi, C., & Vlachos, L. (1998). Comparison of tropisetron and chlorpromazine combinations in the control of nausea and vomiting of patients with advanced cancer. *Journal of Pain Symptom Management 15,* 176-184.
96. Belluomini, J., Little, R.C., Lee, K.A., & Katz, M. (1994). Acupressure for nausea and vomiting of pregnancy: A randomized, blinded study. *Obstetrics & Gynecology 84,* 245-248.
97. Safari, H.R., Fassett, M.J., Souter, I.C., Alsulyman, O.M., & Goodwin, T.M. (1998). The efficacy of methylprednisolone in the treatment of hyperemesis gravidaruim: A randomized, double-blind, controlled study. *American Journal of Obstetrics and Gynecology 179*(4), 921-924.
98. Rees, J.H., Ginsberg, L., & Schapira, A.H. (1997). Two pregnant women with vomiting and fits. *American Journal of Obstetrics and Gynecology 177*(6), 1539-1540.
99. Pole, M., Einarson, A., Pairaudeau, N., Einarson, T., & Koren, G. (2000). Drug labeling and risk perceptions of teratogenicity: A survey of pregnant Canadian women and their health professionals. *Journal of Clinical Pharmacy 40*(6), 573-577.
100. Wilkinson, J.M. (2000). What do we know about herbal morning sickness treatments? A literature survey. *Midwifery 16*(3), 224-228.
101. Gallo, M., Sarkar, M., Au, W., Pietrzak, K., Comas, B., Smith, M., et al. (2000). Pregnancy outcome following gestational exposure to echinacea: A prospective controlled study. *Archives of Internal Medicine 160*(20), 3141-3143.
102. Roila, F., Aapro, M., & Stewart, A. (1998). Optimal selection of antiemetics in children receiving cancer chemotherapy. *Supportive Care in Cancer 6*(3), 215-220.
103. Goodarzi, M. (1998). A double blind comparison of droperidol and ondansetron for prevention of emesis in children undergoing orthopedic surgery. *Pediatric Anesthesia 8*(4), 325-329.
104. Fujii, Y., & Tanake, H. (1999). Granisetron reduces post-operative vomiting in children: A dose-ranging study. *European Journal of Anaesthesia 16*(1), 62-65.

105. Koivuranta, M., Jokela, R., Kiviluoma, K., & Alahuhta, S. (1997). The anti-emetic efficacy of a combination of ondansetron and droperidol. *Anaesthesia 52*(9), 863-868.
106. Pappas, A.L., Sukhani, R., Hotaling, A.J., Mikat-Stevens, M., Javorski, J.J., Donzelli, J., et al. (1998). The effect of preoperative dexamethasone on the immediate and delayed postoperative morbidity in children undergoing adenotonsillectomy. *Anesthesia and Analgesia 87*(1), 57-61.
107. Tang, J., Angelo, R., White, R.F., & Scuderi, P.E. (1998). The efficacy of RS-25259: A long-acting selective 5-HT3 receptor antagonist, for preventing postoperative nausea and vomiting after hysterectomy procedures. *Anesthesia and Analgesia 67*(2), 462-467.
108. Alon, E., Buchser, E., Herrera, E., Christiaens, F., De Pauw, C., Ritter, L., et al. (1998). Tropisetron for treating established postoperative nausea and vomiting: A randomized, double-blind, placebo-controlled study. *Anesthesia and Analgesia 86*(3), 617-623.
109. Osoba, D., Warr, D., Zee, B., Latreille, J., Kaizer, L., & Pater, J. (1995). Pretreatment health-related quality-of-life (HQL) status predicts chemotherapy-induced emesis (CIE). *Proceedings of the Annual Meeting of American Society of Clinical Oncology 14,* A1625.
110. McCabe, M., Smith, F.P., MacDonald, J.S., Woolley, P.V., Goldberg, D., Schein, P.S. (1988). Efficacy of tetrahydrocannabinol in patients refractory to standard antiemetic therapy. *Investigative New Drugs 6*(3), 243-246.
111. Schwartz, R.H., & Beveridge, R.A. (1994). Marijuana as an antiemetic drug: How useful is it today? Opinions from clinical oncologists. *Journal of Addictive Diseases 13*(1), 53-65.
112. Tortorice, P.V., & O'Connell, M.B. (1990). Management of chemotherapy-induced nausea and vomiting [Review]. *Pharmacotherapy 10*(2), 129-145.
113. Gonzales-Rosales, F., & Walsh, D. (1997). Palliative care rounds: Intractable nausea and vomiting due to gastrointestinal mucosal metastases relived by tetrahydrocannabinol. *Journal of Pain Symptom Management 14,* 311-314.
114. Fan, C.F., Tanhui, E., Joshi, S., Trivedi, S., Hong, Y., & Shevde, K. (1997). Acupressure treatment for prevention of postoperative nausea and vomiting. *Anesthesia and Analgesia 84*(4), 821-825.
115. Stein, D.J., Birnbach, D.J., Danzer, B.I., Kuroda, M.M., Grunebaum, A., & Thys, D.M. (1997). Acupressure versus intravenous metoclopramide to prevent nausea and vomiting during spinal anesthesia for cesarean section. *Anesthesia and Analgesia 84*(2), 342-345.
116. Alkaissi, A., Tallnert, M., & Kalman, S. (1999). Effect and placebo effect of acupressure (P6) on nausea and vomiting after outpatient gynaecological surgery. *Acta Anaesthesiologica Scandinavica 43*(3), 270-274.
117. Dibble, S. (1999). Acupressure for nausea. Unpublished manuscript. San Francisco: University of California School of Nursing.
118. Meltzer, D.I. (2000). Selections from current literature. Complementary therapies for nausea and vomiting in early pregnancy. *Family Practice 17*(6), 570-573.
119. Carlsson, C.P.O., Axemo, P., Bodin, A., Carstensen, H., Ehrenroth, B., Madegard-Lind, I., et al. (2000). Manual acupuncture reduces hyperemesis gravidarum: A placebo-controlled, randomized, single-blind, crossover study. *Journal of Pain Symptom Management 20*(4), 273-279.
120. Dundee, J.W., & Yang, J. (1990). Prolongation of the antiemetic action of p6 acupuncture by acupressure in patients having cancer chemotherapy. *Journal of the Royal Society of Medicine 83*(6), 360-362.
121. Dundee, J.W., Ghaly, R.G., Fizpatrick, K.T.J., Abram, W.P., & Lynch, G.A. (1989). Acupuncture prophylaxis of cancer chemotherapy-induced sickness. *Journal of the Royal Society of Medicine 82,* 268-271.
122. Frank, J.M. (1985). The effects of music therapy and guided visual imagery on chemotherapy induced nausea and vomiting. *Oncology Nursing Forum 12*(5), 47-52.
123. Bayuk, L. (1985). Relaxation techniques: An adjunct therapy for cancer patients. *Seminars in Oncology Nursing 1,* 147-150.
124. Cotanch, P.H., & Strum, S. (1987). Progressive muscle relaxation as antiemetic therapy for cancer patients. *Oncology Nursing Forum 14,* 33-37.
125. Morrow, G.R., & Hickok, J.T. (1993). Behavioral treatment of chemotherapy-induced nausea and vomiting. *Oncology 7*(12), 83-97.
126. Arakawa, S. (1997). Relaxation to reduce nausea, vomiting and anxiety induced by chemotherapy in Japanese patients. *Cancer Nursing 20,* 342-349.
127. Scott, D.W., Donahue, D.C., Mastrovito, R.C., Hakes, T.B. (1986). Comparative trial of clinical relaxation and an antiemetic drug regimen in reducing chemotherapy-related nausea and vomiting. *Cancer Nursing 9,* 178-187.
128. Troesch, L.M., Rodehaver, C.B., Delaney, E.A., & Yanes, B. (1993). The influence of guided imagery on chemotherapy-related nausea and vomiting. *Oncology Nursing Forum 20,* 1179-1185.
129. Windle, P.E., Borromeo, A., Robles, H., & Ilacio-Uy, V. (2001). The effects of acupressure on the incidence of postoperative nausea and vomiting in postsurgical patients. *Journal of Perianesthesia Nursing 16*(3), 158-162.
130. Monti, S., & Pokorny, M.E. (2000). Preop fluid bolus reduces risk of post op nausea and vomiting: A pilot study. *Internet Journal of Advanced Nursing Practice 4*(2), 7.
131. Grealish, L., Lomasney, A., & Whiteman, B. (2000). Foot massage: A nursing intervention to modify the distressing symptoms of pain and nausea in patients hospitalized with cancer. *Cancer Nursing 23*(3), 237-243.

SECTION IV

Alterations in Protection

Protection, viewed as a life process, involves numerous complex mechanisms, host-environment interactions, and reactions. Protection as a process results in shielding an individual from stressors or in altering the impact of the stressors. As with the life process regulation, the process of protection encompasses interactions that promote and maintain homeostasis; that is, ensuring an internal environment conducive to the normal functioning of the total organism. Protective mechanisms are physiological, psychological, and sociological. However, the major foci of the chapters in this section are alterations in the physiological mechanisms of protection.

Physiological protective mechanisms are pervasive throughout the body and are the structural and functional defenses that serve to protect the individual against such stressors as physical and chemical injury, mutagens, carcinogens, foreign bodies, and microorganisms. Examples of the wide range of protective mechanisms operating in the body include detoxification of drugs and other potentially harmful chemicals by the liver; the cough reflex, which protects the respiratory tract from foreign bodies; the thick barrier of mucus that protects the stomach against the corrosive effects of hydrochloric acid; the increased production of red blood cells to protect body tissues from hypoxia; the role of platelets in clotting; the chronobiological mechanisms involved in sleep/wake cycles; the finely tuned neuromotor reflexes that remove the body from harmful stimuli to avoid injury; and the first line of defense, the skin, which shields the internal structures from the external environment. Alterations in the body's protective mechanisms can have local or systemic effects, and the consequences can range from minor to fatal.

The six chapters in this section present alterations in protection that manifest wide diversity, effects, and consequences. They are the stress response, immunosuppression, infection, impaired wound healing, altered clotting, and impaired sleep.

The stress response is viewed as an adaptive, protective mechanism that occurs when endogenous or exogenous stimuli are sensed as threatening to the individual. Stimuli include psychological and physiological stressors; a myriad of responses result to allow the individual to respond to danger or to protect adaptive processes.

Immunosuppression can result from many therapies and clinical conditions. Immunocompetence is essential to protect against infectious organisms, foreign bodies or tissue, and antigens. Alterations in immunocompetence can result in serious consequences for the individual. Infection results when protective mechanisms have been compromised. The alterations in protection, that is, etiological explanations for the infection may range from a very simple wound to multiple traumatic injuries.

Impaired wound healing may result from immunosupression, infection, metabolic disorders such as diabetes or poor nutritional or circulatory status. Healing can be delayed, thus putting the individual at risk for infection and sepsis or a chronic nonhealing wound.

Alterations in clotting reflect a state of imbalance in one or more of the multiple factors and processes involved in the mechanisms of hemostasis. Alterations in any of these mechanisms can impair tissue oxygenation and metabolism.

Sleep disturbances are reflected in alterations in the sleep stages; these range from a minor, occasional problem to a severe condition in which the individual becomes dysfunctional or disoriented.

In each chapter, populations at risk for alterations in protection and the risk factors are identified. Professional nurses must be aware of individuals whose protective mechanisms may be impaired and who require therapeutic interventions. The mechanisms for each alteration and the pathological consequences to the individual are presented. Manifestations of the alterations are delineated, and various parameters for monitoring the patient's state of protection and response to therapies over time are identified.

Understanding the mechanisms by which alterations in protection occur provides the means for developing instruments to measure and assess these human responses and for implementing appropriate clinical management strategies. Case studies and selected research are included in these chapters as a way to demonstrate how nursing practice is influenced by the state of knowledge about the phenomena.

CHAPTER

14 Stress Response

GAYLE GIBONEY PAGE & ADA M. LINDSEY

DEFINITION

Much has been written about stress; the primary foci used have included stress as a response to a severe injury, explication of stress and coping paradigms, delineation of stressful life events, and suggestions for stress reduction therapies. In more recently published literature on stress, there has been considerably less confusion about the differences between stressors and the resulting stress response. In earlier reports, these two concepts frequently were described interchangeably. In the nursing literature, there still is a paucity of work describing stress from a physiological response perspective. The focus of this chapter is the stress response as a physiological response to biopsychosocial stressors.

A variety of definitions have been given to the phenomenon; the emphasis depends on the approach or framework being posited. Sociologists, psychologists, physiologists, and nurses have studied the effects of multiple stressors and have used a variety of parameters to determine the resulting stress response. The nature of each of these disciplines and the individual work done have, to some extent, influenced the approaches used, leading to rather disparate bodies of information about stress. Although the intent is to describe the stress response from a physiological perspective, the following definitions of four concepts related to stress will both provide a starting point and minimize the confusion that often accompanies this complicated phenomenon.

Homeostasis, stressor, stress, and adaptive response are the key concepts. Homeostasis is the maintenance of the complex dynamic equilibrium by which life exists; an equilibrium that is constantly challenged by adverse forces, both intrinsic and extrinsic stressors. Thus stress can be defined as a state of threatened homeostasis, a state in which equilibrium, and therefore life, may be at risk. Homeostasis can be reestablished by a complex repertoire of physiological and behavioral adaptive responses of the individual or organism. If the adaptive responses are inadequate or excessive and prolonged, a health steady state is not maintained, and pathological consequences may follow. The responsiveness of the organism to the potency of the stressor, the exacerbating event or events, can be conceptualized as a dose-response curve. The stress response increases with the intensity of the stressor. The curve can shift to the left or right, denoting an excessive or insufficient response, respectively. Multiple factors can affect stress responses of individuals, such as genetics and environmental influences including significant earlier and concurrent life experiences.[1]

PREVALENCE AND POPULATIONS AT RISK

There are no specific reports on the prevalence or incidence of the stress response. Inasmuch as stressors, whether from sociological, psychological, or physiological sources, are ubiquitous (when considering life in general), it becomes obvious that the prevalence of the stress response is great. According to the definition, it is important to acknowledge that although the response generally serves a protective, adaptive function, it is a graded response: there is a point at which it may result in death. What remains somewhat difficult to quantify precisely is the varying magnitudes of these responses and the specific circumstances in which they occur.

Individuals experiencing the situational or developmental stressors described next represent populations at risk. Persons who are at risk for the greater stress response are those who are already compromised in some way. For example, if someone were in a serious auto accident, had multiple traumatic injuries, had undergone surgery, and then developed a wound infection, this subsequent infection might escalate the stress response. By contrast, individuals in whom the hypothalamic-pituitary-adrenal (HPA) axis is not intact or is compromised may have a diminished capacity for responding to stressors. Clinical examples include patients who have adrenal or pituitary gland dysfunction or who have undergone adrenalectomy.

Concurrent sociological, psychological, or pathophysiological problems place the individual at risk for a greater stress response when some other stimulus or insult is encountered. Those with diminished or compromised physiological reserves, such as premature infants, older adults, or people with multiple traumatic injuries or concurrent illness, are at greater risk for having a less than adequate response to significant stressors that are encountered. If the magnitude of the stressors remains great and the existing reserves necessary to mount an adequate stress response are compromised or diminished, death may occur.

RISK FACTORS

Multiple situational stressors are encountered in the day-to-day environment. These can be the daily hassles of finding a parking place, receiving unexpected news, or experiencing a cold environment, or they can be of a more severe nature, such as being involved in an accident, being informed that surgery is necessary, receiving a diagnosis of cancer, or sustaining a burn. Infection, shock, starvation, pain, surgery, emotional arousal, such as fear and anxiety, and even exercise are situational stressors.[2-5]

Events that occur along the developmental or age continuum may be perceived as stressors; for example, the multiple developmental tasks associated with adolescence or the period of adulthood when children leave home or a job change in adulthood may be stressors. Major life events, such as moving, divorce, caring for a spouse with a chronic and debilitating illness, and death of a loved one have been studied as stressors. The individual's perception and interpretation (appraisal) of the stressors influence the magnitude of the response. The response is further modified by a number of other circumstances, such as the individual's age, sex/gender, previous experiences, social support available, and concurrent illness.[6]

One focus of stress-related research uses animals, with the intention of modeling the phenomenon of stress in humans. The responses of animals subjected to a stressful experience can be compared to animals in the same environment without the stressor; in this way, outcomes may be directly attributed to the stressful situation. Stressors used in animal research may be painful or nonpainful. Nonpainful stressors include forced swim stress, restraint stress, and predator exposure stress[7-9]; painful stressors include surgical stress (e.g., laparotomy or hind limb amputation)[10] and footshock or tailshock stress.[11,12]

The prevailing thought is that the human response to stressors is an individual phenomenon. The same stressor does not have the same effect on all individuals subjected to that particular stressor, although some outcomes of some stressors, such as surgery, are similar among individuals.

CLINICAL STATES OR DIAGNOSES

In addition to the examples given, myriad reports have associated other clinical states and stress.[13-22] Some may be viewed as evidence of stress or as pathological consequences of the stress response. These include migraine headaches; peptic and duodenal ulcers; obesity; drug and alcohol abuse; compromised immunocompetence; assorted cardiovascular problems, such as angina and hypertension; and the occurrence or spread of cancer. The extent to which stressors and the stress response contribute to or result in these clinical states remains a circumstance of association; there is no absolute or definitive proof as yet. However, there are data that strongly suggest such relationships.[6]

Other clinical states are viewed as being the stressor that results in a stress response. For example, clinical states that are potent afferent stimuli and that result in increased sympathetic nervous system (SNS) discharge include acute hypovolemia, acute hypoglycemia, and hypoxia.[19] In each of these states, there is a deficiency in a required central nervous system (CNS) substrate. A stress response to emotional arousal, such as fear or anxiety, which may occur with the thought of impending surgery or other circumstances, may augment or exceed the concurrent physiological response to the illness or injury. Some cases of fibrillation following myocardial infarction have been postulated to be the result of a stress response.

Cohen and Williamson[23] proposed two models suggesting the role of stress in influencing infectious disease pathology and illness behaviors. Although acknowledging that there are stressor-induced health-promoting behaviors, they primarily proposed a model to explain stress-induced illness behaviors. They focused on the negative stressful events and affective states and view stress as a state of psychological distress. They suggested that the relationship between stress and susceptibility to infection is mediated through immune system function as modulated via the neuroendocrine hormones that are released in response to stress. Indeed, Cohen et al[24] showed that psychological stress predicts greater expression of illness after exposure to the influenza A virus. On the other hand, compared to individuals who have less diverse social networks, individuals with a more diverse social network, thought to be protective against psychological distress, were significantly less susceptible to developing a common cold and its associated features of production of mucus, ineffective clearing of nasal passages, and viral shedding following introduction of rhinovirus into the nasal mucosa.[25] Taken together, these studies support the suggestion that factors such as social networks and psychological stress affect the host's ability to resist upper respiratory infections.

Another clinical state is risk taking or thrill seeking. Are there pleasurable and enjoyable stressors and, if so, do the responses to these stressors contribute to the same changes that result from unpleasant or harmful stressors? Tache and Selye commented that "it is not what happens to you but how you take it."[26] In support of this hypothesis, parachute jumping has been associated with large increases in ACTH, cortisol, growth hormone, prolactin, thyroid-stimulating hormone (TSH), and circulating catecholamines.[27,28] All hormones except TSH and cortisol returned to normal levels within 1 hour of the jump.[27] The jump was a conscious choice; nevertheless, it is a profound psychological stressor that initiates a marked physiological response.

Teleologically, the stress response has evolved for the benefit it has for survival. Modern society has imposed new values that are perceived by some as important for "survival" and as more or less stressful, for example, achieving greater social or educational status. These new stressors are predominantly psychological in nature, yet they elicit "old world" physiological survival responses. This idea is conveyed by the following quote from Tache and Selye: "Taking an exam does not have the same survival significance as ... facing a pack of wolves, yet we have not learned to respond in a different way to those stressors."[26] Events or hassles encountered every day may not be life threatening, but they still may be perceived as stressors. Pleasurable social occasions also may be stressors.

Finally, perceptions regarding the controllability and predictability of the stressor have been shown to be of some importance in studies examining the effects of stress in animals. Paradigms typically employ three groups: (1) animals able to end stress by exhibiting a learned behavior, such as pushing a lever (controllable stress); (2) animals yoked to group 1 who receive the stressor in the same parameters/dose as the animal to which they are yoked in group 1 but have no control in ending the stressor; and (3) untreated animals. Findings show that whereas there is a significant increase in plasma corticosterone in animals able to control their stress, yoked animals with no control exhibited markedly greater corticosterone levels than the animals able to control their stress.[29,30]

MECHANISMS

The response to a stressor involves multiple mechanisms.[1,19,22,31-39] As noted in the definition, the response is integrated through the hypothalamus and is a graded response, depending on the individual and the magnitude of the afferent signals. The systems participating in the stress response are depicted in Figure 14-1. The process requires many feedback loops (not shown in Figure 14-1), and the response results in an altered physiological equilibrium.

As shown in Figure 14-1, the afferent input that is generated from sensory or psychological stimuli (stressors) is processed locally and then ultimately within the CNS. Neural information is forwarded to the hypothalamus. Through hypothalamic integration, an orderly response is achieved; that is, the hypothalamus coordinates the homeostatic adjustments. Hypothalamic output influences three major responses: (1) SNS discharge via the autonomic nervous system, (2) the release of selected anterior pituitary hormones via stimulation from hypothalamic-releasing or release-inhibiting factors, and (3) release of vasopressin in the posterior pituitary from hypothalamic neurons.

The next level depicted in Figure 14-1 illustrates the importance of recognizing that SNS discharge influences responses in other systems and organs. Increased palmar sweat is an example of an exocrine gland response. There are responses to the sympathetic discharge in several major organs (e.g., liver, pancreas, spleen, bone marrow, and kidney) and in other peripheral tissues enervated with sympathetic nerve endings. The adrenal medulla also responds to sympathetic discharge. Because the processes involved in these responses are multiple and complex, complete explication is beyond the scope of this chapter; they are described simply and briefly.

Release of norepinephrine by the sympathetic nerve endings results in glycogenolysis in the liver (i.e., conversion of stored glycogen to glucose), decrease in insulin and increase in glucagon secretion

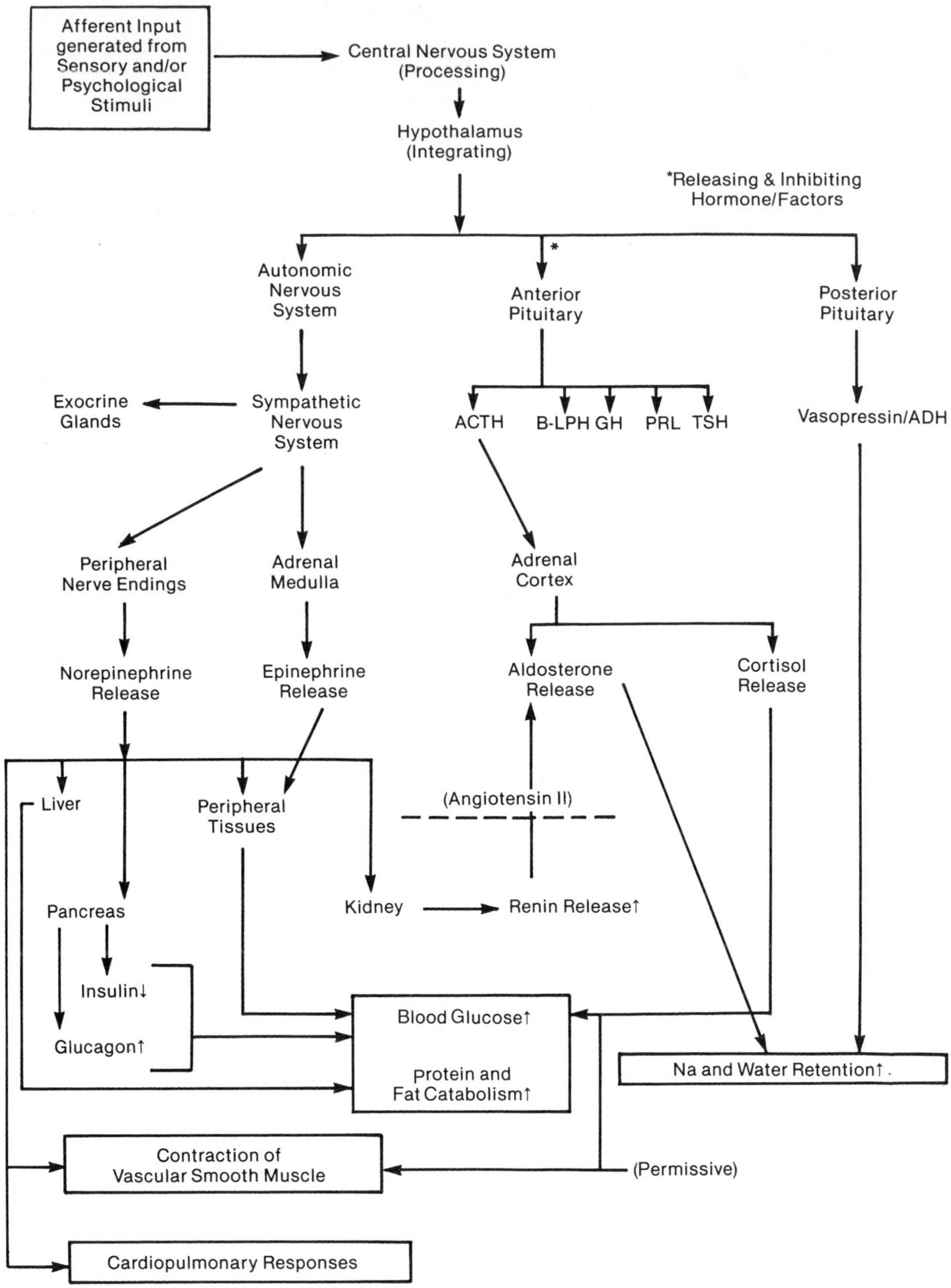

Figure 14-1 Systems participating in the stress response.

in the pancreas, increase in vascular smooth muscle contraction, and a number of other cardiopulmonary responses, including increased heart rate and contractility. Two central concepts are that both substrate and energy metabolism and cardiovascular functions are affected. The net effects of the release of norepinephrine are the increase in blood glucose levels, the peripheral catabolism of protein and fat, and the increase in cardiac output (and consequently increased myocardial oxygen demand), heart rate, respiratory rate, and blood pressure. These changes occur if these systems are not compromised and are capable of responding to the sympathetic discharge.

In response to the sympathetic discharge, epinephrine is released primarily from the adrenal medulla. Circulating epinephrine inhibits the uptake of glucose by peripheral tissues, thus contributing to the increased levels of blood glucose. Epinephrine also promotes the peripheral catabolism of protein and fat for conversion to energy substrate. Epinephrine also contributes to the observed cardiopulmonary responses.

Increased secretion of ACTH from the anterior pituitary is the most dramatic pituitary response. Corticotropin-releasing factor (CRF) is secreted from hypothalamic neurons in response to stressors; in response to CRF, ACTH and other peptides such as beta-lipotropin and its subunit, beta-endorphin, are released from the anterior pituitary. As noted in Figure 14-1, release of other anterior pituitary hormones (growth hormone, prolactin, and TSH) also occurs in the stress response. ACTH primarily stimulates release of cortisol and to a much lesser extent (when ACTH secretion is great) aldosterone from the adrenal cortex. Aldosterone is secreted in response to sodium and potassium levels and to angiotensin II (a product resulting from the action of renin on precursor molecules).

Increased cortisol secretion from the adrenal cortex is the most notable response to increased ACTH. Cortisol influences a great many processes; it has a potentiating effect on the actions of epinephrine and glucagon, with the net effect of an increased blood glucose level. Cortisol exerts a permissive effect, resulting in the sustained vascular smooth muscle response (contraction) to catecholamines (epinephrine and norepinephrine). Without cortisol, this response would not be sustained.

Increased cortisol alters the immune and inflammatory responses. In animals, thymicolymphatic involution, eosinopenia, and immune deficiency have been observed as a response to prolonged, increased cortisol levels. In humans, decreased lymphocytes have been reported in response to minor surgery and psychologically based stress; a decrease in both T cell and B cell lymphocytes has been observed in response to major surgery. Peptide-labeled cytokines are secreted in response to tissue damage or infection; a number of cytokines are under the regulatory influence of glucocorticoids.

Investigators are rapidly gaining knowledge about interactions among the brain, neuroendocrine, and immune systems; research focusing on this issue is at the forefront of psychoneuroimmunology. Evidence suggests that there are extensive communication pathways among the central nervous, endocrine, and immune systems. For example, signals from the brain and neuroendocrine system are transported to the immune system via the autonomic nervous system and hormonal secretion, and the immune system communicates with the brain via inflammatory cytokines.[1,40] There is considerable evidence that the thymus, spleen, and bone marrow are enervated by the autonomic nervous system, the sympathetic branch in particular.[41] The existence of adrenergic receptors on T cells, B cells, and macrophages supports the likely presence of sympathetic innervation of immune organs, although the functional role of such innervation is not clear. Both epinephrine and corticosteroids such as cortisol have been shown to affect both the distribution and activity of immune cells.[33,34,42,43] Cytokines, proteins that are produced by immune cells, can stimulate a number of responses in the CNS, including fever, sleep, and sickness behavior.[34,44]

Target tissue for aldosterone action is the renal tubule cells, with the net result being retention of sodium and excretion of potassium. Vasopressin (antidiuretic hormone [ADH]) is released from hypothalamic neurons terminating in the posterior pituitary. Target tissue for vasopressin action is also renal tubule cells, but the net result is reabsorption of water from the renal tubules. Thus, in the kidneys, secretion of renin in response to the sympathetic discharge, retention of sodium in response to adrenal cortex secretion of aldosterone, and retention of water in response to ADH participate in the net defense of fluid volume.

Table 14-1 summarizes the actions of the glucoregulatory hormones involved in altering substrate metabolism in the stress response. The net effect of insulin is to lower blood glucose levels; however, in response to the sympathetic discharge, less insulin is secreted. In addition, there is an increased secretion of the other glucoregulatory hormones that antagonize the effects of insulin. If the stress is of sufficient magnitude, hyperglycemia results.[14,19,45]

The stress response is a neuroendocrine response that is generally protective and homeostatic. It is a response to threatening external stimuli or to changes originating from the individual's internal environment. There is some evidence that repeated exposure to stressors result in adaptive changes. For example, in rats subjected to repeated stimuli, an increase in adrenal tissue levels of tyrosine hydroxylase occurred.[46] Tyrosine hydroxylase is an enzyme

TABLE 14-1 Glucoregulatory Hormones

HORMONE	ACTION
Insulin*	Inhibits hepatic glucose production Enhances glucose and AA uptake by peripheral tissues Enhances glycogen synthesis
Glucagon	↑ Hepatic glucose production (gluconeogenesis) Glycogenolytic
Catecholamines	↑ Hepatic glucose production Glycogenolytic Inhibits insulin secretion → ↑ AA from muscle Stimulates lipolysis → ↑ FFA ↑ Peripheral uptake of glucose
Cortisol	Potentiates effects of glucagon and catecholamines on hepatic glucose production
Growth hormone (somatotropin)	In periphery, antagonizes effects of insulin Resets response to glucose Stimulates release of FFA

*The net effect of insulin is to lower the blood glucose level. The net effect of other regulatory hormones is to increase the blood glucose level (hyperglycemia). Each of the counterregulatory hormones antagonizes one or more of the effects of insulin.
AA, amino acids; *FFA*, free fatty acids; ↑, increases; →, leads to or results in.

that catalyzes the process of synthesis of norepinephrine and epinephrine; thus, elevated levels of tyrosine hydroxylase increase the capacity for synthesis of the catecholamines involved in the stress response. It is apparent, even from this very cursory overview, that a number of systems and a number of complex, interrelated mechanisms are involved in the stress response. The net effects are the increased availability of energy substrate and maintenance of adequate blood volume and pressure. Table 14-2 summarizes the neuroendocrine responses, metabolic processes, and net results. Stressors elicit integrated neuroendocrine responses involving complex interactions; this stress response is protective and adaptive. Characteristics of the stress response are summarized in Box 14-1.

A reparative phase follows the stress response. Without a change in nitrogen intake, a decrease in the excretion of urinary nitrogen signals the occurrence of the reparative phase. The time for reparation of nitrogen loss depends on the extent of the loss; the rate of restoration is approximately 3 to 5 g of nitrogen per 70 kg/day. After nitrogen balance is achieved, restoration of fat deposits occurs.[19] The entire reparative phase may continue for several weeks to several months. During the reparative phase, there is an anabolic pattern resulting in protein synthesis, cell proliferation, and eventually fat deposition. Table 14-2 summarizes the reparative phase.

One cannot consider the stress response without acknowledgment of the very early work of Hans Selye in describing the "nonspecific" effects of the stress response. From animal experiments, he labeled the responses observed as the *general adaptation syndrome* (GAS); this GAS is characterized by three phases: an alarm reaction, resistance and adaptation, and exhaustion. After an organism is continually exposed to stressors, a triad of pathological consequences occurs: the adrenal glands enlarge, there is involution of the thymus gland, and ulcerations develop in the gastrointestinal tract.[38]

A review of current empirical work provides evidence that refutes many of Selye's theories. Work

BOX 14-1 Characteristics of the Stress Response

- Stress response is natural and generally protective and adaptive.
- There are normal responses to stressors (stressors encountered in everyday circumstances increase catecholamine excretion).
- Physical and emotional stressors trigger similar responses (specificity versus nonspecificity; magnitude and patterns may differ).
- Magnitude and duration of stressors may be so great that homeostatic mechanisms for adjustment fail, leading to death; there are limits in ability to compensate.
- Repeated exposure to stimuli results in adaptive changes, that is, tissue levels of tyrosine hydroxylase increase capacity for synthesis of norepinephrine and epinephrine.
- There are individual differences in response to the same stressors, although some stressors, such as major surgery, result in a very similar pattern of hormonal and immune consequences.

TABLE 14-2 Summary of Neuroendocrine Stress Responses and Resulting Effects

NEUROENDOCRINE	EFFECTS ON METABOLIC PROCESSES	NET RESULTS
↑ Catecholamines ↑ Glucocorticoids ↑ Glucagon ↑ Growth hormone ↓ Insulin	Glycogenolysis Gluconeogenesis Lipolysis Proteolysis	Provision of substrate for energy
↑ Catecholamines ↑ Glucocorticoids ↑ Vasopressin (ADH) ↑ Aldosterone	Sodium and water retention	Defense of fluid volume
Reparative Phase ↑ Insulin ↓ Glucagon ↓ Growth hormone and other growth factors ↑ Thyroid hormones		*Net Results* Protein synthesis Cell proliferation Restoration of fat deposits

↑, Increases; ↓, decreases.

by Mason and others[1,47-52] suggests that the stress response is specific, given the particular properties of the stressful stimulus (i.e., the characteristics of the stress response vary with the type of stressor). This is in contrast to Selye's early work and presents the continuing refinement of the phenomenon. Selye reported his later views on this controversy in the field of stress research.[53] For further examples and explanations of these ideas, refer to the review articles by Mason and others.[47-52]

Moore[19] provided a historical summary of the contributions of early scientists to the current understanding of the homeostatic responses to stressors such as trauma and surgery. These scientists include Charles Darwin, Claude Bernard, Walter Cannon, Harvey Cushing, David Cuthbertson, and Hans Selye. Moore also reviewed the physiological responses that occur with acute injury.

PATHOLOGICAL CONSEQUENCES

Such clinical states as migraine headaches, asthmatic attacks, obesity, atherosclerosis, and hypertension may, in some circumstances, be considered pathological consequences of stress. Direct evidence of pathological causation remains problematic; the evidence to date is rather one of association. There are situations, however, in which pathological consequences do result from the stress response. The response to a severe traumatic injury is an example.[14,19] With moderate to severe trauma, lipolysis, proteolysis, gluconeogenesis, and ureagenesis occur. Amino acids are mobilized primarily from skeletal muscle. The liver converts the carbon fragments to new glucose and forms urea from the nitrogen residues that are excreted as urinary nitrogen. The nitrogen loss is related to the size of the injury and other influencing factors, such as poor nutritional intake and lack of muscle activity. Because glycogen stores in the liver are limited, the gluconeogenesis increases or maintains serum glucose levels. This protective response is requisite to preserve the function of glucose-dependent tissues. With lipolysis of triglycerides, the free fatty acids cannot be converted to glucose, but the glycerol moieties can be used through the Krebs cycle to provide an energy source and the fatty acids can be used as an energy source by some tissues.

With the evolution of advanced lifesaving critical care units and the ability to chronically support nutritional and vital organ function comes a wasting syndrome that appears to be refractory to nutritional supplementation. This syndrome is not associated with any specific disease or trauma, but simply dependent on intensive care support, including mechanical ventilation for at least 7 to 10 days. In general, protein loss from vital organs and tissues continues from degradation and decreased synthesis. Additionally, rather than oxidation, there is reesterification of free fatty acids, which allows fat to accumulate in both adipocytes and organs, such as the liver and pancreas. Current investigations are focusing on changes in the HPA axis. Accompanying this metabolic derangement is immune impairment, rendering the patient susceptible to infection.[54]

An example from animal research illustrates the interaction between hormones and immunity. Rats undergoing painful footshock stress exhibit an analgesic state referred to as stress-induced analgesia (SIA). One measure of the magnitude of SIA is the duration the animal will stand on a hot place (53° C [127° F]) compared with their own pre-SIA state without exhibiting a characteristic hind paw lick, at which time they are removed from the plate. Footshock was found to result in both SIA and suppression of NK cell activity. However, when animals were injected with naltrexone (an opioid antagonist that blocks both morphine analgesia and some forms of SIA) before footshock, they exhibited no SIA and NK cell activity that was equivalent to that of control animals that did not undergo footshock. Additionally, it was found that injection of very large, and very probably stressful, doses of morphine (30 and 50 mg/kg) resulted in NK activity suppression as well. These results support the hypothesis that the immunosuppressive effects of some forms of stress are mediated by opioid peptides.[55]

Surgery is a physiological stressor. The surgical stress response prominently includes neuroendocrine, metabolic, and inflammatory responses to the acute injury. ACTH levels increase markedly by 1 hour after the start of surgery. Further, the plasma concentrations of ACTH and cortisol seem to have no predictable relationship during a typical perioperative period. Peak concentrations of cortisol are reached within a few hours of surgery, and the duration of elevated plasma cortisol levels varies. The magnitude of hypercortisolism generally correlates with the invasiveness of the surgery. Some evidence suggests that the endogenous opioid system plays a role in the stress response to surgery. It is known that the mu-opioid and kappa-opioid receptors affect the HPA axis in surgical stress, and beta-endorphin (coreleased with ACTH at the anterior pituitary) levels may negatively impact homeostasis.[56,57] As can be seen in Figure 14-1, hypothalamic activation of the autonomic nervous system results in a cascade of effects on metabolism and the cardiovascular system.[58,59] The surgically stressed system is thrust into a hypermetabolic state in which there is increased demand for nutrients to promote healing, and there is accelerated metabolism resulting from the physiological stress of surgery. It is important to know that the very young, including neonates, are capable of mounting a stress response to surgery.[60]

Some pain relief interventions have been shown to attenuate, and in some cases, block the surgical stress response. High-dose narcotic anesthesia suppresses the stress response during surgery in adults and neonates as long as blood opiate concentrations remain high; the endocrine and metabolic responses to surgery emerge as opiate concentrations decrease.[61,62] The use of regional anesthesia, such as epidural administration of local anesthetics (e.g., bupivacaine), largely prevents the stress effects of lower abdominal and lower extremity surgery. The endocrine and metabolic responses that are inhibited include the following: levels of ACTH, ADH, thyrotropin-releasing hormone, circulating beta-endorphins, cortisol, aldosterone, renin, and catecholamines. Increased levels of blood glucose and free fatty acid may be attenuated as well, with improvement in plasma nitrogen balance. Regional anesthetic techniques are less successful in inhibiting the stress response resulting from upper abdominal and thoracic surgery.[63-68] Postoperative epidural analgesia administration has been shown to be an effective pain relief strategy; however, no significant modulation of hyperglycemia or hypercortisolism has been demonstrated.[69,70] These findings suggest that some mechanism not dependent on pain is involved in promoting the stress response to surgery.

The immune consequences of stress have been demonstrated in humans and in animals, and there is a growing body of literature reporting this research. Major surgery in humans results in a decrease in the absolute numbers of circulating lymphocyte subpopulations (T, T_h, T_s, T_c, NK, and B) for several days, with normal levels returning by the seventh postoperative day. Although minor surgery results in a similar reduction of lymphocyte subpopulations, these changes are of a lesser magnitude and of shorter duration.[71] Major surgery also significantly depresses both the ability of lymphocytes to proliferate in response to an antigen and NK cell function.[71,72] Several recent studies have shown that the use of spinal or epidural anesthesia and analgesia significantly attenuates the suppression of several immune measures including T cell populations[73] and NK cell activity.[66] Further, other studies have shown that compared with standard anesthesia techniques, the provision of epidural anesthesia and analgesia results in a significant reduction of postoperative complications such as pulmonary and major infectious sequelae.[65,74] (See Chapter 15, Alterations in Immunosuppression, for the functions associated with the above-mentioned cell populations.)

Similar immunosuppression has been demonstrated in animals undergoing surgery.[75-78] A biologically significant outcome unique to animal research is the impact of surgery on tumor metastasis. NK cell activity plays a critical role in the immune defense against metastatic growth.[79-81] Several animal studies have documented the tumor-enhancing effects of surgery.[7,76,82-87] Although both tumor development and immunity are affected by stress, it is not clear that changes in immune function mediate the effect on tumor development; however, a recent study by Ben-Eliyahu et al[7] supports such a causal relationship.[7]

In summary, there are limits to an organism's ability to respond to stressors; if the stressors are sufficiently great, the adaptive mechanisms may fail and death will occur. The response requires energy and metabolic reserves. If these reserves are insufficient or if the response is at the maximum rate of energy production (related to maximum oxygen consumption), and additional stressors such as infection occur, no greater adaptive response may be possible.[1,19,20] Although the stress response is protective, pathological consequences occur when the magnitude of the stressor taxes the homeostatic mechanisms.

RELATED PATHOPHYSIOLOGICAL CONCEPTS

The physiological concepts related to the stress response consist of antecedent conditions, the associated clinical states, or the symptoms reported in association with perceived stress. Examples of conditions antecedent to the stress response and clinical states are multiple traumatic insult, ischemia, hypoxia, burns, surgery, sepsis, loss of a loved one, or some other major sociopsychological loss. But none of these conditions or states constitutes a concept exactly parallel or similar to the stress response. Starvation results in some of the same adaptive mechanisms seen as part of the stress response, but deficient nutrient intake is the antecedent to the response, not the response.

ASSOCIATED PSYCHOSOCIAL CONCEPTS

There are multiple psychosocial concepts that are utilized in studying the physiological stress response. It is beyond the scope of this chapter to provide a thorough review; however, given the increasing evidence of their importance, a few examples are cited. In studies in which the variable of stress is of interest, the most frequently used measures tap the concept of anxiety.[47,88-93] In some cases, the terms *anxiety* and *stress* are used interchangeably. From the perspective of the multiple and complex interrelated mechanisms involved in the stress response, anxiety as a concept does not encompass or convey the same scope of mechanisms. However, emotional arousal does trigger the stress response, which may indeed be a severe response.[13,18,94-97]

Another similarly related concept is work stress. The term *burnout* is used as a concept to convey a response to work stress, now a widely studied chronic life stress with respect to coronary artery disease. There is suggestion of a causal relationship between work-related chronic stress and the development of atherosclerosis. The implicated mechanisms include elevated blood pressure and neurohumoral arousal.[98]

Coping is another psychosocial concept associated with stress.[15,17,88-91,99] Coping patterns, strategies, styles, and behaviors are described variously by the multitude of investigators who are defining the concept and developing instruments to measure it.[15,17,88-91,93,100-104] An individual's coping abilities and resources are perceived to moderate or ameliorate the severity of the perceived stressors and to influence the magnitude of the stress response.

Social support is another focus of stress response research. The opposite, social isolation, has been shown to elevate risk for mortality from all causes, an indication of the strength of a psychosocial factor on physical state. Examples of phenomena in which social support plays a key role in mediating responses to stress can be found in several literatures, including cancer,[105,106] cardiac,[98] and infectious disease.[25]

MANIFESTATIONS

Objective Physiological Manifestations

It is important to recognize that there are differences in the manifestations of the stress response given the many possible characteristics of the stressor itself and the many temporal possibilities for relating the stressor to outcome measures. Different stressors result in different configurations of the stress response, and the success in detecting these objective measures depends on the ability to "capture" the effect by optimally timing measurement of the outcome variable. In other words, different hormonal effects peak at different points in time given the same stressor. For example, ACTH peaks at about 1 hour and cortisol peaks several hours after major surgery.

Equally important is individual variation in reactivity. Most studies report a fairly wide variance in outcomes, which relates to individual responses to stressors.[107] Recent and growing evidence points to a phenomenon that may prove to be a significant factor contributing to such variance—that of SNS hyperresponsivity. In particular, it has been shown that some individuals tend to exhibit exaggerated heart rate and arterial blood pressure responses to stimuli. In the cardiac literature, such hyperresponders exhibit a more rapid progression of atherosclerosis.[98] High stress–related changes in HPA axis activation have been reported to be associated with high cardiac sympathetic reactivity to stress.[108,109]

Hyperglycemia occurs early in the postoperative recovery period after major surgery, and if the response is prolonged, the loss of muscle and adipose tissue becomes obvious and weight loss may occur. Loss of energy may be characterized by slow or weak movements and by difficulty in turning, in getting up, or even in breathing if the response is sufficiently severe and prolonged to involve deterioration of the muscles of respiration, such as the diaphragm and intercostals. With loss of muscle from proteolysis and mobilization of amino acids, an increase in urinary nitrogen excretion is observed.

The most dramatic increases in the hormones participating in the stress response are observed in the plasma levels of ACTH and cortisol (and their metabolites) and catecholamines. In response to increased circulating catecholamines, cardiopulmonary changes, such as increases in blood pressure, heart rate, and respiratory rate, are seen. Many other factors can contribute to changes in these cardiopulmonary parameters, such as alcohol consumption, blood volume, and a variety of pharmacological agents. With regard to these other factors, the cardiopulmonary parameters alone are not reliable indicators of the stress response, but certainly, given probable cause, increases in stress hormone levels and accompanying cardiopulmonary changes are likely manifestations of the stress response. Measurement of multiple parameters is necessary; there is no one direct stress measure, and the context is also of importance in considering the objective measures.[14,31,32,47-49,97]

Measurements of galvanic skin resistance and palmar sweat have been used as indicators of stress. With increased palmar sweat, a decrease in skin resistance is observed. These changes also are indicative of sympathetic discharge; in fact, general diaphoresis or cold hands and feet may be observed. Increased gastric secretions, bronchial and pupil dilation, and tremors are other physiological manifestations of the response.

Timing for collection of the sample also is important. If the sample is from urine, the catecholamine levels obtained will represent a composite or average over the time the urine has been accumulating in the bladder. A plasma sample would more accurately characterize the response to some specific transient stressful event. Timing of the sample collection is not as critical if one is attempting to assess the response to a prolonged or chronic stressor, although circadian rhythm effects must be controlled for.

Cortisol and one of its metabolites, 17-hydroxycorticosteroid (17-OHCS) can be measured in plasma and in urine. These are increased in response to stressors. The magnitude and duration of the response are graded in relation to the magnitude of the stressors and in relation to the individual's characteristics and the physiological state.

The emergence of psychoneuroimmunology has contributed several objective physiological manifestations to the battery of hormonal and metabolic assessments already used. Immune outcomes such as lymphocyte subpopulation distribution, lymphocyte proliferation response to antigenic challenge, NK cell cytotoxicity measurements in vitro, cytokine levels, and resistance to disease and metastatic growth in the whole organism (animal studies) are evident in the literature.

These parameters are only indicators of the response and not a precise direct measure. They are influenced by a variety of other factors, the responses of individuals to the same stimuli (stressors) may be different, and the levels of the various parameters will vary in relation to the progression of the response. For all these reasons, it is important to use a battery or combination of parameters to assess the existence, magnitude, and duration of the stress response. All of the above cited objective manifestations of the stress response are nonspecific responses to stressors. Increased sympathetic activity and adrenomedullary activity result in increased catecholamine secretion, the adrenocortical hyperactivity results in increased glucocorticoids and aldosterone, and the protein catabolism results in increased urinary nitrogen.

Objective Behavioral Manifestations

Some individuals seem to be able to exert more control and others less control over the behavioral responses that are frequently associated with stress. Observable manifestations may be a reflection of the coping behaviors assumed by individuals. Examples of observable behaviors that may suggest the presence of stress are vomiting, fainting, trembling, tapping of fingers, kicking or swinging movement of lower extremities while sitting, sitting on the edge of a chair, clenched fists, other evidence of muscle tension, pitch of voice, speed of talk, crying, pacing, and being immobilized or nonfunctional; perhaps excessive eating, smoking, and drinking may also be indicators. In observing such behaviors, one should not make assumptions about the basis for the behavior. From either a clinical or a research point of view, additional verification of the observed behaviors, the attending circumstances, and other data are necessary.

Subjective Manifestations

In today's world, a number of people freely acknowledge feeling stressed. The feeling is frequently attributed to job demands or the sociopsychological environment or even to the state of physical health. Burnout is a word that has been derived to convey this general feeling of stress. Some report more specific manifestations, such as headaches, nausea, anorexia or hunger, fatigue, problems with sleep and concentration, sensations of uneasiness, and gnawing or burning sensations in the gut; some report palpitations, angina, and difficulty breathing. These reported subjective manifestations may, in fact, suggest stress, or they may be related to some other condition.

Several psychometric instruments have been used as indirect measures to reflect the level of stress or stressors.[47,102,104,110-124] Examples of these instruments include anxiety scales and life event scales. Individuals are requested to complete these scales; their responses are taken as the subjective measure of the variable. Spielberger's State-Trait Anxiety Inventory is designed to determine the individual's anxiety as an inherent trait and anxiety in relation to the current period of time.[120] The Profile of Mood States (POMS) includes anxiety as one of six subscales.[117] A number of other scales have been designed to measure anxiety.[104]

Measurement of psychosocial stressors has included both daily hassles and major life events.[111,112,116,122] The Social Readjustment Rating Scale, developed originally by Holmes and Rahe, has been used as an indicator to quantify the individual's stressful life events.[113,114] This instrument has been revised and has been adapted by a number of other investigators. Sarason and colleagues developed the Life Experiences Survey to capture both positive and negative life events.[118,119]

Recognizing that frequent minor aggravations may contribute to stress, a daily hassles scale has been used.[111,116] Stokes and Gordon developed a 104-item instrument to measure stress in the older adult.[121] They identified stressors from the gerontology literature, from interviews with healthy individuals who were 65 years or older, and from a review of the items by experts in gerontological nursing. The items generated make this instrument most useful in determining psychosocial stressors perceived by elderly individuals.

Benoliel et al[110] developed a 74-item instrument, the nurse stress checklist, to measure the stress of clinically employed nurses. The instrument measures five components of stress: personal reactions, personal concerns, work concerns, role competence, and work completion concerns. This too represents a measure of the individual's perception of stressors and does not measure a physiological response. However, personal reaction items include some behaviors suggestive of physiological alterations.

Standardized instruments (e.g., the Jenkins Activity Scale) are used to classify people's behaviors into what is called type A or type B behaviors.[115] A positive relationship between type A behaviors and proneness to myocardial infarction has been shown.[125-127] This relationship is strengthened when other cardiac risk factors are also present. "Impatient," "time-conscious," "ambitious," "competitive," and "aggressive" are some of the descriptors given to characterize type A behavior. Matthews reviewed, in depth, the work done on characterizing the type A behavior pattern and the measures used in quantifying this coronary-prone behavior.[128] Whether these type A behaviors reflect stress and the extent to which stress results in infarction remains unclear. Type A behavior has also been explored relative to neurohormonal responses to acute stress. There is evidence that type A men exhibit hyperreactive catecholamine responses to psychological stressors.[94]

On the other hand, others propose that there should be doubt regarding the clinical robustness of type A behavior. Several confounding variables have been suggested including social support and hostility. A major attribute of the type A behavior pattern, hostility is a rather broad construct of negativity toward interpersonal relationships, which may include such traits as anger, cynicism and mistrust. Several studies have positively associated hostility with cardiac events. Given that hostility is also associated with other lifestyle patterns such as smoking, increased alcohol consumption, poor diet and obesity, social isolation may also be present[98]; thus illustrating the incredible complexity of such psychosocial characterizations.

There are, of course, other measures. These are all indirect measures used to tap the subjective dimensions, that is, the person's perception of the variable being measured. None of these are designed specifically to measure the stress response but to tap characteristics reflective of or associated with the phenomenon.

SURVEILLANCE AND MEASUREMENT

From a broad perspective, surveillance includes identification of and, if possible, assessment of the intensity of the stressors over time. From a narrower perspective, surveillance of the stress response includes consideration of the multiple parameters specified above. The professional nurse can have a primary role in monitoring parameters associated with both the stressors and the stress response. Insulin and blood glucose levels, urinary excretion of nitrogen, nitrogen balance, indicators of loss of muscle, ACTH and cortisol levels, heart rate, respiratory rate, and blood pressure are the more commonly monitored parameters reflecting changes in the stress response. Immune function may become an important parameter to consider. Subjectively reported sensations also need to be noted (see Manifestations).

Given that the nature of the stress response is generally protective, adaptive, and homeostatic, if the stressor is transient and the individual's resources are adequate, with time the response diminishes and normal values for the parameters are observed. The professional nurse should be alert to changes in urinary excretion of nitrogen as well as other indicators of loss of muscle protein, such as specific behaviors reflecting muscle weakness. Noting either an increase or a decrease in these parameters is an important nursing observation. If the response has been prolonged owing to the magnitude of the stressors, a decrease in excretion of urinary nitrogen is the signal indicating the reparative phase. If the response results from more chronic or psychological stressors, surveillance of the behavioral manifestations and the subjectively reported sensations may be the more important parameters for the professional nurse to use in surveillance of the stress response. Evidence of compromise in immune status may be another critical indicator of the presence of a stress response. (See the more detailed descriptions of these parameters in Manifestations.) Several reviews provide additional information on psychological and neuroendocrinological measures to monitor the stress response.[47,95,118,122,129,130]

CLINICAL MANAGEMENT

An immediate therapeutic goal is to eliminate, ameliorate, or diminish the stressors. This presumes that the stressors are known or identifiable and that they are more than a transitory event. In some instances, however, the precipitating stressors may be an event, such as a traumatic accident or loss of a loved one. Therapies used to decrease the stressor are as variable as the stressors. They can be directed very specifically to eliminate the stressor, such as use of an antibiotic selected for its effectiveness in the treatment of an infection from a specific causative organism, or the therapies can be more general, such as patient education to enhance coping abilities, use of resources, or stress management techniques.

If the magnitude of the stressors and the stress response is great (e.g., multiple traumatic injuries), subsequent therapeutic goals include provision of substrate and maintenance of fluid volume to complement the adequacy of the response. Following the more immediate phases of the response, therapies are directed toward restoration of tissue and of the individual. The professional nurse has an important role in all of these therapies.

Current therapies include (1) administration of glucose, potassium, and insulin intravenously; (2) administration of blood, blood components, or other fluids; (3) administration of glucocorticoids; (4) administration of total parenteral nutrition; (5) use of protective environments; and (6) use of technologically developed life-supporting systems. The specific role of the nurse is dependent on the nature of the stressors, the extent of the stress response, and the therapies instituted. Therapies for a variety of circumstances precipitating the stress response are reviewed by others.[19,131-135]

For those with a more psychologically derived stress response, therapies are designed to assist the individual in dealing with the stress-producing situations, to enhance stress management techniques such as guided imagery and relaxation strategies, and to develop coping behaviors to ameliorate the stress-producing effects of various situations.* Biofeedback has been used with some success as a therapy in diminishing the stress response.[137,138] There is no best or definitive therapy that is effective for preventing the response to sociopsychological stressors or for treating the response. The characteristics of persons for which specific therapies would be most effective are also unknown. Therapies are explored primarily

*References 15, 17, 89, 90, 93, 101, 104-106, 136.

on an individual trial basis. To date, there are insufficient data available about the effectiveness of these therapies and the treatments have not been standardized across studies. Thus comparison of findings with the potential for deriving practice implications remains problematic. Professional nurses can continue to make contributions to this field as they investigate the effectiveness of the therapies in diminishing the stress response.

CASE STUDY

The course of Mr. F's illness illustrates the changes that occur during an acute physiological stress response. Mr. F, a 55-year-old executive, was driving home on a rainy, stormy evening, having left his office after an argument with one of his associates. Tired, worried, and under much psychological stress in the last month because of a business failure, Mr. F was driving faster than the freeway speed limit in a hurry to get home. Suddenly, a car swerved in front of him, he was unable to react quickly enough, and his car crashed into the other car. Not wearing a seat belt, he was thrown from the car onto the freeway. Mr. F had multiple fractures, lacerations, and a lacerated spleen. After being transported to the emergency department by paramedics, he was taken to surgery, where he underwent an exploratory laparotomy and repair of the ruptured spleen and fractures. Postoperatively, Mr. F was admitted to the surgical intensive care unit. During the first 24 hours of recovery, vital signs and laboratory values exemplified those changes expected to occur during a physiological stress response.

For the first 24 hours, Mr. F's heart and respiratory rates and temperature were elevated, accompanied by slight hypotension. These responses (except hypotension) demonstrated the increased secretion of both epinephrine and norepinephrine. Serum sodium levels were moderately elevated with decreasing sodium excretion in the urine; there also was evidence of conservation of the extracellular fluid volume. The blood loss had augmented aldosterone secretion normally seen with stress as well as the release of vasopressin, the antidiuretic hormone. Serum potassium, phosphate, and sulfate levels were decreased, reflecting the loss of electrolytes and other cellular contents resulting from cell lysis. Increased levels of urine creatine, creatinine, and urea nitrogen occurred, and with a decreased intake, a negative nitrogen balance resulted. A dramatic initial finding was the hyperglycemia resulting from the net effects of norepinephrine, epinephrine, and cortisol secretion. There was a decrease in insulin secretion and an increase in glucagon secretion. Under normal circumstances, insulin secretion would be increased in response to hyperglycemia, but under conditions of stress, insulin secretion is suppressed, resulting in a net hyperglycemia with a decreased ability for glucose utilization. Mr. F's increased blood cortisol and 17-hydroxycorticosteroid levels were evidence that ACTH had stimulated the adrenal cortex to produce glucocorticoids, typical of the stress response following traumatic injury. Although Mr. F was a candidate for hypoxemia resulting from ventilation-perfusion abnormalities with abdominal incisional pain and multiple fractures, he was in the expected mixed state of metabolic and respiratory alkalosis with hyperventilation.

Over the next 7 days, Mr. F was treated with vigorous respiratory therapy and intravenous fluids. Despite the use of parenteral substrates, he continued to remain in an acute catabolic state. He lost 5 pounds and continued to lose phosphorus and nitrogen and showed consistent elevated levels of urine creatine and creatinine. Serum sodium levels also remained elevated. With treatment, the potassium and phosphorus levels were only slightly decreased. A wound infection developed that contributed to a persistent slightly elevated temperature. Levels of plasma and urinary corticosteroids remained increased. In several days, Mr. F was given a high-protein, high-caloric oral diet, and his intake progressively approached his caloric expenditure.

During the next 2 weeks, metabolic and electrolyte values returned to normal. Following augmented antibiotic therapy, the abdominal wound healed; the patient began walking with crutches and was discharged home on a high-protein and high-caloric diet. With the complex compensatory physiological stress response to a multiple traumatic injury, homeostatic balance was restored. Table 14-3 is a summary of the metabolic changes following Mr. F's accident.

The professional nurse has many responsibilities in caring for an individual such as Mr. F. This case example

TABLE 14-3 Summary of Metabolic Changes Observed in a Patient (Mr. F)

	POSTOPERATIVE PERIOD		
	24 HOURS	7 DAYS	24 DAYS
Temperature	↑	↑	↔
Glucose (blood)	↑	↑	↔
Potassium (serum)	↓	↓ ↔	↔
Sodium (serum)	↑	↑	↔
Phosphorus (serum)	↓	↓	↔
Urine creatine, creatinine, and nitrogen	↑	↑	↔
Cortisol	↑	↑	↔
17-Hydroxycortico-steroid	↑	↑	↔
Weight	↔	↓	↓

↑ = increased; ↓ = decreased; ↔ = normal.

is only a summarization of the more characteristic changes that occur as a result of an acute stress response. The important parameters to be monitored were included as well as examples of the direction of change to be expected in similar clinical circumstances. In addition, there were nursing responsibilities inherent in the therapies administered, in managing pain, wound care and in assisting Mr. F in interpersonal and physical activities associated with his clinical state and recovery process.

SELECTED RESEARCH

Numerous studies about stressors and stress responses have been reported. The approaches used are as varied as the stressor examined. The following briefly described examples only begin to characterize the range of studies.

Characterizing the stressful nature of exercise is a major focus in recent studies. The impact of exercise upon neuroendocrine and immune activity largely depends on the intensity of the exercise, whether the exercise intensity and duration serve as a source of physiological stress.[5,140,141] Exercise of sufficiently high intensity and duration has been shown to result in elevated cortisol levels (e.g., following 2.5 hours of high intensity running in a trained individual,[141] or running or cycling to exhaustion).[142,143] Similarly, levels of circulating beta-endorphin have been shown to be significantly increased following as little as 3 minutes of maximal exercise or more prolonged intensive exercise,[5,145] or after exhaustive exercise.[142,145] Low work loads have not been associated with elevated serum or plasma levels of cortisol or beta-endorphin.[5,140] NK cell activity has been shown to be suppressed following prolonged and intense exercise in highly trained individuals, but less so in the untrained.[140,141] This difference in responses between trained and untrained individuals appears to relate to the significantly greater NK cytotoxic activity observed at baseline in those that are trained, both young[141] and old.[146] The biological significance of the previously mentioned hormonal or immune changes in response to exercise is not well studied. Two studies conducted by Nieman et al[146,147] offer a hint of possible physical benefits of a regular program of brisk walking. Young women walkers (45 minutes/day, 5 days/week) noted upper respiratory tract symptoms one-half of the number of days compared to sedentary control subjects throughout the 15-week program.[147] Among elderly women, the incidence of the common cold during a 12-week walking program (5 days/week) was 21% among the walkers and 50% among the sedentary controls.[141]

Animal studies provide a highly controlled environment in which to test exercise effects on HPA axis and immune function, and also provide a means by which to assess the biological significance of an immune outcome not measurable in humans, such as resistance to infection or cancer. In mice, treadmill running to voluntary fatigue followed by intranasal administration of herpes simplex type 1 virus (HSV-1) resulted in greater illnesses and death compared to both sedentary animals and those limited to 30 minutes of running, suggesting that antiviral resistance is compromised following such a stressor.[148] Two studies in rats provide an indication of the possible beneficial effects of exercise training on an in vivo measure of NK cytotoxicity, the clearance of radiolabeled lymphoma cells from the lungs. Five weeks of voluntary wheel running increased host ability to clear the lymphoma cells from their lungs compared to sedentary controls, and this finding was accompanied by an increase in the concentration of splenic NK cells in the trained rats.[149]

Studies that implicate the biological significance of neuroendocrine and immune changes are valuable in that they provide a means by which to evaluate the morbidity/mortality potential that might be associated with a given stressor; or on the other hand, possible benefits gained from an intervention. As illustrated in the exercise studies, much can be learned in this regard by employing one or more of a broad array of animal models of disease or infection, or careful investigation of the more limited outcomes within acceptable ethical practices for human investigation. Examples already presented in this chapter include the work by Cohen et al[24,25] regarding relationships between social support networks or psychological stress and susceptibility to upper respiratory infection; the provision of epidural anesthesia for surgery and reductions in postoperative pulmonary and infectious sequelae[65,74]; and relationships between work-related chronic stress and the development of atherosclerosis.[98]

Life stresses such as university examinations have proved to be fertile ground for exploring the impact of common situational stressors on neuroendocrine and immune function. Seminal work on medical students' responses to examinations has shown transient changes in multiple immune parameters, indicating a down regulation of immune function around exam time as opposed to nonexam times. Additional studies noted increased self-reported symptoms of infectious illness during examination periods. The timing of seroconversion in response to hepatitis B inoculations was shown to be associated with medical student anxiety levels and social support: low levels of anxiety and high levels of social support were related to earlier seroconversion.[150,151] Using the same examination paradigm in dental students, the healing of a small (3.5-mm) oral mucosal biopsy wound was compared within subjects during summer vacation versus 3 days before the first major examination of the term. Without exception, wound healing time was greater during the examination period, an average of 3 days longer over an average course of 9 days to healing.[152]

Given the mounting evidence of decrements in immune function associated with aging, life stressors and their physiological sequelae in the elderly have become important areas of study.[153] An increasingly prominent life stressor among older populations is providing long-term care for a spouse with dementia. Caregiving was shown to be associated with decrements in cellular immunity and significantly more days of infectious illness compared to sociodemographically matched control subjects. Additionally, availability of social support was a factor; decreased social support available to the caregiver was associated with greater distress by dementia-related behaviors exhibited by the spouse and larger immune decrements.[151] Two studies by different groups showed that when compared to matched control subjects, caregivers exhibited a poorer antibody response to influenza vaccines.[154,155] Additionally, caregivers exhibited greater salivary cortisol levels compared to matched control subjects.[154] Finally, compared to healthy matched controls, caregivers exhibited significant delays in healing 3.5-mm cutaneous biopsy wounds (48.7 versus 39.3 days).[156]

With chronic repeated periods of immobilization (restraint stress) in rats, increased adrenal medulla tissue levels of the enzyme tyrosine hydroxylase were found.[46] This enzyme catalyzes the rate-limiting step in the synthesis of catecholamines. This adaptive response of increasing tyrosine hydroxylase levels enhances the capacity for synthesis of the catecholamines. Other studies in mice have shown restraint stress to depress antiviral cellular immunity and IL-2 secretion, rendered stressed animals more susceptible to influenza virus,[157] and a delay of both the early inflammatory response to cutaneous wounding and complete healing.[160]

Intervention studies in individuals with cancer directed toward stress reduction have suggested such strategies are beneficial not only with regard to improvements in psychosocial outcomes, but enhancement of some immune measures and even survival. An important preface in these studies is that psychological interventions were in addition to medical care and subjects in the control group also received optimum medical care. A seminal study conducted by Spiegel et al[159] compared standard treatment to a weekly psychological support group for a year in individuals with metastatic breast cancer. Group meetings emphasized emotional support, sharing of fears and self-disclosure. Psychosocial outcomes such as tension, fatigue, confusion, and vigor were significantly improved in the treatment group. At 10 years after the study, all but 3 of the 86 original participants had died. Although not originally an objective, analysis of death records indicated that survival time was improved in the treatment group, 36.3 months versus 18.9 months in the standard care group.[160] Although no neurohumoral or immune outcomes were assessed at the time of the study, the powerful evidence of enhanced survival by the addition of psychological support prompted several studies, which incorporated the assessment of these physiological measures.

One such study by Fawzy et al[161] investigated possible benefits of providing a 6-week structured group intervention encompassing health education, stress management, coping skills and group psychotherapy in newly diagnosed malignant melanoma patients following surgical treatment. The treatment group exhibited significantly lower levels of distress than the untreated controls and increases in some immune cell populations.[162] At 6 years, there was a significantly greater death rate in control subjects compared to treated individuals.[163] This and the study mentioned earlier only represent the many intervention studies that have addressed issues related to stress in the vulnerable cancer population.[105,106]

Recent findings validate that surgery enhances metastatic growth in rats and suggest a role for pain in mediating these effects; Page et al[87] used a mammary adenocarcinoma tumor (MADB106) syngeneic to the inbred Fischer 344 rat. This tumor metastasizes to the lungs when injected intravenously and is sensitive to NK cell activity for the first day following injection. These characteristics match what is known about the process of metastatic growth in humans and therefore make this model useful for studying the impact of stress on metastatic spread. The findings of this research demonstrate that rats undergoing standard abdominal surgery under halothane anesthesia exhibit a twofold increase in the number of pulmonary metastases compared with untreated controls or animals given halothane anesthesia only.[87] Further, analgesic doses of morphine attenuated the surgery-induced increased susceptibility to metastasis.[10,87] This finding suggests that pain does play a role in mediating surgery-induced enhanced metastasis. If similar relationships among pain, stress, and metastasis occur in humans, then pain control must be considered a vital component of postoperative care.

These few examples of studies were selected to illustrate the diverse nature of research on stress, to include some studies conducted by nurse investigators, to cross clinical areas of interest, to acknowledge work completed, and to recognize the scope of work yet to be accomplished in the field of stress. Critical analysis of these studies is beyond the scope of this chapter. Finally, taken together, these examples provide evidence suggesting that there are illness, and possibly even mortality, risks associated with the physiological arousal associated with stress, whether it is of psychological, sociological, or physiological origin. There is a hint that it is possible to attenuate such consequences by providing psychological or physiological therapies.

QUESTIONS FOR FUTURE STUDY

One notable observation is that findings in these sample studies cannot be compared; the purposes are different, samples are different, measures used to quantify the variables of interest are different, the interventions are different, and even the conceptualization of the stress response is described differently. This observation provides the basis for considering the implications for further research.

Lowrey[164] presented some theoretical and methodological issues confronting researchers studying stress. Primarily, she made a case for the need for nurse researchers to examine carefully the articulation and relevance of the framework, physiological variables, and measures selected. To develop the knowledge base for the field, similar studies need to be conducted using similar samples with a sufficient number of subjects, similar interventions, and similar measures. Future studies need to extend the work of previous studies. Currently there are too few examples in the stress field in which this systematic building is occurring. There are more specific and sensitive biochemical assays available for measurement of levels of catecholamines and other hormones and metabolites in blood and urine samples; thus, the study of the stress response now can be more precise and reliable. It is also possible to consider using several of the immune function measures as indicators or to examine stress response relationships. It is obvious, even from the few studies included as examples, that considerably more research is required to achieve the understanding of stress necessary to establish clinically appropriate and effective interventions. Considering the very broad range of stressors, their ubiquitous nature, and the influence of the individual's characteristics on the response, it is not a simple problem; there are and will continue to be multiple and diverse findings.

REFERENCES

1. Chrousos, G.P. (1998). Stressors, stress, and neuroendocrine integration of the adaptive response. The 1997 Hans Selye Memorial Lecture. *Annals of the New York Academy of Science 851,* 311-335.
2. Kiecolt-Glaser, J.K., & Glaser, R. (1999). Psychoneuroimmunology and cancer: Fact or fiction? *European Journal of Cancer 35,* 1603-1607.
3. Yang, E.V., & Glaser, R. (2000). Stress-induced immunomodulation: Impact on immune defenses against infectious disease. *Biomedicine & Pharmacotherapy 54,* 245-250.
4. Page, G.G., & Ben-Eliyahu, S. (1997). The immune-suppressive nature of pain. *Seminars in Oncology Nursing 13,* 10-15.
5. Pedersen, B.K., Bruunsgaard, H., Klokker, M., Kappel, M., MacLean, D.A., Nielsen, H.B., et al. (1997). Exercise-induced immunomodulation—possible roles of neuroendocrine and metabolic factors. *International Journal of Sports Medicine 18,* S2-S7.
6. Fava, G.A., & Sonino, N. (2000). Psychosomatic medicine: Emerging trends and perspectives. *Psychotherapy and Psychosomatics 69,* 184-197.
7. Ben-Eliyahu, S., Page, G.G., Yirmiya, R., & Shakhar, G. (1999). Evidence that stress and surgical interventions promote tumor development by suppressing natural killer cell activity. *International Journal of Cancer 80,* 880-888.
8. Stefanski, V., & Ben-Eliyahu, S. (1996). Social confrontation and tumor metastasis in rats: Defeat and beta-adrenergic mechanisms. *Physiology & Behavior 60,* 277-282.
9. Ben-Eliyahu, S., Yirmiya, R., Liebeskind, J.C., Taylor, A.N., & Gale, R.P. (1991). Stress increases metastatic spread of a mammary tumor in rats: Evidence for mediation by the immune system. *Brain, Behavior, and Immunity 5,* 193-205.
10. Page, G.G., McDonald, J.S., & Ben-Eliyahu, S. (1998). Pre-operative versus postoperative administration of morphine: Impact on the neuroendocrine, behavioural, and metastatic-enhancing effects of surgery. *British Journal of Anaesthesiology 81,* 216-223.
11. Sacerdote, P., Manfredi, B., Bianchi, M., & Panerai, A.E. (1994). Intermittent but not continuous inescapable footshock stress affects immune responses and immunocyte beta-endorphin concentrations in the rat. *Brain, Behavior, and Immunity 8,* 251-260.
12. Fleshner, M., Bellgrau, D., Watkins, L.R., Laudenslager, M.L., & Maier, S.F. (1995). Stress-induced reduction in the rat mixed lymphocyte reaction is due to macrophages and not to changes in T cell phenotypes. *Journal of Neuroimmunology 56,* 45-52.

13. Frankenhaeuser, M. (1975). *Sympathetic-adrenomedullary activity, behavior and the psychosocial environment. Research in psychophysiology.* New York: John Wiley.
14. Ganong, W.F. (1981). Neuroendocrine responses to injury and shock. *Advances in Physiological Sciences 26,* 35-44.
15. Holroyd, A., & Lazarus, R.S. (1982). Stress, coping and somatic adaptation. In L. Goldberger, & S. Breznitz (eds.), *Handbook of stress, theoretical and clinical aspects* (pp. 21-25). New York: Free Press.
16. Hyman, R., & Woog, P. (1982). Stressful life events and illness onset: A review of crucial variables. *Research in Nursing and Health 5,* 163.
17. Lazarus, R. (1974). Psychological stress and coping in adaptation and illness. *International Journal of Psychiatry in Medicine 5,* 321-333.
18. Mason, J.W. (1975). Psychologic stress and endocrine function. In E.J. Sachar (ed.), *Topics in Psychoneuroendocrinology.* New York: Grune & Stratton.
19. Moore, F.D. (1977). Homeostasis: Bodily changes in trauma and surgery. In D.C. Sabiston (ed.), *Textbook of Surgery.* Philadelphia: W.B. Saunders.
20. Schumer, W. (1976). Metabolism during sepsis and shock. *Heart & Lung 5,* 416-421.
21. Sparacino, J. (1982). Blood pressure, stress and mental health. *Nursing Research 31,* 89-94.
22. Wilmore, D.W., Long, J.M., Mason, A.D., & Pruitt, B.A. (1976). Stress in surgical patients as a neurophysiologic reflex response. *Surgery, Gynecology & Obstetrics 142,* 257-269.
23. Cohen, S., & Williamson, G.M. (1991). Stress and infectious disease in humans. *Psychology Bulletin 109,* 5-24.
24. Cohen, S., Doyle, W.J., & Skoner, D.P. (1999). Psychological stress, cytokine production, and severity of upper respiratory illness. *Psychosomatic Medicine 61,* 175-180.
25. Cohen, S., Doyle, W.J., Skoner, D.P., Rabin, B.S., & Gwaltney, J.M. (1997). Social ties and susceptibility to the common cold. *Journal of the American Medical Association 277,* 1940-1944.
26. Tache, J., & Selye, H. (1978). On stress and coping mechanisms. *Stress Anxiety 5,* 3-24.
27. Richter, S.D., Schurmeyer, T.H., Schedlowski, M., Hadicke, A., Tewes, U., Schmidt, R.E., et al. (1996). Time kinetics of the endocrine response to acute psychological stress. *Journal of Clinical Endocrinology and Metabolism 81,* 1956-1960.
28. Oberbeck, R., Schurmeyer, T.H., Jacobs, R., Benschop, R.J., Sommer, B., Schmidt, R.E., et al. (1998). Effects of beta-adrenoceptor-blockade on stress-induced adrenocorticotrophin release in humans. *European Journal of Applied Physiology 77,* 523-526.
29. Kant, G.J., Bauman, R.A., Anderson, S.M., & Mougey, E.H. (1992). Effects of controllable vs. uncontrollable chronic stress on stress-responsive plasma hormones. *Physiology & Behavior 51,* 1285-1288.
30. Anderson, S.M., Saviolakis, G.A., Bauman, R.A., Chu, K.Y., Ghosh, S., & Kant, G.J. (1996). Effects of chronic stress on food acquisition, plasma hormones, and the estrous cycle of female rats. *Physiology & Behavior 60,* 325-329.
31. Rowbottom, D.G., & Green, K.J. (2000). Acute exercise effects on the immune system. *Medicine and Science in Sports and Exercise 32,* S396-S405.
32. Ciaranello, R., & Lipton, M. (1982). *Panel report on biological substrates of stress. Stress and human health: A study by the Institute of Medicine/National Academy of Sciences* (pp. 189-254). New York: Springer.
33. Dantzer, R., & Kelley, K.W. (1989). Stress and immunity: An integrated view of relationships between the brain and the immune system. *Life Sciences 44,* 1995-2008.
34. Dunn, A.J. (1989). Psychoneuroimmunology for the psychoneuroendocrinologist: A review of animal studies of nervous system-immune system interactions. *Psychoneuroendocrinology 14,* 251-274.
35. Ganong, W.F. (1980). Participation of brain monoamines in the regulation of neuroendocrine activity under stress. In E. Usdin, R. Kvetnansky, & I.J. Kopin (eds.), *Catecholamines and stress* (pp. 115-124). New York: Elsevier.
36. Kopin, E.J. (1976). Catecholamines, adrenal hormones, and stress. *Hospital Practice 11,* 49-55.
37. Selye, H. (1956). A syndrome produced by diverse noxious agents. *Nature 72,* 138.
38. Selye, H. (1956). *The Stress of life.* New York: McGraw-Hill.
39. Dantzer, R., & Kelly, K.W. (1989). Stress and immunity: An integrated view of relationships between the brain and the immune system. *Life Science 44,* 1995-2008.
40. Watkins, L.R., & Maier, S.F. (1999). Implications of immune-to-brain communication for sickness and pain. *Annals of the New York Academy of Science 96,* 7710-7713.
41. Felten, S.Y., Madden, K.S., Bellinger, D.L., Kruszewska, B., Moynihan, J.A., & Felten, D.L. (1998). The role of the sympathetic nervous system in the modulation of immune responses. *Advances in Pharmacology 42,* 583-586.
42. Dhabhar, F.S., Miller, A.H., McEwen, B.S., & Spencer, R.L. (1995). Effects of stress on immune cell distribution: Dynamics and hormonal mechanisms. *Journal of Immunology 154,* 5511-5527.
43. Schedlowski, M., Hosch, W., Oberbeck, R., Benschop, R.J., Jacobs, R., Raab, H.R., et al. (1996). Catecholamines modulate human NK cell circulation and function via spleen-independent β_2-adrenergic mechanisms. *Journal of Immunology 156,* 93-99.
44. Sternberg, E.M. (1997). Neural-immune interactions in health and disease. *Journal of Clinical Investigations 100,* 2641-2647.
45. DeFronzo, R.A., Sherwin, R.S., & Felig, P. (1980). Synergistic interactions of counter-regulatory hormones: A mechanism for stress hyperglycemia. *Acta Chirurgica Scandinavica Supplementum 498,* 33-42.
46. Kvetnansky, R., Weise, V.K., & Kopin, I.J. (1970). Elevation of adrenal tyrosine hydroxylase and phenylethanolamine-N-methyl transferase by repeated immobilization of rats. *Endocrinology 87,* 744-749.
47. Baum, A., Grunberg, N., & Singer, J. (1982). The use of psychological and neuroendocrinological measurements in the study of stress. *Health Psychology 1,* 217-236.
48. Lenox, R., Kant, G., Sessions, G., Pennington, L., Mougey, E., & Meyerhoff, J. (1980). Specific hormonal and neurochemical responses to different stressors. *Neuroendocrinology 30,* 300-308.
49. Mason, J. (1974). Specificity in the organization of neuroendocrine response profiles. In *Frontiers in neurology and neuroscience research* (pp. 68-80). First International Symposium of the Neuroscience Institute, University of Toronto. Toronto: Canada.
50. Mason, J.W. (1975). A historical view of the stress field. Part I. *Human Stress 1,* 6-12.

51. Mason, J.W. (1975). A historical view of the stress field. Part II. *Journal of Human Stress 1,* 22-36.
52. Munck, A., Guyre, P.M., & Holbrook, N.J. (1984). Physiological functions of glucocorticoids in stress and their relations to pharmacological actions. *Endocrine Reviews 5,* 25-44.
53. Selye, H. (1975). Confusion and controversy in the stress field. *Journal of Human Stress 1,* 37-44.
54. Van den Berghe, G.H.A. (1999). The neuroendocrine stress response and modern intensive care: The concept revisited. *Burns 25,* 7-16.
55. Shavit, Y., Lewis, J.W., Terman, G.W., Gale, R.P., & Liebeskind, J.C. (1984). Opioid peptides mediate the suppressive effect of stress on natural killer cell cytotoxicity. *Science 223,* 188-190.
56. Cover, P.O., & Buckingham, J.C. (1989). Effects of selective opioid-receptor blockade on the hypothalamo-pituitary-adrenocortical responses to surgical trauma in the rat. *Journal of Endocrinology 121,* 213-220.
57. Giuffre, K.A., Udelsman, R., Listwak, S.C., & Chrousos, G.P. (1988). Effects of immune neutralization of corticotropin-releasing hormone, adrenocorticotropin, and β-endorphin in the surgically stressed rat. *Endocrinology 122,* 306-310.
58. Anand, K.J. (1986). The stress response to surgical trauma: From physiological basis to therapeutic implications. *Progress in Food & Nutrition Science 10,* 67-132.
59. O'Neal, K., & Waxman, K. (1987). Mediators of altered perioperative physiology. *Critical Care Clinics 3,* 359-371.
60. Anand, K.J., Brown, M.J., Causon, R.C., Christofides, N.D., Bloom, S.R., & Aynsley-Green, A. (1985). Can the human neonate mount an endocrine and metabolic response to surgery? *Journal of Pediatric Surgery 20,* 41-48.
61. Anand, K.J.S., & Hickey, P.R. (1992). Halothane-morphine compared with high-dose sufentanil for anesthesia and postoperative analgesia in neonatal cardiac surgery. *New England Journal of Medicine 326,* 1-9.
62. Kehlet, H. (1984). The stress response to anaesthesia and surgery: Release mechanisms and modifying factors. *Clinical Anaesthesiology 2,* 315-339.
63. Tsuji, H., Shirasaka, C., Asoh, T., & Uchida, I. (1987). Effects of epidural administration of local anaesthetics or morphine on postoperative nitrogen loss and catabolic hormones. *British Journal of Surgery 74,* 421-425.
64. Salomäki, T.E., Leppäluoto, J., Laitinen, J.O., Vuolteenaho, O., & Nuutinen, L.S. (1993). Epidural versus intravenous fentanyl for reducing hormonal, metabolic, and physiologic responses after thoracotomy. *Anesthesiology 79,* 672-679.
65. Yeager, M.P., Glass, D.D., Neff, R.K., & Brinck-Johnsen, T. (1987). Epidural anesthesia and analgesia in high-risk surgical patients. *Anesthesiology 66,* 729-736.
66. Koltun, W.A., Bloomer, M.M., Tilberg, A.F., Seaton, J.F., Ilahi, O., Rung, G., et al. (1996). Awake epidural anesthesia is associated with improved natural killer cell cytotoxicity and reduced stress response. *American Journal of Surgery 171,* 68-73.
67. Kehlet, H. (1998). The stress response to surgery: Release mechanisms and the modifying effect of pain release. *Acta Chirurgica Scandinavica 550,* 22-28.
68. Kehlet, H. (1989). Surgical stress: The role of pain and analgesia. *British Journal of Anaesthesiology 63,* 189-195.
69. Schulze, S., Roikjaer, O., Hasselstrøm, L., Jensen, N.H., & Kehlet, H. (1988). Epidural bupivacaine and morphine plus systemic indomethacin eliminates pain but not systemic response and convalescence after cholecystectomy. *Surgery 103,* 321-327.
70. Scott, N.B., Mogensen, T., Bigler, D., Lund, C., & Kehlet, H. (1989). Continuous thoracic extradural 0.5% bupivacaine with or without morphine: Effect on quality of blockade, lung function and the surgical stress response. *British Journal of Anaesthesiology 62,* 253-257.
71. Tønnesen, E., Brinklov, M.M., Christensen, N.J., Olesen, A.S., & Madsen, T. (1987). Natural killer cell activity and lymphocyte function during and after coronary artery bypass grafting in relation to the endocrine stress response. *Anesthesiology 67,* 523-533.
72. Tønnesen, E. (1989). Immunological aspects of anaesthesia and surgery – with special reference to NK cells. *Danish Medical Bulletin 36,* 263-281.
73. Le Cras, A.E., Galley, H.F., & Webster, N.R. (1998). Spinal but not general anesthesia increases the ratio of T helper 1 to T helper 2 cell subsets in patients undergoing transurethral resection of the prostate. *Anesthesia and Analgesia 87,* 1421-1425.
74. Cuschieri, R.J., Morran, C.G., Howie, J.C., & McArdle, C.S. (1985). Postoperative pain and pulmonary complications: Comparison of three analgesic regimens. *British Journal of Surgery 72,* 495-498.
75. Pollock, R.E., & Lotzová, E. (1987). Surgical-stress-related suppression of natural killer cell activity: A possible role in tumor metastasis. *Natural Immunity and Cell Growth Regulation 6,* 269-278.
76. Saba, T.M., & Antikatzides, T.G. (1976). Decreased resistance to intravenous tumour-cell challenge during reticuloendothelial depression following surgery. *British Journal of Cancer 34,* 381-389.
77. Page, G.G., Ben-Eliyahu, S., & Liebeskind, J.C. (1994). The roll of LGL/NK cells in surgery-induced promotion of metastasis and its attenuation by morphine. *Brain, Behavior, and Immunity 8,* 241-250.
78. Saba, T.M., & Antikatzides, T.G. (1976). Decreased resistance to intravenous tumour-cell challenge during reticuloendothelial depression following surgery. *British Journal of Cancer 34,* 381-389.
79. Gorelik, E., Wiltrout, R.H., Okumura, K., Habu, S., & Herberman, R.B. (1982). Role of NK cells in the control of metastatic spread and growth of tumor cells in mice. *International Journal of Cancer 30,* 107-112.
80. Hanna, N. (1985). The role of natural killer cells in the control of tumor growth and metastasis. *Biochimica et Biophysica Acta 780,* 213-226.
81. Wiltrout, R.H., Herberman, R.B., Zhang, S., Chirigos, M.A., Ortaldo, J.R., Green, K.M., et al. (1985). Role of organ-associated NK cells in decreased formation of experimental metastases in lung and liver. *Journal of Immunology 134,* 4267-4275.
82. Buinauskas, P., McDonald, G.O., & Cole, W.H. (1958). Role of operative stress on the resistance of the experimental animal to inoculated cancer cells. *Annals of Surgery 148,* 642-645.
83. Hattori, T., Hamai, Y., Harada, T., Ikeda, H., & Ikeda, T. (1977). Enhancing effect of thoracotomy and/or laparotomy on the growth of ascitic tumors in rats. *Japanese Journal of Surgery 7,* 258-262.
84. Hattori, T., Hamai, Y., Harada, T., Ikeda, H., & Ikeda, T. (1977). Enhancing effect of thoracotomy and/or laparotomy on the development of the lung metastases in rats after intravenous inoculation of tumor cells. *Japanese Journal of Surgery 7,* 263-268.

85. Lewis, M.R., & Cole, W.H. (1958). Experimental increase of lung metastases after operative trauma (amputation of limb with tumor). *Archives of Surgery 77,* 621-626.
86. Lundy, J., Lovett, E.J., Hamilton, S., & Conran, P. (1978). Halothane, surgery, immunosuppression and artificial pulmonary metastases. *Cytopathology 41,* 827-830.
87. Page, G.G., Ben-Eliyahu, S., Yirmiya, R., & Liebeskind, J.C. (1993). Morphine attenuates surgery-induced enhancement of metastatic colonization in rats. *Pain 54,* 21-28.
88. Folkman, S., & Lazarus, R.S. (1980). An analysis of coping in a middle-aged community sample. *Health and Social Behavior 21,* 219-239.
89. Folkman, S., Schaefer, C., & Lazarus, R.S. (1980). Cognitive processes as mediators of stress and coping. In V. Hamilton, & D.M. Warburton (eds.), *Human stress and cognition: An information processing approach* (pp. 265-298). New York: John Wiley & Sons.
90. Lazarus, R.S. (1981). The stress and coping paradigm. In C. Eisdorfer, D. Cohen, A. Kleinman, & P. Maxim (eds.), *Models for psychopathology* (pp. 173-209). New York: Spectrum.
91. Pearlin, L.I., & Schooler, C. (1978). The structure of coping. *Journal of Health and Social Behavior 19,* 2-21.
92. Sczekalla, R.M. Stress reactions of CCU patients to resuscitation procedures on other patients. *Nursing Research 22,* 65-69.
93. Weinberger, D., Schwartz, G., & Davidson, R. (1979). Low-anxious, high-anxious, and repressive coping styles: Psychometric patterns and behavioral and physiological responses to stress. *Journal of Abnormal Psychology 88,* 369-380.
94. Biondi, M., & Picardi, A. (1999). Psychological stress and neuroendocrine function in humans: The last two decades of research. *Psychotherapy and Psychosomatics 68,* 114-150.
95. Frankenhaeuser, M. (1975). Experimental approaches to the study of catecholamines and emotion. In L. Levi (ed.), *Emotions: Their parameters and measurement.* New York: Raven Press.
96. Dimsdale, J., & Moss, J. (1980). Short-term catecholamine response to psychological stress. *Psychosomatic Medicine 42,* 493-497.
97. Dimsdale, J., & Herd, J. (1992). Variability of plasma lipids in response to emotional arousal. *Psychosomatic Medicine 44,* 413-430.
98. Rozanski, A., Blumenthal, J.A., & Kaplan, J. (1999). Impact of psychological factors on the pathogenesis of cardiovascular disease and implications for therapy. *Circulation 99,* 2192-2217.
99. Robinson, L. (1990). Stress and anxiety. *Nursing Clinics of North America 25,* 935-943.
100. Cohen, S. (1980). After effects of stress on human performance and social behavior: A review of research and theory. *Psychology Bulletin 87,* 578-604.
101. Gal, E., & Lazarus, R.S. (1975). The role of activity in anticipating and confronting stressful situations. *Journal of Human Stress 1,* 4-19.
102. Jalowiec, A., & Powers, M.J. (1981). Stress and coping in hypertensive and emergency room patients. *Nursing Research 30,* 10-15.
103. Lazarus, R., & Launier, R. (1978). Stress-related transactions between person and environment. In A. Pervin, & M. Lewis (eds.), *Perspectives in interactional psychology.* New York: Plenum Press.
104. Stone, C.G., Cohen, F., & Adler, N. (1979). *Health psychology: A handbook.* San Francisco: Jossey Bass.
105. Spiegel, D., Sephton, S.E., Terr, I.A., & Stites, D.P. (1998). Effects of psychosocial treatment in prolonging cancer survival may be mediated by neuroimmune pathways. *Annals of the New York Academy of Science 840,* 674-683.
106. Fawzy, F.I., & Fawzy, N.W. (1998). Group therapy in the cancer setting. *Journal of Psychosomatic Research 45,* 191-200.
107. Kemeny, M.E., & Laudenslager, M.L. (1999). Beyond stress: The role of individual difference factors in psychoneuroimmunology. *Brain, Behavior, and Immunity 13,* 73-75.
108. Cacioppo, J.T., Berntson, G.G., Malarkey, W.B., Kiecolt-Glaser, J.K., Sheridan, J.F., Poehlmann, K.M., et al. (1998). Autonomic, neuroendocrine, and immune responses to psychological stress: The reactivity hypothesis. *Annals of the New York Academy of Science 840,* 640-673.
109. Cacioppo, J.T., Malarkey, W.B., Kiecolt-Glaser, J.K., Uchino, B.N., Sgoutas-Emch, S.A., Sheridan, J.F., Berntson, G.G., & Glaser, R. (1995). Heterogeneity in neuroendocrine and immune responses to brief psychological stressors as a function of autonomic cardiac activation. *Psychosomatic Medicine 57,* 154-164.
110. Benoliel, J.Q., McCorkle, R., Denton, T., & Spitzer, A. (1990). Measurement of stress in clinical nursing. *Cancer Nursing 13,* 221-228.
111. Delongis, A., Coyne, J.C., Dakof, G., Folkman, S., & Lazarus, R.S. (1982). Relationship of daily hassles, uplifts, and major life events to health status. *Health Psychology 1,* 119-136.
112. Dohrenwend, B.S., & Dohrenwend, B.P. (1974). *Stressful life events: Their nature and effects.* New York: John Wiley.
113. Holmes, T., & Rahe, R. (1967). The social readjustment rating scale. *Journal of Psychosomatic Research 11,* 218.
114. Holmes, T., & Masuda, M. (1974). Life change and illness susceptibility. In B.S. Dohrenwend, & B.P. Dohrenwend (eds.), *Stressful life events: Their nature and effect.* New York: John Wiley.
115. Jenkins, C.D., Rosenman, R.H., & Friedman, M. (1967). Development of an objective psychological test for the determination of the coronary prone behavior pattern in employed men. *Journal of Chronic Disease 20,* 371-379.
116. Kanner, A.D., Coyne, J.C., Schaefer, C., & Lazarus, R.S. (1981). Comparison of two modes of stress measurement: Daily hassles and uplifts versus major life events. *Journal of Behavioral Medicine 4,* 1-39.
117. McNair, D.M., Lorr, M., & Droppleman, L.F. (1971). *POMS manual for profile of mood states.* San Diego: Educational and Industrial Testing Service.
118. Sarason, I., deMonchaux, C., & Hunt, T. (1975). Methodological issues in the assessment of life stress. In L. Levi (ed.), *Emotions: Their parameters and measurement.* New York: Raven.
119. Sarason, I.G., Johnson, J.H., & Siegel, J.M. (1978). Assessing the impact of life changes: Development of the life experiences survey. *Journal of Consulting and Clinical Psychology 46,* 932-943.
120. Spielberger, C.D., Gorsuch, R.L., & Lushene, R.E. (1970). *STAI manual for the State-Trait Anxiety Inventory.* Palo Alto, Calif.: Consulting Psychologists Press.
121. Stokes, S.A., & Gordon, S.E. (1988). Development of an instrument to measure stress in the older adult. *Nursing Research 37,* 16-19.

122. Tausig, M. (1982). Measuring life events. *Journal of Health and Social Behavior 23,* 52-64.
123. Volicer, B.J., & Bohannon, M.W. (1975). A hospital stress rating scale. *Nursing Research 24,* 352-359.
124. Volicer, B.J. (1975). Stress factors in the experience of hospitalization. *Community Nursing Research 8,* 53-67.
125. Rosenman, R.H., Braud, R.V., Sholtz, R.I., & Friedman, M. (1976). Multivariate prediction of coronary heart disease during 8.5 year follow-up in the Western Collaborative Group Study. *American Journal of Cardiology 37,* 903-910.
126. Jenkins, C.D. (1976). Recent evidence supporting pyschologic and social risk factors for coronary disease, Part 1. *New England Journal of Medicine 294,* 987-994.
127. Jenkins, C.D. (1976). Recent evidence supporting psychologic and social risk factors for coronary disease, Part 2. *New England Journal of Medicine 294,* 1033-1038.
128. Matthews, K.A. (1982). Psychological perspectives on the type A behavior pattern. *Psychology Bulletin 91,* 293-323.
129. Weiner, H. (1992). *Perturbing the organism: The biology of stressful experience.* Chicago: University of Chicago Press.
130. Plotnikoff, N.P., Faith, R.E., Murgo, A.J., & Good, R.A. (eds.). (1998). *Cytokines: Stress and immunity.* Boca Raton: CRC Press.
131. Long, C., & Blakemore, W. (1979). Energy and protein requirements in the hospitalized patient. *Journal of Parenteral and Enteral Nutrition 3,* 69-71.
132. Brennan, M. (1981). Total parenteral nutrition in the cancer patient. *New England Journal of Medicine 305,* 375-382.
133. Wilmore, D. (1976). Alimentation in injured and septic patients. *Heart & Lung 5,* 792.
134. Blackburn, G. (1979). Hyperalimentation in the critically ill patient. *Heart & Lung 8,* 67-70.
135. Lumb, P., Dalton, B., Bryan-Brown, C., & Donnelly, C. (1979). Aggressive approach to intravenous feeding to the critically ill. *Heart & Lung 8,* 71-80.
136. Donovan, M. (1981). Study of the impact of relaxation with guided imagery on stress among cancer nurses. *Cancer Nursing 4,* 121-126.
137. Meichenbaum, D., & Jaremko, M.E. (1983). *Stress reduction and prevention.* New York: Plenum Press.
138. Anchor, K.N., Beck, S.E., Sievking, N., & Adkins, J. (1982). A history of clinical biofeedback. *American Journal of Clinical Biofeedback 5,* 3-16.
139. Tvede, N., Kappel, M., Klarlund, K., Duhn, S., Halkjaer-Kristensen, J., Kjaer, M., et al. (1994). Evidence that the effect of bicycle exercise on blood mononuclear cell proliferative responses and subsets is mediated by epinephrine. *International Journal of Sports Medicine 15,* 100-104.
140. Nieman, D.C. (1997). Exercise immunology: Practical applications. *International Journal of Sports Medicine Supplement 11,* S91-S100.
141. Nieman, D.C., Ahle, J.C., Henson, D.A., Warren, B.J., Suttles, J., Davis, J.M., et al. (1995). Indomethacin does not alter natural killer cell response to 2.5 h of running. *Journal of Applied Physiology 79,* 748-755.
142. Kraemer, W.J., Patton, J.F., Knuttgen, H.G., Marchitelli, L.J., Cruthirds, C., Damokosh, A., et al. (1989). Hypothalamic-pituitary adrenal responses to short duration high-intensity cycle exercise. *Journal of Applied Physiology 66,* 161-166.
143. Baum, M., Muller-Steinhardt, M., Liesen, H., & Kirchner, H. (1997). Moderate and exhaustive endurance exercise influences the interferon-gamma levels in whole-blood culture supernatants. *European Journal of Applied Physiology 76,* 165-169.
144. Goldfarb, A.H., Jamurtas, A.Z., Kamimori, G.H., Hegde, S., Otterstetter, R., & Brown, D.A. (1998). Gender effect on beta-endorphin response to exercise. *Medicine and Science in Sports and Exercise 30,* 1672-1676.
145. Rupprecht, M., Salzer, B., Raum, B., Hornstein, O.P., Koch, H.U., Riederer, P., et al. (1997). Physical stress-induced secretion of adrenal and pituitary hormones in patients with atopic eczema compared with normal controls. *Experimental and Clinical Endocrinology and Diabetes 105,* 39-45.
146. Nieman, D.C., Henson, D.A., Gusewitch, G., Warren, B.J., Dotson, R.C., Butterworth, D.E., et al. (1993). Physical activity and immune function in elderly women. *Medicine and Science in Sports and Exercise 25,* 823-831.
147. Nieman, D.C. (1990). The effects of moderate exercise training on natural killer cells. *International Journal of Sports Medicine 11,* 467-473.
148. Davis, J.M., Kohut, M.L., Colbert, L.H., Jackson, D.A., Ghaffar, A., & Mayer, E.P. (1997). Exercise, alveolar macrophage function, and susceptibility to respiratory infection. *Journal of Applied Physiology 83,* 1461-1466.
149. Jonsdottir, I.H., Asea, A., Hoffmann, P., Dahlgren, U.I., Andersson, B., Hellstrand, K., & Thoren, P. (1996). Voluntary chronic exercise augments in vivo natural immunity in rats. *Journal of Applied Physiology 80,* 1799-1803.
150. Glaser, R., Kiecolt-Glaser, J.K., Malarkey, W.B., & Sheridan, J.F. (1998). The influence of psychological stress on the immune response to vaccines. *Annals of the New York Academy of Science 840,* 649-655.
151. Kiecolt-Glaser, J.K. (1999). Stress, personal relationships, and immune function: Health implications. *Brain, Behavior, and Immunity 13,* 61-72.
152. Marucha, P.T., Kiecolt-Glaser, J.K., & Favagehi, M. (1998). Mucosal wound healing is impaired by examination stress. *Psychosomatic Medicine 60,* 362.
153. Guidi, L., Tricerri, A., Frasca, D., Vangeli, M., Errani, A.R., & Bartoloni, C. (1998). Psychoneuroimmunology and aging. *Gerontology 44,* 247-261.
154. Vedhara, K., Cox, N.K., Wilcock, G.K., Perks, P., Hunt, M., Anderson, S., et al. (1999). Chronic stress in elderly carers of dementia patients and antibody response to influenza vaccination. *Lancet 353,* 627-631.
155. Kiecolt-Glaser, J.K., Glaser, R., Gravenstein, S., Malarkey, W.B., & Sheridan, J.F. (1996). Chronic stress alters the immune response to influenza virus vaccine in older adults. *Proceedings of the National Academy of Science of the United States of America 93,* 3043-3047.
156. Kiecolt-Glaser, J.K., Marucha, P.T., Malarkey, W.B., Mercado, A.M., & Glaser, R. (1995). Slowing of wound healing by psychological stress. *Lancet 346,* 1194-1196.
157. Sheridan, J.F., Ningguo, F., Bonneau, R.H., Allen, C.M., Huneycutt, B.S., & Glaser, R. (1991). Restraint stress differentially affects anti-viral cellular and humoral immune responses in mice. *Journal of Neuroimmunology 31,* 245-255.
158. Padgett, D.A., Marucha, P.T., & Sheridan, J.F. (1998). Restraint stress slows cutaneous wound healing in mice. *Brain, Behavior, and Immunity 12,* 64-73.
159. Spiegel, D., Bloom, S.R., & Yalom, I. (1981). Group support for patients with metastatic cancer. *Archives of General Psychiatry 38,* 527-533.

160. Spiegel, D., Bloom, S.R., Kraemer, H.C., & Gottheil, E. (1989). Effect of psychosocial treatment on survival of patients with metastatic breast cancer. *Lancet 2,* 889-891.
161. Fawzy, F.I., Cousins, N., Fawzy, N.W., Kemeny, M.E., Elashoff, R., & Morton, D.L. (1990). A structured psychiatric intervention for cancer patients: I. Changes over time in methods of coping and affective disturbance. *Archives of General Psychiatry 47,* 720-725.
162. Fawzy, F.I., Kemeny, M.E., Fawzy, N.W., Elashoff, R., Morton, D.L., Cousins, N., et al. (1990). A structured psychiatric intervention for cancer patients: II. Changes over time in immunological measures. *Archives of General Psychiatry 47,* 729-735.
163. Fawzy, F.I., Fawzy, N.W., Hyun, S.C., Elashoff, R., Guthrie, D., Fahey, J.L., et al. (1993). Effects of an early structured psychiatric intervention, coping, and affective state on recurrence and survival 6 years later. *Archives of General Psychiatry 50,* 681-689.
164. Lowrey, B. (1987). Stress research: Some theoretical and methodological issues. *Image—the Journal of Nursing Scholarship 19,* 42-46

CHAPTER

15 Alterations in Immunocompetence

MARILYN SAWYER SOMMERS

DEFINITION

Immunocompetence is the ability of an individual's immune system to support life by defending the body against internal and external threats to health. Threats can occur from the body's own cells if they mutate into tumor cells or if autoantibodies form against body cells. External threats occur from pathogenic organisms, such as bacteria or viruses. The function of the immune system, therefore, may be viewed broadly as the ability to differentiate the body's own cells (self) from invading agents or mutating cells (nonself).[1,2] Immunosuppression is the prevention of an immune response; immunocompromise, by comparison, is the state of having an immune system incapable of reacting to an immune challenge, such as pathogens or tissue damage.[2] Immunocompromise results from an alteration in immune function in any of the four main components of the immune system: B cell deficiency, T cell deficiency, complement (C) deficiency, and phagocyte deficiency.

The Social Policy Statement from the American Nurses' Association describes the human response as an area of concern to nurses.[3] The responses to an immune challenge, whether these are the normal responses to pregnancy and carrying a fetus (nonself), the response to a blood transfusion or an organ transplant, the response to mutated self cells, or the response to a fulminating bacterial infection, are relevant to nursing practice and amenable to nursing interventions. Nursing interventions can be focused on individuals across the life span, because immunocompetence is a phenomenon that is needed for health in people of all ages. The very young and the very old, however, are particularly vulnerable to alterations in immunocompetence.[4-7]

Questions exist about the nature of the relatively poor immune response in the very young, but newborns appear to have inadequate lymphocyte function, with T cell impairment (see Mechanisms) in particular. Newborns rely on passive immunity to maintain immunocompetence as they receive immunoglobulins through the transfer of maternal IgG across the placenta before birth. In addition, as newborns begin to nurse, they receive a large quantity of IgA in colostrum, which provides protection from respiratory and gastrointestinal infections. Fetuses and newborns have the capacity for some immunoglobulin production, particularly the most primitive immunoglobulin, IgM. After birth, newborns begin to produce IgG and IgA; levels of these immunoglobulins progressively increase throughout the first 6 months of life.[4,5]

At the other end of the life span, elders have a decreased ability to maintain immunocompetence, but the reasons for this diminished capacity are uncertain. Scientists report that elders have a decreased ability to produce IgG, have fewer T cells, and a delayed hypersensitivity response.[4,5] As people age, they develop increased levels of circulating autoantibodies and decreased surveillance against mutating cells, thereby increasing the risk of tumor proliferation. Elders therefore become less immunocompetent and are at higher risk than middle-aged adults for the emergence of malignancies and neoplasms.[1,4,5]

Pregnancy has long been associated with an altered susceptibility to infection. Before 1950, the single most common indication for therapeutic abortion was tuberculosis.[7] Diseases caused by viruses, intracellular bacteria, fungi, and protozoa have greater virulence during pregnancy. Pregnant women who contract hepatitis A, hepatitis B, and influenza have worse health outcomes than their nonpregnant counterparts.[7] B cell immunity, however, appears to be maintained at prepregnancy levels with normal serum immunoglobulin production, whereas T cell immunity changes. The precise mechanisms for altered immunocompetence during pregnancy are unknown, but scientists understand some of the reasons for modulation of the immune response. Current theories of reduced immunocompetence during pregnancy suggest the following changes: increased production of steroid hormones leads to suppression of lymphocytes and macrophages; alpha-fetoprotein secreted by the fetal liver depresses proliferative T cell responses; CD4+ (helper T) cells decrease in number and CD8+ (cytotoxic T) cells increase in number; and thymic involution occurs.[1,5,7]

Therefore alterations in immunocompetence may result from different and complex mechanisms that are related to pathological and natural causes. No single alteration can explain the complex interactions that occur when immunocompetence and overall general health are threatened.

PREVALENCE AND POPULATIONS AT RISK

Although no statistics represent the prevalence of all cases of alterations in immunocompetence, the global phenomenon of the human immunodeficiency virus infection/acquired immunodeficiency syndrome (HIV/AIDS) pandemic has received a great deal of attention from experts in public health. The National Center for Health Statistics report that more than 600,000 people have been diagnosed with AIDS in the United States since the disease was first recognized.[8] From 650,000 to 900,000 Americans are infected with HIV, a rate of 310 to 420 per 100,000 population.[8,9] HIV was the fourteenth leading cause of death overall in the United States, the fifth leading cause of death in people ages 25 to 44 in 1997 (down from the leading cause of death in this age group in 1995),[10] and fourth leading cause of death globally.[11]

Although the incidence of HIV/AIDS appears to be on the decline in the United States, the continent of Africa in particular is coping with an epidemic that experts believe is prematurely killing a generation of adults. In Zimbabwe, approximately 25% of the population carries the virus, and nearly 40% of women who present for HIV counseling test positive for HIV.[12] Experts estimate that more than 21 million people were living with HIV or AIDS in Sub-Saharan Africa in 1997.[13] The U.S. Public Health Service identified four populations at risk for HIV/AIDS: men who have sex with men, injecting drug users, infants of untreated or undetected HIV-positive women, and heterosexual persons with high-risk sexual practices and/or who use addictive substances such as crack cocaine.[8,14] The HIV/AIDS pandemic has contributed to what is called global *human poverty* because of its effects on life expectancy, human development, and global economics. The effects of the pandemic cut across cultures and economies. Although Africa has the lowest quality of life indices in the world, the United States has the highest level of "human poverty" among industrialized nations.[15] In 1997, South and Southeast Asia had 6 million people infected with HIV/AIDS and Latin America had 1.3 million.[13]

Despite the extent and severity of the HIV/AIDS pandemic, the largest populations at risk for alterations in immunocompetence are those of developing nations. The World Health Organization (WHO) estimates that 174 million children under the age of 5 are malnourished, as indicated by low weight for age, and 230 million have stunted development. In developing countries, approximately half of all children who die before the age of 5 are malnourished.[16] Malnutrition affects adults as well as children. Worldwide, more than 800 million people cannot meet basic energy needs, and over 2 billion lack essential micronutrients.[16] Poor nutrition causes decreased immunoglobulin production and phagocyte activity as well as reduced integrity of the skin and mucous membranes.[4-7] For these reasons, the populations of developing nations are at risk for alterations in immunocompetence, a risk that is increased by the lack of resources for primary prevention of illness. Malnutrition is not only an international problem, however; the U.S. Department of Agriculture reported in September 2000 that children and African American families made up a disproportionate number of Americans who went hungry in the previous year. This report indicates that 12 million American children faced hunger, with several million starving.[17] This poor nutritional status increases the risk for immunocompromise.

Infectious diseases other than HIV/AIDS place children and young adults in particular at risk for severe health-related problems. Four of the leading ten causes of global mortality are infectious diseases: acute lower respiratory infections third, HIV/AIDS fourth, diarrheal diseases sixth, and tuberculosis (TB) eighth.[11] Infectious diseases are the world's biggest killer of children and young adults and account for more than 13 million deaths a year. Just six infectious diseases—TB, malaria, HIV/AIDS, pneumonia, diarrheal diseases, and measles—account for 90% of all infectious diseases[18] (Figure 15-1). Morbidity and mortality rates climb when individuals have altered immunocompetence because of poor nutrition and extremes of age coupled with poverty and inadequate health care resources.

Other populations at risk for alterations in immune system function exist as well. Individuals with disease or clinical states such as diabetes mellitus, alcohol dependence, liver failure, and severe

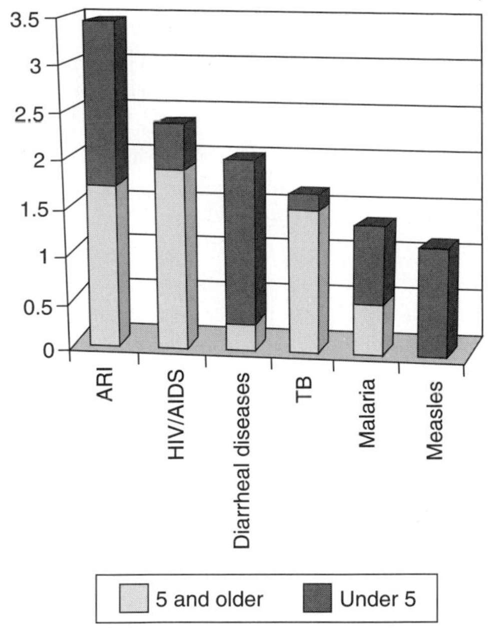

Figure 15-1 Millions of deaths worldwide in 1998 from the six leading causes of death from infectious diseases. *ARI,* Acute respiratory infections; *HIV/AIDS,* human immunodeficiency virus/acquired immunodeficiency syndrome; *TB,* tuberculosis. (Adapted from Heyman, D.L. [2000]. The urgency of a massive effort against infectious diseases. World Health Organization statement before the Committee on International Relations, U.S. House of Representatives, June, 29, 2000. www.who.int [accessed September 9, 2000].)

injury or burns have a reduced immune response. Congenital immunodeficiencies, although rare, exist as well and can involve any of the four main components of the immune system: B cell deficiencies, T cell deficiencies, C deficiencies, and phagocyte deficiencies. Examples of these disorders include X-linked hypogammaglobulinemia, thymic aplasia, and severe combined immunodeficiency disease (SCID).[4,7]

Therefore immunocompetence gives populations at risk protection against infectious diseases. The discipline of nursing has recognized the importance of human responses, such as immunocompetence, as an area of concern for nursing interventions.[1,3] Nursing interventions are critical if we are to limit epidemics that threaten vulnerable populations and limit the personal cost of infectious disease and immunosuppression to individuals. Vulnerable populations of concern to nurses exist not only in North America but globally as well. Sigma Theta Tau International (STTI), the honor society of nursing, recognizes the need for nursing to lead in global health care issues.[19] A global focus for preventive and restorative nursing interventions is essential if nurses are to meet the challenge of maintaining immunocompetence in at-risk populations.

RISK FACTORS

In addition to the risk factors identified in the Definition section, other factors also influence immunocompetence. A person's ability to respond to foreign invaders depends on past exposure to ultraviolet radiation (an environmental factor), as well as personal factors, such as an increased corticosteroid level and exposure to anesthesia or alcohol. Sun exposure is thought to induce immune suppression and reduce the effectiveness of immunization.[20] Ultraviolet light is thought to cause replication of viruses by blocking viral repressor proteins.[4] Inhalation agents and epidural anesthesia are known to cause altered cytokine function and altered white blood cell counts, although the precise immune mechanisms and outcomes are unclear.[21,22] Although the precise mechanism of action for the corticosteroid influence on immune system function is uncertain, corticosteroids are known to cause lysis of lymphocytes, decreased recruitment of monocytes, inhibition of cytokines (interferon in particular), and stabilization of lysosomes.[1,4,7]

Acute and chronic alcohol use can impair immune function. Binge drinking and acute alcohol intoxication are associated with unintentional injuries. Acutely intoxicated people who are injured have more than twice the number of infections than do those who do not consume alcohol.[23] Acute alcohol consumption before an injury, as compared with abstinence, is associated with decreased tumor necrosis factor production, posttraumatic immunosuppression, and impaired cell-mediated immunity.[23,24] Chronic drinking leads to alterations in both phagocytic cells and lymphocytes. Phagocytic cells have decreased adhesion and chemotaxis, with a decreased ability to ingest and breakdown bacteria. Dependent drinkers also have lower-than-normal numbers of circulating T cells, elevated levels of immunoglobulins with altered proliferation of B cells, and reduced numbers of natural killer (NK) cells.[24]

In addition to the extremes of age and life span events, such as pregnancy, a variety of factors can place a person at risk for immunocompromise. By recognizing these factors, clinicians can initiate interventions to support immunocompetence and begin protective measures to limit the risk of infection.

MECHANISMS

The body has several nonimmunological defenses against infection. Surface defenses include mucus, coughing, peristalsis, epithelial cell turnover, local disinfectants, such as gastric acid and skin lipids, and normal microbial flora on the skin and in the GI tract.[7] The primary barriers to invading pathogens (the skin and mucous membranes) are largely nonspecific and nonimmunological. Normal skin is almost completely resistant to infection unless it is disrupted by injury. Skin prevents pathogen invasion because of its dry, acidic environment, antibacterial fatty acids, and normal flora. Within the mucous membranes of the body, the mucous layer of epithelial cells prevents microorganisms from attaching to the cell surface. The action of cilia moves the microorganisms trapped in the mucus out of the body.[7]

Immunocompetence is maintained by cell-mediated immunity and antibody-mediated (humoral) immunity with the interaction of two other essential components of the immune system: Complement (C) and phagocytic cells. Cell-mediated and humoral immunity produces a specific response that protects against a specific organism, whereas phagocytes produce a more general, nonspecific defense against pathogens. The C system completes or enhances immune reactions. If an organism maintains immunocompetence, three primary functions are maintained: defense, surveillance, and homeostasis. An immunocompetent individual defends self from nonself by providing resistance to invaders, such as microorganisms, whereas the role of surveillance is to identify and destroy the body's own cells that have mutated and have the potential to form neoplasms. Homeostasis supports the removal of cellular debris so that cell types and cell lines remain uniform and unchanged over the life of the individual.[1,4]

Nonspecific Defense: The Phagocytes

Although all the cells of the blood are derived from pluripotential hemopoietic stem cells, those most involved in nonspecific defenses are the phagocytes, neutrophils, and macrophages (Figure 15-2). Neutrophils are stimulated by a limited number of chemical stimuli such as fibrin and collagen fragments, C, and platelet activating factors. These chemotactic stimuli are present with any type of tissue injury (e.g., acute trauma, thermal or chemical burns, bacterial infections, and foreign bodies) and ensure that neutrophils can respond to tissue injury

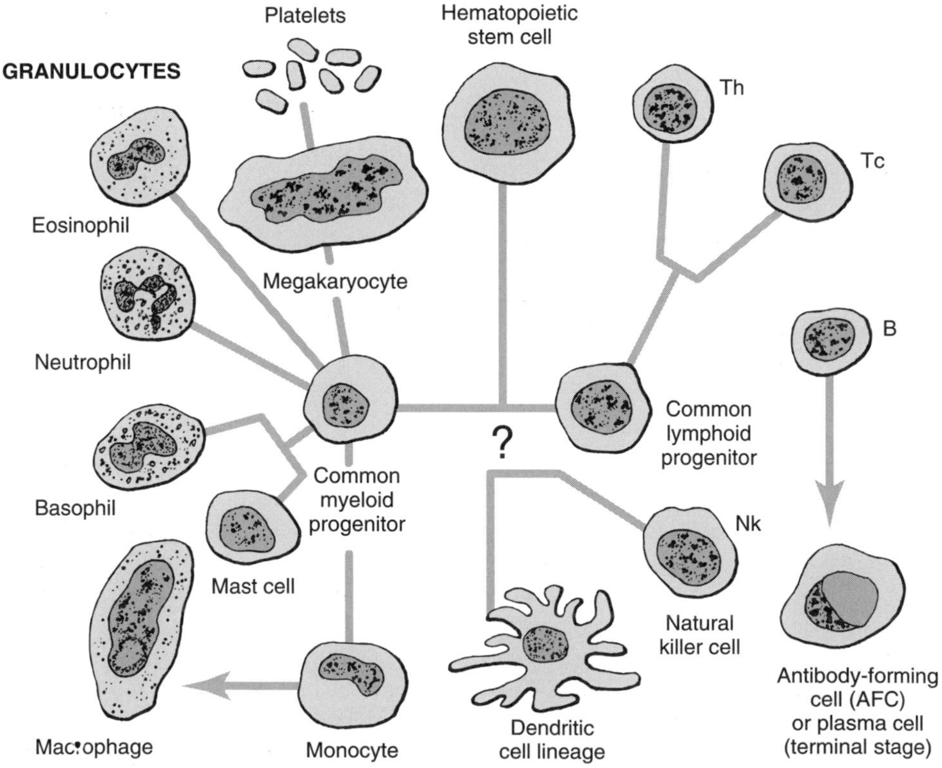

Figure 15-2 Family of cells derived from the pluripotential hemopoietic stem cells. (From Price, S.A., & Wilson, L.M. [1997]. *Pathophysiology* [5th ed., p. 63]. St Louis: Mosby.)

no matter what the cause (a nonspecific defense). Neutrophils comprise approximately 60% of the circulating white blood cells and spend 5 to 6 days maturing in the bone marrow before they are released into the blood. Once in the circulation, they are programmed to die by apoptosis 12 hours after entering the blood. An immunocompetent adult has approximately 50 billion neutrophils in the circulation at all times, and to maintain these levels, over 100 billion neutrophils are produced each day.[5,7] A defense system based solely on neutrophils, however, would expose an organism to many potentially injurious pathogens, such as proteinaceous toxins and individual viral particles. Neutrophils are also unable to modify their responses on the basis of past experience with agents. Some of these deficits are shored up immunologically by monocytes and macrophages.[7]

In comparison to neutrophils, macrophages can live for months or even years in body tissues, organs, and serosal cavities. Tissue-associated phagocytic cells (macrophages), regardless of location, are derived from circulating monocytes and belong to a single lineage, the mononuclear phagocyte system. Phagocytosis is an important function of these cells and a form of endocytosis, the uptake by a cell of material from its surrounding environment. In phagocytosis, the cell's plasma membrane surrounds a particle to form large vesicles called phagosomes. Phagosomes fuse with lysosomes, which release enzymes into the phagosomes that ultimately digest and destroy the particles.[5]

Activated macrophages are avid phagocytes, are larger than neutrophils, and can engulf entire senescent or damaged host cells.[5,7] Neutrophil and macrophage activity is complementary. Macrophage phagocytosis tends to be slower than that of neutrophils but allows for ingestion of whole cells, whereas the oxidative burst of neutrophils tends to be more vigorous and is toxic to bacteria. Neutrophils play the greatest role in acute pyrogenic infections whereas macrophages are more prevalent in chronic or granulomatous infections.[4,7] Activated macrophages not only function as phagocytes but also secrete over 100 enzymes, mediators, C components, coagulation factors, and reactive oxygen species. The secretory products of macrophages direct the actions of lymphocyte responses and, by doing so, place macrophages among the most important components of immunocompetence.[1,5,7]

Specific Defenses

The human body's system of defense-related phagocytosis works together with the lymphoid system, which defends against invaders through two arms of the immune system: cell-mediated immunity and antibody-mediated (humoral) immunity.

Cell-mediated immunity is the immune response primarily carried out by T lymphocytes, or T cells. When the body is exposed to a pathogen, the T cells proliferate and direct cellular interactions specific to the antigen that triggers the response. An *epitope* (antigenic determinant) is a small chemical group, usually 5 amino acids or sugars in size, on the antigen that can elicit and react with an immunoglobulin (antibody).[1,7] Antibody-mediated immunity, on the other hand, is specific immunity mediated by the production of immunoglobulins by B lymphocytes in response to an antigen. The definition of an antigen (cells that react with immunoglobulins) differs subtly from that of an immunogen, which are molecules or cells that induce an immune response.[1] In most situations, antigens are immunogens and the terms are used interchangeably. A hapten is an exception, however. *Haptens* are molecules that are not immunogenic by themselves but can react with a specific antibody. They only become immunogenic when they bind with a carrier protein. Common haptens include penicillin and the oil in plants that cause poison ivy.[4]

Stem cells are the source of three cell types of lymphocytes: T cells, B cells, and natural killer (NK) cells. NK cells are lymphocytes with some T cell markers; however, NK cells and T cells differ from each other because NK cells are *prethymic;* that is, they do not pass through the thymus to mature, as do T cells. T cells have several subsets that are differentiated from each other by a cluster of differentiation (CD) protein on the cell surface. T cells also have surface proteins, T cell receptors (TCR), that are able to detect the presence of foreign antigens and interact with them when invaders are cleaved by phagocytic cells and presented as antigenic determinants.[1,4]

Cell-Mediated Immunity. The two most important subsets of T lymphocytes are identified by a CD: CD4+ cells and CD8+ cells. The CD4+, or helper T, cells perform a regulator function by releasing cytokines (small molecular weight proteins that are secreted by lymphocytes and other cells of the immune system). Cytokines from CD4+ cells regulate immune processes, such as the production of immunoglobulins by B cells and the activation of T cells and tissue macrophages.[1,5] CD8+, or cytotoxic, T cells perform two primary effector functions: delayed hypersensitivity reactions and cytotoxic reactions.[1,7] Delayed hypersensitivity occurs when immunogens of intracellular organisms cause an allergic response. Cytotoxic reactions, by contrast, occur with destruction of virally infected cells, tissue grafts, and tumor cells.[1] In cytotoxic reactions, CD8+ cells release perforins, toxic chemicals that damage the infected cell's outer membrane. Perforins create a pore through the cell membrane, allow extracellular fluid to enter, and cause the cell to lyse. In the setting of organ or tissue transplantation, the recipient's CD8+ cells recognize that the donor cells are not "self." With the help of regulator CD4+ cells, the CD8+ cells develop a clone of cells specific to the destruction of the nonself transplanted antigens. The CD8+ cells kill the cells in the donor tissue by the release of perforins. A final subset of T lymphocytes are memory T cells, which are CD4+ cells that have multiplied into a clone of cells following an initial exposure to an antigen. Memory T cells are capable of rapid activation upon reexposure.[1,6,7]

Antibody-Mediated (Humoral) Immunity. B cells arise from stem cells in the bone marrow and make up approximately 20% of the circulating lymphocyte population.[1,4] As they mature in the bone marrow, B cells begin to express immunoglobulins on their surface. The first immunoglobulins produced are independent of an antigen, unrelated to reaction with an epitope, and of the immunoglobulin M (IgM) class. The second stage of B cell maturation is an antigen-dependent phase, in which B cells interact with an antigen and become activated. B cell activation occurs as the B cell acts as an antigen-presenting cell (APC). The pathogen binds with the monomer form of IgM that is expressed on the B cell's surface. The aggregated immunoglobulin–epitope complex undergoes endocytosis, after which the antigen is processed and presented on the B cell's surface.[1] The processed antigen complex is recognized by a CD4+ lymphocyte, which produces interleukins that stimulate growth and differentiation of the B cell and formation of a clone that produces immunoglobulins specific to the antigen. Immunoglobulin classifications and functions are outlined in Table 15-1.

Some of these activated B cells become plasma cells, the effector cells of the B cell lineage. Plasma cells produce thousands of immunoglobulins per second for a specific epitope. After several days, immunoglobulin production ceases and the plasma cell dies.[1] Other activated B cells become memory B cells, which are rapidly activated when reexposure

TABLE 15-1 Immunoglobulins

CLASS	% TOTAL Ig IN SERUM	PRIMARY SITES IN BODY	STRUCTURE	MAJOR FUNCTIONS
IgA	15%	Secretions: saliva; colostrums; tears; mucus of respiratory, genitourinary, and gastrointestinal tracts	Monomer or dimer	Neutralizes toxins in the blood Provides defense against microorganisms in the mucous membranes
IgD	0.2%	Serum Surface of B cells	Monomer	Uncertain role May act as antigen receptor or have a role in B cell differentiation
IgE	0.004%	Serum, interstitial fluid, exocrine secretions	Monomer	Fixes to receptors on mast cells and basophils in allergic response leading to release of histamine Type I hypersensitivity reactions Defense in parasitic infections
IgG	75%	Blood and interstitial fluid Only Ig that can cross placenta	Monomer	Produces the secondary response Provides passive immunity in newborn C fixation, opsonization, precipitation, agglutination
IgM	10%	Serum Surface of B cells	Monomer or pentamer	**Functions:** Effective in causing agglutination and C fixation Acts as a B cell receptor on cell surface

to the antigen occurs. Most memory cells express immunoglobulin G (IgG) on their surface, but others express IgM.[1,4]

Natural Killer Cells. NK cells, the third major classification of lymphocytes, have some T cell markers but are considered prethymic cells (they do not pass through the thymus gland for maturation). NK cells were initially identified by their ability to kill certain tumors and virally infected cells.[7] Although NK cells are derived from the same stem cell precursor as all blood cells, little is known about their growth and development. Although they compose only 5% to 15% of circulating lymphocytes, large numbers of NK cells are also found in the spleen, lung, intestine, and liver. NK cells specialize in destroying virus-infected cells and neoplasms by the perforin mechanism similar to those produced by CD8+ cells. Unlike CD8+ cells, NK activation does not require previous sensitization by an antigen.

Differentiating Self From Nonself. The major histocompatibility complex (MHC) is a single gene cluster on the short arm of the 6th chromosome. The MHC controls the production of one particular set of protein molecules (MHC molecules) that serve as cellular antigens, or "self-markers." Recognition of the MHC molecule by the body's own immune system causes the development of self tolerance, the ability of the body to restrain from attacking its own cells. MHC molecules are found on the surface of virtually all nucleated cells and are divided into three classes. Class I MHC molecules, found on the surface of all nucleated cells and platelets except spermatozoa and ova, interact with virally infected cells. When a cell becomes virally infected, the viral epitope is displayed on the surface of the cell by MHC class I molecules. Therefore class I molecules interact with microorganisms that are replicated intracellularly.[1,4] The class II MHC molecule is involved in types of cellular reactions originating from pathogens that replicate outside the cell, such as bacteria. When an antigen-presenting cell (APC) such as a macrophage or neutrophil uses phagocytosis to kill bacteria or other extracellular microorganisms, one product of phagocytosis is a processed antigen, or epitope. The class II MHC molecule presents the processed antigen on its surface. Class II MHC molecules are found on monocytes, macrophages, B cells, and some activated T cells.[1,4-7]

Class III MHC molecules are actually part of the C cascade. The term *complement* (C) was initially used by Paul Ehrlich to describe serum activity that augmented the ability of specific immunoglobulins to cause lysis of bacteria.[4] The C system consists of more than 25 proteins found in human serum and tissue fluids. The C system has four major biological roles: (1) opsonization, which prepares microorganisms for phagocytosis by coating them with C fragments; (2) generation of peptide fragments that activate phagocytes; (3) lysis of antigens such as bacteria, allografts, and tumor cells; and (4) production of immune mediators. The overall role of the C system is to act as an amplifier of all the immune reactions occurring in response to a microorganism.[1,7]

The role of the MHC class molecules is important to the activation of the immune system cells and, in particular, T cells. T cells recognize antigens only when they are broken down into smaller peptides in the form of epitopes. When a cell is infected with a virus, proteolytic enzymes digest the virus whose antigenic determinants bind with an MHC class I molecule. The proteins present the processed antigen on the surface of the cell as a complex, which attracts cytotoxic T and leads to lysis of the infected cell. By comparison, MHC class II molecules interact with APCs (macrophages, monocytes, B cells) during antigen processing.[7] After phagocytosis, degranulation (storage granules with a variety of enzymes such as lysozyme and collagenase empty their contents into the phagosome to degrade the pathogen) by macrophages results in a processed antigen. It is then presented on the cell surface by an MHC class II molecule. CD4+ T cells recognize peptide-MHC complexes and initiate B cell antibody responses.

Immunocompetence: The Integrated Immune Response

Cell-mediated immunity is the arm of the immune response carried out primarily by T cells. When the body is exposed to a pathogen, T cells proliferate and direct a host of cellular and subcellular interactions against the specific epitope. Cell-mediated immunity has four functions:[1,4]

1. Cytotoxic reactions: CD8+ cells cause direct cell death of virally infected cells or tumor cells. Binding occurs with the virally infected cell, which is killed when the CD8+ cell releases perforins. NK cells also cause nonspecific cytotoxic functions.
2. Delayed hypersensitivity reactions: Inflammation results when T cells produce cytokines, which not only affect tissues but also activate other cells, such as APCs.
3. Memory function: A subset of T cells, or memory T cells, allows for an accelerated

immune response the second time the body is exposed to an immunogen.

4. Regulator function: CD4+ and CD8+ lymphocytes facilitate and suppress cell-mediated and humoral immune responses.

Humoral immunity consists of the responses mediated by immunoglobulins in body fluids.[4] B cells both differentiate into plasma cells that produce immunoglobulins and serve as antigen-presenting cells. Immunoglobulins, which make up approximately 20% to 25% of the protein content in the plasma,[1,4,7] are also found in tears, saliva, mucosal secretions of the respiratory, GI, and GU tract, and in colostrum. When immunoglobulins on the surface of B cells bind with an antigen, they initiate a cascade of events: B cell activation, proliferation of a clone of B cells, and maturation of plasma cells. Other functions of immunoglobulins include C activation, opsonization, and intracellular signal transduction.

Immunoglobulins initiate their biological actions through agglutination, neutralization, and precipitation. During agglutination, an antibody-antigen reaction causes antigens to clump together and form a lattice with a soluble immunoglobulin. The lattice formation leads to neutralization, inactivation, or lysis of the antigen. Neutralization is a biological inactivation of microorganisms or bacterial toxins resulting from immunoglobulin binding. Immunoglobulin-toxin complexes then undergo precipitation, the reaction between soluble immunoglobulin and antigen or toxin that causes the complexes to fall out of solution. The products of these processes are destroyed by phagocytic cells.

The humoral response takes the form of a primary response during the first encounter with an antigen, followed by a secondary response. The primary response occurs when surface receptors (IgM or IgD) on a B cell bind with an epitope that shows the best "fit" with the immunoglobulin. After binding, the B cell is stimulated to proliferate. A clone of cells forms; these mature into plasma cells able to synthesize immunoglobulins with specificity to the pathogen. During the secondary response, the antigen, or one closely related, is encountered a second time. With a second exposure to the antigen, a secondary response occurs. The secondary response, which allows for a rapid antibody response in 3 to 5 days, occurs because antigen-sensitive memory B cells initiate and sustain immunoglobulin production. Immunoglobulins produced from the secondary response tend to bind antigen more firmly and dissociate less easily than those from the primary response.[1,7]

To maintain immunocompetence, the body's physiological response is a complex interaction between APCs, T and B lymphocytes, and other proteins, such as C and cytokines (Figure 15-3). APCs can ingest microorganisms without opsonization (when an antigen is coated with C or immunoglobulin). However, binding occurs more quickly with opsonization and the process of phagocytosis is amplified. When an MHC molecule from either an APC or a virally infected cell presents an epitope on the cell surface, T cells bind with the MHC-epitope complex. MHC class I and II molecules not only present the epitope but also stabilize the cell-to-cell interaction. Following T cell activation and production of Interleukin-1 by APC, a clone of either CD8+ or CD4+ T cells results. The antigen is destroyed because of the action of perforins from cytotoxic CD8+ cells. Interleukins stimulate B cells to produce immunoglobulins, whose interactions with the antigen or toxin lead to agglutination, neutralization, and precipitation. C amplifies the interactions, leading to further antigen lysis and destruction. Memory T and B lymphocytes proliferate to provide a more rapid secondary response to the antigen when it is next encountered.[1,4-7]

Pathological Conditions Affecting the Immune System

When pathological conditions affect immunocompetence, an individual develops risk to both short-term and long-term health. Some conditions, such as viral or bacterial infections, hypersensitivity reactions, and cancer, lead to activation of the immune system. Other conditions, such as HIV/AIDS and traumatic injuries, lead to a blunted immune response.

Acute Infections. Microorganisms are pathogens if they are capable of causing a disease; these include bacteria, viruses, and protozoa. The two main mechanisms by which bacteria cause disease are inflammation from tissue invasion and production of toxins. Humans have an immune response—inflammation—to both mechanisms. Two types of inflammation occur: pyrogenic and granulomatous. In pyrogenic, or pus-forming inflammation, neutrophils are the predominant cells involved in the immune response. The mature, segmented neutrophils with a multi-lobed nucleus, or "segs," constitute 50% to 60% of circulating white blood cells and move immediately to the infected area, where they perform their phagocytic function and are destroyed. Immature neutrophils with a nonsegmented nucleus, or "bands," normally compose 8%

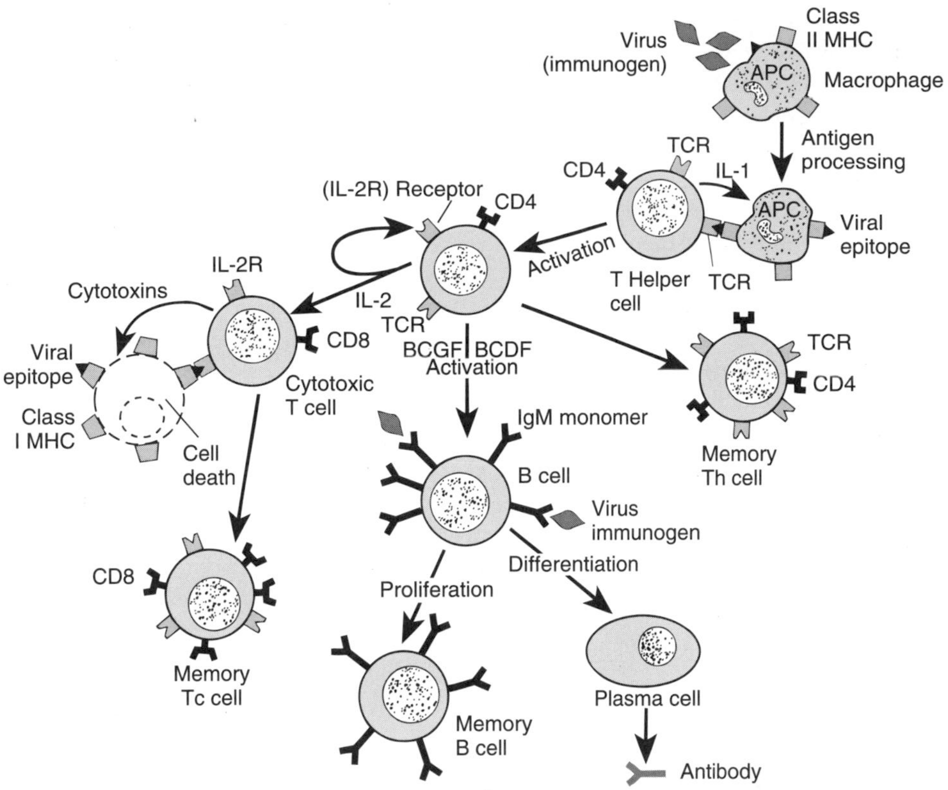

Figure 15-3 Process of cell-mediated and humoral responses during viral invasion of body cells. (From Price, S.A., & Wilson, L.M. [1997]. *Pathophysiology* [5th ed., p. 63]. St. Louis: Mosby.)

or less of total white blood cells. In serious infections, the life span of a neutrophil is shortened to only a few hours. When immature cells are released to replace them, higher than normal levels of bands occur. An increase in bands is called *shift to the left*.[1,4,7] In granulomatous inflammation, the cell-mediated immune system with T cells and macrophages predominates. Bacterial antigens stimulate T cell activity and phagocytosis by macrophages occurs.

Bacteria also cause disease through the production of endotoxins and exotoxins. Exotoxins are produced by gram-negative and gram-positive bacteria and lead to such diseases as diphtheria *(Corynebacterium diphtheriae)*, tetanus *(Clostridium tetani)*, botulism *(Clostridium botulinum)*, cholera *(Vibrio cholerae)*, gas gangrene *(Clostridium perfringens)*, and toxic shock syndrome *(Staphylococcus aureus)*. Exotoxins, which are secreted by bacteria, are among the most toxic substances known.[4] Exotoxins bind to the cell membrane, are transported across the membrane, and through enzyme activity disrupt cell functioning or kill the cell. Endotoxins, on the other hand, are a component of the bacteria cell wall released with bacterial cell death; they are present only in gram-negative bacteria. Endotoxin production can lead to the clinical syndrome of septic shock with fever, coagulation defects, hypotensive shock, and impaired organ perfusion mediated by a cascade of cytokines.[25,26] Immunoglobulins, which defend against toxins by neutralizing them, bind these antigenic proteins and directly inactivate them by steric (by affecting the spatial arrangement of atoms) effects.[7]

Acute viral infections trigger immune responses that differ from bacterial infections. Viruses and double-stranded RNAs (thought to be synthesized during viral replication) induce a nonspecific response through the production of interferons, a group of glycoproteins. The interferons inhibit viral growth by blocking the translation of viral proteins.[4] Other nonspecific responses used to defend against viruses are macrophage phagocytosis, fever, and mucociliary clearance. Defenses specific to the virus include both humoral and cell-mediated immunity.

Infectious mononucleosis is a disease that not only triggers an immune response but also affects immunocompetence. It is usually a benign, self-limiting lymphoproliferative disease caused by Epstein-Barr virus (EBV). Clinical symptoms include fever, lymphadenopathy, splenomegaly, and sore throat.[27,28] When the EBV enters the cytoplasm of epithelial cells, usually by close human contact, such as through saliva transmission during kissing, the virus spreads from nasopharyngeal, oropharyngeal, and salivary epithelial cells to the underlying lymphoid tissues and to B lymphocytes. B cells then shed antibodies, usually IgM initially and then IgG. A large number of CD8+ cells are also released, which are not specific for EBV-infected B cells, but their role is unclear. In addition, virus-specific CD8+ cells are also produced. The nonspecific CD8+ cells (many of which are large, atypical lymphocytes) elevate the total white blood cell count, which shows absolute lymphocytosis, with a total count of between 12,000 and 18,000 cells/mm^3, more than 60% of which are lymphocytes.[28] Serious complications include hepatic dysfunction, rupture of the spleen, and B cell proliferation leading to lymphoma.[27,28]

Hypersensitivity Reactions. Contact with antigens leads not only to induction of an immune response but also to potentially damaging reactions. Exogenous antigens, such as dust, pollen, medications, foods, and chemicals may result in an immune response ranging from trivial to potentially lethal.[29-32] The triggered immune response to exogenous and endogenous antigens are known collectively as hypersensitivity reactions (Table 15-2) and can be initiated either by a humoral or cell-mediated response. Hypersensitivity reactions include not only auto-immune disorders[31,32] but also reactions to transplanted tissues and organs.[33,34]

Malignant Neoplasms. A large number of both DNA and RNA viruses have been associated with cancer in humans and animals. Four DNA viruses have been implicated in the causation of human cancer: papillomaviruses, Epstein-Barr virus, hepatitis B virus, and Kaposi's sarcoma herpes virus. The

TABLE 15-2 The Immune Response to Exogenous Antigens: Hypersensitivity Reactions

TYPE	DESCRIPTION	DISORDERS	PATHOPHYSIOLOGICAL MECHANISMS
Type I reaction	Rapidly developing immunological reaction that occurs over a period of minutes May occur with a minute quantity of antigen Antigen-antibody complexes bind to mast cells or basophils in a previously-sensitized individual[28] Epidemiology: Occurs at rate of 0.4 cases per million per year in general population and 0.6 per 1000 in hospitalized patients[29] Clinical presentation: Urticaria, angioedema, hyperinflation of lungs, hypersecretion of bronchial submucosal glands, submucosal edema, mucus plugging of airways, hypotension	Local reaction Cutaneous swelling Allergic rhinitis or conjunctivitis Bronchial asthma Hay fever Systemic reaction Anaphylaxis—acute, generalized reaction with multi-organ involvement Anaphylactic shock—anaphylaxis with hypotension	Formation of IgE. Immediate release of vasoactive amines (such as histamine and adenosine), chemotactic factors, enzymes, and proteoglycans (such as heparin) from mast cells and basophils.[28] Recruitment of other inflammatory cells.
Type II reaction	Mediated by antibodies directed toward antigenic determinants (on self-cells or exogenous antigens such as drug metabolites absorbed on the cell surface[28] Results from binding of antibodies to normal or altered cell-surface antigens Epidemiology and presentation vary by disease	Goodpasture syndrome Bullous pemphigoid Pernicious anemia Acute rheumatic fever	Three different mechanisms 1. Complement (C)-dependent—direct lysis and opsonization occurs from C activation. 2. Antibody-dependent, cell-mediated cytotoxicity-target are killed by cells lysis with an interaction with nonspecific cells such as NK cells. 3. Antibody-mediated cellular dysfunction—antibodies directed against cell surface lead to impaired cellular function.[28]

TABLE 15-2 The Immune Response to Exogenous Antigens: Hypersensitivity Reactions—cont'd

TYPE	DESCRIPTION	DISORDERS	PATHOPHYSIOLOGICAL MECHANISMS
Type III reaction	Induced by antigen-antibody complexes that produce tissue damage through activation of the C system Toxic reaction occurs either with circulation or at extravascular sites where immune complexes have been deposited Epidemiology and presentation vary by disease	Exogenous Glomerulonephritis (from *Streptococci* or heroin), infective endocarditis (from *Streptococci*), arthritis (from *Yersinia enterocolitica*), Polyarteritis nodosa (from hepatitis B or cytomegalovirus), serum sickness (from foreign serum), hemolytic anemia (from quinidine) Endogenous Systemic lupus erythematosus (from nuclear antigens)[29,30] Rheumatoid arthritis (from immunoglobulins) Glomerulonephritis (from tumor antigens)[28]	Antigen-antibody complexes activate C and attract neutrophils. Neutrophils release lysosomal enzymes and prostaglandins, vasodilator peptides, and chemotactic substances. Tissue damage results from free oxygen radicals. Immune complexes also lead to platelet aggregation and activation of Hageman factor, resulting in inflammation and formation of microemboli.[28] Vasodilation, edema, and tissue necrosis result.
Type IV reaction	Cell-mediated type of hypersensitivity reaction initiated by sensitized T cells Delayed-type hypersensitivity initiated by CD4+ cells Direct cell cytotoxicity mediated by CD8+ cells (cytotoxic T cell response) Epidemiology and presentation vary by disease	Tuberculosis (delayed type) Contact dermatitis (delayed type) Rejection of tissue and organ transplantation[32,33] (delayed type and cytotoxic response)	Delayed-type hypersensitivity—accumulation of mononuclear cells around small veins and venules with lymphocyte "cuffing" around vessels, dermal edema, and deposits of fibrin in interstitium. Cytotoxic response—target cells are killed through the release of perforins and granzyme, which perforate cell membranes. Ligand-depending killing also leads to apoptosis of target cells.[28] Transplant rejection—complex process involving both cell-mediated and humoral immunity. T cells of recipient recognize MHC molecule on donated organ as "foreign." Recipient releases cytokines, lymphocytes and macrophages accumulate, and CD8+ cells cause lysis of donated tissue. Preformed antidonor antibodies may also exist in the serum and contribute to an immediate rejection.[28]

human T cell leukemia virus is also known to cause cancer following transmission through sexual intercourse, blood products, and breastfeeding.[35]

The immune system also plays an important role in tumor immunity. Immune surveillance is defined as the body's ability to recognize and destroy nonself tumor cells when they appear. Because cancers do appear, immune surveillance is imperfect, although it has an essential function for maintaining immunocompetence.[35] Both tumor-specific antigens [TSA] (antigens present only on tumor cells and not on normal cells) and tumor-associated antigens [TAA] (antigens present on both tumors as well as normal cells) have been identified. TSAs are derived from peptides that are uniquely present within tumor cells and presented on the cell surface by class I MHC molecules. They are encoded by genes that are silent in normal human cells but are expressed by tumor cells. TAAs are also recognized as nonself; cell-mediated reactions attach the nonself cells and limit their proliferation. Tumor antigens also elicit the development of specific antibodies, which may either be cytotoxic or tumor enhancing. Other tumors contain antigens that normally occur in fetal but not adult cells, such as carcinoembryonic antigen, which sometimes occurs with carcinoma of the colon, pancreas, breast, or liver. Alpha-fetoprotein, normally produced by the fetal liver, is also present at elevated levels in some individuals with liver cancer.[4]

Immunocompetence includes surveillance to detect and eliminate newly arising clones of neoplastic cells. The role of the immune system to prevent or control tumors in humans is uncertain[4] but is thought to include NK cells, which act through nonspecific responses without immunoglobulins, CD8+ cytotoxic T cells, and activated macrophages. Cytotoxic T cells play a protective role against virus-associated neoplasms, whereas macrophages may kill tumor cells through the release of reactive oxygen metabolites. The strongest argument for the existence of immunosurveillance is the increased frequency of cancers in immunodeficient and immunosuppressed individuals. Approximately 5% of people with congenital immunodeficiencies develop cancer, a rate 200 times the expected prevalence.[35] Individuals who are maintained on immuno-suppressive therapy following organ transplantation and people with HIV/AIDS also have higher rates of cancer (lymphoma in particular) than the general population.[35,36]

Most cancers, however, occur in immunocompetent individuals[35] and therefore the tumors have developed a mechanism to escape or evade surveillance. Some tumor cells escape surveillance by modulation. Others internalize the surface antigen so that the cells no longer present a target for surveillance and immune attack. Other mechanisms occur as well. As tumors progress, they may fail to express MHC class I molecules, they may stop producing co-stimulating molecules that T cells need to proliferate, or they may kill CD8+ cells that come in contact with the tumor.[35]

HIV/AIDS. The human immunodeficiency virus (HIV), a human T cell lymphotrophic retrovirus, is the cause of acquired immunodeficiency syndrome (AIDS). Although both HIV-1 and HIV-2 have been identified, the HIV-1 virus is found worldwide, whereas HIV-2 is found primarily in West Africa.[4] HIV infects and kills CD4+ T lymphocytes, leading to the loss of cell-mediated immunity and thereby the loss of immunocompetence. Other immune cells that have the CD4 proteins on their surfaces, such as macrophages and monocytes, can also be infected. The HIV has a high-affinity interaction between the coat protein of HIV-1 and the cell-surface CD4 protein. After the virus gains entrance to the CD4+ T cell through the assistance of a co-receptor CXCR4, the RNA genome of the virus is reverse transcribed and a cDNA copy, or provirus, is integrated into the cell's genome.[5] The integrated provirus is transcribed, viral RNA messages spliced and translated into proteins, and new viral particles are formed.

An immunocompetent individual has an appropriate, integrated response of all components of the immune system with both specific and nonspecific protection for the body against invaders and unhealthy cells.[37] Immunocompetence is dependent on T and B cell functioning to establish and maintain a healthy body environment. The loss of any component or function of the immune system has a negative impact on immunocompetence and places the individual at risk for severe pathological consequences.

PATHOLOGICAL CONSEQUENCES

When an internal or external threat is not successfully challenged and overcome by the immune system, immunocompetence is lost and pathological consequences occur. The infecting organism that leads to the most severe immunocompromise is the HIV, whose replication has profound consequences. With HIV infection, completed viral particles bud from the T cell membrane, leading to viral replication, extensive budding, cell death, and severe CD4+ cell depletion. Early in the course of the disease, HIV colonizes the spleen, lymph nodes, and tonsils, which become reservoirs of infected cells.[29] Immunocompetence is also affected by the loss of immature precursors of CD4+ T cells by direct infection of thymic progenitor cells or accessory cells that secrete cytokines. Other mechanisms that reduce immunocompetence are fusion of infected and non-infected cells and apoptosis of uninfected CD4+ T cells by aberrant signaling.[4-7] The ultimate effects include the following:[4-7,29,36]

- Lymphopenia resulting from selective loss of CD4+ helper–induced T cells, with an inversion of the CD4:CD8 cell ratio (normally 2:1)
- Decreased T cell function with loss of memory T cells and decreased delayed-type hypersensitivity reaction
- Decreased proliferative response to antigens, decreased cytotoxicity, and decreased production of interleukin-2 and interferon
- Inability to mount an immunoglobulin response to a new antigen and hypergammaglobulinemia
- Decreased phagocytosis, chemotaxis, and MCH class II molecule expression

Clinical features of HIV/AIDS range from acute illness with fever, weight loss, diarrhea, and generalized lymphadenopathy to severe disease with multiple opportunistic infections, neurological disease, and neoplasms such as Kaposi's sarcoma and lymphoma. Opportunistic infections rarely cause disease in immunocompetent individuals but can cause serious infection when people are immunocompromised.[4] Since 1992, a decrease in the incidence of opportunistic infections (OI) associated with HIV/AIDS has occurred, particularly in the most common forms (*Pneumocystis carinii* pneumonia, esophageal candidiasis, and disseminated *Mycobacterium avium* complex disease). This decrease is thought to have occurred primarily because of highly active antiretroviral therapy (HAART).[38] Although decreasing because of pharmacological therapy, opportunistic infections account for approximately 80% of deaths in patients with AIDS.[29] Despite the progress made with newer forms of therapy, the prognosis remains dismal. From its emergence in 1981 to the end of 1997, more than 12 million people died from HIV/AIDS.[29]

During HIV infection, immunocompromise results and the individual becomes more susceptible to pathogens than before the infection. Other conditions, such as traumatic injuries, stress, and some forms of cancer also lead to immunocompromise and pathological consequences.

Traumatic Injuries

Injuries such as thermal or chemical burns, profound hemorrhage, crush and blunt injuries, and penetrating wounds, lead to immunosuppression and immunocompromise.[39-42] Multiple organ failure with overwhelming infection is the most frequent cause of death for people who survive an initial trauma resuscitation after severe injury.[40] Immunosuppression and increased susceptibility to infection are known to persist for up to 10 days after the initial injury; many people also experience an increased susceptibility to sepsis and septic shock.[41] Following trauma, immunocompromise occurs because of impaired T cell activity with altered CD4/CD8 ratios, decreased production of cytokines, decreased T cell proliferation, and decreased antibody-dependent cell-mediated cytotoxicity.[39,41] In addition, macrophage function is impaired with decreased antigen presentation[39] and cytokine release with decreased production of TNFαinterleukin-6, and prostaglandin E_2.[43] The immune suppression experienced by individuals with multiple traumas is exacerbated by transfusions of blood products, a therapeutic intervention to manage hypovolemia and tissue hypoxia following injury. Numerous investigators have found that days and weeks after blood transfusion, a decrease occurs in the secretion of cytokines needed for immune reactions (interleukin-2, colony-stimulating factor, tumor necrosis factor, and interferon).[44-47] Other immune responses to blood transfusion include increased production of prostaglandin E by macrophages (an immunosuppressant that reduces macrophage differentiation and phagocytosis), diminished macrophage migration, and decreased CD4/CD8 ratios. Therefore the combination of multiple injuries and blood transfusions places the individual at risk for severe immunocompromise at the very time that resistance to invaders is paramount.

Stress

The pathological consequences of stress and the role of stress in immunocompromise are areas of ongoing investigation. Immune function, particularly NK cell activity, lymphocyte function, and immunoglobulin A function, are all diminished in stressed and depressed patients. It is still difficult, however, to specify the conditions under which stress diminishes immunocompetence, and empirical evidence is missing to support a causal relationship between stress and altered immune function in humans.[48,49] Nurse scientists, however, have found significant, positive relationships between psychological distress in women with suspected breast cancer and TNF. TNF is a chemical released by cells of the immune system during the inflammatory process and activation of the immune response. The investigators conclude that symptom distress and symptom occurrence has a relationship to immunocompetence, although the specific effects have yet to be elucidated.

Cancer

Some types of cancer can lead to immunocompromise. Multiple myeloma, a plasma cell neoplasm, causes increased cytokine production and decreased immunoglobulin production. Recurrent bacterial infections are common due to suppression of humoral immunity.[50] Lymphoid neoplasms, such as Hodgkin's disease and non-Hodgkin's lymphomas, and the leukemias lead to a broad array of immune dysfunction, with deficits in white blood cell formation and function and underproduction or overproduction of the products of white blood cells that are essential for immunocompetence.[50]

In short, a variety of conditions are associated with immunocompromise. These conditions may render the individual unable to respond to an immune challenge or a foreign invader. In addition, treatments such as radiotherapy, chemotherapy, and pharmacological immunosuppression following organ transplantation may render an individual immunocompromised. Without immunocompetence, an individual has significant and serious risks to health and requires expert nursing care to manage immunocompromise.

RELATED PATHOPHYSIOLOGICAL CONCEPTS/DIFFERENTIAL DIAGNOSIS

A pathophysiological concept related to but also distinct from alterations in immunocompetence is infection (see Chapter 16). Infection is defined as the state or condition in which the body is invaded by a pathogenic agent that, under favorable conditions, multiplies and produces injury.[2] Infections can lead to alterations in any system of the body. For example, patients with herpes simplex may have encephalitis, esophagitis, keratitis, or a genital infection; symptoms from these infections range from blurred vision to dysphagia and from corneal ulcers to perirectal lesions. Patients with AIDS may have pneumocystic pneumonia, with shortness of breath and cough or cachexia and fever.

Several considerations are important in determining the source of an infection and in analyzing options for a differential diagnosis. The type of microorganism, the degree of immunocompetence of the individual or host, and the portal of entry are important considerations. Some microorganisms are highly pathogenic and others cause disease rarely. Virulence is a quantitative measure of pathogenicity and is measured by the number of microorganisms needed to cause disease. The infectious dose required to cause disease varies greatly across organisms. The infectious dose of *Shigella* is less than 100 organisms, whereas *Salmonella,* which causes diarrhea by infecting the GI tract just as *Shigella* does, requires approximately 100,000 organisms.[4] Portals of entry include mucous membranes, the blood, open wounds and sores, and the respiratory tract.

A huge number of microorganisms can cause illness. A wide range of organs and tissues are involved in immune diseases. A broad continuum of immune responses, from immunocompetence to immunocompromise to immunosuppression, exists in humans. For these reasons, no single algorithm works successfully to determine the patient's underlying disease. A general discussion, however, of strategies for assessment to determine manifestations of immune dysfunction and surveillance follows.

MANIFESTATIONS AND SURVEILLANCE

A person's appearance provides important information about immunocompetence. An individual who has a competent immune response to an acute viral or bacterial infection has such symptoms as diaphoresis and flushed skin. Because of the immunocompromise that accompanies aging, elders may have acute infections with few overt symptoms or subtle symptoms, such as listlessness and mild hypothermia. A chronic illness and accompanying immunocompromise may lead to pallor, gauntness, emaciation, listlessness, and an appearance older than the stated age.[51] Other signs of immunocompromise after at least a week of a local wound infection include poor healing, drainage, or induration. For acutely ill individuals who require hospitalization because of immunocompromise, daily surveillance by nurses of all skin surfaces, wounds, and body systems with portals of entry such as the mouth and genitourinary track is essential to determine the response to a pathogen.

Normal lymph nodes are an indicator of immunocompetence. Important aspects of the lymph node examination include size, shape, symmetry, mobility, tenderness, and temperature.[51,52] Lymph nodes that are large, fixed, inflamed, tender, or "matted" (enlargement that feels as if the nodes are a mass rather than discrete nodes) warrant further investigation. If a node is inflamed or fixed and immobile, involvement of the regional lymph nodes may have occurred as well. Immunocompromise may also be indicated with splenic enlargement, which occurs when cell overproduction occurs in immune disorders and acute infections.

When immunocompromise is suspected, serial laboratory assessments are warranted. Generally physicians or nurse practitioners will follow the complete blood count, differential, and erythrocyte sedimentation rate. To identify the source of an unknown inflammatory response, the C-reactive protein (an acute-phase protein present after tissue trauma, cellular necrosis, inflammation, and infection) level, serum C levels, and C fixation tests are often obtained. Practitioners also evaluate the results of bacterial cultures and sensitivities of pertinent body fluids or drainage from wounds. Laboratory determination of enzyme-linked immunosorbent assay is used to measure immunoglobulin levels as well as antibodies to HIV. Other diagnostic tests may include bone marrow aspiration, lymphangiogram, and skin testing.

CLINICAL MANAGEMENT

Clinical management of disorders of immunocompetence depends on the nature of the immune challenge. Many disorders are managed pharmacologically[53,54] and others by symptom management.[55,56] Regardless of the type of immune disorder, interventions that support illness prevention and health promotion are essential. Table 15-3 outlines management strategies for common immune disorders. Because of the severity and extent of illness from HIV infections, it is important, in addition to a review of Table 15-3, to consider several of the important management issues for this immunocompromised population.

The most promising management strategy to date for individuals infected with HIV has been highly active antiretroviral therapy (HAART), which has been shown to partially restore CD4+ cell counts and reduce HIV-related morbidity and mortality.[57,58] However, many issues remain for treatment when individuals are receiving HAART. In particular, little is known about the need for prophylaxis against opportunistic infections during HAART, and the role of HAART in actually restoring immune function is uncertain. What is known is that during HAART, viral loads decrease and health status and quality of life improve.[58,59]

Despite these advances, however, HAART has led to two important nursing care concerns: some individuals may relapse to unsafe sexual behaviors,[59] and some may have difficulty adhering to unprecedented levels of medication adherence.[60] The need exists for continued use of condoms after initiation of HAART, because seminal cells can potentially transmit HIV.[59] Therefore nurses need to reinforce teachings about safe-sex behaviors despite the improvements seen with HAART. The second concern, that of medication adherence, has been addressed by a nursing intervention based on a framework developed by Ickovics and Meisler[61] and refined by Holzemer et al.[60] The Client Adherence Profiling-Intervention Tailoring (CAP-IT) intervention is an innovative, structured nursing assessment and care-planning activity. CAP-IT interventions allow a standardized assessment of client needs and tailored HAART adherence intervention strategies. Following an in-depth assessment of client characteristics such as knowledge related to HIV infection, personal medication regimen, reasons for missing medications, and social support, an individualized plan of care is developed to enhance adherence. Holzemer et al[60] reported that not only do clients find the protocol acceptable, but that it also is feasible to use in a case manager's practice. In the future the investigators plan to test CAP-IT in a randomized clinical trial to determine its effectiveness.

Another salient issue of concern for management of individuals with alterations in immunocompetence is that of antibiotic resistance. A growing concern exists that antimicrobial therapy is leading to increasing antibiotic resistance. The two primary factors thought to cause antibiotic resistance are the prevalence of resistance genes and the extent of antibiotic use. Actions that are recommended to limit resistance include good handwashing techniques for all health care providers, limiting prescriptions for unneeded antibiotics, prescribing antibiotics that target only a narrow range of bacteria, isolating hospital patients with multi–drug-resistant infections, and maintaining familiarity with local data on antibiotic resistance.[62]

The management of individuals with altered immunocompetence is a collaborative effort that encompasses pharmacotherapy, interventions to enhance health promotion and disease prevention, and strategies to stress the importance of adherence to the management plan. Individuals with immunocompromise present a complex set of circumstances to expert nurses and advanced practitioners, and creative and innovative interventions are essential.

CONCEPTUAL MODELS

Physiological models explain immunocompetence and immunocompromise. The theory of *clonal*

TABLE 15-3 Management Consideration for Disorders of Immunocompetence

DISORDER	MANAGEMENT STRATEGIES	CLINICAL OUTCOMES
Bacterial infections	Pharmacotherapy—cultures and sensitivities dictate appropriate antimicrobial therapy. Possible approaches include beta-lactam antimicrobials such as penicillins; macrolide and azalide antimicrobials such as erythromycin; vancomycin; tetracyclines; chloramphenicol; aminoglycoside antimicrobial agents; inhibitors of folic acid metabolism, such as sulfonamides; fluroquinolones; and metronidazole[53,54] Oral or parenteral fluids Fever reduction with antipyretics such as acetaminophen Teaching—prevention strategies, medication management, prevention of antibiotic resistance, nutritional management	Maintenance of airway breathing, circulation Eradication of infection Normothermia Hydration Knowledge of treatment regimen[55] Knowledge of prevention strategies
Hypersensitivity reactions	Airway/breathing management; subcutaneous epinephrine if type I reaction threatens airway and breathing; endotracheal intubation and mechanical ventilation as needed Support of circulation—volume expansion and vasopressors as needed Other pharmacotherapy—beta-adrenergic agonist inhaled therapy, glucagons, glucocorticoids, antihistamines, topical preparations Observation Teaching—prevention strategies, self-administration of epinephrine	Maintenence of airway, breathing, circulation[49] Hydration Knowledge of treatment regimen Knowledge of prevention strategies
Cancer	Surgical removal of tumors; radiotherapy; chemotherapy[52,54] Nutritional management Maintenance of quality of life through exercise, meditation, support groups If treatment is not successful, hospice care If treatment is successful, teach ongoing cancer surveillance	Eradication of cancer cells Protection from infection (hand washing, reducing contact with others with infections) Stable body weight Comfort
HIV/AIDS	Pharmacological therapy—highly active antiretroviral therapy (HAART)—(nucleoside analog reverse transcriptase inhibitors [NRTIs]), nonnucleoside analog reverse transcriptase inhibitors [NNRTIs], protease inhibitors [PIs])[54] Prophylaxis against opportunistic infections—antiviral medications, antibiotics, antifungal medications Analgesia Maintenance of quality of life through exercise, medication management meditation, support groups, nutritional management Teaching—prevention strategies, therapeutic regimen	Suppression of HIV replication Prevention of infection Comfort Stable body weight Knowledge of treatment regimen Knowledge of prevention of transmission strategies
Traumatic injuries	Airway/breathing management; endotracheal intubation and mechanical ventilation as needed Support of circulation—volume expansion with fluids and blood products Surgical exploration and repair of injuries Pharmacotherapy as needed—antimicrobials, vasopressors, histamine$_2$ blockers, analgesia Observation Teaching—prevention strategies, management of substance abuse problems, therapeutic regimen	Maintenance of airway, breathing, circulation Wound healing Comfort Prevention of infection Stable body weight

deletion explains that immature T cells, which have no TCR, CD4, or CD8 protein, migrate to the thymus from the bone marrow. The role of the TCR in a mature T cell is to bind an antigenic determinant or epitope, whereas the role of the CD4 or CD8 proteins in a mature T cell is to stabilize the interaction between a T cell and other cells. A mature T cell leaving the thymus therefore has both a functioning receptor to bind with an epitope and either a CD4 or CD8 protein. If the T cell is to be functional when it leaves the thymus, it needs both to recognize nonself epitopes and develop functional CD4 or CD8 proteins.[1] Cells that cannot perform these functions are deleted within the thymus, where they are either killed by other cells or made to undergo apoptosis (programmed cell death). The theory of clonal deletion postulates that the clone of cells that cannot recognize nonself cells are useless and therefore deleted. Cells that cannot recognize self cells, which are harmful, are also deleted. The remaining clone is able to differentiate between self and nonself and proliferates to maintain immunocompetence.[63]

The B cell role in humoral immunity is explained by the theory of clonal selection. An individual has a pool of approximately 10 million B cells, each of which has IgM or IgD on its surface. The immunoglobulins can react to one antigen (or a closely related group of antigens).[1,7] The theory postulates that an antigen interacts with the B cell that shows the best "fit" with the immunoglobulins on its surface. When the B cell is activated by the antigen-immunoglobulin reaction, it proliferates and forms a clone of cells. The clone cells mature into plasma cells, which secrete an immunoglobulin specific for the antigen that initiated this sequence.

A third physiological model applicable to the phenomenon of immunocompetence is the theory of psychoneuroimmunology. In this theory, stress is postulated as a state of disharmony or threatened homeostatis provoked by a psychological, environmental, or physiological stressor.[63] Stress leads to thoughts and emotions that influence the brain and the immune system, activating a bidirectional circuit between the two systems. (For additional information, see Chapter 14, Stress Response.) The mechanism for this interaction occurs via the hypothalamic-pituitary-adrenal (HPA) axis, which initiates a cascade of reactions throughout the individual. These reactions upregulate or downregulate the immune system in the response to stress by increasing or decreasing levels of neurotransmitters and hormones.[63-65]

The stress response begins with corticotropin releasing factor (CRF) stimulating the HPA axis as serotonin, norepinephrine, and acetylcholine activate the hypothalamus. Elevation of chemicals such as norepinephrine, epinephrine, corticosteroids, opiates, and dopamine leads to immunosuppression. Growth hormone and prolactin decline after the initiation of stress and contribute to downregulation of the immune system. Chemicals also cue CRF to change corticosteroid and norepinephrine metabolism.[63-65]

The psychoneuroimmunology framework has been used as a model for a number of research studies. For example, Robinson, Mathews, and Witek-Janusek[66] provide a review of 10 intervention studies using a psychoneuroimmunology framework with HIV-infected participants. The authors concluded that despite small sample sizes, the results of the studies provide support for a positive effect of various interventions on immunological and health-related indices in HIV-infected individuals. Therefore multiple frameworks exist that can provide the basis of testing interventions for individuals with alterations in immunocompetence.

CASE STUDY

Immunocompetence is illustrated by the case study of a young man who experiences an acute but temporary illness. KP is a 20-year-old college senior who came to the health center with a history of a worsening sore throat over 3 days. He reported accompanying fatigue, generalized weakness, a sense of being chilled, headache, and anorexia. On physical examination, he appeared acutely ill, with an intensely red, swollen pharynx and oropharynx with yellow exudates on both tonsils. His vital signs were these: temperature, 38.5° C (101.4° F); blood pressure, 122/68; heart rate, 102 beats/min; and respiratory rate, 18 breaths/min. Examination of his neck revealed several enlarged and painful cervical lymph nodes, but he had no meningeal irritation and his heart and chest examination yielded normal findings. His abdomen was flat but he had a tender liver edge felt 1.5 cm below the costal margin and his spleen tip was palpable. His laboratory profile was as follows: white blood cell count, 14,000 mm^3; hematocrit, 39%; differential, 51% polymorphonuclear neutrophils (polys), 45% lymphocytes (lymphs), 3% monocytes (monos), and platelets 100,000 mm^3.

The clinical examination illustrated symptoms typical of infectious mononucleosis caused by Epstein-Barr virus (EBV).[7] Differential diagnoses included infections with other pathogens, such as herpes simplex viruses, cytomegalovirus, and adenoviruses, as well as

Streptococcus pyogenes and *Neisseria gonorrhoeae,* but these conditions, as well as viral hepatitis, usually do not cause severe pharyngitis. Laboratory tests confirmed the diagnosis with a throat culture revealing alpha-hemolytic streptococci and 4 days later, a positive Monospot test result indicated 3% atypical lymphocytes. In addition, transaminases were elevated, bilirubin was normal, and the white blood cell count had increased to 17,000 mm^3, with a differential of 3% bands, 62% polymorphonuclear neutrophils (polys), 31% lymphocytes (lymphs), and 4% monocytes (monos).

KP was admitted to the infirmary for a week, where he received warm saline gargles and oral analgesia to manage his sore throat. Swallowing was difficult, and he was therefore placed on a full liquid diet. Adequacy of hydration was managed with oral fluids and by monitoring his urine output. He was sequestered from other students with acute infections to prevent a secondary infection. When he returned to his dormitory, he was counseled to rest and avoid contact sports that might cause trauma to his liver or spleen. Because EBV is transmitted through saliva, it was explained to him to avoid kissing and sharing utensils for several weeks. No antiviral medications are available to treat EBV. Because KP was immunocompetent before exposure to the virus, spontaneous recovery occurred 4 weeks after his presentation to the health center.

SELECTED RESEARCH

Most of the published research in the nursing literature use descriptive methods with variables that describe an individual's immunocompetence or the human response to HIV/AIDS. The immune response has been explored during the stress of final examinations in adolescents,[67] in abused and non-abused women,[68] during epidural analgesia during labor,[21] during diagnostic procedures for breast cancer,[49] following burn injuries,[69] and during the postpartum period.[70] The results of these studies generally support the theory of psychoneuroimmunology but do not test the effectiveness of interventions. However, the methods of physiological research are becoming more sophisticated. These methods may lay the foundation for clinical trials to test the effect of interventions on immunocompetence. An example of such a study is McCarthy et al's research on the effect of meperidine on cytokine release. The authors postulate that because meperidine decreased secretion of interleukin-1 beta, the drug may decrease rigors and chills during therapies such as amphotericin-B.[71]

The nursing research literature exploring the immune response in people with HIV/AIDS is better developed than the literature on immunocompetence. In a classic article published in 1988, Larson reviewed the nursing literature on HIV/AIDS from January 1983 through 1987 and found that none of the 36 articles published were research-based.[72] Goldrick et al[73] found in a more recent analysis that, over the past decade, almost 250 research articles studying HIV/AIDS have been published in the nursing literature.[73] They reported that 36% were classified in the psychological domain, 26% in the physiological domain, 10% in the behavioral domain, 10% in the social domain, 7% in the quality of life domain, and 11% in the stage of disease domain. The authors described the study design for 53% as correlational, 35% as descriptive, and 12% as experimental.[73]

In addition to descriptive studies of individuals with HIV/AIDS, investigators are focusing more on symptom management and prevention. Grady, Anderson, and Chase[74] described the extent and severity of fatigue in HIV-infected men who were participating in a clinical trial of interleukin-2 therapy. They found that the therapy was associated with a dramatic increase in fatigue that, although transient, severely affected quality of life. Crosby et al[75] studied HIV prevention strategies of low-income women in a large sample in Missouri. They found that only half the women used prevention strategies; most common strategies were HIV testing and questioning partners about their sexual history. In one of the few intervention studies in the nursing literature, Nicholas and Webster[76] found that a behavioral intervention focusing on the mind-body interaction in persons with HIV did not improve immune function. Intervention studies, however, are not the only type of studies to have current relevance. Withell[77] published a small descriptive study investigating the experiences of Ugandan women living with HIV/AIDS that can guide interventions for practitioners supporting the health of the African people.

QUESTIONS FOR FUTURE STUDY

The study of the immune response is in its infancy in nursing for several reasons. First, nurse scientists are just beginning to gain the requisite scientific laboratory skills to test the cellular and subcellular reactions that lead to immunocompetence. Second, many investigators have implemented descriptive studies rather than clinical trials testing nursing interventions. The dearth of intervention studies is evident in Goldrick et al's review[63] and in electronic literature searches. One of the most promising areas for investigation is symptoms management. People with an immune challenge often experience fatigue, fever, anorexia, and tissue breakdown as a result of their disorder. Testing interventions that assist people to manage these symptoms successfully while maintaining quality of life is a fertile area for research. Nurses also have an imperative to discover strategies to help people change their risk-taking behaviors that expose them to the risk of HIV/AIDS. A whole generation of young people are at risk around the world if health care providers are unable to encourage protective ("safe") sexual practices. Equally important are behavioral interventions that lead to decreases in illicit intravenous drug use.

Wherever research questions lead nurse-scientists, we know that immunocompetence is necessary for life. Through research and interventions, nurses can support immunocompetence, assist people to manage immune challenges, and limit immunocompromise.

REFERENCES

1. Sommers, M.S. (1998). Immunological clinical physiology. In M.R. Kinney, S.B. Dunbar, J.A. Brooks-Brunn, N. Molter, & J.M. Vitello-Cicciu (eds.), *AACN Clinical Reference for Critical Care Nursing* (4th ed., pp. 917-933). St Louis: Mosby.
2. Thomas, C.L. (1997). *Taber's cyclopedic medical dictionary* (18th ed.). Philadelphia: F.A. Davis.
3. American Nurses Association. (1995). *Nursing: A social policy statement.* Kansas City, Mo.: Author.
4. Levinson, W.F., & Jawetz, E. (2000). *Medical microbiology and immunology* (6th ed.). New York: Lange/McGraw-Hill.
5. Goldsby, R.A., Kindt, T.J., & Osborne, B.A. (2000). *Kuby immunology* (4th ed.). New York: W.H. Freedman.
6. Janeway, C.A., Travers, P., Walport, M., & Capra, J.D. (1999). *Immunobiology: Immune system in health and disease* (4th ed.) New York: Garland.
7. Stites, D.P., Terr, A.I., & Parslow, T.G. (1997). *Medical immunology* (9th ed.). Norwalk, Conn.: Appleton & Lange.
8. National Center for Health Statistics. (1999). *Healthy people 2000 review, 1998-1999.* Hyattsville, Md.: Public Health Service.
9. Karon, J.M., Rosenberg, P.S., McQuillan, G., Khare, M., Gwinn, M., & Petersen, L.R. (1996). Prevalence of HIV infection in the United States, 1984-1992. *Journal of the American Medical Association 276,* 126-131.
10. Hoyert, D.L., Kochanek, K.D., & Murphy, S.L. and Centers for Disease Control and Prevention. (1999). Deaths: Final data for 1997. Centers for Disease Control and Prevention, National Vital Statistics Reports 47(19), 1-105. http://www.cdc.gov (accessed September 9, 2000).
11. World Health Organization. (2000). Leading causes of global mortality, 1998. http://www.who.int (accessed September 9, 2000).
12. Ezzell, C. (2000). Care for a dying continent. *Scientific American 282*(5), 96-105.
13. Mann, J.M., & Tarantola, D.J. (1998). HIV 1998: The global picture. *Scientific American 279*(1), 82-83.
14. Centers for Disease Control and Prevention. (2000). HIV/AIDS among men who have sex with men and inject drugs—United States, 1985-1998. *MMWR 49,* 465-470.
15. Moulson, G. (2000). AIDS, wars take toll on quality of life in Africa, report says. USA Today, June 30, 2000, 16A.
16. World Health Organization. (1996). Child malnutrition: Fact Sheet 119. http://www.who.int (accessed September 9, 2000).
17. World Health Organization. (2000). Millions still going hungry in the United States, report finds. New York Times, Sunday, September 10, 2000, A20.
18. Heyman, D.L. (2000). The urgency of a massive effort against infectious diseases, World Health Organization, statement before the Committee on International Relations, U.S. House of Representatives, June 29, 2000. http://www.who.int (accessed September 9, 2000).
19. Sigma Theta Tau International. (1999). Strategic plan 2005. http://www.nursingsociety.org/stratplan (accessed September 10, 2000).
20. World Health Organization. (1999). Solar radiation and human health: Fact Sheet 227. http://www.who.int (accessed September 9, 2000).
21. Fehder, W.P., & Gennaro, S. (1998). Immune alterations associated with epidural analgesia for labor and delivery. *MCN: The Journal of Maternal Child Nursing 23,* 292-299.
22. Biddle, C. (1998). The long-term consequences of anesthesia. *Current Reviews for Nurse Anesthetists 21*(2), 15-20.
23. Gentilello, L.M., Cobean, R.A., Walker, A.P., Moore, E.E., Wertz, M.J., & Dellinger, E.P. (1993). Acute ethanol intoxication increases the risk of infection following penetrating abdominal trauma. *Journal of Trauma 34,* 669-675.
24. Szabo, G. (1997). Alcohol's contribution to compromised immunity. *Alcohol Health and Research World 21,* 30-41.
25. Oberholzer, A., Oberholzer, C., & Moldawer, L.L. (2000). Cytokine signaling—regulation of the immune response in normal and critically ill states. *Critical Care Medicine 28*(S4), N3-N12.
26. Keane, M.P., & Strieter, R.M. (2000). Chemokine signaling in inflammation. *Critical Care Medicine 28*(S4), N13-N26.
27. Godshall, S.E., & Kirchner, J.T. (2000). Infectious mononucleosis: Complexities of a common syndrome. *Postgraduate Medicine 107*(7), 175-186.
28. Samuelson, J. (1999). Infectious diseases. In R.S. Cotran, V. Kumar, & T. Collins (eds.), *Robbins pathologic basis of disease* (6th ed., pp. 329-402). Philadelphia: W.B. Saunders.
29. Cotran, R.S., Kumar, V., & Collins, T. (1999). Diseases of immunity. In R.S. Cotran, V. Kumar, & T. Collins (eds.), *Robbins Pathologic Basis of Disease* (6th ed., pp. 188-259). Philadelphia: W.B. Saunders.
30. Terr, A. (1997). Anaphylaxis and urticaria. In D.P. Stites, A.I. Terr, & T.G. Parslow (eds.), *Medical immunology* (9th ed., pp. 409-418). Norwalk, Conn.: Appleton & Lange.
31. D'Cruz, D. (2000). Autoimmune diseases associated with drugs, chemicals and environmental factors. *Toxicology Letters 112-113,* 421-432.
32. Carroll, M.C. (2000). A protective role for innate immunity in autoimmune disease. *Clinical Immunology 95*(1 Part 2), S30-S38.
33. Tolkoff-Rubin, N.E., & Rubin, R.H. (2000). Recent advances in the diagnosis and management of infection

in the organ transplant recipient. *Seminars in Nephrology 20*(2), 148-163.
34. Lanza, R.P., Cooper, D.K., & Chick, W.L. (1997). Xenotransplantation. *Scientific American 277*(1), 54-59.
35. Cotran, R.S., Kumar, V., & Collins, T. (1999). Neoplasia. In R.S. Cotran, V. Kumar, & T. Collins (eds.), *Robbins pathologic basis of disease* (6th ed., pp. 260-338). Philadelphia: W.B. Saunders.
36. Cruikshank, W.W., Kornfeld, H., & Center, D.M. (2000). Interleukin-16. *Journal of Leukocyte Biology 67*(6), 757-766.
37. Workman. L.M. (2000). The lymphoid system and its role in maintaining immunocompetence. *Seminars in Oncology Nursing 14*(4), 248-255.
38. Kaplan, J.E., Hanson, D., Dworkin, M.S., Frederick, T., Bertolli, J., Lindegren, M.L., et al. (2000). Epidemiology of human immunodeficiency virus-associated opportunistic infections in the United States in the era of highly active antiretroviral therapy. *Clinical Infectious Diseases 30*(S1), S5-S14.
39. Xu, Y.X., Ayala, A., & Chaudry, I.H. (1998). Prolonged immunosuppression after trauma and hemorrhagic shock. *Journal of Trauma 44,* 335-341.
40. Puyana, J.C., Pellegrini, J.D., De, A.K., Kodys, K., Silva, W.E., & Miller, C.L. (1998). Both T helper-1 and T helper-2 type lymphokines are depressed in posttrauma anergy. *Journal of Trauma 44,* 1037-1046.
41. Knoferl, M.W., Angele, M.K., Ayala, A., Cioffi, W.G., Bland, K.I., & Chaudry, I.H. (1999). Do different rates of fluid resuscitation adversely or beneficially influence immune responses after trauma-hemorrhage? *Journal of Trauma 46,* 23-33.
42. Nolan, B., Collette, H., Baker, S., Duffy, A., De, M., Miller, C., et al. (2000). Inhibition of neutrophil apoptosis after severe trauma is NFκβ dependent. *Journal of Trauma 48,* 599-605.
43. McCarter, M.D., Mack, V.E., Daly, J.M., Naama, H.A., & Calvano, S.E. (1998). Trauma-induced alterations in macrophage function. *Surgery 123,* 96-101.
44. Scorza, L.B., Waymack, J.P., & Pruitt, B.A. (1990). The effect of transfusions on the incidence of bacterial infection. *Military Medicine 155,* 337-339.
45. Fernandez, L.A., MacSween, J.M., You, C.K., & Gorelick, M. (1992). Immunologic changes after blood transfusion in patients undergoing vascular surgery. *American Journal of Surgery 163,* 262-269.
46. Kao, K.J. (2000). Mechanisms and new approaches for the allogeneic blood transfusion-induced immunomodulatory effects. *Transfusion Medicine Reviews 14,* 12-22.
47. Kirkley, S.A. (1999). Proposed mechanisms of transfusion-induced immunomodulation. *Clinical and Diagnostic Laboratory Immunology 6,* 652-657.
48. Kaye, J., Morton, J., Bowcutt, M., & Maupin, D. (2000). Stress, depression, and psychoneuroimmunology. *Journal of Neuroscience Nursing 32*(2), 93-100.
49. DeKeyser, F.G., Wainstock, J.M., Rose, L., Converse, P.J., & Dooley, W. (1998). Distress, symptom distress, and immune function in women with suspected breast cancer. *Oncology Nursing Forum 25*(8), 1415-1421.
50. Aster, J., & Kumar, V. (1999). White cells, lymph nodes, spleen, and thymus. In R.S. Cotran, V. Kumar, & T. Collins (eds.), *Robbins pathologic basis of disease* (6th ed., pp. 645-695). Philadelphia: W.B. Saunders.
51. Sommers, M.S. (1998). Immunological patient assessment. In M.R. Kinney, S.B. Dunbar, J.A. Brooks-Brunn, N. Molter, & J.M. Vitello-Cicciu (eds.), *AACN clinical reference for critical care nursing* (4th ed., pp. 935-946). St Louis: Mosby.
52. Bates, B. (1995). *A guide to physical examination and history taking* (6th ed.). Philadelphia: Lippincott.
53. Carey, C.F., Lee, H.H., & Woeltje, K.F. (1998). *The Washington manual of medical therapeutics* (29th ed.). Philadelphia: Lippincott-Raven.
54. Dipiro, J.T., Talbert, R.L., Yee, G.C., Matzke, G.R., Wells, B.G., & Posey, L.M. (1999). *Pharmacotherapy: A pathophysiologic approach* (4th ed.) Stamford, Conn.: Appleton & Lange.
55. McCloskey, J.C., & Bulechek, G.M. (1996). *Nursing interventions classification* (2nd ed.). St Louis: Mosby.
56. Sommers, M.S., & Johnson, S. (1997). *Nursing therapeutics for diseases and disorders.* Philadelphia: F.A. Davis.
57. Chaisson, R.E. (1999). Natural history of HIV infection in the era of combination antiretroviral therapy. *AIDS 13*(14), 1933-1942.
58. Agnoli, M.M. (2000). Immune reconstitution in the HAART era, Part 1: Immune abnormalities in HIV/AIDS. *Journal of the Association of Nurses in AIDS Care 11*(1), 78-81.
59. Agnoli, M.M. (2000). Immune reconstitution in the HAART era, Part 2: Implications for practice. HIV/AIDS. *Journal of the Association of Nurses in AIDS Care 11*(2), 97-99.
60. Holzemer, W.L., Henry, S.B., Portillo, C.J., & Miramontes, H. (2000). The client adherence profiling-intervention tailoring (CAP-IT) intervention for enhancing adherence to HIV/AIDS medications: A pilot study. *Journal of the Association of Nurses in AIDS Care 11*(1), 36-44.
61. Ickovics, J.R., & Meisler, A.W. (1997). Adherence in AIDS clinical trials: A framework for clinical research and clinical care. *Journal of Clinical Epidemiology 50*(4), 385-391.
62. Levy, S.B. (1998). The challenge of antibiotic resistance. *Scientific American 278*(3), 46-53.
63. von Boehmer, H., & Kisielow, P. (1991). How the immune system learns about self. *Scientific American 265*(4), 74-81.
64. Black, P.H. (1995). Psychoneuroimmunology: Brain and immunity. *Scientific American 2*(6), 16-25.
65. Blalock, J.E. (1994). The syntax of immune-neuroendocrine communication. *Immunology Today 15,* 504-511.
66. Robinson, F.P., Mathews, H.L., & Witek-Janusek, L. Stress reduction and HIV disease: A review of intervention studies using a psychoneuroimmunology framework. *Journal of the Association of Nurses in AIDS Care 11*(2), 87-96.
67. Kang, D., Coe, C.L., McCarthy, D.O., & Ershler, W.B. (1997). Immune responses to final exams in healthy and asthmatic adolescents. *Nursing Research 46,* 12-19.
68. Constantino, R.E., Sekula, L.K., Rabin, B., & Stone, C. (2000). Negative live experiences, depression, and immune function in abused and nonabused women. *Biological Research for Nursing 1,* 190-198.
69. DeKeyser, F.G., Winchruch, R.A., & Munster, A. (1996). Interactions of ACTH and TGF beta on monocyte proliferation: Implications for trauma and burn patients. *Research in Nursing & Health 19,* 511-516.
70. Gennaro, S., Fehder, W.P., York, R., & Douglas, S.D. (1997). Weight, nutrition, and immune status in postpartal women. *Nursing Research 46,* 20-25.
71. McCarthy, D.O., Murray, S., Galagan, D., Gern, J.E., & Hutson, P.R. (1998). Meperidine attenuates the secretion but not the transcription of interleukin 1β in human mononuclear leukocytes. *Nursing Research 47,* 19-24.
72. Larson, E. (1988). Nursing research and AIDS. *Nursing Research 37,* 60-62.

73. Goldrick, B.A., Baigis, J.A., Larsen, J., & Lemert, J.L. (2000). Nursing research and HIV infection: State-of-the-science. *Image–the Journal of Nursing Scholarship 32,* 233-237.
74. Grady, C., Anderson, R., & Chase, G.A. (1998). Fatigue in HIV-infected men receiving investigational interleukin-2. *Nursing Research 47,* 227-234.
75. Crosby, R.A., Yarber, W.L., & Meyerson, B. (2000). Prevention strategies other than male condoms employed by low-income women to prevent HIV infection. *Public Health Nursing 17,* 53-60.
76. Nicholas, P.K., & Webster, A. (1996). A behavioral medicine intervention in persons with HIV. *Clinical Nursing Research 5,* 391-406.
77. Withell, B. (2000). A study of the experiences of women living with HIV/AIDS in Uganda. *International Journal of Palliative Nursing 6,* 234-244.

CHAPTER 16 Infection

JOSEPH J. GAUTHIER & JOAN G. TURNER

DEFINITION

An infectious disease is one in which a pathogen invades a susceptible host and causes damage. Infection is the invasion of the body by microorganisms or viruses, whereas disease implies a negative change in the state of health. A pathogen is an infectious agent (microorganism or virus) that is capable of causing disease. Some pathogens are highly virulent and can cause disease when only a few invade, whereas others are weakly virulent and cause disease only when they enter the body in large numbers. Opportunistic pathogens cause disease only when they enter a normally uninhabited area of the body or when the host is in a compromised state.

Individuals are continuously exposed to microorganisms throughout their lives; significant numbers of microorganisms make up the normal flora of the human body. These microorganisms usually cause no harm and may actually be of benefit by competing with incoming pathogens for nutrients and creating adverse environments for invaders. Of particular concern in nursing care is when the balance between normal flora and pathogens is upset, such as when broad-spectrum antibiotics suppress the normal bacterial flora and permit the growth of opportunistic pathogens that would otherwise be held in check.

For infectious disease to occur, there must be a source or reservoir of the infectious agent.[1] Reservoirs may be human, animal, or nonliving (soil, food, and water). Humans are a major reservoir of infectious agents. Although people with signs and symptoms of disease are easily recognized as being able to transmit disease, healthy people and those who no longer show signs and symptoms (carriers) can also harbor and transmit pathogens. Animals may carry and/or transmit disease. Rabies and Lyme disease are classic examples. Soil and water harbor a variety of pathogens. *Clostridia,* which cause tetanus and botulism, are common soil inhabitants. Water that has been contaminated with human waste can carry the cholera bacillus and other agents that cause intestinal diseases. Many foods are potential sources of infectious agents. Beef is notorious as a source of pathogenic *Escherichia coli* (O157:H7), and poultry is often contaminated with *Salmonella.*[2] Diseases are transmitted by direct contact, vehicles, and vectors (fingers, flies, and fomites). Preventing transmission represents an import method of controlling the spread of disease.

To cause disease, infectious agents must overcome the body's three lines of defense.[1] The primary line of defense is the skin and mucous membranes. Such characteristics as integrity of skin, normal function of mucous membranes and cilia, stomach acidity and digestive enzymes, and antimicrobal chemicals, such as lactoferrin, lysozyme, and cytokines, provide substantial defense against invading microbes. The secondary line is the inflammatory response and phagocytosis. Signs and symptoms of infectious disease are often associated with manifestations of this response. Pathogens that survive the primary and secondary lines of defense must finally deal with the tertiary line of defense which is the immune system. Humoral and cell-mediated immunity work together to protect us against pathogens. (For more detail on immunity, see Chapter 15, Alterations in Immunocompetence.) Patients whose defenses are compromised by state of health, invasive procedures, or immunosuppressive drugs have increased susceptibility diseases.[3-6]

With the availability of antibiotics after the Second World War and the continual development of new vaccines, it was thought that infectious diseases could eventually be brought under control. However, they remain a leading cause of morbidity and mortality in the United States and throughout the world. New pathogens are continually emerging (e.g., HIV, hantavirus, and ebola virus) and diseases thought to be under control are reemerging (e.g., tuberculosis and pertussis).[7-9] Factors that contribute to new and emerging diseases include increased human exposure to new geographic areas because of world travel, climate changes that affect levels and exposure to infectious agents, and genetic changes in infectious agents. Efforts to treat and prevent infectious disease must be supported and will require continued research, surveillance, interventions, and education.

PREVALENCE AND POPULATIONS AT RISK

Infectious diseases continue to menace people regardless of gender, age, ethnicity, or socioeconomic status. They cause suffering and death and impose an enormous financial burden on society as a whole. Table 16-1 lists the major notifiable diseases and their incidence for 1998 in the United States.

The incidence of certain specific diseases is notable. In 1998, 604,420 cases of genital chlamydial infection were reported, the highest rate (237/100,000) reported since this disease was added to the list in 1995. A total of 3793 cases of cryptosporidiosis were reported. This disease continues to be underreported as a result of improper diagnosis and lack of routine testing of stool specimens. There were 355,642 cases of gonorrhea, an 8.9% increase over 1997. Of the 30 cases of hantavirus pulmonary syndrome reported in 12 states, 9 cases were fatal (30%). In the United States, most cases of postdiarrheal hemolytic uremic syndrome (HUS) are caused by *Escherichia coli* O157:H7. In 1998, 90 cases of postdiarrheal HUS were reported. Hepatitis C infection is the most common chronic bloodborne infection in the United States. Persons may be unaware that they are infected, but they may transmit the virus to others, and they are at risk for chronic liver disease and liver cancer. The number of Lyme disease cases reported for 1998 was the highest ever reported. This could be a result of increased human contact with infected ticks as well as enhanced reporting. For the last several years the number of reported cases of pertussis has increased. Reasons for this may be increased awareness of pertussis among health care workers, better diagnostic methods, and better reporting. Approximately 10,200 cases of invasive group A streptococcal disease were reported in 1998, with a fatality rate of 12.2%. Toxic shock syndrome and necrotizing fasciitis each accounted for approximately 5% of invasive cases.

Most of the deaths from infectious disease occur in developing countries, where approximately one in

TABLE 16-1 Summary of Incidence of Notifiable Diseases in the United States During 1998

DISEASE	CASES	DISEASE	CASES
AIDS	46,521	Meningococcal disease	2,725
Botulism, total	116	Mumps	666
Brucellosis	79	Pertussis (whooping cough)	7,405
Chancroid	189	Plague	9
Chlamydia	604,420	Poliomyelitis, paralytic	1
Cholera	17	Psittacosis	47
Cryptosporidiosis	3,793	Rabies, animal	7,259
Diphtheria	1	Rabies, human	1
Encephalitis, California serogroup viral	97	Rocky Mountain spotted fever	365
Eastern equine	4	Rubella (German measles)	364
St. Louis	24	Rubella, congenital syndrome	7
Escherichia coli O157:H7	3,161	Salmonellosis	43,694
Gonorrhea	355,642	Shigellosis	23,626
Haemophilus influenzae, invasive disease	1,194	Syphilis, total (all stages)	37,977
Hansen's disease (leprosy)	108	Primary and secondary	6,993
Hepatitis A	23,229	Congenital	801
Hepatitis B	10,258	Tetanus	41
Hepatitis C; non-A, non-B	3,518	Toxic-shock syndrome	138
Legionellosis	1,355	Trichinosis	19
Lyme disease	16,801	Tuberculosis	18,361
Malaria	1,611	Typhoid fever	375
Measles (rubeola)	100	Varicella (chickenpox)	82,455

Centers for Disease Control and Prevention. (1999). Summary of notifiable diseases in the United States, 1998. *MMWR*, 47(53).

three children is malnourished and one in five is not immunized. These problems are exacerbated by mass population movements brought about by regional wars and by growth of densely populated cities with unsafe water, poor sanitation, and poverty. Worldwide, six infectious diseases, pneumonia, tuberculosis, diarrhea, malaria, measles, and AIDS, account for more than half of the premature deaths.[10] Pneumonia often affects children with low birthweight or those weakened by malnutrition. More than 33 million people worldwide have AIDS. Most will not be able to afford the expensive treatment regimens that are available in developed countries. Limited supplies of newer immunomodulators and anti-retrovirals are available if the individual has the money to pay for them. Diarrheal diseases occur in 1.5 billion children under 5 years of age each year and they claim the lives of nearly 2 million young children each year. Tuberculosis, which was once thought to be under control, has reemerged and is killing 1.5 million people a year. Nearly one third of the world's population has latent TB infection. Malaria kills more than 1 million people each year, most of them young children. Measles, the most contagious disease known to mankind, accounts for about 900,000 deaths among children each year.

In general, populations at risk for infectious disease include the very young and the very old. Malnutrition significantly increases susceptibility to infectious agents and crowded conditions associated with poverty or military installations increase the likelihood of the spread of disease. Lack of good sanitation and drug abuse are also significant contributors. Severely immunocompromised persons (e.g., organ transplant patients, patients undergoing chemotherapy and in radiation therapy, and persons with HIV-related infection) are also at higher risk for infectious diseases.

RISK FACTORS

Risk factors for infectious diseases can be personal, environmental, or developmental. A variety of circumstances can influence susceptibility. Chronic diseases such as cancer, renal disorders, diabetes, liver disease, and respiratory disorders create conditions for infectious disease by interfering with body defenses. For example, diabetes can lead to neuropathy, glycosuria, and poor circulation. Other pathophysiological conditions, including alcoholism, immunosuppression, impaired circulation, obesity, hormonal factors, and splenectomy are contributors.

Many treatment-related factors increase susceptibility. Examples include medications, such as antibiotics, steroids, antiviral agents, insulin, tranquilizers, immunosuppressants, and antacids; surgery; dialysis; parenteral nutrition; chemotherapy; the presence of invasive lines (circulatory, gastrointestinal, respiratory, urinary); intubation; and organ transplants. Other personal factors that influence susceptibility are a history of infections, smoking, prolonged immobility, trauma (accidental or intentional), being in the postpartum period, prolonged length of hospital stay, and burns.

Environmental factors include exposure to infectious agents, animal or insect bites, and environmental stresses. Developmental factors that influence susceptibility of newborns and young children include lack of maternal antibodies and/or immunizations, lack of normal flora, open wounds (e.g., umbilical, circumcision), an immature immune system, and malnutrition. Elderly persons may be susceptible to infectious disease as a result of debilitation, poor nutrition, diminished immune system function, or chronic disease.

MECHANISMS

Many pathogens initiate disease by entering the body through a preferred portal of entry.[1] Major portals of entry include the respiratory tract, GI tract, urogenital tract, the skin and mucous membranes, and the parenteral route. Disease usually is the result of the microorganism's entry into the host, attachment to host tissues, evasion of the host defenses, and damage to tissues. Some pathogens produce damage without penetrating the body. For example, dental caries are caused by *Streptococcus mutans;* the bacteria attach to the surface of the tooth and produce acid, resulting in dissolution of the enamel. Other pathogens cause damage by production of exotoxins in food. *Clostridium botulinum* and certain species of *Staphylococcus* are examples of these.

The relationship between microorganism and host can take many forms, with the result of an infectious agent causing damage to the host. If the agent becomes established and resides in or on the body but does not cause damage, this is called *colonization.* Asymptomatic carriers are individuals who are infected but do not show signs and symptoms of disease. However, they are capable of shedding the infectious agent and can often spread infection.

Infectious agents possess a variety of virulence factors that influence their ability to overcome host defenses and cause disease (Table 16-2). These virulence factors either promote colonization and invasion or they cause damage to the host. The first

TABLE 16-2 Virulence Traits of Infectious Agents

VIRULENCE FACTOR	ACTION PROMOTED
Fimbrae	Attachment to mucosal cells
Nonfimbral proteins	Attachment to host cells
Chemotaxis	Movement to areas for subsequent attachment
IgA proteases	Breakdown of secretory IgA
Chelins	Allow organism to acquire iron
Lactoferrin protease	Allow organism to acquire iron
Capsule	Protection against phagocytosis
Endotoxin	Weakens host
Exotoxins	Variety of types of damage to host
Ability to vary surface structures	Evasion of the immune system

step in the disease process is often attachment to host cells. This is especially important where surfaces are washed by fluids (e.g., the urinary tract). Attachment is mediated by specific structures on the surfaces of the infectious agent called *adhesins.* Adhesins may be rod-shaped protein tubules called *fimbrae* or cell surface proteins called *afimbral adhesins.* For example, *Streptococcus pyogenes* has a nonfimbral adhesin that binds to the fibronectin and allows it to bind to host cell surfaces.[11]

Some bacteria are able to gain entrance to cells that are normally nonphagocytic. Attachment to specific receptors on the host cell via bacterial surface proteins, called *invasions,* results in changes in the host cytoskeleton and engulfment of the bacterium.[12] Some invasions bind to host surface proteins *(integrins)* located on the basolateral surfaces of mucosal cells. It is believed that binding to integrins may allow pathogens to evade phagocytosis. The constant flow of fluids protect some mucosal surfaces from bacterial colonization. Bacteria that are motile and can move toward the mucosal surface by chemotaxis have an advantage. Chemotactic strains of pathogenic *E. coli* have been shown to be more virulent than nonchemotactic strains.[13,14] Secretory immunoglobulin A (IgA) attaches bacterial cells to the mucin covering mucosal membranes and thus facilitates their removal. Some bacteria escape this entrapment by producing an IgA protease that cleaves IgA and releases the bacterial cell. A part of the body's defense against infectious disease is to sequester iron by binding it to proteins such as lactoferrin, transferrin, and hemin. Successful pathogens must obtain iron. Mechanisms for iron acquisition include production of siderophores (chelators with high affinity for iron) or by degrading iron-containing molecules such as lactoferrin[15-17] (see Table 16-2).

A capsule is a layer of polysaccharide or protein that covers the bacterial surface and protects the cell against phagocytosis. Capsules prevent complement activation. Although vaccines using capsular material have been successful in some cases, certain bacteria evade the immune response by incorporating molecules such as sialic acid into the capsule. This causes the surface of the microorganism to resemble host surfaces. Capsules containing sialic acid residues are not immunogenic.

Some bacteria have developed ways to survive inside of phagocytic cells, such as macrophages and granulocytes. Examples of survival strategies include escaping the phagosome, preventing phagosome-lysosome fusion, and production of a chemical to prevent the harmful effects of lysosome toxins. Other survival mechanisms include changing surface proteins during the course of infection to evade the immune system and coating of the bacterial cell surface with fibronectin to make it seem to be host material.

Exotoxins are toxic proteins that are excreted by a variety of bacteria. These proteins attack different types of cells (neurotoxin, leukotoxin, hepatotoxin, cardiotoxin) and act upon these cells by different mechanisms. Representative exotoxins and their targets are listed in Table 16-3.

An important class of exotoxins are the superantigens. These proteins bind indiscriminately to the

TABLE 16-3 Bacterial Exotoxins and Their Physical Actions on the Host

EXOTOXIN	EFFECT
Cholera toxin	Profuse diarrhea
Diphtheria toxin	Inhibition of protein synthesis and damage to organs
Tetanus toxin	Spastic paralysis
Botulinum toxin	Paralysis
Listeriotoxin	Escape from phagosomes
Gangrene toxin	Death of phagocytes
Toxic shock toxin	Toxic shock syndrome

class II major histocompatibility complex proteins (MHCs) of macrophages and the T cell receptors on cytotoxic T cells, resulting in excessive stimulation of the T cells. This causes production and release of high levels of interleukin and other cytokines, resulting in a variety of symptoms including nausea, vomiting, malaise, and fever.[12]

Exotoxins can be produced in food before it is ingested (e.g., staphylococcal exotoxin). The organism that produces the toxin may not be able to colonize the host, and the damage is done by the toxin alone. Antibiotic treatment would therefore be useless in these cases.

Bacteria that colonize a wound or mucosal surface may produce an exotoxin that acts locally (cholera exotoxin) or enters the bloodstream (diphtheris exotoxin). If the exotoxin acts locally to cause tissue damage, the damage may reduce blood circulation to the area and make it inaccessible to antibodies and immune system cells. Many pathogenic bacteria produce proteases, lipases, hyaluronidases, and other enzymes that provide nutrients for the invading organisms and causes tissue damage.

Endotoxin is the lipopolysaccharide found in the outer membrane of gram-negative bacteria that is released from the cells when they lyse. Lysis results from the action of complement, phagocytosis or antibiotics.[1] If enough endotoxin is released, the result can be septic shock. Some gram-positive bacteria produce proteins that have the same effect as endotoxin. Septic shock can lead to collapse of the circulatory system, multiple organ system failure, and death. Examples of situations that can result in sepsis include bladder infections associated with indwelling urinary catheters and the use of contaminated intravenous fluids. Signs of septic shock include elevated temperature, increased rate of heartbeat and respiration, and an increase in polymorphonuclear leukocytes (PMNs) in the blood. Risk factors include immunosuppressive chemotherapy, burns, diabetes, AIDS, and extremes of age (young or old).

The onset of septic shock is often rapid, and it is difficult to diagnose in the early stages. Therefore the best prevention is early antibiotic treatment. Unfortunately, it is dangerous if antibiotic treatment is begun after high levels of bacteria in the blood have been reached, because it can lead to release of more endotoxin.

Some bacteria have antigens that stimulate production of antibodies that cross-react with antigens of the host. This can result in serious damage to host organs and tissues. For example, *S. pyogenes* produces antigens that induce the production of antibodies and T cells that cross react with heart tissue and cause an inflammatory response that damages the heart.[12] Heat shock proteins are another class of bacterial antigens that stimulate cross-reactions. When host cells are stressed, they display similar heat shock proteins on their surfaces, and the subsequent immune reaction to the bacterial antigens causes damage to these cells.[18]

PATHOLOGICAL CONSEQUENCES

When bacterial pathogens invade body tissue, they usually encounter phagocytes (e.g., monocytes and macrophages). If they can overcome this line of defense, they can cause damage in several ways. One is to cause direct damage by destroying cells. The pathogen may also enter nonphagocytic cells by a process that is induced by the pathogen and resembles phagocytosis.[12] Once inside, the pathogen reproduces and then invades neighboring cells.

Many pathogens produce toxins that are transported by blood (toxemia) and lymph to other parts of the body where damage is caused. Some produce exotoxins which are proteins that kill host cells (cytotoxins), interfere with nerve impulse transmission (neurotoxins) or affect cells of the gastrointestinal tract (enterotoxins) (Table 16-4). Superantigens interact nonspecifically with immune cells and cause overproduction of cytokines, resulting in a systemic inflammatory response.

Endotoxin is a lipopolysaccharide found in the outer membrane of gram-negative bacteria and released when these cells die. Endotoxin causes the same signs and symptoms, regardless of the organism: chills, fever, weakness, and aches. Endotoxin can also cause shock and disseminated intravascular coagulation (DIC), characterized by formation of

TABLE 16-4 Various Exotoxins and Their Cellular Effects

EXOTOXIN	EFFECT
Diphtheria toxin	Inhibits protein synthesis
Erythrogenic toxins	Damage blood capillaries (red rash)
Botulism toxin	Prevents transmission of impulses from nerves to muscles
Tetanus toxin	Blocks relaxation pathway resulting in uncontrollable muscle contraction
Cholera toxin	Affects transport of ions in intestinal cells

clots throughout the micro-circulation, resulting in depletion of clotting factors and a tendency to bleed.

Other infectious agents have specific mechanisms for damaging the host. Viruses attach to specific receptors and enter host cells. Reproduction of the virus causes damage or destruction of the host cell. Virulence factors are less clearly understood in fungi; it is known, however, that many fungi produce toxins and many are allergenic. Some are known to produce proteases and others form a capsule that protects them against phagocytosis. Protozoa possess a variety of virulence mechanisms. *Plasmodium,* the malaria parasite, invades the host cell and grows within it, whereas *Giardia lamblia* attaches to host cells and digests them.

RELATED PATHOPHYSIOLOGICAL CONCEPTS

A characteristic that many infectious diseases share with other noninfectious diseases is inflammation. For example, peritonitis may be caused by rupture of the gut or it may be the result of ingestion of a poisonous chemical. Hepatitis may be caused by alcoholism or by a hepatitis virus. Aspiration pneumonia exhibits symptoms similar to infectious disease. The inflammatory response may also be initiated by an allergen such as penicillin or pollen, with no involvement of an infectious agent.

Differential diagnosis usually involves isolation and identification of the infectious agent. Identification had traditionally involved obtaining the causative agent in pure culture using selective and differential media, followed by staining techniques, biochemical tests, and/or immunological methods. More modern procedures employ nucleic acid amplification methods and nucleic acid probes. In the near future, DNA chips (microarrays) will become an important diagnostic tool.[19-21]

MANIFESTATIONS AND SURVEILLANCE

The most common manifestations of infectious disease are the signs and symptoms associated with inflammation. Information that is important to obtain can be assessed from these few questions. Does the patient complain of fever (continuous or intermittent)? Is there a history of previous infections (urinary tract, pneumonia, surgical wounds, respiratory tract, blood, bone and joint, cardiovascular, central nervous system, eye, ear, nose, throat, mouth, systemic, gastrointestinal)? Is there pain or swelling? An exposure history can provide important clues as to the cause of a particular infectious disease. Travel, especially outside the United States, may result in exposure to new pathogens or pathogens found in inadequately treated water. Such diseases as chickenpox and respiratory tuberculosis are contracted via the airborne route. Exposure to vectors may result in Lyme disease, rabies, or bubonic plague. Many infectious agents such as *Legionella, Giardia,* and *Cryptosporidium* can be contracted through water.

CLINICAL MANAGEMENT AND SURVEILLANCE

The best management of infectious disease is, of course, prevention. Preventive measures for inpatients or persons in the community begin with an assessment of susceptibility factors, such as age, immune deficiency, substance abuse, nutritional deficit, presence of surgical incisions, puncture wounds, and the loss of skin integrity.

After surgery, the incision must be routinely assessed and the patient monitored for signs and symptoms of inflammation. For patients with indwelling urinary catheters, it is important to note the color and odor of the urine as well as any urinary frequency, urgency, or dysuria. To reduce the chances or severity of pneumonia, breath sounds should be assessed every 8 hours and sputum samples evaluated for purulence, blood, and odor, so that antibiotic therapy can be initiated if infection is suspected. Suctioning should be employed if the patient is unable to clear secretions and strict adherence to aseptic technique is essential for all invasive procedures and the changing of ventilator tubing. Sites of invasive lines should be routinely monitored for inflammation. Patients who are immunocompromised require special care. They should be placed in a private room with visitors limited and all visitors required to wash their hands. To the extent possible, the use of invasive devices should be limited. Susceptibility to infectious disease can be reduced by proper and timely immunizations and by maintaining sufficient and proper nutrition. To avoid the development of resistance by organisms, antibiotic use should be monitored so these are neither overused nor underused for inpatients and outpatients. Patients and their families should be carefully instructed about the causes, risks, and communicability of infections as well as proper antibiotic use.

Home health care patients are at risk for developing nosocomial and vancomycin-resistant enterococcal (VRE) infections, because such patients are often immunocompromised, debilitated, and/or receiving multiple courses of antibiotics.[22] Prevention is the key to managing the spread of VRE infections, and strategies should focus on careful selection of antibiotics, proper hand washing, and infection-control practices in the home.

Nurses are at risk for acquiring communicable diseases both at work and at home. Methods to protect nurses, their patients, and their families from acquiring or spreading some of the more common communicable diseases include obtaining pertinent immunizations, using universal or disease-specific precautions, and compliance with postexposure prophylaxis. The special concerns of pregnant nurses must also be considered.[23]

CONCEPTUAL MODEL

The conceptual approach used to support this content on infection is the natural history of disease model first described by Leavell and Clark[24] in the early 1950s. By applying the components of this model, health care professionals can clearly identify priorities for preventive activity for any health problem in virtually any population located in any care setting. The natural history model may be defined as follows: "A narrative and schematic representation which portrays a chronological sequencing of departures from health. The sequence begins with the factors that promote health, but the model also addresses the very first forces that inaugurate pathological departures. An innate function of this model is to describe various approaches to prevent and control pathological processes, and this function is known collectively as the levels of prevention."[25]

The natural history of any given disease can be visualized as potentially occurring in four stages. In the *stage of susceptibility,* the host (person or persons affected), the agent (causative organism in the case of infectious diseases), and the environmental risk factors are *present but not yet interacting* to cause disease. The host, agent, and environment are often abbreviated H-A-E. If there is complete success with primary prevention, the disease will not occur, because the components of the H-A-E will not interact. Interventions such as disease-specific immunization are said to provide "specific protection," whereas more general interventions are called *general health promotion* strategies.

The stage of susceptibility ends and the *presymptomatic stage* begins when the H-A-E begin to interact at the cellular level. Actually, the stage of presymptomatic disease correlates with that period of time called the *incubation period* in infectious diseases. This is a relatively "silent" stage in that no diagnosis is yet possible. There is no corresponding level of prevention in the presymptomatic stage, and no nursing intervention strategies are possible to slow or halt the progression of disease. As diagnostic procedures are continually refined, the length of time any given patient spends in this stage shortens.

The presymptomatic stage, regardless of duration, ends when signs or symptoms make a diagnosis possible. At this point, the disease is in the *clinical stage* of development. Nursing management in the clinical stage is centered around secondary prevention strategies. Early diagnosis and treatment play a very significant role in those diseases for which there is a very effective treatment in the early clinical course. For example, as will be seen in the case study on ventilator-associated pneumonia, it is crucial to obtain a proper specimen for culture and sensitivity and then treat the patient as early as possible with an empiric antibiotic regimen. Also a part of secondary prevention are disability limitation strategies; that is, use of interventions that would prevent disabling sequelae or further morbidity or mortality.

The *stage of disability* begins when management strategies used by the entire health care team have been ineffective in preventing an irreversible pathological condition, which includes undesirable clinical outcomes ranging from psychomotor impairment to chronic sensory deficits or death. These changes do not occur if secondary prevention strategies have been effective. Tertiary prevention strategies are used in this stage and include interventions such as those designed to maximize remaining potential or even providing appropriate end-of-life care.

CASE STUDY

Ventilator-Associated Pneumonia. EM is an 81-year-old ambulatory male, community-dwelling resident. He was admitted to the hospital after developing severe right quadrant pain and altered mental status. He has had six hospital admissions in the previous 5 years. His medical history includes hypertension, chronic obstructive pulmonary disease (COPD), and sleep apnea. He was admitted to the surgical intensive care unit (SICU) in a large teaching hospital, where a pulmonary artery catheter was placed for hemodynamic monitoring.

Mr. M was suspected of having a bowel obstruction, and the day after admission, he underwent an exploratory laparotomy. The surgeon found carcinoma of the cecum with associated bowel necrosis and performed a right hemicolectomy. After surgery, Mr. M was returned to the SICU supported by a mechanical ventilator, a pulmonary artery catheter, a nasogastric tube, and an indwelling catheter.

Mr. M's postoperative course was complicated by the fact that his endotracheal tube extended into his right mainstem bronchus. Subsequently he developed a right middle lobe atelectasis. The endotracheal tube was repositioned, but he required repeated bronchoscopies for the removal of mucous plugs. He extubated himself on postoperative day 3 and tolerated extubation for 48 hours. Two days later, he was noted to be increasingly lethargic. Blood gas measurement demonstrated respiratory acidosis, and he was reintubated for ventilatory support.

Eight days after surgery, Mr. M was febrile and his sputum had become purulent. Gram stain of a sputum specimen obtained by tracheal aspirate revealed 50 polymorphonuclear leukocytes (polys) per low-power microscopic field, 2+ gram-positive cocci in clusters, 4+ gram-negative rods, and 1+ gram-negative coccobacilli. The cultures grew 2+ *S. aureus* and 4+ *Klebsiella pneumoniae* resistant to ampicillin and gentamicin but sensitive to other aminoglycoside antibiotics. Mr. M's white blood cell count was 26,000/mm^3, with 70% polys, 10% bands, and 20% lymphocytes. Additional cultures obtained the next day grew the same organisms, plus *Acinetobacter wolffii.*

With appropriate antibiotic therapy and nursing management, Mr. M's temperature returned to normal and his respiratory status improved. He was weaned from the respirator 2 weeks after surgery. Despite a urinary tract infection with *Candida albicans,* Mr. M was transferred from the SICU to the surgical aftercare floor 18 days after surgery. He continued to progress well, and on postoperative day 23, he was discharged with home care.

The Host-Agent-Environment Interaction

The case study illustrates factors that place an individual at higher risk of ventilator-associated pneumonia (VAP): advanced age, a history of COPD, immune deficiencies often associated with cancer, and abdominal or thoracic surgery. Additional factors include a depressed level of consciousness, a prior episode of a large-volume aspiration, stress-bleeding prophylaxis with cimetidine, with or without an antacid, 24-hour ventilator-circuit changes, fall-winter season, presence of a nasogastric tube, recent bronchoscopy, and administration of antimicrobial agents.[26]

SELECTED RESEARCH

Although pharmaceutical companies continue to work to develop new antibiotics and vaccines, nursing research has focused on interventions for treating patient responses to infectious disease and for preventing its spread.

It is well known that malnourished individuals are more susceptible to infectious diseases.[27] Black[28] investigated zinc deficiency and increased risk of diarrhea, pneumonia, and malaria and found that zinc supplementation decreases both duration and incidence of these diseases. Ensuring that patients receive proper nutrition is an important aspect of improving health.[29]

There is clearly a need for continued education about immunizations. Blair et al[30] reported that although many factors are believed to influence caregivers' decisions to vaccinate their children, few studies focus on caregiver understanding of childhood diseases and vaccination. The purpose of the study was to profile caregivers who presented their children for vaccination at public health clinics regarding their level of understanding of childhood vaccine preventable diseases. They found a very low level of knowledge among these caregivers: 23% had no knowledge regarding the vaccinations that their children were receiving and the disease for which the vaccination was administered. Many were unsure of the relationship between vaccination and the likelihood of their children contacting an infectious disease.

Gingerich[31] provided an overview of the importance of the community health and public health care delivery system in the study, prevention, and treatment of infectious disease, as well as resources that can assist health care professionals in the identification, care, and treatment of infectious diseases. There is a need for continued research on methods of surveillance and reporting, as well as methods to promote cooperation among persons with different roles in the public health community.

Research has also focused on risk assessment of specific patient groups. For example, Schell[32] investigated the risks for cardiovascular (CV) infections, which include reduced immunocompetence of the host, preexisting cardiac conditions, and exposure to infectious organisms. For example, devices such as indwelling central venous catheters, prosthetic valves/devices, and conditions that create turbulent blood flow increase risk for CV infections. Schell pointed out that an understanding of risk factors for CV infections helps guide a CV nurse's plan of care related to assessment and interventions for prevention and treatment of CV infections. Nosocomial bacterial meningitis and cerebrospinal fluid (CSF) shunt infections result in considerable morbidity and mortality, necessitating an organized and thoughtful approach to prevention, diagnosis, and management. Morris and Low[6] suggested that prophylactic antibiotics appear to reduce the rate of postcraniotomy meningitis often caused by *S. aureus.* On the other hand, prophylactic antibiotics do not appear to reduce the risk of developing a CSF shunt infection. CSF shunt infections usually require shunt removal and antimicrobial chemotherapy to effect a successful outcome.

Kollef et al[33] evaluated the relationship between inadequate antimicrobial treatment of infections (both community-acquired and nosocomial) and hospital mortality for 2000 patients requiring admission to intensive care units. One hundred sixty-nine infected patients (8.5%) received inadequate antimicrobial treatment of their infections. This represented 25.8% of the 655 patients assessed to have either community-acquired or nosocomial infections. The occurrence of inadequate antimicrobial treatment of infection was most common among patients with nosocomial infections which developed after treatment of a community-acquired infection (45.2%), followed by patients with nosocomial infections alone (34.3%) and patients with community-acquired infections alone (17.1%). Because inadequate treatment of infections among patients requiring ICU admission appears to be an important determinant of hospital mortality, it was suggested that clinical efforts to reduce the occurrence of inadequate antimicrobial treatment could improve the outcomes of critically ill patients and that prior antimicrobial therapy should be recognized as an important risk factor for the administration of inadequate antimicrobial treatment among ICU patients with clinically suspected infections. These few studies illustrate the need for additional research to provide a basis for prevention and/or care of individuals with an infection.

QUESTIONS FOR FUTURE STUDY

Control and prevention of infectious disease will require research efforts on several fronts. The emergence of new infectious diseases can be attributed to changes in the characteristics and risk factors of patients, the widespread use of antibiotics, changes in the environment, the role of xenotransplantation, and international travel.[2] In the United States, the incidences of *C. difficile, E. coli* gastroenteritis, hantavirus, hepatitis C virus infection, and Lyme disease have increased significantly during the past two decades. Antibiotic-resistant enterococci, *S. aureus, S. pneumoniae,* and *M. tuberculosis* have also emerged as signficant disease-causing agents. Identifying, treating, and controlling emerging infectious diseases and pathogens have created enormous challenges for future research, both medical and nursing. As new and better treatments turn some acute diseases such as AIDS into chronic conditions, research is needed on better ways to manage the long-term manifestations of these diseases.

Many diseases, such as Lyme disease[34] and pulmonary infections with nontuberculous mycobacteria,[7] are difficult to diagnose, and recognition of the causative agent may be delayed for long periods after onset of infection. Because isolation and identification are key components of diagnosis, molecular techniques for *Borrelia,* nontuberculous mycobacteria, and other infectious agents are emerging. Continued evaluation of the efficacy of current, multidrug regimens and of new generations of antibiotics for treatment of these infections will be needed to improve treatment results. Nurses will play a key role on research teams for evaluation of the efficacy of new treatments and may be initiators of research on the management of patients subjected to new treatments. For instance, new ideas are needed to improve patient compliance with multidrug regimens for tuberculosis and HIV infections.

Control of communicable diseases imported from other countries has been based on a model of exclusion, isolation, and quarantine. This policy is inconsistent with current commerce and travel and ignores the potential for rapid spread of infectious disease worldwide. To deal realistically with conditions as they exist in the world today, control of communicable diseases must involve monitoring and investigations of disease emergence, vector transmission, reservoir patterns, and factors that influence pathogen movement. The public health system must be organized with international cooperation to ensure adequate surveillance, prevention, control, and education.[8] National and local contingency plans must be developed, with international cooperation, for dealing with emerging infectious diseases.

Education continues to be a key tool in the fight against infectious disease. Research into the best methods of making people aware of prevention methods is needed. Our understanding of the relation between specific nutritional factors and susceptibility to disease is limited. Future studies on nutritional factors that protect us from infectious disease will lead to more economical disease prevention.

Another area in which nursing research is needed is that of protection of health care workers. Many studies have been done to promote health care workers' judicious use of hand washing, as well as barrier and other isolation techniques, and to modify the environment (e.g., with the use of self-shielding needles) to lessen the chance of work-related infection. However, the incidence of needlesticks and other occupational exposures remains too high.[35,36]

Infectious diseases continue to be the major cause of morbidity and mortality throughout the world, and will remain so in the foreseeable future.[9] Research leading to recognition of and interventions for emerging infectious diseases, identification of mechanisms of resistance to antimicrobial agents, and development of prevention strategies is essential.

REFERENCES

1. Tortora, G.J., Funcke, B.R., & Case, C.L. (1998). Microbiology, *An Introduction.* Menlo Park, Calif.: Addison Wesley Longman.
2. Chou, T. (1999). Emerging infectious diseases and pathogens. *Nursing Clinics of North America 34*(2), 427-442.
3. Allman, R.M., Goode, P.S., Burst, N., Bartolucci, A.A., & Thomas, D.R. (1999). Pressure ulcers, hospital complications, and disease severity. Impact on hospital costs and length of stay. *Advances in Wound Care: the Journal for Prevention & Healing 12*(1), 22-30.
4. Bond, G. (1999). Infection control assessment in the perioperative setting. *Seminars in Perioperative Nursing 8*(1), 24-33.
5. Li, C.H., Tzeng, C.M., Chen, H.W., & Lie, W.S. (1999). Risk factors of nosocomial infection in pediatric intensive care units. *Journal of Nursing (China) 46*(1), 37-46.
6. Morris, A., & Low, D.E. (1999). Nosocomial bacterial meningitis, including central nervous system shunt infections. *Infectious Disease Clinics of North America 13*(3), 735-750.
7. Cook, J.L. (1999). Focus: Respiratory tract infections. Pulmonary nontuberculosis mycobacterial infections in immunocompetent patients. *Clinical Laboratory Science 12*(5), 302-308.
8. Forrest, D.M. (1996). Control of imported communicable diseases: Preparation and response. *Canadian Journal of Public Health 87*(6), 368-372.
9. Jackson, M.M., Rickman, L.S., & Pugliese, G. (1999). Pathogens, old and new: An update for cardiovascular nurses. *Journal of Cardiovascular Nursing 13*(2), 1-22.
10. Grundtland, G.H. (1999). *WHO Infectious Diseases Report.* Available: http://www.who.int/infectious-disease-report/index-rpt99.html.
11. Joh, D., Speziale, P., Gurusiddappa, S., Manor, J., & Hook, M. (1998). Multiple specificities of the staphylococcal and streptococcal fibronectin-binding microbial surface components recognizing adhesive matrix molecules. *European Journal of Biochemistry 258*(2), 897-905.
12. Salyers, A.A., & Whitt, D.D., (1994). Bacterial Pathogenesis: A molecular approach. Washington, D. C.: ASM Press.
13. Beeken, W., Fabian, J., & Fenwick, J. (1995): The chemotactic response of blood neutrophils and monocytes to strains of *Escherichia coli* with different virulence characteristics. *Journal of Medical Microbiology 42*(3), 196-199.
14. Savkovic, S.D., Koutsouris, A., & Hecht, G. (1996). Attachment of a noninvasive enteric pathogen, enteropathogenic *Escherichia coli,* to cultured human intestinal epithelial monolayers induces transmigration of neutrophils. *Infection & Immunity 64*(11), 4480-4487.
15. Braun, V., & Killmann, H. (1999). Bacterial solutions to the iron-supply problem. *Trends in Biochemical Sciences 24*(3), 104-109.
16. Schryvers, A.B., & Stojiljkovic, I. (1999). Iron acquisition systems in the pathogenic *Neisseria. Molecular Microbiology 32*(6), 1117-1123.
17. Xiao, R., & Kisaalita, W.S. (1997). Iron acquisition from transferrin and lactoferrin by *Pseudomonas aeruginosa pyoverdin. Microbiology 143*(Part 7), 2509-2515.
18. LaVerda, D., Kalayoglu, M.V., & Byrne, G.I. (1999). Chlamydial heat shock proteins and disease pathology: New paradigms for old problems? *Infectious Diseases in Obstetrics and Gynecology 7*(1-2), 64-71.
19. Edman, C.F., Mehta, P., Press, R., Spargo, C.A., Walker, G.T., & Nerenberg, M. (2000). Pathogen analysis and genetic predisposition testing using microelectronic arrays and isothermal amplification. *Journal of Investigative Medicine 48*(2), 93-101.
20. Pollack, J.R., Perou, C.M., Alizadeh, A.A., Eisen, M.B., Pergamenschikov, A., Williams, C.F., et al. (1999). Genome-wide analysis of DNA copy-number changes using cDNA microarrays. *Nature Genetics 23*(1), 41-46.
21. Zweiger, G. (1999). Knowledge discovery in gene-expression-microarray data: Mining the information output of the genome. *Trends in Biotechnology 17*(11), 429-436.
22. Millhelm, E.T., Woodward, M., Jennings, H., & Evans, M.E. (1999). Managing vancomycin-resistant enterococci in the home care setting. *Home Healthcare Consultant 6*(8), 16-17.
23. Bertin, M.L. (1999). Communicable diseases: Infection prevention for nurses at work and at home. *Nursing Clinics of North America 34*(2), 509-526.
24. Leavell, H.R., & Clark, E.G. (1953). *Preventive medicine for the doctor and his community.* New York: McGraw-Hill.
25. Turner, J.G., & Chavigny, K.H. (1988). *Community health nursing: An epidemiologic perspective through the nursing process.* Philadelphia: Lippincott.
26. Tablan, O.C., Anderson, L.J., Arden, N.H., Breiman, R.F., Butler, J.C., & McNeil, M.M. (1994). Guideline for prevention of nosocomial pneumonia. *Infection Control and Hospital Epidemiology 15*(9), 587-627.
27. Grundtland, G.H. (1999). Removing obstacles to healthy development. *WHO Infectious Diseases Report.* Available: http://www.who.int/infectious-disease-report/index-rpt99.html.
28. Black, R.E. (1998). Therapeutic and preventive effects of zinc on serious childhood infectious diseases in developing countries. Zinc for child health. Proceedings of a Symposium held in Baltimore, Md., November 17-19, 1996. *American Journal of Clinical Nutrition 68*(Suppl 2), 476S-479S.
29. Jacob, E. (1999). Making the transition from hospital to home: Caring for the newly diagnosed child with cancer. *Home Care Provider 4*(2), 67-75.
30. Blair, A., Davies, E., Nebauer, M., Pirozzo, S., Saba, S., & Turner, C. (1997). Why immunise: Care giver understanding of childhood immunisation. *Collegian: Journal of the Royal College of Nursing 4*(3), 10-17.
31. Gingerich, B.S. (1999). Epidemiology of infectious disease. *Home Healthcare Consultant 6*(8), 24-26.
32. Schell, H.M. (1999). The immunocompromised host and risk for cardiovascular infection. *Journal of Cardiovascular Nursing 13*(2), 31-48.

33. Kollef, M.H., Sherman, G., Ward, S., & Fraser, V.J. (1999). Inadequate antimicrobial treatment of infections: A risk factor for hospital mortality among critically ill patients. *Chest: the Cardiopulmonary Journal 115*(2), 462-474.
34. McKay, L. (1998). Lyme disease: Presentation, diagnosis, and treatment recertification series. *Physician Assistant 22*(6), 27-28.
35. Jagger, J., & Perry, J. (1999). Exposure safety. Averting needle sticks. *Nursing 29*(8), 28.
36. Pruett, S. (1998). CE update—phlebotomy IV. Needlestick safety for phlebotomists. *Laboratory Medicine 29*(12), 754-761.

CHAPTER

17 Impaired Wound Healing

NANCY A. STOTTS

DEFINITION

A wound is a disruption of normal tissue structure and function that results from a pathological process or external force. Healing is defined by the Wound Healing Society (WHS) as restoration of normal anatomical structure and function.[1] Impaired healing is disruption or delay in the normal processes of healing, resulting in derangement of normal anatomical structure and function. Impairment is manifested primarily as delayed healing, infection, and abnormal scar formation. This WHS definition was validated using slides of wounds that were healed or not healed.[2] Plastic surgeons (n = 16) were asked to use their clinical judgment to determine whether the wounds were healed or not healed based on the WHS definition. Data were compared against the attending physician's knowledge of the patient's status. Data showed good interrater reliability (Kappa 0.68), a sensitivity of 0.84, specificity of 0.92, and a positive predictive validity of 0.93. These findings support the construct validity of the definition and indicate that it can reliably be used in clinical practice.

CLASSIFICATION OF WOUNDS

Wounds are classified by their depth, acuity, or closure technique[3] (Table 17-1). The depth classification categorizes wounds as partial-thickness or full-thickness. Partial-thickness injuries penetrate into the epidermis and dermis; full-thickness injuries extend into the subcutaneous tissue and muscle or bone. Examples of partial-thickness injuries are abrasions and skin graft donor sites; examples of full-thickness wounds are surgical incisions and pressure ulcers.

Acute wounds proceed through the healing process in an orderly and timely manner, resulting in return of anatomical structure and function of the injured area. Classic acute wounds are surgical and traumatic wounds. Chronic wounds, by contrast, do not proceed to healing in an orderly and timely manner or do not result in anatomical and functional integrity.[1] Chronic wounds include pressure ulcers, vascular ulcers, and diabetic wounds. All chronic wounds manifest some level of impaired healing, but only a small proportion of acute wounds become chronic wounds.

Closure technique is used to describe healing of full-thickness injuries. Wounds heal by primary intention when the wound is clean, there is little loss of tissue, and the edges are neatly approximated and closed with sutures, staples, or tissue adhesive. An example of a wound healing by primary intention is a surgical incision. Healing by secondary intention is used when the wound is contaminated, the tissue loss is irregular, and the wound is allowed to remain open to granulate, contract, and epithelialize. An example of a wound healing by secondary intention is a venous leg ulcer. In healing by tertiary intention, the wound initially is left open for 4 or 5 days because of the high bacterial count and then closed by primary intention when the bacterial load drops to a normal level.[3] An example of healing by tertiary intention is an appendix that has ruptured and been removed; the appendectomy incision is left open for several days and then closed surgically.

PREVALENCE AND POPULATIONS AT RISK

The prevalence of impaired healing can be addressed by looking at subpopulations of patients with wounds, specifically surgical incisions, pressure ulcers, venous ulcers, and diabetic ulcers. Impaired healing does not have a discrete ICD-10 code, so its prevalence cannot be tracked by auditing ICD codes.

Surgical incisions are the most frequent acute wounds, and infection of these wounds represents the major mechanism of impairment. Approximately 27 million surgical procedures are performed in the United States annually.[4] The rate of infection varies by surgical wound classification (clean, clean contaminated, contaminated, and dirty infected)—from

TABLE 17-1 Wound Classifications and Examples of Each

CLASSIFICATION	EXAMPLE
Depth	
Partial-thickness	Abrasion; skin tear
Full-thickness	Incision; stage III pressure ulcer
Acuity	
Acute wound	Surgery; trauma
Chronic wound	Venous ulcer
Closure Technique	
Primary intention	Surgical incision
Secondary intention	Pressure ulcer
Tertiary intention	Colostomy takedown

1.5% to 15.8% in clean wounds to more than 45% in dirty infected wounds. The impact of surgical infection is significant: it is the third most frequent nosocomial infection, accounting for 14% to 15% of all nosocomial infections.[5]

Venous, pressure, and diabetic ulcers constitute the bulk of chronic wounds. Given the lack of a uniform standard for tracking chronic wounds, the number of each type of chronic wound is at best an estimation. Venous ulcers occur in more than 600,000 Americans.[6] Impaired mobility, negative emotions (fear, social isolation, anger, and depression), increased care burden, and loss of time from work for those employed are associated with venous ulcers and wounds. Pressure ulcer prevalence across settings is high, ranging from 11% to 21%.[7,8] The annual cost of pressure ulcer treatment is estimated at between $2.2 and $3.6 billion.[9] Diabetic ulcers occur in 15% to 20% of the 18 million Americans with diabetes mellitus. Foot ulceration is associated with the neuropathy of diabetes and contributes to the more than 67,000 lower extremity amputations performed annually in diabetic patients.[10]

RISK FACTORS

Risk factors can be conceptualized from a mechanism perspective. From this viewpoint, major risk factors for impaired healing are repetitive injuries, ischemia, excessive inflammation, and senescent cells.[11] These four categories are not mutually exclusive, and often persons have several of these processes taking place concurrently. Understanding who is at risk is important, because it allows the provider to plan preventive activities and appropriate therapy.

Repetitive injury occurs when trauma causes reinjury in healed wounds. Because most healing involves scar formation and scar is not as robust as uninjured tissue, repeated injury often results in delayed healing and/or infection. Persons who are insensate (lack an intact sensory portion of the peripheral nervous system), such as diabetic patients and persons with spinal cord injury, are prone to repetitive injuries.[12] They are not aware of tissue injury when it occurs and so continue their activities, causing more damage and more severe injury. Repetitive injury also is seen in persons with intact sensation, such as patients with vascular ulcers and pressure ulcers.

Ischemia is another major cause of impaired healing. Oxygen and nutrients needed for repair cannot get to injured tissue. This situation is seen with arterial disease, tissue edema, vasospastic disease, and the use of beta-blockers.[13] Ischemia and its deleterious effects may be aggravated by stress,[13] cold,[14] pain,[15] and smoking.[16] (See Chapter 21, Ischemia.)

Inflammatory conditions also increase the risk of impaired healing. Systemic conditions, such as scleroderma and pyoderma gangrenosa, result in antioxidants being produced with associated pathological conditions.[11] Similarly, with ischemic-reperfusion injuries, such as venous ulcers and pressure ulcers, excess antioxidants are produced and cause local tissue damage.[17]

Senescent cells also contribute to the risk of impaired healing. These "old cells" do not respond to growth factors and cytokines as do younger cells, and this compromises the healing process. Older persons and those with chronic wounds often have senescent cells.[11] Debridement of these old cells results in restoration of a normal healing trajectory.[18]

Moving from a conceptual perspective to a more pragmatic clinical perspective, researchers report a long list of risk factors for impaired healing. There are different sets of risk factors, depending on the researcher's framework for examining factors, the type of wound, the operational definition of variables, the study methods, and the sample employed. This variability in research methods has resulted in a dramatic lack of agreement among studies measuring risk factors for impaired healing. For example, predictors of increased risk of nonhealing venous leg ulcers include a history of vein ligation or stripping, hip or knee surgery, an ankle-brachial index (ABI) of less than 0.8, yellow fibrin covering more than half the ulcer, a large-sized ulcer, and an ulcer of long duration.[19] In contrast, patient risk factors for surgical site infection include old age, poor nutritional status, diabetes, smoking, obesity, infection at a remote site in the body, colonization with microorganisms, altered immune response, and prolonged preoperative hospital stay.[5]

The variability in findings among studies may reflect the heterogeneity of the conditions included in impaired healing, a lack of complete understanding of the physiology of impaired healing, and inadequate instruments to measure disruption in healing. A list of generic risk factors for impaired healing can, however, be used to screen patients across populations. Factors frequently related to impaired healing across populations include old age, insufficient oxygen or perfusion, increased bacterial burden, old wound tissue, excess interface pressure on the site, psychophysiological stress, malnutrition, having specific diseases, and adverse effects of therapy.[20,21]

MECHANISMS

Healing is initiated whenever there is tissue damage to the body. Understanding impaired healing depends on knowledge of normal healing. Thus normal healing will be discussed first, followed by impaired healing.

Normal Healing

Partial-thickness wounds heal primarily by epithelialization. Initiation of the inflammatory process results in release of epidermal growth factor, which stimulates mitosis of epidermal cells. Subsequently, epidermal cells arise from the edges of the wound as well as the hair follicles and sweat glands. The epidermal cells that arise from the hair follicles and base of the glands give rise to "tufts" of epidermal cells that look white or skin colored and are located in the base of the wound. The epithelial cells proceed to elongate and divide until a single layer covers the wound and then a second layer is produced. Epithelial cells migrate most efficiently over a clean, moist surface.[20]

Full-thickness injury initiates a cascade of processes that are overlapping; however, they usually are described as occurring in three phases: the inflammatory, proliferative, and remodeling stages. The inflammatory phase prepares the area for new tissue formation; the proliferative phase is focused on new tissue formation; and the remodeling phase is the period during which wound tensile strength is developed (Box 17-1).

Healing is initiated with injury and damage to blood vessels. Vasoconstriction occurs, platelets are activated, and the coagulation cascade is initiated. The combination results in a loose clot formation. Platelets interact with the damaged tissue and thrombin is released, which converts fibrinogen to fibrin, resulting in a secure clot[20] (see Chapter 18, Altered Clotting). Growth factors released from the alpha granules of the platelets include platelet-derived growth factor (PDGF), epidermal growth factor (EGF), insulinlike growth factor I (IGF-I), and transforming growth factor-beta (TGF-beta). These contribute to mitotic activity and initiation of the various cellular activities that result in repair. Simultaneously, chemotactic activity is initiated by the TGF-beta that is released from the platelets and the tumor necrosis factor-alpha (TNF-alpha) from the endothelial damage. As a result, neutrophils and fibroblasts are called to the area.

BOX 17-1 Three Phases of Healing and Major Events in Each

Inflammatory Phase
Hemostasis
Growth factor release
Wound clean-up

Proliferative Phase
New vessel formation
Collagen production
Contraction

Remodeling Phase
Tensile strength increases

Neutrophils are the principal white blood cell in acute inflammation. They come rapidly to the area of injury, have a short life (24 to 48 hours), and overall are the predominate inflammatory cell in the wound for the first 3 days. Neutrophils phagocytose bacteria and release the proteases elastase and collagenase that help to break down damaged extracellular matrix.[22]

Monocytes, also signaled by TGF-beta or fragments of fibronectin, are activated and become macrophages that secrete growth factors and act to phagocytose foreign material through the remainder of the healing process. Growth factors synthesized and released from macrophages include TGF-beta, TGF-alpha, leukocyte-derived growth factor, and heparin-binding epidermal growth factor.[23] These growth factors stimulate the migration of fibroblasts, epithelial cells, and vascular endothelial cells into the wound. In addition, fibroblasts in adjacent tissue express integrin receptors that recognize fibrin. Fibroblasts then recognize the integrin receptors and move into the matrix of the clot that has formed. Fibroblasts, vascular endothelial cells, and keratinocytes proliferate and release growth factors.

The growth factors support angiogenesis and the synthesis of extracellular matrix. Fibroblasts are responsible for the synthesis of the extracellular matrix including collagen, elastin, and proteoglycans. Over time, collagen and ground substance (combination of glycosaminoglycans and proteoglycans) fill the wound space as scar tissue. Remodeling of this tissue continues for months to years; however, angiogenesis and cell proliferation stop. During this period, a balance is achieved between collagen synthesis and lysis.[20]

Thus most healing occurs by repair, and scar tissue replaces injured tissue. Regeneration occurs only in the liver and the epithelium. Wound healing in the fetus, regardless of its location, also occurs by a scarless process that parallels regeneration. Although the mechanism of fetal healing is not well understood, a number of factors have been related to scarless fetal healing, including minimal inflammatory reaction, little cytokine production, and the almost complete absence of transforming growth factor beta (TGF-beta) that is seen in a fibrotic wound scar in an adult.[24]

Impaired Healing

Healing that is impaired does not occur in the expected fashion. Impaired healing is seen primarily as delayed healing, infection, and abnormal scar formation. Delayed healing may occur secondary to an underlying pathological condition (e.g., venous disease, and ischemia from unrelieved pressure). It also may occur secondary to dehiscence or evisceration or from hematoma or seroma formation. Infection occurs when the microbial burden overwhelms the host's immune capacity. Abnormal scar formation is seen in genetically predisposed populations and in others after massive tissue injury such as burns and crush injuries.

Delayed Healing. Delayed healing is the sine qua non of chronic wounds, although chronic wounds also are characterized by lack of structural integrity, delay in the formation of granulation tissue, and ultimately by the formation of more abundant scar tissue.[22] The biological processes that lead to chronic wounds are not entirely understood; however, Mast and Shultz[23] hypothesized that there is a common pathophysiology and that the usual inflammatory process associated with injury goes astray. Repeated trauma, ischemia, or low levels of bacterial contamination act as an inflammatory stimulus that persists in chronic wounds. A cycle is set up wherein TNF-alpha and interleukin-1 are produced and result in a positive feedback system. These factors result in increased levels of matrix metalloproteases (MMP) and reduced levels of tissue inhibitors of metalloproteases (TIMPs). The cycle that is established results in degradation of growth factors and receptors that contribute to delayed healing. The most frequent types of chronic wounds are venous ulcers, pressure ulcers, and diabetic foot ulcers.

Venous Ulcers. Two systems of veins in the lower extremity, a deep system and a superficial system, connected by a communicating system, contribute to the cause of venous ulcers. Normal venous return is accomplished primarily through contraction of the calf muscles, pushing the flow proximally with the valves in the veins preventing retrograde flow. When the valves become incompetent, calf muscle contraction pushes blood flow both proximally and distally. The distally displaced blood flows into the superficial veins, and venous pressure increases. The increased venous pressure causes leakage of fluids into the tissues, increasing leg edema and fibrin deposition. Mechanical trauma to the edematous leg results in the development of ulcers.

Two theories are proposed to explain the pathophysiology of venous ulcers and response to injury: the fibrin cuff theory[25] and the white blood cell (WBC) trapping theory.[26] The fibrin cuff theory suggests that fibrin forms an impermeable barrier around the capillary sphincters, and nutrients and oxygen cannot get from the capillary bed to the tissues, so cells die. By contrast, the WBC trapping theory states that WBCs that are trapped in the postcapillary venules are activated and release chemicals that result in cell damage and death. Although some data support each theory, neither theory has yet been substantiated by controlled scientific research studies.[27]

Pressure Ulcers. Pressure ulcers are thought to arise from three sources: vertical pressure over a bony prominence, friction and shear resulting in horizontal pressure damage to the vasculature of the skin and subcutaneous tissue, and ischemia-reperfusion injury.[26,28,29] The classic vertical pressure theory purports that unrelieved pressure on the skin over a bone causes high pressures next to the bone and lower pressure near the skin. The pressure distribution results in a cone shaped necrosis that is largest next to the bone and smallest at the skin level. Pressure exerted vertically may present as necrosis days or weeks after the initial insult.

In contrast to vertical pressure causing tissue deformation, friction and shear result in the tissue architecture being distorted with horizontal pressure.

This is seen primarily on the posterior body on the sacrum and heels. Friction occurs when patients are moved across the bed surface. Shear is seen when people slide down in bed when the head of the bed is elevated.[17] This causes the superficial and deeper tissue layers to move in opposing directions, resulting in stretching and rupture of small blood vessels.

Recent work suggests that pressure ulcers result from repetitive ischemia-reperfusion injury.[28] The ischemia-reperfusion theory suggests that repeated periods of ischemia result in the release of the by-products of anaerobic metabolism, resulting in damage to tissue. Reperfusion results in increased production of free radicals, leukocyte recruitment, endothelial cell swelling, reduction in arteriolar diameter, and increased resistance in the microcirculation.[28]

It is not clear whether these three proposed mechanisms are manifested independently or whether they interact in pressure ulcers that are seen clinically. Further work is needed to sort out this issue, largely so interventions can be proposed that address the specific mechanism. To date, most attention has been focused on vertical pressure as an etiological factor.

Diabetic Foot Ulcers. People who have had diabetes for a number of years frequently develop ulcers of the feet. The etiology of the ulcer is usually related to reduced blood supply, nerve damage, elevated glucose levels, or a combination of these problems.[12] Trauma results in ulcer development and healing is impaired because of the combination of reduced blood supply, neuropathy, and increased glucose levels.

Arteriosclerotic disease in large and small vessels develops over time in diabetes, following the same pattern as in nondiabetics. There is increased involvement of the vessels below the knee, particularly the tibial and peroneal arteries.[30] Data show that arterioles become sclerotic, blocking blood flow to capillaries, resulting in ischemia.

The cause of neuropathy in diabetics is related to increased sorbitol pathway activity, reduced axonal transport, and microvascular ischemia.[27] Neuropathy in the person with diabetes may present as sensory, motor, autonomic, or a combination of these dysfunctions.

Persons with sensory loss cause trauma to their feet from repetitive use and their inability to sense damage when it occurs. Small nerve fiber sensory loss causes loss of pain sensation, touch, and temperature sensation. Large fiber involvement results in loss of vibratory sensation and proprioception. In persons with normal sensation, the pain associated with the injury alerts the person to the problem and he or she stops the activity. The diabetic with sensory neuropathy is not aware of the damage and so often will continue the activity, compounding the initial injury.

Motor neuropathy leads to loss of small muscles so an imbalance is created between the extensor and flexor muscles. This problem is manifested as clawing of toes, prominent metatarsal heads, anterior displacement of foot pads, and gait disturbances.[12] Motor neuropathy causes foot deformity as the muscles of the foot lack the innervation needed for muscle tone that maintains the usual foot architecture. Changes in the bony structure occur and pressure points for weight-bearing are shifted, often resulting in ulceration due to excess pressure over bony prominences.

Autonomic neuropathy alters blood flow to the foot as well as the usual skin sweating and moisturizing of the skin. Cracks may develop in the feet, allowing microorganisms to enter the tissue.[27]

High glucose levels also contribute to impaired healing in diabetes. White blood cells do not function as effectively in high glucose environments. Data show that infection rates in persons with diabetes are higher than in nondiabetics.[12]

Infection. Infection of a wound is present when organisms invade the tissues and produce a systemic response.[31] It occurs when the host-environment relationship is disrupted and the organism predominates. People have an elegant and redundant system for protection against microorganisms; infection occurs when the system breaks down or becomes overwhelmed with the bacterial load.

High levels of bacteria (10^5 organisms or more per gram of tissue) lead to high levels of proinflammatory cytokines, increased MMP, decreased TIMPs, and decreased levels of growth factors.[32] Controlling bacteria in the wound is the goal of care so the wound can be closed surgically or by contraction.[33]

Abnormal Scar Formation. Abnormal scar formation, called *fibroproliferative disease,* is manifested as keloid and hypertrophic scar tissue.[34] Keloids are scars that extend beyond the margin of the original wound. Hypertrophic scars are erythematous, fibrous tissue that typically do not extend beyond the initial wound. Keloids usually retain their original size, whereas hypertrophic scars usually get smaller over time.

Keloids can develop from any injury and seem to have a genetic basis. In contrast, hypertrophic scar results from full-thickness injury and histologically, this scar tissue has nodules present.[35] In neither case is the mechanisms by which they develop entirely understood. Both are associated with increased inflammation, high levels of cytokines, and abnormal remodeling of new tissue.[34]

PATHOLOGICAL CONSEQUENCES

The pathological consequences of impaired healing are broad and include physiological and psychosocial dimensions. Amputation is among the physiological consequences seen in persons with diabetes and those with peripheral vascular disease.[10,30] Infection of wounds may lead to bacteremia and sepsis and often involve long hospitalization. These systemic problems are serious and may even result in death.[5] Pain may limit activity, resulting in decreased quality of life, self-imposed social isolation, and physical deconditioning.[15] The odor associated with some wounds and the activity restriction may lead to body image alterations and isolation.[27] Excessive scar formation is related to functional as well as cosmetic alterations.[11,34]

RELATED PATHOLOGICAL CONCEPTS

Wound healing impairment is associated with several concepts including immunoincompetence, ischemia, uncontrolled pain, body image disturbance, and psychological stress. Immunoincompetence and ischemia are mechanisms by which impairment in healing occurs. Uncontrolled pain may contribute to the development of a wound through vasoconstriction or may result from tissue disruption. Usually body image disturbance and psychological stress are outcomes of a wound, but they may become part of a positive feedback system by which the person with the wound has so much stress because of body image or psychological stress that vasoconstriction occurs, causing ischemia and resulting in deterioration of the wound.

MANIFESTATIONS AND SURVEILLANCE

Ongoing assessment is critical to identify whether healing is progressing as expected or is impaired. Assessment is done with every dressing change, minimally on a weekly basis. Wounds that are acute and those whose treatment has changed need to be assessed most frequently, usually daily or when the dressing is changed. The parameters used to assess healing are outlined in Table 17-2. As can be seen in the table, there is little consensus on the parameters that are recommended to be included in surveillance. Currently scientific data do not indicate what parameters need to be monitored. Until such time as data on the most appropriate parameters are available, institutions need to develop a protocol for surveillance in clinical practice that addresses their specific populations so consistent data can be collected to track the trajectory of repair.

A number of tools have been developed to monitor healing in full-thickness wounds. Most of these were developed for use with pressure ulcers and include the Pressure Sore Status Tool (PSST),[36,37] the Sessing Scale,[38] the Sussman Tool,[39] and the Pressure Ulcer Scale for Healing.[40,41] All of these scales provide a score that is the sum of individual items. Scores over time can be plotted to indicate the direction of change and the user can conclude whether the wound is healing or experiencing some disruption in the healing process. Further instrument development is needed to determine whether a specific scale score can be used to differentiate healing from impaired healing. In clinical practice and in research studies, clinical parameters are used to diagnose healing in both partial-thickness and full-thickness wounds. Such signs as wound size and change in size over time, amount of inflammation, and wound drainage, as well as symptoms such as the amount of pain and "itchiness" of the wound, are used to evaluate healing. Laboratory values such as hematocrit and hemoglobin levels, a white blood cell count, and hemoglobin A1C are used to evaluate factors known to support healing or contribute to impaired healing.

Delayed Healing

Delayed healing of a partial-thickness injury is usually manifested as a wound size that does not decrease or that increases. The wound does not fill in from the wound edges or the skin appendages (hair follicles and glands) in the base of the wound.[3]

With full-thickness injury that is healing by primary intention, the wound edges may not be well approximated. There may be continuous drainage of fluid from the incision line for more than 48 to 72 hours after the closure. The wound drainage may be discolored rather than clear (tan, yellow, green, or serosanguenous) and malodorous. Inflammation may not appear with the initial injury, or it may continue after the first 5 days. The wound does not develop a healing ridge in the first 7 to 9 days after closure.[42]

Wound disruption, dehiscence, and evisceration of an acute wound result in delayed healing.[43] Wound disruption is often seen after a hematoma or seroma forms in wounds healing by primary

TABLE 17-2 Comparison of Wound Surveillance Parameters Proposed by a Professional Organization (WHS) and Governmental Body (Agency for Health Care Policy Research)

PARAMETER	WOUND HEALING SOCIETY*	PRESSURE ULCER TREATMENT GUIDELINE†
Extent of wound	Tissue levels	Size
	Perimeter/area (length × width)	Sinus tracts
	Volume	Tunneling
	Undermining	Undermining
Associated attributes of wound	Location	Location
	Tissue viability	Stage
	Duration	Exudate
	Blood flow	Necrotic tissue
	Oxygenation	Presence of granulation
	Infection	Epithelialization
	Odor	
	Exudate	
	Edema	
	Inflammation	
	Repetitive trauma/insult	
	Innervation	
	Wound metabolism	
Host factors	Nutrition	Nutrition
	Prior wound manipulation	Pain
	Pain	Psychosocial health
		Physical health
		Complications
Environmental factors	Demographics	
	Systemic agents	
	Systemic disorders	

*Lazarus, G.S., Cooper, D.M., Knighton, D.R., Margolis, D.J., Pecoraro, R.E., Rodeheaver, G., Robson, M.C. (1994). Definitions and guidelines for assessment of wounds and evaluation of healing. *Archives of Dermatology 130,* 489-493.
†Bergstrom, N., Bennett, M.A., Carlson, C.E., et al. (1994). *Treatment of pressure ulcers: Clinical practice guideline, No. 15*. Rockville, Md.: U.S. Department of Health and Human Services, Public Health Services, Agency for Health Care Policy and Research. AHCPR Publication No. 95-0652.

intention. Blood or serum accumulates in the wound space. This increases the distance across which new vessels must grow. Increased levels of proteases are needed to create a canal or opening for the new vessels. Evisceration and dehiscence usually occur in the first 7 days after primary closure and after sutures are removed; however, they may occur at any time between days 1 and 21. Abdominal or thoracic pressure is increased with coughing, vomiting, or abdominal distention. When the cavity pressure exceeds the tensile strength of the incision, the incision will open. Data indicate that a serosanguineous drainage is present before evisceration or dehiscence in some proportion of cases (23% to 84%) and may be a sign of potential incisional disruption.[43]

In wounds healing by secondary intention, a key parameter in diagnosing delayed healing is that the wound does not get smaller; in fact, sometimes wound size even increases. In clinical practice, wound size is measured with a disposable ruler. The longest dimension of the wound, the length, is measured and then the widest part of the wound that is perpendicular to the length, the width, is evaluated.[44,45] The length is multiplied by the width to obtain a gross measure of surface area. Measurement of surface area using length times width is based on measurement of the area of a rectangle, and although most wounds are not rectangular, this measure allows reasonable estimation of surface area in practice.

Other methods of measuring surface area include tracing the wound perimeter onto an acetate sheet and measuring its area with planimetry,[46,47] tracing the wound onto graph paper and counting the number of squares,[47] and stereophotography.[48] These techniques are more exact and have been used in research. Although they are more precise, they may be too complicated or time consuming for clinical practice.

Depth also is measured,[1,49] usually with a rigid probe at the deepest portion of the wound. Delayed healing is characterized by no decrease in depth or an increase in depth. In pressure ulcers, depth is described categorically in terms of stages: stage I is the most superficial and stage IV the deepest (Box 17-2). Although it is expected that depth will be measured as part of routine wound assessment, depth has not been shown to be correlated with healing in pressure ulcers.[37,41]

Depth and area are sometimes used to estimate wound volume. There is agreement in the literature that volume is difficult to measure and that it would be good to know, but that a gross estimate is sufficient for most clinical practice decisions.

Other approaches used when volume is to be evaluated include covering the wound with a transparent dressing and filling the volume with normal saline solution,[50] filling the wound with dental impression material,[51,52] and using stereophotography.[48] These methods are reserved for use in research, because they are complicated and time and resource intensive.

The nature of tissue is also used to evaluate impairment.[3,53] The quality of granulation tissue is evaluated. Clinically, this may be manifested as pale tissue that does not progress from pale pink to the beefy red that characterizes granulation tissue. Failure of this color progression is a reflection of impaired angiogenesis (and subsequent flow of blood through new vessels). Concomitantly, the normal grainy texture of the granulation tissue is not present or is muted, so the tissue looks almost smooth. At times with delayed healing, granulation tissue looks somewhat transparent or "jellylike."

Some wounds are undermined (i.e., the tissue loss beneath the skin is greater in size than the skin opening of the wound). It is important to document the dimensions of the undermining so change in size can be appreciated. Usually a stiff probe is inserted into the wound in all directions and the distance of undermining noted. Some practitioners record the wound size by describing the wound as though it were on a clock face: "The wound is 2 cm deep; opening is round and 2 cm in diameter; at the 3 o'clock position it is undermined 4 cm."

Another sign of delayed healing is the presence of exudate in the wound. Exudate is a by-product of bacteria and their phagocytosis and digestion by WBCs. Exudate varies in color, depending on the organism present (e.g., *Pseudomonas* produces a thick, green drainage). The degree of hydration of the exudate also affects its color: dryer exudate is darker in color. In acute inflammation, exudate is usually liquid, whereas in chronic wounds it has more of a fibrous character.

Sometimes the wound is totally filled with necrotic tissue or slough. Necrotic tissue is dark in color, usually black, and indicates the tissue is dead. Dead tissue supports growth of microorganisms, especially gram-negative organisms. Often odor is associated with necrotic tissue; the odor clears as the number of gram-negative organisms decreases.[3] Slough usually is yellow to yellow-brown, depending on its state of hydration. It is produced with chronic inflammation and is predominantly fibrous.

Wounds healing by tertiary intention are assessed as those healing by secondary intention when they are open. After their bacterial load drops and they are closed with sutures or staples, these wounds are evaluated as any other wounds healing by primary intention.

BOX 17-2 Depth Classification for Pressure Ulcers: Staging

Partial-Thickness

Stage I: Pressure ulcer involves only nonblanchable erythema. In persons with darkly pigmented skin, signs that may be seen are induration, warmth, discoloration as well as the symptom of pain.

Stage II: Pressure ulcer involves partial-thickness injury.

Full-Thickness

Stage III: Pressure ulcer extends into the subcutaneous tissue but not through the fascia.

Stage IV: Pressure ulcer extends through the fascia into the muscle and may involve tendon or bone.

Infection

Infection is a major manifestation of impaired healing. In persons with an intact immune system, the local response to infection is inflammation and pus formation. Odor may accompany the tissue invasion, a sign that gram-negative organisms are present. Systemically, fever and leukocytosis occur. The standard diagnostic test for infection is wound culture, ideally via a tissue biopsy. Infection is defined as 10^5 organisms or more per gram of tissue, or fewer if very virulent organisms such as beta-hemolytic streptococci are found.[31]

In surgical wounds, wound infection has been called *surgical site infection* (SSI). It is described by depth of tissue and categorized as superficial, deep, and organ/space (Figure 17-1). Superficial SSI involves only the skin or subcutaneous tissue at the incision. Deep SSI extends into the deep soft tissues of the incision, including the fascia and muscles. Organ/space SSI involves any organ/space other than the incision.[5] Although infection is defined by the results of tissue culture (10^5 organisms or more with the likelihood ratio per gram of tissue), most often infection is diagnosed based on clinical signs. Criteria to diagnose SSI are shown in Figure 17-1.

Infection in chronic wounds, while having many similar manifestations as in acute wounds, has been said to be characterized by the presence of inflammation and pus.[31] Granulation tissue also characterizes chronic wounds, however the bacterial level cannot be determined merely by the presence of granulation tissue. Recent work by Gardner et al[54] explored the validity of clinical signs and symptoms of local chronic wound infection in persons with chronic wounds. With a sample (n = 36) of persons with various types of chronic wounds, they evaluated the clinical presentation of the wound under controlled circumstances and compared it with whether the wound was infected as determined by tissue biopsy. The classic signs of infection (pain, erythema, edema, heat, and purulent exudate) as well as signs specific to chronic wounds (serous exudate with concurrent inflammation, delayed healing, discoloration, friable granulation tissue, foul odor, wound breakdown) were systematically evaluated. The likelihood ratio showed that the signs and symptoms with the greatest discriminatory power were friable granulation tissue, foul odor, edema, delayed healing, and serous exudate with concurrent inflammation. Pain and wound breakdown could not be evaluated with the likelihood ratio, because the statistic will not permit division by zero. These preliminary data open the door to thinking differently about clinical signs of chronic wound infection. The manifestations of infection in chronic wounds are found in Box 17-3.

CLINICAL MANAGEMENT

The goal of care for patients with impaired healing is to interrupt the impaired healing cycle and reestablish a positive healing trajectory. For patients with delayed healing, an optimal environment is needed to support healing: a moist wound bed, maximal oxygenation and perfusion, substrates and nutrients needed for repair, and minimal bacterial burden. For patients with infected wounds, the emphasis is on control of bacterial burden (also referred to as "bioburden") and then, later, promoting healing. For persons with keloids or

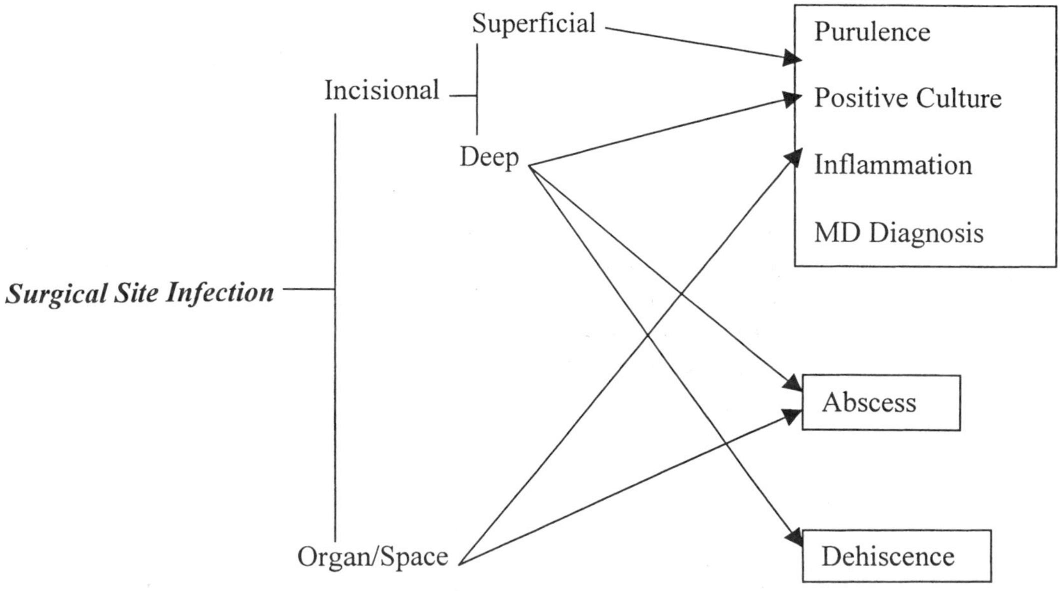

Figure 17-1 Criteria for diagnosis of surgical site infection.

BOX 17-3 Manifestations of Chronic Wound Infection*

- Inflammation (erythema, pain, edema, and induration) surrounding the wound that extends from the wound edge >0.5 cm
- Drainage increases or changes in color or odor
- Pain at the site or change in sensation for those with neuropathy
- Lack of or poor quality granulation tissue
- No improvement in healing in 2 weeks in a clean wound

*In diabetes, unexplained high serum glucose levels may also be present.

hypertrophic scar tissue, the focus of treatment is to reduce the structural and/or cosmetic consequences of the scar tissue using some combination of compression garments, silicone gel sheets, injection of steroid agents, and surgery.

The classic work on a moist environment was reported in 1962 by Winter,[55] who showed that healing occurred more rapidly in a moist occlusive environment than in a dry one. Although use of a moist environment is the usual practice today, this was a radical assertion at the time, and research findings opened the door to the development of a wide range of dressings and truly revolutionized wound care. Transparent dressings, hydrocolloids, alginates, foam dressings, and combinations of these dressings all have been developed and marketed. An excellent review of the literature on dressings has been published in evidence-based review articles.[56,57]

Maximizing blood flow has long been recognized as important to healing. Blood flow brings oxygen and substrates for repair to cells and has recently been recognized as pivotal to healing. Adequate intravascular volume is important in providing needed substrates to wounds.[58-60] Also, because the sympathetic nervous system mediates subcutaneous blood flow, factors that affect sympathetic outflow directly affect healing.[13] Recognized as significant in reducing blood flow are inadequate intravascular volume,[58-60] pain,[15] cold temperature,[14] stress,[13] and medications that cause peripheral vasoconstriction.[13]

Because of the importance of oxygen in normal healing and the fact that the hemoglobin carries the majority of the body's oxygen content, anemia has been implicated as a factor that may result in impaired healing. However, animal and human studies show that anemia is not a threat to healing until the values are very low (hematocrit below 20%), decreased intravascular volume is present, or the patient is unable to compensate by increasing cardiac output.[61,62]

Appropriate substrates and nutrients need to be present for healing. Protein, carbohydrates, fats, multivitamins, zinc, copper, and magnesium are essential for healing.[63] Normally these are ingested orally, or are provided by the enteral or parenteral route. The required amounts vary, based on the patient's body size, degree of injury, and metabolic state, as well as the individual's ability to absorb and utilize what is provided. Specific defects in healing can occur when individual nutrients are decreased. For example, a deficiency in vitamin C results in decreased collagen synthesis, and that allows collagen catabolism to exceed anabolism so that the wound breaks down. For the most part in the United States, deficits are not of a specific nutrient but rather are manifested as protein-calorie malnutrition.

Control of bacterial burden is central to the prevention and treatment of delayed healing and infection.[33] Bioburden is reduced by cleansing, debridement, use of topical antibacterial agents, administration of antibiotics, and systemic support of immune function by providing adequate blood flow, optimal oxygenation, and the nutrients needed for repair.

Cleansing is the use of a solution to remove debris, contaminants, exudates, and metabolic waste products from the surface of the wound. This practice has been accepted as the standard of care for all chronic wounds since the publication of the Agency for Health Care Policy and Research's Clinical Practice Guideline: Treatment of Pressure Ulcers.[64] Cleansing has been shown to reduce bacterial burden in wounds, although no studies have been reported that examined the effect of irrigation or cleansing on wound infection, and studies have not been reported that examine the effect of irrigation on other aspects of the healing environment. Some researchers have sought to examine wound fluid to understand the optimal environment for healing,[65] yet it is not clear whether irrigation at each dressing change supports or hinders healing.

Data show that cleansing with isotonic fluid at moderate pressures is better able to remove contaminants than when either low pressure or high pressure is used. The solution used should be isotonic, because skin cleansers and antiseptics are toxic to cells.[66,67] Low pressure lacks the force to remove the contaminants, and high pressure pushes fluid into the tissues, creating a potential nidus for infection.[68,69] This translates clinically into the use of normal saline solution with a 35-ml syringe and with an 18-gauge angiocath or the use of a commercial irrigation machine set to pressures between 4 and 15 psi.[49] The volume of fluid needed to thoroughly cleanse the wound has not been reported. In addition, recent data show that pressures generated with a syringe vary greatly in a simulated wound irrigation situation,[70] suggesting that standardized training needs to be done or commercially available machines used to create standard pressure.

Cleansing with a solution, rather than removal of debris with gauze or a surgical scrub brush, is recommended. The rationale for this strategy is that mechanical pressure causes additional trauma to the area and increases the risk of infection.[69]

For wounds that have debris, necrotic tissue, or slough in them, debridement is a mainstay of treatment to remove nonviable tissue. Necrotic tissue is a natural breeding ground for microorganisms and the level of organisms falls as dead tissue is removed.[64] The type of debridement selected (autolytic, chemical, mechanical, or surgical) depends on the desired degree of selectivity and speed of removal. The availability of trained personnel to perform the appropriate treatment also is an issue in some situations. (This topic is discussed in depth in a review article by Falabella.[71]) It should be noted that the value of debridement was reaffirmed when accelerated healing was seen in studies where aggressive surgical debridement alone or in combination with growth factors was used.[18]

The use of topical antiseptics to reduce bioburden is controversial, because topical antiseptics may cause more harm than good. Data from a series of studies show that topical agents in fact do kill various cells, including fibroblasts.[72] Based on these data, the AHCPR Pressure Ulcer Treatment Panel recommended that antiseptics not be used.[49] However, much of the research supporting this recommendation was done in vitro, raising the question of whether it could be generalized to clinical practice with humans. One of the issues is the form of the antiseptic. For example, iodine has been identified as a solution that causes harm to tissue and therefore is an undesirable topical agent. Data show that elemental iodine is toxic, and iodine solution mixed with a surfactant (e.g., povidone-iodine) retards healing. By contrast, cadeximer iodine gel traps the bacteria in biodegradable microsperes, where the organisms die.[72] The issue of whether to use topical antiseptics requires further exploration.

CONCEPTUAL MODEL

A variety of models have been used to guide the investigation of wound healing.[13,28,65,73,74] Models serve to clarify thinking, stimulate new hypotheses, and assist with analysis and synthesis of knowledge in a field. Gottrup et al[73] suggested that the choice of the model is driven by the problem under investigation, the method to be used, whether the study is animal or human, the variability of the phenomena being studied, the outcomes of interest, and the recruitment criteria. They stated that the major concerns are the question to be answered and the degree of sophistication or simplification desired. Current review articles address the various animal

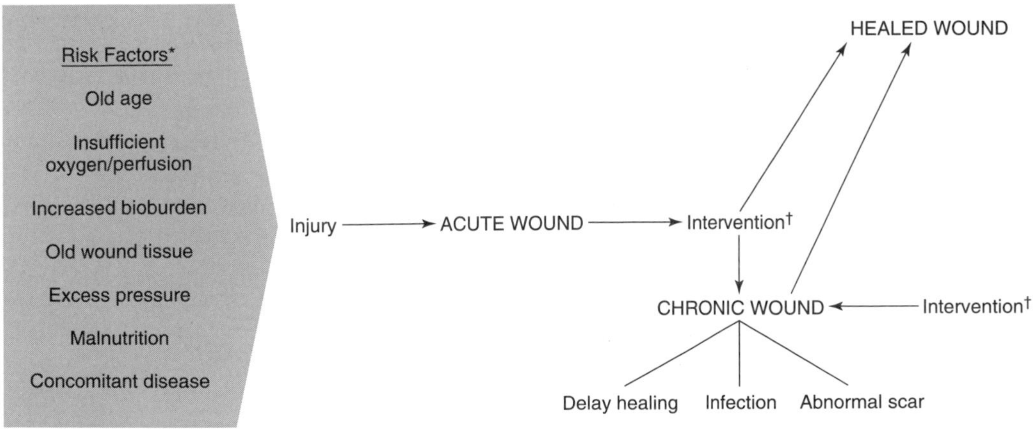

* Risk factors apply not only to the injury, but also throughout the healing/impaired healing process.
† Includes most local wound environment, oxygenation/perfusion, provision of substrates/nutrition, control of pain, temperature and stress, etc.

Figure 17-2 Conceptual model of impaired healing.

models available[74] as well as the in vitro and in vivo models available to examine soft tissue injury.[73]

This author proposes a conceptual model that addresses the factors involved in impaired healing (Figure 17-2). The initiating factor for all wounds is injury. The injury disrupts tissue. The risk factors interact with the injury to initially create an acute wound. With routine intervention, most acute wounds heal without impairment. However, some acute wounds become chronic wounds, and there is delayed healing, infection, or abnormal scar tissue formation. In this model the healing status is reevaluated and interventions are undertaken that lead to healing or to continuation of a chronic wound.

CASE STUDIES

CASE STUDY 1

Mr. C is a 58-year-old African American man with chronic obstructive pulmonary disease and chronic heart failure. Mr. C has been living at home and was admitted to the hospital with pneumonia. Now, a week after his admission to the nursing home for rehabilitation, Mr. C is oxygen and prednisone dependent and remains in bed with the head of the bed at a 70-degree angle. He is anxious, and his blood becomes desaturated with nearly any activity.

He has contractures of the hips and knees (maximal extension, 120 degrees) and must be transferred from the bed to a chair with a mechanical lift. His heels have areas of necrosis present that after debridement each are 9 cm in diameter. Complete debridement was not possible because the patient could not tolerate having the head of the bed lowered to position him for debridement. Topical enzymes were applied to the heels, and both edematous legs were wrapped to the knees with Ace bandages. Splints were used to remove pressure from the heels because his contractures, respiratory status, and anxiety prevented pressure removal from the heels with positioning.

Support for healing was provided with the moist wound environment supplied by the enzymatic debridement medication, maximizing blood flow to the tissues by ensuring appropriate intravascular volume and the use of the Ace bandages to reduce leg edema, and reducing bacterial burden with the debridement. The heel tissue was dead, but not infected, so there was no indication for systemic antibiotics. After a week, the wound was clean and beginning to decrease in size. The use of an Unna boot was considered to maintain compression from the knees to the toes and yet reduce the number of dressing changes, because the patient became anxious and combative when the dressings were changed daily. Twice a week, Unna boot changes were used initially, because the wound still was heavily exudative and its status needed to be monitored.

Approximately 10 days later, respiratory compromise was identified, and the patient was readmitted to the acute care unit for intubation, therapeutic paralysis, and ventilation. On his return to the long-term care facility, his leg edema had abated and heel ulcer size had decreased to 6 cm in diameter. The wounds were clean. Unna boots were continued and changed weekly until the wounds closed, then compression stockings were used to mitigate the effects of his underlying venous disease.

CASE STUDY 2

Mrs. K is a 58-year-old housewife who presented in the emergency department with a 1- or 2-day history of pain and swelling of the left leg. Some discoloration of the leg was noted, beginning the morning of admission; the discoloration increased during the day. Mrs. K reported chills but no fever, and decreased urination despite increased intake. In the emergency department, her blood pressure (BP) was 80/36, heart rate 130, respiratory rate 40, and temperature 97.2° F (36.2° C). Her condition was managed with fluid boluses, but she continued to be anuretic. She was started on renal dose dopamine. Her past medical history was noncontributory. She was admitted to the ICU because of the cellulitis of her left lower leg and her severe acidosis. She was started on antibiotic therapy, and a vascular surgeon was consulted to rule out compartment syndrome.

Mrs. K was diagnosed with necrotizing fasciitis at the bedside (after two incisions were made in the left lower leg showing necrotic tissue). The patient was taken to the operating room and underwent left guillotine above-the-knee amputation, with extensive debridement of necrotic tissue on her medial thigh.

Her postoperative course was notable for the following:

1. Hypotension, probably secondary to sepsis: A phenylephrine hydrochloride (Neosynephrine) drip with epinephrine and norepinephrine (Levophed) were used to maintain a mean arterial BP of 50–60. The low BP was likely caused by continued sepsis despite an antibiotic regimen of gentamycin, vancomycin, and piperacillin (Zosyn). Wound and blood cultures later revealed gram-negative rods, specifically *Escherichia coli,* which was adequately covered with antibiotics. Fever began to develop 12 hours after debridement and remained present through the remainder of her hospital course.

2. Acute renal failure (ARF): The course was also complicated with ARF with anuria, continued azotemia, a base deficit of −13, elevated creatinine to a level of 2.6, and evidence of fluid overload.

3. Progressive necrotizing fasciitis: By late on the day of surgery, the patient also had evidence of

continuing necrotizing fasciitis, with discoloration and development of blisters on the left lateral thigh, above the site of the amputation. The patient also had developed mottling on the right lower extremity, initially attributed to ischemia from vasoconstriction secondary to maximal vasopressor support. However, there was suspicion of necrotizing fasciitis, and the patient later developed blistering on the right leg as well.

This woman's case illustrates the complex and serious diagnostic and treatment issues that are seen with tissue infection. Careful history indicated that she scratched herself on the leg while working in the garden planting new flowers. It was hypothesized that the organism *(E. coli)* entered her system at that time. The localized cellulitis rapidly became infection and systemic sepsis. Surveillance was critical to early diagnosis and treatment.

SELECTED RESEARCH

Winter's work[55] on moist healing ushered in an era of prolific research in wound healing. Scientific expansion has been vast, spanning every aspect of healing and employing methods from the bench to the bedside. Nursing research in wound healing has made major inroads in several areas. Selected studies of significance to nursing will be reviewed here.

Braden's and Bergstom's development of a scale to predict pressure ulcer development in persons in long term care probably is one of the most important works of the last quarter century.[75] This instrument is a model for others to use in identifying high-risk patients. It is easy to use and inexpensive. It has high levels of validity and reliability across populations and settings.[9,76-79] Its wide adaptation after the publication of the Pressure Ulcer Prevention Guidelines[80] has revolutionized care for high-risk patients. Whether the prevalence of ulcers has decreased since the wide dissemination of the Pressure Ulcer Prevention Guideline is difficult to assess as a result of lack of comparative data because of differences in definition of terms and research methods used in conducting the research.[81]

The use of pressure ulcer risk assessment was studied in a group of elderly hip fracture patients.[82] In a retrospective chart audit of a stratified random sample (n = 545) from a target sample of 1 calendar year of California Medicare hip fracture patients (n = 17,402), medical record abstraction showed that pressure ulcer risk assessment was documented in only 44%. Of the cases in which risk assessment was performed, only 20% were assessed using an instrument with established validity and reliability. Of significance is the fact that 19% of the sample developed pressure ulcers, but the ulcers were unrelated to the documented risk status at hospital admission. These data indicate that although the instruments have been developed to provide evidence-based care, they are not used consistently.

Nutrition is an important component in the care of persons at risk for wound impairment. Guenter et al[83] examined the nutritional status of hospitalized patients (n = 120) with stage III or IV pressure ulcers. Most subjects had a neurological diagnosis. This descriptive correlational study showed that at admis-sion the mean albumin level was low (2.65 g/dl±0.56). Less than 10% of patients had a normal albumin level, yet mean body weight was 91% ± 11 of usual body weight, indicating these persons probably had protein malnutrition. In addition, patients had a low prealbumin level (11.03 mg/dl ± 6.09), indicating that their preadmission intake was not adequate for them to be anabolic. These data show that pressure ulcer patients were admitted to the hospital with seriously decreased protein intake. Why this situation exists and how nursing factors in the situation were not addressed in this study.

Psychosocial issues also are important in patients with impaired healing. Pieper, Szczepaniak, and Templin[84] explored psychosocial adjustment, coping, and quality of life in persons (n = 32) with venous ulcers and a history of intravenous drug use, most commonly heroin. Data from this cross-sectional study showed that ulcers had been present more than 10 years (mean 10.68 ± 3.39) with a mean ulcer size of 35.9 cm^2 ± 47.13. The wound area was positively correlated with psychological distress (r = 0.38) and pain intensity (r = 0.44), and inversely correlated with quality of life (r = –0.52). Thus big wounds are associated with distress, pain, and poor quality of life. Coping scores were quite variable ($p < 0.001$) and not significantly related to wound area. This work is a beginning in understanding the impact of venous ulcers on the life of persons who are former intravenous drug users. Further work is needed in this area, especially in light of the large proportion of the population who has a history of intravenous drug use and our limited knowledge about pain management in this population.

Nurses are doing important work in extending the understanding of the mechanisms of impaired healing. In a study conducted at the Wound Healing Laboratory at the National Institute of Nursing Research, Wysocki et al[85] explored the balance of proteases and their inhibitors in acute and chronic wounds to understand their role in the development of new extracellular matrix, cell migration, and remodeling. Using wound fluid from mastectomy wounds (acute wounds) and venous ulcers (chronic wounds) and sera from healthy volunteers, they explored the expression and temporal sequence of plasminogen activators and inhibitors. The investigators measured urokinase plasminogen activator (uPA), plasminogen activator inhibitor-1 (PAI-1), and gelatinase-B (metalloproteinase-9). Data showed that the chronic wounds had higher levels of uPA that decreased as the wounds healed and approached those of acute wounds. Also, as the wound healed, there was a balance reached between the activator (uPA) and the inhibitor (PAI-1). These findings suggest that a proteolytic cascade is initiated by the PA-plasmin system and that the imbalance between with activator and inhibitor plus the presence of metalloprotease-9 contributes to delayed healing in chronic wounds. These data also indicate that biological markers are useful in assessing the balance between the proteases and their inhibitors.

The mechanism by which treatment enhances healing of chronic wounds also has been explored. Leg elevation, long the mainstay of treatment in venous disease, and its effect on oxygenation and perfusion were explored by Wipke-Tevis et al.[86] Subjects (n = 20) with venous ulcers had transcutaneous oxygen measured on the ulcer leg when positioned (1) supine, (2) with leg elevation at 30 degrees, (3) sitting, and (4) standing. Minimal changes occurred when subjects breathed room air. After an oxygen challenge, perfusion was again measured. Findings showed that with the oxygen challenge, when compared with supine positioning, perfusion was lower during leg elevation, sitting and standing ($p < 0.05$). Further work is needed to determine whether the very basic treatment of venous ulcers with leg elevation and positioning is, in fact, beneficial.

QUESTIONS FOR FUTURE STUDY

An array of research questions surround the concept of impaired healing. They can be thought of as related to mechanisms, risk factors, surveillance, and treatment. There are basic questions as to the mechanisms of impairment, such as the role of reperfusion injury in the development of pressure ulcers and the appropriate role of proteases in various phases. Much research remains to identify populations at risk and mechanisms of impaired healing. It is not clear what the best system is for surveillance of these wounds. In fact, further work is needed to define the dimensions that constitute healing. The work of Gardner et al,[54] documents the need to think more inclusively about how to diagnose infection. A parsimonious model to track pressure ulcer healing has been proposed with only three dimensions of assessment. It needs prospective verification before it can be widely used in care.[41]

Further work remains to clarify the therapy or cluster of therapies that best prevent impaired healing or interrupt the cycle of impairment. Systemic support for healing is seen as fundamental to reversing the impaired healing cycle and major areas of research on systemic therapies include hydration, nutritional support, and oxygenation/perfusion. Research in this area is in its early stages.

It is not known what volume of fluid is needed to prevent impaired healing and return healing to its normal pace. Data are lacking on the rate at which fluids should be given and whether fluids high in some specific substrate need to be provided (e.g., normal saline solution versus Ringer's lactate). Yet it is recognized that the balance needs to be found between reversing impaired healing and causing iatrogenic problems (e.g., congestive heart failure).

Nutrition is a major factor in preventing impaired healing and its sequelae and is universally accepted as critical to healing. Basic issues, such as the number of calories required for healing, remain to be resolved. There are estimates of the amount of protein required to reverse impaired healing, but again, these are only estimates. In addition, the specific combination of vitamins and minerals needed to support healing has only been estimated. Innovative therapies, such as anabolic therapy and the use of specific substrates such as arginine, have been examined in some populations. Further work is needed to determine their applicability across the various populations with impaired healing.

Early studies established that oxygen and perfusion are pivotal to healing; yet how to manipulate oxygen and perfusion and the role of analgesia in supporting oxygenation-perfusion and healing. Much more work remains to be done in examining how pain can be modulated to influence oxygenation-perfusion in patients with delayed healing and wound infection.

The role of temperature modulation as an adjunct to oxygenation-perfusion in maximizing perfusion has not been well examined. The effects of simple therapies, such as warm stockings for chronic foot wounds or additional blankets for those with sacral wounds, have not been explored. How to modulate autonomic nervous system stimulation and its concomitant vasoconstriction deserves additional attention. For example, the role of strategies to mitigate physical or emotional stress and anxiety on oxygenation-perfusion has largely been neglected from a scientific perspective.

Extensive research in local therapies has led to innovative product development and cutting-edge therapies in treating wounds. Dressings, topical therapies, and support surfaces have improved. Topical therapies for reversal of impaired healing need additional study. The issue of growth factors, antioxidants, and various cytokines in the prevention and treatment of impaired healing needs additional attention. What substrates should be applied to the wound at what dose and what frequency remain questions that need explication.

Fundamental issues require further exploration, such as the type of cleansing that is most efficacious, the frequency with which it should be done, and the amount of fluid or duration of cleansing that needs to be undertaken. There also is the question of what topical agent, if any, to use to control bacteria, how long to use it, and under what circumstances. There are basic issues of support surfaces for persons confined to bed or wheelchair; the optimal interface pressure is not known, and the frequency of turning and pressure relief has not been scientifically determined. The literature does not indicate whether the level of pressure relief needed depends on body weight or composition (e.g., thin persons compared with obese persons).

Finally, little work has been done on the psychosocial effects of healing. There is a need to understand the responses to impaired healing and how to modulate them.

Impaired healing remains an area rich in researchable questions. Only with further scientific study can the prevention of impaired healing and treatment of persons with these wounds approach the ideal of evidence-based care.

REFERENCES

1. Lazarus, G.S., Cooper, D.M., Knighton, D.R., Margolis, D.J., Pecoraro, R.E., Rodeheaver, G., Robson, M.C. (1994). Definitions and guidelines for assessment of wounds and evaluation of healing. *Archives of Dermatology 130,* 489-493.
2. Margolis, D.J., Berlin, J.A., & Strom, B.L. (1996). Interobserver agreement, sensitivity, and specificity of a "healed" chronic wound. *Wound Repair and Regeneration 4,* 335-338.
3. Stotts, N.A., & Cavanaugh, C.E. (1999). Assessing the patient with a wound. *Home Healthcare Nurse 17*(1), 27-35.
4. Centers for Disease Control and Prevention, National Center for Health Statistics. (1997). Vital and Health Statistics, Detailed Diagnoses and Procedures, National Hospital Discharge Survey, 1994. Vol. 127. Hyattsville, Md.: DHHS Publications.
5. Mangram, A.J., Horan, T.C., Pearson, M.L., Silver, L.C., & Jarvis, W.R. (1999). Guideline for prevention of surgical site infection, 1999. *Infection Control Hospital Epidemiology 20,* 250-278.
6. Phillips, T., Stanton, B., Provan, A., & Lew, R. (1994). A study of the impact of leg ulcers on quality of life: Financial, social, and psychologic implications. *Journal of the American Academy of Dermatology 31,* 49-53.
7. Barczak, C.A., Barnett, R.I., Childs, E.J., & Bosley, L.M. (1997). Fourth National Pressure Ulcer Prevalence Survey. *Advances in Wound Care 10*(4), 18-26.
8. Brandeis, G.H., Morris, J.N., Nash, D.J., & Lipsitz, L.A. (1990). The epidemiology and natural history of pressure ulcers in elderly nursing home residents. *Journal of the American Medical Association 264*(22), 2905-2909.
9. Bergstrom, N., Braden, B., Kemp, M., Champagne, M., & Ruby, E. (1996). Multi-site study of incidence of pressure ulcers and the relationship between risk level, demographic characteristics, diagnoses, and prescription of preventive interventions. *Journal of the American Geriatrics Society 44*(1), 22-30.
10. National Diabetes Fact Sheet: National estimates and general information of diabetes in the United States. Accessed at www.cdc.gov/diabetes/pubs/facts98/htm.
11. Hunt, T.K. (2000). Why wounds fail to heal. In G.L. Moneta (ed.), *New approaches in wound healing: Novel surgical techniques and advances in tissue engineering* (pp. 9-13). Littleton, Colo.: Postgraduate Institute for Medicine.
12. Economides, P.A., & Veves, A. (2000). Etiopathogenesis of foot ulceration in wounds. *WOUNDS 12*(6 Suppl B), 3-6.
13. Hunt, T.K., & Hopf, H.W. (1997). Wound healing and wound infection: What surgeons and anesthesiologists can do. *Surgical Clinics of North America 77*(3), 587-606.
14. Kurz, A., Sessler, D.I., & Lenhardt, R. (1996). Perioperative normothermia to reduce the incidence of surgical-wound infection and shorten hospitalization. Study of Wound Infection and Temperature Group [see comments]. *New England Journal of Medicine 334*(19), 1209-1215.
15. Krasner, D. (1998). Painful venous ulcers: Themes and stories about their impact on quality of life. *Ostomy/Wound Management 44*(9), 38-42, 44, 46, passum.
16. Jorgensen, L.N., Kallehave, F., Christensen, E., Siana, J.E., & Gottrup, F. (1998). Less collagen production in smokers. *Surgery 123*(4), 450-455.
17. Nixon, J. (2001). The pathophysiology and aetiogy of pressure ulcers. In M.J. Morison (ed.), *The prevention and treatment of pressure ulcers* (pp. 17-36). St Louis: Mosby.
18. Steed, D.L. (1995). Clinical evaluation of recombinant human platelet-derived growth factor for the treatment of lower extremity diabetic foot ulcers. Diabetic ulcer study group. *Journal of Vascular Surgery 21,* 71-78, discussion 79-81.
19. Margolis, D.J., Berlin, J.A., & Strom, B.L. (1999). Risk factors associated with the failure of a venous leg ulcer to heal. *Archives of Dermatology 135*(8), 920-926.
20. Waldrop, J., & Doughty, D. (2001). Wound-healing physiology. In R.A. Bryant (ed.), *Acute and chronic*

wounds: Nursing management (2nd ed., pp. 17-39). St Louis: Mosby.

21. Stotts, N.A., & Wipke-Tevis, D.D. (2001). In D.L. Krasner, G.T. Rodeheaver, R.G. Sibbald (eds.), *Co-factors in impaired healing. Chronic wound care: A clinical source book for healthcare professionals* (3rd ed.). Wayne, Pa.: HMP Communications.
22. Stadelmann, W.K., Digenis, A.G., & Tobin, G.R. (1998). Physiology and healing dynamics of chronic cutaneous wounds. *American Journal of Surgery 176*(Suppl 2A), 26S-38S.
23. Mast, B.A., & Schultz, G.S. (1996). Interactions of cytokines, growth factors, and proteases in acute and chronic wounds. *Wound Repair and Regeneration 4,* 411-414.
24. Adzick, N.S., & Lorenz, H.P. (1994). Cells, matrix, growth factors, and the surgeon. The biology of scarless fetal wound repair. *Annals of Surgery 220,* 10-18.
25. Browse, N.L., Burnand, K.G. (1982). The cause of venous ulceration. *Lancet 2,* 243-245.
26. Coleridge Smith, P.D., Thomas, P., Scurr, J.H., Dormandy, J.A. (1988). Causes of venous ulceration: A new hypothesis. *British Medical Journal 296,* 1726-1727.
27. Sandeman, D., & Shearman, C.P. (1999). Clinical aspects of lower limb ulceration. In R. Mani, V. Falanga, C.P. Shearman, & D. Sandeman (eds.), *Chronic wound healing* (pp. 4-25). Philadelphia: W.B. Saunders.
28. Peirce, S.M., Skalak, T.C., Rodeheaver, G.T. (2000). Ischemia-reperfusion injury in chronic pressure ulcer formation: A skin model in the rat. *Wound Repair and Regeneration 8,* 68-76.
29. Kosiak, M. (1959). Etiology and pathology of ischemic ulcers. *Archives Physical Medicine and Rehabilitation 40,* 62-69.
30. Boulton, A.J.M., Vileikyte, L. (2000). Pathogenesis of diabetic foot ulceration and measurement of neuropathy. *WOUNDS 12*(6 Suppl B), 12B-18B.
31. Robson, M. (1997). Wound infection: A failure of wound healing caused by an imbalance of bacteria. *Surgical Clinics of North America 77*(3), 637-650.
32. Tarnazzer, R.W., & Shultz, G.S. (1996). Biochemical analysis of acute and chronic wound environments. *Wound Repair and Regeneration 4,* 321-325.
33. Robson, M. (1999). Award recipient address: Lessons learned from the sport of wound watching. *Wound Repair and Regeneration 7*(1), 2-6.
34. Tredget, E.E., Nedelec, B., Scott, P.C., & Ghahary, A. (1997). Hypertrophic scar, keloids, and contractures. The cellular and molecular basis for therapy. *Surgical Clinics of North America 77*(3), 701-730.
35. Ehrlich, H.P. (1998). The physiology of wound healing. A summary of normal and abnormal wound healing processes. *Advances in Wound Care 11*(7), 326-328.
36. Bates-Jensen, B.M., Vredevoe, D.L., & Brecht, M.L. (1992). Validity and reliability of the Pressure Ulcer Status Tool. *Decubitus 5*(6), 20-28.
37. Bates-Jensen, B.M. (1997). The Pressure Ulcer Status Tool a few thousand assessments later. *Advances in Wound Care 10*(5), 65-73.
38. Ferrell, B.A., Artinian, B.M., & Sessing, D. (1995). The Sessing Scale for assessment of pressure ulcers healing. *Journal of the American Geriatric Society 43,* 37-40.
39. Sussman, C., & Swanson, G. (1997). Utility of the Sussman Wound Healing Tool in predicting wound healing outcomes in physical therapy. *Advances in Wound Care 10*(5), 74-77.
40. Thomas, D., Rodcheaver, G.T., Bartolucci, A.A., Frantz, R.A., Sussman, C., Ferrell, B.A., et al. (1997). Pressure ulcer scale for healing: Derivation and validation of the PUSH tool. *Advances in Wound Care 10*(5), 96-101.
41. Stotts, N.A., Rodeheaver, G.T., Thomas, D.R., Frantz, R.A., Bartolucci, A.A., Sussman, C., et al. (2001). An instrument to measure healing in pressure ulcers: Development and validation of the Pressure Ulcer Scale for Healing (PUSH). *Journals of Gerontology. Series A: Biological Sciences and Medical Sciences 56*(12), M795-799.
42. Pareira, M.D., & Serkes, K.D. (1962). Predictors of wound disruption by use of the healing ridge. *Surgery, Gynecology, and Obstetrics 115,* 72.
43. Carlson, M.A. (1997). Acute wound failure. *Surgical Clinics of North America 77*(3), 607-636.
44. Feedar, J.A., Kloth, L.C., & Gentzkow, G.D. (1991). Chronic dermal ulcer healing enhanced with monophasic pulsed electrical stimulation. *Physical Therapy 71*(9), 639-649.
45. Brown-Etris, M. (1995). Measuring healing in wounds. *Advances in Wound Care 8*(4), 535-585.
46. Thomas, A.C., & Wysocki, A.B. (1990). The healing wound: A comparison of three clinically useful methods of measurement. *Decubitus 3*(1), 18-25.
47. Schubert, V. (1997). Measuring the area of chronic wounds for consistent documentation in clinical practice. *WOUNDS 9*(5), 153-159.
48. Frantz, R.A., & Johnson, D.A. (1992). Stereophotography and computerized image analysis: A three-dimensional method for measuring wound healing. *Wounds 4*(2), 58-62.
49. Bergstrom, N., Bennett, M.A., Carlson, C.E., et al. (1994). *Treatment of pressure ulcers: Clinical practice guideline, No. 15.* Rockville, Md.: U.S. Department of Health and Human Services. Public Health Services, Agency for Health Care Policy and Research. AHCPR Publication No. 95-0652.
50. Plassman, P., Melhuish, J.M., & Harding, K.G. (1994). Methods of measuring wound size: A comparative study. *Wounds 6*(2), 54-61.
51. Resch, C.S., Kerner, E., Robson, M.C., Heggers, J.P., Scherer, M., Boertman, J.A., et al. (1988). Pressure sore volume measurement: A technique to document and record wound healing. *Journal of the American Geriatric Society 36,* 444-446.
52. Stotts, N.A., Salazar, M.J., Wipke-Tevis, D., & McAdoo, E. (1996). Accuracy of alginate molds for measuring wound volumes when prepared and stored under varying conditions. *WOUNDS 8*(5), 158-164.
53. Van Rijswijk, L., Braden, B.J. (1999). Pressure ulcer patient and wound assessment: An AHCPR clinical practice guideline update. *Ostomy/Wound Management 45*(1A Suppl), 56-67.
54. Gardner, S.E., Frantz, R.A., Doebbeling, B.N. (2001). The validity of the clinical signs and symptoms used to identify localized chronic wound infection. *Wound Repair and Regeneration 9*(3), 178-186.
55. Winter, G. (1962). Formation of the scab and the rate of epithelialization of superficial wounds in the skin of the young domestic pig. *Nature 193,* 293-294.
56. Ovington, L.G. (1998). The well-dressed wound: An overview of dressing types. *WOUNDS 10*(Suppl A), 1A-11A.
57. Baranoski, S. (1999). Wound dressings: Challenging decisions. *Home Healthcare Nurse 17*(1), 19-25.

58. Jonsson, K., Jensen, J.A., Goodson, W.H. 3rd, West, J.M., & Hunt, T.K. (1987). Assessment of perfusion in postoperative patients using tissue oxygen measurements. *British Journal of Surgery 74*(4), 263-267.
59. Jonsson, K., Jensen, J.A., Goodson, W.H. 3rd, Scheuenstuhl, H., West, J., Hopf, H.W. (1991). Tissue oxygenation, anemia, and perfusion in relation to wound healing in surgical patients. *Annals of Surgery 214*(5), 605-613.
60. Hartmann, M., Jonsson, K., Zederfeldt, B. (1992). Effect of tissue perfusion and oxygenation on accumulation of collagen in healing wounds. Randomized study in patients after major abdominal operations. *European Journal of Surgery 158,* 521-526.
61. Heughan, C., Grislis, G., & Hunt, T.K. (1974). The effect of anemia on wound healing. *Annals of Surgery 179*(2), 163-167.
62. Jensen, J.A., Goodson, W.H. 3rd, Vasconez, L.O. & Hunt, T.K. (1986). Wound healing in anemia. *Western Journal of Medicine 144*(4), 465-467.
63. Thomas, D.R. (1997). Specific nutritional factors in wound healing. *Advances in Wound Care 10*(4), 40-43.
64. Rodeheaver, G.T. (1999). Pressure ulcer debridement and cleansing: A review of current literature. *Ostomy/Wound Management 45*(Suppl 1A), 805-855.
65. Witte, M.B., & Barbul, A. (1997). General principles of wound healing. *Surgical Clinics of North America 77*(3), 509-528.
66. Rodeheaver, G.T., Kurtz, L., Kicher, B.J., & Edlich, R.F. (1980). Pluronic F-68: A promising new skin wound cleaner. *Annals of Emergency Medicine 9*(11), 572-576.
67. Foresman, P.A., Payne, D.S., Becker, D., Lewis, D., & Rodeheaver, G.T. (1993). A relative toxicity index for wound cleansers. *WOUNDS 5*(5), 226-231.
68. Green, V.A., Carlson, H.C., Briggs, R.L., & Stewart, J.L. (1971). A comparison of the efficacy of pulsed mechanical lavage with that of rubber-bulb syringe irrigation in removal of debris from avulsive wounds. *Oral Surgery, Oral Medicine, and Oral Pathology 32*(1), 158-164.
69. Rodeheaver, G.T., Petty, D., Thacker, J.G.AX, Edgerton, M.T., & Edlich, R.F. (1975). Wound cleansing by high pressure irrigation. *Surgery, Gynecology & Obstetrics 141*(3), 357-362.
70. Campany, E., Johnson, R.W., & Whitney, J.D. (2000). Nurses' knowledge of wound irrigation and pressures generated during simulated wound irrigation. *Journal of Wound, Ostomy and Continence Nursing 27*(6), 296-303.
71. Falabella, A. (1998). Debridement of wounds. *WOUNDS 10*(Suppl C), 1-9.
72. Eaglstein, W.H., & Falanga, V. (1997). Chronic wounds. *Surgical Clinics of North America 77*(3), 689-700.
73. Gottrup, F., Agren, M.S., & Karlsmark, T. (2000). Models for use in wound healing research: A survey focusing on in vitro and in vivo adult soft tissue [see comments]. *Wound Repair and Regeneration 8*(2), 83-96.
74. Davidson, J.M. (2001). Experimental animal wound models. *WOUNDS 13*(1), 9-23.
75. Braden, B., & Bergstrom, N. (1987). A conceptual schemata for the study of the etiology of pressure sores. *Rehabilitation Nursing 12*(1), 8-12.
76. Bergstrom, N., Braden, B.J., Laguzza, A., & Holman, V. (1987). The Braden Scale for Predicting Pressure Sore Risk. *Nursing Research 36*(4), 205-210.
77. Bergstrom, N., Demuth, P.J., & Braden, B.J. (1987). A clinical trial of the Braden Scale for Predicting Pressure Sore Risk. *Nursing Clinics of North America 22*(2), 417-428.
78. Braden, B.J., & Bergstrom, N. (1994). Predictive validity of the Braden Scale for pressure sore risk in a nursing home population. *Research in Nursing and Health 17*(6), 459-470.
79. Bergstrom, N., Braden, B., Kemp, M., Champagne, M., & Ruby, E. (1998). Predicting pressure ulcer risk: A multisite study of the predictive validity of the Braden Scale. *Nursing Research 47*(5), 261-269.
80. Panel for the Prediction and Prevention of Pressure Ulcers in Adults. (1992). *Pressure ulcers in adults: Prediction and prevention.* Rockville, Md.: U.S. Department of Health and Human Services. Public Health services, Agency for Health Care Policy and Research, Publication 92-0047.
81. National Pressure Ulcer Advisory Panel: Cuddigan, J., Ayello, E.A., & Sussman, C. (eds.), (2001). Pressure ulcers in America: Prevalence, incidence, and implications for the future. Reston, Va.: NPUAP.
82. Stotts, N.A., Deosaransingh, K., Roll, F.J., & Newman, J. (1998). Underutilization of pressure ulcer risk assessment in hip fracture patients. *Advances in Wound Care 11*(1), 32-38.
83. Guenter, P., Malyszek, R., Bliss, D.Z., Steffe, T., O'Hara, D., LaVan, F., et al. (2000). Survey of nutritional status in newly hospitalized patients with stage III or stage IV pressure ulcers. *Advances in Wound Care 13*(4), 164-168.
84. Pieper, B., Szczepaniak, K., & Templin, T. (2000). Psychosocial adjustment, coping, and quality of life in persons with venous ulcers and a history of intravenous drug use. *Journal of Wound, Ostomy and Continence Nursing 27,* 227-237.
85. Wysocki, A., Kusakabe, A.O., Change, S., & Tuan, T.L. (1999). Temporal expression of urokinase plasminogen activator, plasminogen activator inhibitor and gelatinase-B in chronic wound fluid switches from a chronic to acute wound profile with progression to healing. *Wound Repair and Regeneration 7,* 154-165.
86. Wipke-Tevis, D.D., Stotts, N.A., Williams, D.A., Froelicher, E.S., & Hunt, T.K. (2001). Tissue oxygenation, perfusion, and position in patients with venous leg ulcers. *Nursing Research 50*(1), 24-32.

CHAPTER 18 Altered Clotting

JANICE D. NUNNELEE

DEFINITION

Altered clotting is the state in which the body does not respond appropriately to factors related to coagulation of blood. This reflects a state of disequilibrium in hemostasis, occurring in the regulation of clot formation, retraction and/or lysis of the clot. Coagulation depends on the interaction of the classic triad of vessel wall injury, activation of coagulation factors, and the body's fibrinolytic system. Alteration of any portion of this interaction or system can result in hemorrhage, thrombosis, or changes in laboratory values that are of no clinical significance. Clinically, the extremes are bleeding and clotting.

PREVALENCE AND POPULATIONS AT RISK

Altered clotting can occur as a result of inherited factors or acquired factors. The incidence of inherited clotting problems is low. Recent research, however, has uncovered new inherited factors, which are more common than previously suspected.[1] Inherited coagulopathies that may result in a hypercoagulable state include antithrombin III (ATIII), protein C and S deficiencies, antiphospholipid antibody syndrome (anticardiolipin, or aCL, lupus anticoagulant),[2] G20210A prothrombin mutation,[3] inherited homocysteinemia,[4] and factor V Leiden.[1,5] Recent research indicates that high plasma levels of factor VII increase the risk of recurrent thrombosis. The most common inherited bleeding disorders are hemophilia A and von Willebrand's disease. The incidence of each disorder is listed in Table 18-1.

Altered clotting can occur in all patients across the life span. The elderly and very young children are at high risk for mortality and morbidity resulting from the complications due to altered clotting. Additionally, patients with critical illness, injury, pregnancy, or other comorbidities are at higher risk for developing altered clotting.

Although the reason for some bleeding or hypercoagulable states may be unexplained,[7] acquired disorders account for most significant bleeding or clotting occurrences. Acquired disorders often occur in conjunction with multiple disorders[8] and this makes the diagnosis and interpretation of laboratory data difficult. Patients with liver disease may have vitamin K deficiencies, which result in decreased production of factors II, V, VII, IX, X, and ATIII. Additionally liver disease may contribute to thrombocytopenia and altered fibrinolytic activity. Deep venous thrombosis (DVT), pulmonary embolism (PE), bleeding, heparin induced thrombocytopenia (HIT), and disseminated intravascular coagulation (DIC) are examples of the results of altered clotting.[7,9]

DVT is a common acquired clotting abnormality with variable prevalence rates depending on the population. For example, in the general surgical population, the prevalence is 19 percent to 25 percent. The prevalence increases to 50 percent to 60 percent in the orthopedic surgical population undergoing repair for a fractured hip, or receiving total hip or knee arthroplasty. The prevalence in persons who've sustained a spinal cord injury is 67 percent to 100 percent.[10]

RISK FACTORS

Environmental, Personal, and Developmental Factors

Thrombotic States. Virchow's classic thrombosis triad of stasis, vessel wall injury, and alteration in coagulable state[11] occurs because of specific events. It is believed that stasis alone does not result in thrombosis.

Stressors that contribute to stasis and a resultant decrease in blood flow velocity are immobility, bed rest, obesity, dehydration, and hypotension. Stasis allows clotting factors to stay in one area and form a clot; however, platelets do not adhere to an intact endothelium. Stasis further increases the risk of clot formation because of decreased circulation to the liver and reticuloendothelial system, which have a role in clearing activated clotting factors from circulation.

TABLE 18-1 Incidence of Inherited Coagulopathies

TYPE	INCIDENCE
ATIII	1:2000–5000
Protein C	1:16,000
Protein S	1:16,000
Antiphospholipid/ anticardiolipin	Not clearly known
Factor V Leiden	5% of whites; <2% in other groups
G20221 0a mutation	± 8% of whites[3]
Homocysteinemia	12% of population[4]
Hemophilia A (factor VIIIC)	1:5000 male births[6]
Hemophilia B (factor IX)	1:30,000 male births[6]
von Willebrand's disease	4:100,000 to 5:1000 (depending on type, some subtypes only found within families)

Data from Twardowski, P., & Green, D. (1999). Thrombotic disorders in vascular patients. In V. Fahey (ed.), *Vascular Nursing* (3rd ed.). Philadelphia: W.B. Saunders; and Eichinger, S., Minar, E., Hirschl, M., Bialonczyk, C., Stain, M., Mannhalter, C., et al. (1999). The risk of early recurrent venous thromboembolism after oral anticoagulant therapy in patients with G20210A transition in the prothrombin gene. *Thrombosis and Hemostasis 81*(1), 14-17; and Arun, B., & Kessler, C.M. (2001). Clinical manifestations and therapy of the hemophilias. In R. Colman, J. Hirsch, V. Marder, A. Clowes, & J. George (eds.), *Hemostasis and thrombosis: Basic principles and clinical practice* (pp. 815-824). Philadelphia: Lippincott Williams & Wilkins.

Vessel wall injury allows clotting factors to adhere to the endothelium. A primitive response to injury is constriction of the vessel, but more subtle injury results in activation of the coagulation cascade. Vessel wall injury may result from overdistention of the vessel, pressure, trauma, shear stress, or irritating medications. Disruption of a vessel wall activates the coagulation system, and a clot is the result.

Coagulation status is the third factor that can result in thrombosis. Coagulation factors are produced in the liver; therefore diseases such as cirrhosis, hepatitis, and vitamin K deficiency affect clotting. Large tumors are commonly associated with thrombus formation and some studies have noted that almost half of these patients develop thromboses.[12] Carcinoma can cause a hypercoagulable state as a result of decreased coagulation inhibitors (ATIII, proteins C and S) and release of tissue thromboplastin[13] as well as a low grade localized intravascular coagulation. Deep venous thrombosis (DVT) occurs because of alterations in one or more of these three factors. Important risk factors for DVT are increasing age, prolonged immobility, cancer, orthopedic surgeries such as repair of hip fracture and knee and hip arthroplasty, abdominal surgery, major trauma, spinal cord injury, stroke, and history of thromboembolic events.[10]

Developmentally, there are ages at which altered clotting is more common. Each type of altered clotting that will be discussed has a typical age of onset. Elderly persons may be at higher risk for thromboembolism because of their medications, decreased mobility, increased rate of injury, the presence of comorbidities, or other phenomena. Younger persons (under the age of 50) in whom thromboses occur should be screened for coagulopathies.[13] Infants who have serious illness are at higher risk for thrombosis. Studies in children and neonates with thrombosis have found that more than 80% have more than two risk factors for thrombosis.[14,15] In families in which children are found to have thrombotic disease, the adults and other children should be screened for inherited disorders. Often investigation of the adults (parents) supplies the diagnosis, as interpretation of tests in infants is difficult.[16]

Bleeding States. Bleeding disorders fall into four categories, according to their causative factors: vascular disorders, platelet disorders, abnormalities in the platelet adhesive protein (von Willebrand's disease),[8] and coagulation disorders (hemophilia A and B and other factor deficiencies). These can be divided further into genetic disorders and acquired disorders.

In vascular disorders, bleeding can occur because of injured, inflamed, or otherwise damaged vessels or from abnormal permeability of the vessel wall. These states can be a result of inherited diseases such as Ehlers-Danlos syndrome, Rendu-Osler-Weber syndrome, and other disorders or acquired problems, such as Cushing syndrome, Henoch-Schönlein's purpura,[17] dietary deficiencies (e.g., scurvy), infections, and medications.

Platelet disorders result from decreased platelet production or from increased platelet destruction.[8] Inherited disorders of platelet production often end in early death,[12] and patients who live past childhood often have infections as causes of death. Causes of decreased platelet production include aplastic anemia, bone marrow diseases (e.g., Hodgkin's disease and leukemia), bone marrow depression secondary to drugs (e.g., chemotherapy, gold, and nonsteroidal antiinflammatory medications), liver failure, renal failure, and vitamin deficiencies, such as B_{12} or folate. Increased platelet destruction can result from preeclampsia (hemolysis, elevated liver enzymes, low platelet [HELLP] syndrome), hemolytic-uremic syndrome (female to male ratio 3:1),[12] renal disease, thrombotic thrombocytopenic purpura (TTP), and DIC.[9]

A category of platelet bleeding disorders is von Willebrand's disease. This is a congenital defect found on chromosome 12. The coagulation disorders of hemophilia A and B are sex-linked disorders that are graded by severity.

MECHANISMS

Normal Clotting

Blood clotting is initiated through the extrinsic or intrinsic system; the critical component is a tissue factor (i.e., thromboplastin, which is an intracellular lipoprotein) (Figure 18-1). (For a full discussion of normal clotting, see Coleman et al.[18]) The most important plasma component is factor VII. Additional factors in the clotting cascade include factors IX and X, prothrombin, proteins C and S. All of these factors exist in the blood and vascular system (including the liver). Vessel injury results in the exposure of tissue thromboplastin to blood and the initiation of the clotting cascade (extrinsic system). This process allows activated factor VIIa and phospholipid to activate factor IX to IXa. In turn, factor IXa converts factor X to Xa. The intrinsic system works in tandem with the extrinsic system. The intrinsic system exists entirely within the vascular system and also includes the contact activation of factor XI to XIa, which, in the presence of Ca^{++}, converts IX to IXa. This latter conversion begins a pathway for blood coagulation (the common pathway) that does not depend on factor VII—namely, the activation of factor X to Xa. Factor Xa converts prothrombin to thrombin. Thrombin then cleaves fibrinopeptides from fibrinogen and converts factor XIII to XIIIa, which links the fibrin clot (see Figure 18-1).

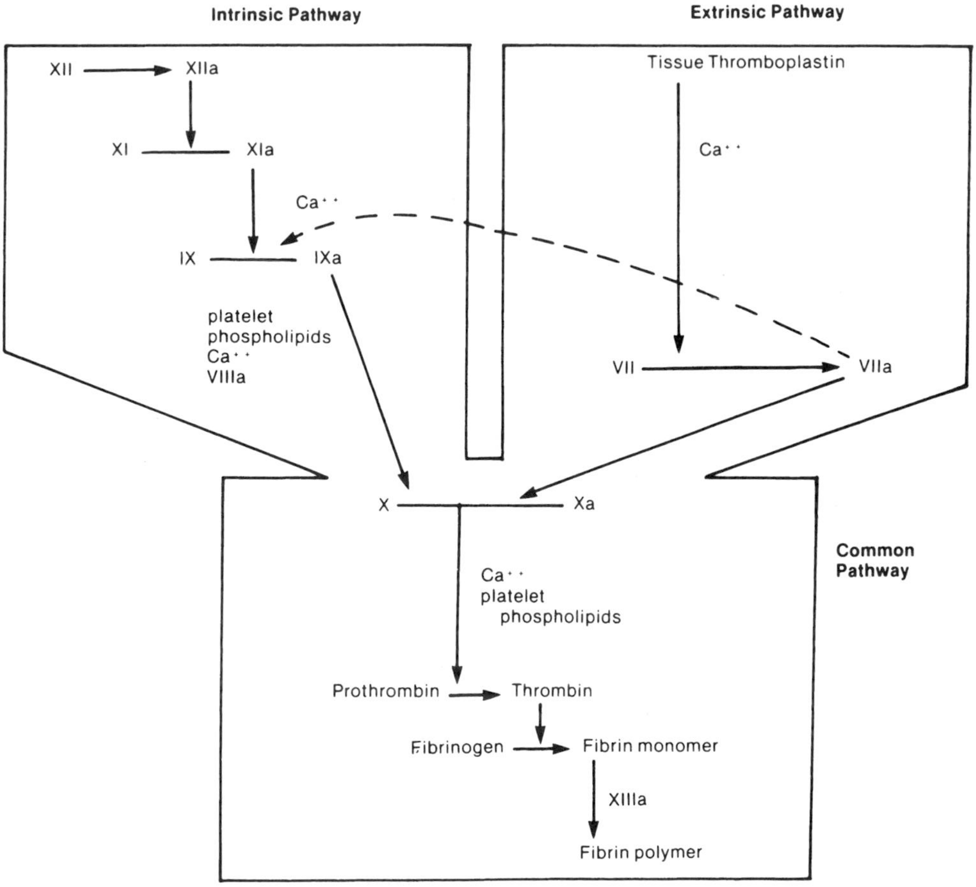

Figure 18-1 Coagulation processes: intrinsic, extrinsic, and the common pathways. (Adapted from Hirsch, J., & Brain, E.A. [1983]. *Homeostasis and thrombosis: A conceptual approach* [2nd ed.]. New York: Churchill Livingstone.)

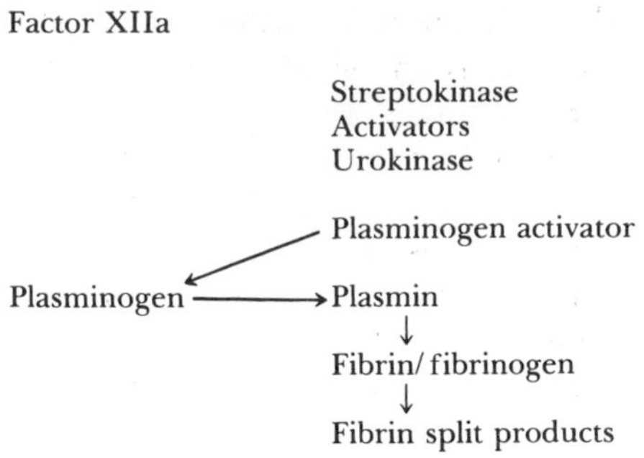

Figure 18-2 Fibrinolytic pathway.

Thrombin actually acts on multiple parts of the system, including fibrinogen, factors XIII, V, and VIII, platelet membrane proteins, and proteins S and C. Additionally, thrombin helps to recruit platelets to the site of the clot, depending on how active the intrinsic and extrinsic pathways are.

Fibrin aggregation occurs in the second stage of hemostasis (the first stage is the platelet aggregate). The resulting fibrin mass holds platelets together and attaches them to the vessel wall.

A number of forces keeps clots from extending and maintains hemostasis. First, normal blood flow disrupts the clot, and the platelets that are not strongly adherent to the clot are washed free. Second, thrombin in the hemostatic plug ultimately inactivates those factors that it was potentiating.[18] Third, soluble activated coagulation proteins (e.g., thrombin, factor Xa) may diffuse away from the clot and bind to inhibiting proteins, such as ATIII. Fourth, fibrinolysis occurs as a result of the fibrinolytic system. Plasminogen is converted to plasmin, a protease active enzyme. The process of conversion is controlled by factor XIIa, thrombin, and plasminogen activators.[18] Tissue plasminogen activator (t-PA) is produced by the endothelial cells along with prourokinase, and both have the ability to convert plasminogen to plasmin. Plasmin digests fibrin as well as factors V and VIII, creating fibrin degradation products (FDPs), which bind with fibrin monomers and prevent further clot formation. The clot is gradually reduced. During clot breakdown, the FDPs have unique subsets such as the D-dimer, which provides a serum marker for fibrinolysis (Figure 18-2).

Altered Clotting

Mechanisms of altered clotting involve the abnormal factors that impair the normal mechanisms of hemostasis, resulting in bleeding or thrombosis. The mechanisms of normal hemostasis must work against both thrombosis and hemorrhage; they depend on a balance of the procoagulant system and inhibitors and the fibrinolytic system and its inhibitors. Primary inhibitors include ATIII, proteins C and S, heparin cofactor II, and others. Examples of the types and the activity affected by the coagulopathies are seen in Boxes 18-1 and 18-2.

PATHOLOGICAL CONSEQUENCES

The pathological consequences of altered clotting are bleeding, arterial or venous thrombosis, and DIC. Bleeding may be caused by injury, a defect, or a deficiency in coagulation factors.

Venous thrombosis is a serious and sometimes fatal consequence of altered clotting. Generally clots occur in valve pockets where activated clotting factors and platelets accumulate (especially with stasis). Thrombus is formed in the normal coagulation cascade, and the thrombus (DVT) grows and extends into the lumen of the vessel, occluding it. The body's normal fibrinolytic system attempts to contain the clot, but in the presence of defective or limited enzymes, the clot extends. A piece of the clot may break off and travel to the lungs, becoming a PE. If the clot stays in one spot, it will eventually lyse, but the valve and vein wall are permanently damaged. This may result in post-thrombotic leg, (i.e., chronic venous insufficiency), characterized by: edema, hemosiderin deposits (ankle), skin liposclerosis, and eventually venous ulcers.[24-26]

If the venous thrombosis is massive, severe edema will result and cause arterial compromise and ischemia, with possible gangrene and loss of the limb, a condition known as phlegmasia cerula dolens.[27]

A PE may result from a fragment of DVT, a right-sided heart thrombus,[12] or a clot from a subclavian vein catheter. The embolism blocks the pulmonary arterial tree and chemically induces arterial and bronchial constriction. The embolism activates platelets, which release thromboxane A_2 (a powerful vasoconstrictor) and serotonin (a powerful vasoconstrictor and bronchoconstrictor). The results of this event are pulmonary hypertension, bronchoconstriction (with dyspnea), and hypoxemia.[12] The size and location of the PE determine whether the patient is symptomatic and whether the PE is fatal. Thrombi in the pelvic veins may be larger than those in the distal leg and have a greater potential for causing a fatal PE. Persons undergoing pelvic surgery or sustaining an injury, pregnant or postpartum women, and persons with carcinoma are at risk for pelvic thrombi.

Chronic PE may result in severe permanent damage to the lungs with resultant chronic

BOX 18-1 Effects of Selected Inherited Clotting Disorders on Coagulation

Antithrombin III Deficiency

ATIII counteracts thrombin and other proteases involved in coagulation. Without use of heparin, ATIII inactivates thrombin and other proteases. Moderate decreases in ATIII result in an increased risk of thrombosis.

Factor V Leiden

The mutation on the factor V gene is known as the factor V Leiden. It is an inherited mutation resulting in the inability of activated protein C (APC) to cleave the factor V protein. Factor V works to coagulate blood while protein C normally acts to inhibit coagulation:[1,19] This increases the incidence of thrombosis.

Protein C Deficiency (PC)

Protein C is a vitamin K–dependent anticoagulant protein that acts by cleaving activated coagulation factors V and VIII:C.[20] Protein C is inhibited somewhat by warfarin,[21] but it is not clinically significant. Protein S increases the action of protein C. Protein C deficiency can be congenital and may be more common than ATIII deficiency,[12] or may occur with acute DIC, massive deep venous thrombosis (DVT), pulmonary emboli, or severe liver disease. With a protein C deficiency, thrombosis increases.

Protein S Deficiency (PS)

Protein S is a cofactor for the inactivation of factor V and platelet factor V. Additionally, it is a cofactor with protein C for increased fibrinolysis. Protein S is decreased in the presence of warfarin. Protein S is decreased in type I diabetes mellitus and increased in type II. Levels of protein S decrease in pregnancy and may account for increased thromboses at the end of pregnancy and postpartum.

Antiphospholipid Antibody Syndrome

There are two types of antiphospholipid antibody syndrome—that which is induced by the lupus anticoagulant (LA) and those induced by the anticardiolipin antibodies.[2] LA results in thrombosis.[12] Patients with lupus (10%) and other autoimmune disorders, cancer, infections, Crohn's disease, thrombocytopenic purpura, and patients taking some medications, such as hydralazine and procainamide, may be affected.

There are three types of anticardiolipin antibodies (aCL): IgA, IgG, and IgM. These antibodies are associated with thrombosis but the exact mechanism of action with aCL and LA is unknown. It is hypothesized that the antibodies have an affinity for the phospholipids involved in many points in the coagulation process. The main hallmark of the syndrome is a histopathological lesion (thrombosis) without inflammation.[22] It predisposes to thrombosis and recurrent thrombosis. The mechanism of action is related to the inappropriate prothrombin interaction in the coagulation process.

G202210a Transition in the Prothrombin Gene

This transition is a genetic tendency that is a variation at the nucleotide position on the gene.[3] It predisposes an individual to thrombosis and recurrent thrombosis. The mechanism of action is related to the inappropriate prothrombin interaction in the coagulation process.

Inherited Homocysteinemia

In the process of folate metabolism the amino acid homocysteine is formed. Elevated homocysteine levels injure endothelium, decrease the activation of protein C and increase the binding of lipoprotein to fibrin. All of this increases the risk of DVT, arterial thromboses, stroke, and heart disease, particularly in younger patients.[4]

Adapted from Page, M. (1998). Factor V Leiden mutation: A nursing perspective. *Journal of Vascular Nursing 16*(4), 73-77; and Brenner, Z., & Myer, S. (2000). Antiphospholipid antibody syndrome: Implications for nursing practice. *Heart & Lung 29*(5), 331-339; and Eichinger, S., Minar, E., Hirschl, M., Bialonczyk, C., Stain, M., Mannhalter, C., et al. (1999). The risk of early recurrent venous thromboembolism after oral anticoagulant therapy in patients with G20221 0A transition in the prothrombin gene. *Thrombosis and Hemostasis 81(1)*, 14-17; and Twardowski, P., & Green, D. (1999). Thrombotic disorders in vascular patients. In V. Fahey (ed.), *Vascular Nursing* (3rd ed.). Philadelphia: W.B. Saunders; and Bick, R. (1992). *Disorders of thrombosis and hemostasis*. Chicago: ASCP Press; and Hoerl, H., Tabares, A., & Kottke-Marchang, K. (1996). The diagnosis and clinical manifestations of activated protein C resistance, a case report and review of the literature. *Vascular Medicine 1*, 275-280; and Stenflo, J. (1984). Structure and function of protein C. *Seminars in Thrombosis and Hemostasis 10*, 104-109; and Lubetsky, A., Seligsohn, U., Ezra, D., & Halkin, H. (1992). The effect of the plasma levels of proteins C&S on the prediction of warfarin maintenance dose requirements. *Clinical Pharmacology and Therapeutics 52*, 42-49; and Kharnashta, M., Cuadrado, M., Mujic, F., Taub, N., Hirsh, B., and Hughes, G. (1995). The management of thrombosis in the antiphospholipid syndrome. *New England Journal of Medicine, 332*, 993-997.

BOX 18-2 Effects of Selected Inherited Bleeding Disorders on Coagulation

Hemophilia A

Factor VIII:C is responsible for the procoagulant activity in the conversion of factor X to Xa.[12] Hemophilia A is an inherited sex-linked recessive trait characterized by a deficiency or defect of VIII:C.

Hemophilia B (Christmas Disease)

Hemophilia B is also a sex-linked recessive trait. It is a deficiency of factor IX:C or a defective factor. It also affects platelet function in its severest form.[12]

von Willebrand's Disease

von Willebrand's disease is caused by low factor VIII levels and an absence of an antigen, factor VIII:vWF:Ag. The antigen (vWF) is responsible for the activity that is necessary for normal platelet aggregation, normal platelet adhesion to subendothelial surfaces and for normal platelet-endothelial interaction.[23] vWF may induce the synthesis or release of factor VIII:C. von Willebrand's disease is an inherited dominant trait.[12]

Bick, R. (1992). *Disorders of thrombosis and hemostasis*. Chicago: ASCP Press; and Fowler, W., Fretto, L., & Hamilton, K. (1985). Substructure of human von Willebrand factor. *Journal of Clinical Investigation 76,* 4468-4471.

hypoxemia, dyspnea, right sided heart failure, and disability.

DIC is not an independent occurrence; it is a mechanism of disease (or syndrome) associated with both hemorrhage and thrombosis. DIC occurs as a result of a triggering event, such as sepsis (Box 18-3). Thrombin is released and degrades fibrinopeptides A and B from fibrinogen. This forms a clot or clots in the microcirculation and leads to diffuse thrombosis. Because the clots are in the microcirculation, platelets become trapped and thrombocytopenia occurs.[12] Fibrinogen degrades into FDPs. The FDPs interfere with fibrin polymerization and platelet function, which leads to hemorrhage. At the same time, plasmin is circulating and induces lysis of many of the clotting factors, resulting in hemorrhage.

Accompanying all of these actions is granulocyte release, activation of factor XII to XIIa, platelet release, and endothelial damage.[28] Activation of the kinin system by plasmin causes systemic vasodilation and increased capillary permeability. There is a shift of plasma proteins and fluid to the interstitial space, resulting in hypotension and shock. Death may result from shock, or irreversible organ damage may occur from the microemboli in the kidneys, liver, lungs, adrenal glands, or other vital organs.

BOX 18-3 Precipitating Events Associated With DIC

Obstetrical Events
- Abortion
- Amniotic fluid embolism
- Eclampsia
- HELLP syndrome
- Placental abruption
- Retained fetus syndrome

Cardiovascular Disease
- Acute myocardial infarction
- Peripheral arterial disease

Others
- Burns
- Hemolysis (and massive transfusion)
- Malignancy
- Septicemia

RELATED PATHOPHYSIOLOGICAL CONCEPTS

The pathophysiological concept most closely related to altered clotting is ischemia. Either bleeding or clotting may result in decreased oxygen supply to organs or tissues. The resulting tissue damage is ischemia. If metabolic needs are not met, eventually tissue death occurs (see Chapter 21, Ischemia).

MANIFESTATIONS AND SURVEILLANCE

Manifestations of altered clotting may be bleeding or clotting. Often the presence or absence of a defect in hemostasis can be documented with a thorough history and physical examination. The emphasis of the assessment should be on the site, severity and type of bleeding, or careful history of family coagulation defects, use of medications, smoking, drug use, surgeries, rare disorders, and previous history of clotting. Each inherited disorder has a pattern. Acquired bleeding disorders tend to present themselves in the presence of other medical conditions, such as carcinoma, chemotherapy, infections, and other stressors.

TABLE 18-2 Manifestations of Bleeding

OBJECTIVE	SUBJECTIVE
Decreased hematocrit	Dyspnea
Decreased hemoglobin	Fatigue
Epistaxis	Headaches
Gingival bleeding	Menorrhagia
Hemarthrosis	Nausea
Hematoma	Pain
Hypotension	Visual disturbances
Intracranial hemorrhage	Weakness
Mucosal bleeding	
Gastrointestinal	
Melena	
Hematemesis	
Genitourinary	
Hematuria	
Hemoptysis	
Oliguria or anuria	
Oozing from skin or puncture sites	
Pallor	
Petechiae	
Purpura	
Spontaneous bruising	
Tachycardia	

Frank bleeding is easy to identify; internal bleeding is less obvious. The person assessing the patient may have to rely on indirect indicators, such as falling blood pressure, tachycardia, and dizziness. Rapidly dropping hemoglobin and hematocrit levels will confirm blood loss. The presence of a rising reticulocyte count will confirm the bone marrow's attempt to replace lost blood. Table 18-2 is a comprehensive list of the manifestations of bleeding.

Bleeding coagulopathies have predictable patterns if they are inherited. The bleeding tendency of hemophilia A reflects the amount of circulating factor VIII:C. Persons with less than 5% of factor VIII:C have spontaneous severe bleeding early in childhood. These may occur when the child scrapes himself and bleeds profusely. Mild (10% to 40%) and moderate (5% to 10%) quantities of factor VIII:C may protect against spontaneous bleeding but may cause hemorrhage with trauma. Patients with mild hemophilia A may not be diagnosed until trauma or surgery occurs. Hemophilia B has similar incidences. von Willebrand's disease often presents early in childhood with purpura, easy bruising, mucosal bleeding, genitourinary bleeding, and severe epistaxis.

DIC signs and symptoms vary widely and depend on the bleeding or thrombotic complications of the syndrome. Commonly, bleeding occurs from at least three unrelated sites.[12] Other signs may include shock, fever, proteinuria, and hypoxia.[12] Organ damage symptoms depend upon the organ affected.

Most common thrombotic coagulopathies (see Box 18-1) result in venous thrombosis but others predispose to arterial thrombosis. ATIII deficiencies result in venous thromboses at an early age. Most primary events occur in the midteens to late teens, and sites include the lower extremities and the mesenteric veins.[12] In addition to early occurrence, recurrent DVT is common. Factor V Leiden is highly correlated with the use of oral contraceptives or hormone replacement therapy.[1] Additionally, pregnancy increases the risk of DVT significantly.

Protein C (PC) deficiency presents with clotting and often pulmonary emboli in the teenage years. Skin necrosis with use of warfarin is common in patients with PC deficiency. Some evidence indicates that PC may be more common in persons from the Arab Middle East.[29] Acquired PC deficiency is seen in patients with DIC, massive DVT, and severe liver disease.[30]

Protein S (PS) deficiency may result in both arterial and venous thrombosis. Thromboses generally occur for the first time in persons under the age of 45 and may occur at unusual sites.[31] A first presentation may be a superficial phlebitis in a patient who is young and has no other risk factors. Recurrent thromboses within a year are reported to be between 13% and 17%.[32]

Antiphospholipid syndrome affects both the arterial and venous system (DVT is most common).[2] Arterial manifestations may include early myocardial infarctions, frequent bypass graft occlusions, early ischemic stroke or transient ischemic attacks, early angioplasty, and intracardiac thrombi.[2,22] In the aCL form of antiphospholipid syndrome, early and recurrent fetal loss (miscarriage before 12 weeks' gestation) may be common. Lupus anticoagulant is often associated with prothrombin deficiency and contributes to the incidence of significant bleeding instead of clotting.[33]

Venous thrombosis symptoms vary from none present, the erythema associated with a superficial phlebitis, to the collapse from a pulmonary embolus. The number one sign of venous thrombosis is acute unilateral leg edema. Homan's sign, although often used, is notoriously inaccurate. Some patients have slight temperature elevations, tenderness in the area involved, or superficial dilation of the veins. Duplex imaging and Doppler ultrasonography are the modalities of diagnosis; venography is rarely used.

In patients with massive thrombosis and edema, venous thrombosis may result in arterial compromise and phlegmasia cerula dolens.[27] Symptoms are severe pain, blueish color, and edema.

Arterial thrombotic occlusion symptomatology depends on the acuteness of the occlusion, the vessels affected, the degree of collateral circulation, and the amount of ischemia. Signs of major acute arterial occlusions are known as the "6 *Ps*:" pain (often intractable), pallor (waxy white, from lack of blood flow), pulselessness (an occluded vessel has no pulse), polar sensation (cold) paralysis, and parasthesias.[34] Once an occlusion has occurred, the limb may become mottled and blue below the level of the occlusion. Loss of sensation and movement rapidly become worse as the amount of ischemic time increases. In a patient who has atherosclerosis, the symptoms may be more subtle because of the presence of collateral circulation. In these patients, claudication (pain or cramping in a muscle group with exercise, which is relieved by rest and is reproducible) may become worse. This may progress to rest pain, which is severe pain caused by inadequate blood supply, even at rest. Rest pain generally occurs in the toes or forefoot when the patient is recumbent and improves with ambulation. This rest pain may progress to ulceration or gangrene.[34] Color changes with smaller arterial emboli may present with patchy blue or purple discoloration on the foot or plantar surface of the foot.

The manifestations of pulmonary embolism depend upon the size of the clot and the area of lung compromised. Small emboli may go undetected; massive PE may cause collapse and sudden death. Intermediate size pulmonary emboli present with pleuritic pain, dyspnea, anxiety, restlessness, hypoxemia, and hemodynamic instability. The most common symptoms are dyspnea and tachycardia.[35] A ventilation-perfusion (VQ) lung scan or pulmonary angiography is used to confirm PE.

Occlusions in the cerebrovascular system present as neurological changes. Smaller emboli may result in transient ischemic attacks (TIAs) and larger ones may cause a complete occlusion of the carotid or other major vessel and a resultant stroke. Bruits may be detectable in one or both carotid arteries, indicating turbulent or narrowed blood flow.

SURVEILLANCE

Laboratory tests may be the first and continued indicators of altered clotting. Screening tests may be needed to define the disorder. Patients with bleeding disorders require at a minimum: prothrombin time (PT), measured as the international normalized ratio (INR), activated partial thromboplastin time (APTT), bleeding time, liver panel, blood urea nitrogen (BUN), creatinine, and complete blood cell count with platelet count. Normal bleeding time is 9 minutes or less. Prolongation of bleeding time may indicate a platelet disorder or inherited clotting abnormality. Once a family history of bleeding has been identified, the appropriate disorder must be investigated (identifying a defect or a deficiency of a clotting factor). A prolonged prothrombin time may indicate a problem in the extrinsic pathway or anticoagulation (appropriate factors should be checked). A prolonged APTT may reflect anticoagulants or abnormalities in factors VII, IX, X, XI, and XII as well as fibrinogen and prothrombin. In clotting disorders the same tests must be performed, with assessment of arterial blood gases if PE is suspected or urine myoglobin if limb ischemia or trauma is present. These are all assessed on initial presentation.

Platelet counts normally range from 150,000 to 350,000/mm^3.[36] Bleeding may occur below 40,000/mm^3 if there are other coagulation disorders present. Spontaneous bleeding occurs below 10,000/mm^3. In the presence of unfractionated heparin, these should be assessed in 3 days and then daily with a fall below 100,000/mm^3, indicating possible heparin-induced thrombocytopenia (HITT).[9] This syndrome is marked by thrombosis rather than bleeding and requires cessation of heparin.

Syndromes such as HITT and DIC will have markedly abnormal screening laboratory results. Further studies may be required such as FDPs, D-dimer, protamine sulfate test, and platelet aggregation tests. A combination of tests to identify D-dimer and FDPs has highly predictive value in diagnosing DIC.[37]

Inherited thrombotic coagulopathy requires vigilance in monitoring the patient for recurrence. Education in the signs of thrombosis, especially in sites other than the first experienced is essential. Current recommendations are for screening for inherited thrombophelia only in patients with a positive family history of thrombosis, those with thromboses receiving anticoagulation medication that is at therapeutic level, and in patients who develop a thrombosis before age 45.[13,38]

Many DVTs and PEs are clinically silent and they go undetected and untreated. Routine surveillance for DVT with duplex ultrasonography or impedance plethysmography has not been shown to be effective in reducing the prevalence of symptomatic

DVT or fatal PE.[10] Prevention of these serious and potentially fatal problems, therefore, is critical.

CLINICAL MANAGEMENT

Prevention of bleeding is a primary goal of therapy in patients at risk for bleeding. In patients who have bled, identification of the cause, stabilization of the patient, prevention of tissue loss, replacement of blood components, and maintenance of body image are paramount.

Counseling for patients with bleeding disorders may include information about signs of bleeding and genetic and pregnancy counseling. Nursing is often instrumental in education as well as monitoring the patient's response to blood and blood products. Nurses are generally responsible for surveillance of laboratory values and must be aware of normal ranges in the patient and the population.

The studies of the various methods of DVT prophylaxis are numerous and the reader is referred to several major reviews and meta-analyses exploring both physical methods (e.g., graduated compression stockings and pneumatic compression devices) and anticoagulation.[10,39,40] A summary of the thromboembolism prevention guidelines developed by the American College of Chest Physicians[10] for several moderate and high risk populations is provided in Table 18-3. In general, graduated compression stockings or pneumatic pressure devices are effective in preventing DVT and non-fatal PE when used alone in moderate and high risk populations.[10,39,40] In very high risk populations, these methods should be used in combination with anticoagulation with low-dose unfractionated heparin (LDUH) or low-molecular weight heparin (LMWH) since they may confer additional benefit. When anticoagulation is contraindicated, physical methods should be used instead.[10,39] Correct fit and application of compression stockings and devices are essential in order to be effective and to prevent complications of their use, such as leg edema, DVT, and arterial occlusion.[10]

Studies comparing the effectiveness of LDUH and LMWH found them to be comparable in reducing DVT and subsequent non-fatal PE; but there

TABLE 18-3 Guidelines for DVT Prophylaxis*

RISK GROUP	PROPHYLAXIS
1. General Surgery	
Moderate risk minor procedures with additional risk factors (e.g., > age 60, previous thromboembolic event, immobility, etc.); nonmajor surgery, age 40-60 with no other major surgeries, age <40 with no other risk factors.	LDUH, LMWH, or use of GCS or pnuematic compression devices.
High risk nonmajor surgery, age >60 or with additional risk factors: major surger, age >40 or with additonal risk factors.	LDUH, LMWH, or pneumatic compression devices.
Very high risk	LDUH or LMWH is combination with GCS or pneumatic compression devices.
2. Hip Fracture Surgery	LDUH or LMWH, or adjusted dose warfarin. Alternately, pneumatic compression device if high risk of bleeding.
3. Spinal Cord Injury	
Acute	LMWH or adjusted dose heparin for a mininum of 3 months or until completion of rehabilitation.
Rehabilitation	Continuation of LMWH or conversion to adjusted dose warfarin (INR target 2.5, with range of 2.0-3.0).
4. Ischemic Stroke	LDUH or LMWH. Alternately, GCS or pneumatic compression device if high risk of bleeding.

Legend: LDUH=Low-dose unfractionated heparin; LMWH=low molecular weight heparin; GCS=graduated compression stockings; INR=international normalized ratio.

*Compiled from: 10. Geerts, W.H., Heit, J.A., Clagett, G.P., Pineo, G.F., Colwell, C.W., Anderson, Jr., F.A., et al. (2001). Prevention of thromboembolism. *Chest,* 119, 132S-175S. 41. Estrada, C.A., Mansfield, C.J., & Heudebert, G.R. (2000). Cost-effectiveness of low-molecular weight heparin in the treatment of proximal deep vein thrombosis. *Journal of General Internal Medicine,* 15, 108-115.

is insufficient data to determine if these heparins prevent fatal PE and post-thrombotic leg.[10] LMWH, however, causes less bleeding and HITT than unfractionated heparin (UH), can be used in the outpatient setting in ambulatory patients, and does not require laboratory monitoring. For these reasons, LMWH can be more cost-effective than UH,[41,42] especially if DVT prophylaxis must continue for several weeks or months. In a patient with thrombosis, warfarin therapy is started at the same time as heparin. The INR is the test for monitoring warfarin; the level should be between 2 and 3. Complications of warfarin include bleeding, skin necrosis, and interactions with many other medications (e.g., trimethoprim-sulfamethoxazole, and fluconazole; consult a pharmacology text for a complete list). Patients should wear an identification bracelet or necklace stating that they are receiving warfarin and should have complete discharge instructions on the medication. Anticoagulation therapy is continued for at least 3 to 6 months after a first episode, although this is still in question. In patients with known recurrence and an inherited clotting disorder, most practitioners prescribe lifelong anticoagulation medications. However, recent research indicates that 1 to 3 years may be adequate. After that, the implication is that the risks of warfarin therapy outweigh the benefits.[32] Other researchers recommend lifetime anticoagulation for a life-threatening thrombotic event.[43] If a patient has a PE while receiving heparin or warfarin, interruption of the vena cava with an inferior vena cava filter is generally performed.[35] Acute arterial occlusion may be treated with thrombectomy, thrombolytic therapy, or observation and anticoagulation therapy, depending on the degree of tissue involvement.

DIC treatment is controversial. Antithrombotic therapy may be necessary. Supportive measures (e.g., fluid resuscitation and pain management), platelet transfusion, fresh frozen plasma, vitamin K, folic acid, and cryoprecipitate may be given.[37] Treatment of the underlying disorder is imperative.

CASE STUDIES

The following case studies illustrate two conditions of altered clotting.

CASE STUDY 1

Ms. JL is an 18-year-old woman who has been extremely healthy all her life. She was recently placed on low-dose birth control pills for dysmenorrhea. Following this, she developed a warm, red, painful area in her medial calf. She and her mother were seen by an adult nurse practitioner.

Examination revealed a cord in a superficial vein branch of the greater saphenous vein. Duplex imaging revealed a superficial phlebitis. CBC, INR, and a PTT were within normal range. The nurse practitioner instructed the patient on the regular use of NSAIDs, the need to be ambulatory and to make a follow-up appointment in 1 week in the office. The patient was not referred.

The mother had had two previous superficial phlebitis episodes while under the care of another health care provider, and no therapy or testing had been recommended. Several first-degree relatives of the mother had a history of DVT and PE. All relatives had had their first episode before age 30.

Testing for inherited coagulopathy revealed a protein S deficiency. The mother requested testing for herself and the rest of the children, all adults. Counseling from the nurse practitioner included the following: abstinence from birth control pills for JL, recommendations for alternate forms of contraception, education about the signs and symptoms of DVT and other thrombotic events, and copies of records be forwarded to present (and future) gynecologists. JL's mother and one brother also had a protein S deficiency. All family members were counseled to carry a card identifying their deficiency to alert any future caregivers, and to obtain genetic counseling before any planned pregnancies. Family members were urged to be seen by their health care provider on a regular basis to maintain optimal health.

CASE STUDY 2

Mr. FD is a 76-year-old man with metastatic colon cancer (Duke's C on initial surgery) who is undergoing chemotherapy (5 flurourocil [5-FU]). He presented with multiple ecchymoses, fatigue, and a history of several melanotic stools. His platelet count was 35,000/mm^3, hemoglobin 7 g/dl, and hematocrit 21%. He had previously required erythropoetin for anemia during his chemotherapy. He is married and well aware of his diagnosis. He is cognitively intact.

After 2 units of packed cells, his condition was stable and his fatigue was lessened. An evaluation during the hospitalization revealed multiple liver metastases. Discussion by the oncology nurse practitioner (ONP) with the patient and his wife allowed them to understand the combination risk of future bleeding episodes due to chemotherapy and decreased liver function.

The patient and his wife decided that further chemotherapy was futile and of more risk than benefit. Accordingly, they composed an advance directive and discontinued further intervention. The unit nurse and family services provided them with information on the advance directive implications. Hospice was contacted and supportive care was instituted. Hospice nursing and an advance directive allowed the patient and his wife to be comfortable and supported, with less fear of bleeding complications. The hospice nurse monitored the stools for guaiac and the hematocrit level weekly. Before discharge, the hospital nurse educated FD and his wife about the signs of bleeding. They were instructed to call the oncologist or the ONP with any signs of bleeding.

These two case studies demonstrate the educational, emotional, and physical needs of very different patients with altered clotting. Both cases illustrate the critical role nurses play in education and support, as well as evaluation of the patient.

SELECTED RESEARCH

The literature related to coagulopathies, especially the inherited types, is limited by small sample sizes and retrospective designs. The total number of patients seen is small in most institutions, except in those with large hemostasis and thrombosis centers. However, much can be learned from such studies. They often provide important questions out of which larger, prospective, randomized studies are conceptualized and conducted. An important retrospective study was reported by Khamashta et al.[22] who described their experience treating 147 patients with antiphospholipid–antibody syndrome seen in their lupus clinic over a 10-year period. The sample was comprised primarily of women (84%) with a median age of 32 years. Of the 147 patients, 101 had 186 episodes of recurrent venous or arterial thrombosis during the follow-up period. The median length of time from the initial thrombosis to the first recurrence was 12 months. In 54% of the patients, their first episode was a venous thrombosis, 76% of which were DVTs. The remaining 46% experienced an arterial thrombosis as their first thrombotic event, most of which were strokes or transient ischemic attacks. Anticoagulation therapies consisted of: low-dose aspirin only (75 mg daily), warfarin categorized according to high intensity (INR ≥ 3) and low intensity (INR <3) therapy and further categorized by whether aspirin accompanied the treatment, and none (meaning no therapy administered).

The 101 patients who had recurrences were followed a median of 82 months after the initial thrombotic event; the 46 patients who had only a single thrombotic event were followed a median of 60 months. The results indicated that high intensity warfarin plus aspirin resulted in no recurrences during the 39.8 patient years of treatment, which was a lower rate than those who received no treatment ($p < 0.001$) and the lowest rate of all other treatments. However, the first 6 months after cessation of warfarin had the highest recurrence rate (1.30 events per 16.2 patient years). The median time to the first recurrence after cessation of warfarin was 2 months (range, 0.5 to 6). Bleeding episodes occurred in 29 patients, all of whom had INR >3 at the time of the bleed; 7 of these were also receiving aspirin. Of the 29 patients with bleeding, 7 were severe, a rate of 0.071 episodes per patient year. In 4 of these 7 patients, warfarin could be restarted and no further episodes of bleeding occurred during follow-up. This study raised a number of questions to be answered by prospective studies of the recurrence rates of thrombosis after a first event and RCTs of secondary prevention of thrombosis in patients with antiphospholipid-antibody syndrome.

The Pulmonary Embolism Prevention (PEP) Trial Collaboration Group[44] conducted a large, multicenter, randomized, placebo-controlled study of the effectiveness of aspirin in preventing DVT and PE in 13,356 patients undergoing surgery for hip fracture and 2648 patients having elective hip or knee arthroplasty. The investigators hoped to definitively answer the question of aspirin's effectiveness in these groups. The study end points were mortality from all causes up to day 35 and in-hospital occurrence of DVT, PE, myocardial infarction, stroke, and bleeding episodes. There was no routine screening for thromboembolic events during the hospital stay; diagnostic evaluation took place only if clinically indicated.

In the hip fracture patients DVT occurred in 1.0% of the aspirin group and in 1.5% of the placebo group ($p = 0.03$), representing a reduction of 29% in the aspirin group. Also, in these patients, definite or probable PE occurred in 0.7% in the aspirin group and in 1.2% of those assigned to the placebo group ($p = 0.002$), representing a reduction of 43% with aspirin. Fatal PE also was significantly lower in the aspirin group compared to the placebo group (0.3% vs. 0.6%, respectively; $p = 0.002$). Similar reductions in DVT and PE occurred in the patients undergoing elective hip or knee arthroplasty. In the hip fracture patients, non-fatal MI and deaths from ischemic heart disease were significantly higher in the aspirin group (1.6%) than the placebo group (1.2%). The investigators did not speculate about why this may have occurred.

During the immediate post-operative period, aspirin caused 6 bleeding episodes per 1000 patients that required transfusion and a mean drop in hemoglobin of 0.2 gram overall. There were no differences between the groups in fatal, cerebral, or disabling bleeding episodes. Bleeding and other thrombotic events (MI and stroke) were not reported for the hip and knee arthroplasty patients.

Despite the apparent benefit of aspirin on decreasing the recurrences of DVT and PE, the investigators did not control for important confounding variables. Large numbers of patients in both groups received additional anticoagulation such as unfractionated heparin (n = 2432) and LMWH (n = 3424). When the patients receiving both LMWH and aspirin (n = 1761) were compared with patients receiving only LMWH (n = 1,663) there was no significant difference in the occurrences of thromboembolic events between the two groups. Thus, the addition of aspirin provided no benefit above that conferred by LMWH, a finding that must be considered along with the significant increase in bleeding that occurred in the aspirin group. Also, an unspecified number of patients received other prophylactic interventions, such as GCS, pneumatic pressure devices, and a variety of different mobilization therapies. How many of these patients were receiving more than one prophylactic modality in addition to aspirin or placebo was not reported. Hence, the true effect of aspirin could not be determined reliably in this study.

A number of small clinical trials attempted to determine the most effective length of anticoagulation therapy after a first occurrence of venous thromboembolism, but their small sample sizes and design flaws precluded a conclusive answer.[10] Hoping to eliminate some of the major drawbacks of these earlier trials, Schulman et al.[45] conducted a multi-center randomized trial to compare the effectiveness of 6 weeks and 6 months of warfarin or dicoumarol therapy in preventing recurrence of venous thromboembolism in patients over 15 years of age (n = 892) who had a first episode of DVT or PE. Patients were screened for and excluded if they had a hereditary coagulopathy or were receiving anticoagulation therapy for another reason. Concurrently with initial treatment with unfractionated or low-molecular weight heparin, oral anticoagulation was prescribed to achieve an INR of 2.0-2.85 for the duration of the study period. End points of the study were recurrent DVT and/or PE that could be objectively confirmed, major hemorrhage during oral anticoagulation, and death. Patients were followed at 1.5, 3, 6, 9, 12, and 24 months after the therapeutic INR was achieved. The investigators found a 50% reduction in recurrence of venous thromboembolism in the 6-month group (9.5%) compared with the 6-week group (18.1%). This reduction was found consistently in almost all of the subgroups of patients (e.g., those with temporary or permanent risk factors, distal or proximal DVT, presence or absence of family history of venous thromboembolism). After termination of oral anticoagulation, both groups experienced an increase in the incidence of venous thromboembolism recurrences, which persisted for the 2 years of follow-up. The latter finding indicates that the thromboembolic process increases the risk of recurrence for an indefinite period, and reinforces the need for patients to be well educated about taking their oral anticoagulants for 6 months continuously as prescribed. Oral anticoagulation is clearly more effective than 6 weeks of the same therapy in reducing DVT and PE after a first occurrence. However, the optimum duration of oral anticoagulation after a first event is still to be determined, as is the length of time the increased risk of recurrent thromboembolism continues after anticoagulation is discontinued.

QUESTIONS FOR FUTURE STUDY

Research in large multicenter trials is needed to establish optimal treatment (type and duration) for patients with inherited coagulopathy. This data will also provide a basis for developing patient education programs for each disorder.

Studies of treatment options and antigen-antibody reactions are needed in hemophilia and other, much less common disorders of bleeding. Studies in families with clotting disorders who have not had their type identified may reveal the presence of other clotting disorders. This knowledge could be helpful for screening patients with recurrent thrombosis, those who have a family history of thrombosis, or who have recurrent thrombosis while being treated.

In regard to DVT prophylaxis, large, randomized clinical trials (RCTs) are needed to test the effectiveness of physical methods (i.e., GCS and pneumatic pressure devices) in specific populations, such as patients with malignancies and hypercoagulable states, and to compare physical methods with each other and with anticoagulation therapy in medical and surgical populations. Systematic evaluation of the complications of physical methods is essential in order to know their true risk-benefit ratio.[39] Large RCTs also are needed to evaluate several important outcomes we have little reliable data on; (i.e., fatal PE, post-thrombotic leg, chronic post-embolic pulmonary disease, and side effects of anticoagulation, including local wound complications).[40] Longitudinal studies are needed in order to clarify the length of time patients are at risk for recurrence of thrombosis after a venous or thrombotic event and the optimal duration of anticoagulation.[40]

Nursing studies of patient understanding of the disease states may assist in devising teaching plans that fit within the patient illness model. There is some evidence that greater congruence between patient and provider understanding enhances adherence to therapy.[46,47]

Hirudin, a new direct thrombin inhibitor, is among many new heparins and heparinoids that are currently being developed that may have fewer complications than UH and LMWH.[48] Large RCTs must be conducted comparing their effectiveness against UH and LMWH in medical and surgical populations.

Studies in hemophilia and other rarer factor disorders of bleeding are necessary. Treatment options and antigen-antibody reactions need to be studied and standardized.

These are rich areas for nurse researchers to direct their efforts and for advanced practice nurses to lend their clinical expertise. As a profession, nurses are in a prime position to disseminate new knowledge to other health care providers and patients.

REFERENCES

1. Page, M. (1998). Factor V Leiden mutation: A nursing perspective. *Journal of Vascular Nursing 16*(4), 73-77.
2. Brenner, Z., & Myer, S. (2000). Antiphospholipid antibody syndrome: Implications for nursing practice. *Heart & Lung 29*(5), 331-339.
3. Eichinger, S., Minar, E., Hirschl, M., Bialonczyk, C., Stain, M., Mannhalter, C., et al. (1999). The risk of early recurrent venous thromboembolism after oral anticoagulant therapy in patients with G202210A transition in the prothrombin gene. *Thrombosis and Hemostasis 81(1)*, 14-17.
4. Twardowski, P., & Green, D. (1999). Thrombotic disorders in vascular patients. In V. Fahey (ed.), *Vascular Nursing* (3rd ed.). Philadelphia: W.B. Saunders.
5. Kryel, P., Minar, E., Hirschl, M., Bialonczyk, C., Stain, M., Schneider, B., et al. (2000). High plasma levels of factor VIII and the risk of recurrent venous thromboembolism. *New England Journal of Medicine 343*(7), 457-462.
6. Arun, B., & Kessler, C.M. (2001). Clinical manifestations and therapy of the hemophilias. In R. Colman, J. Hirsch, V. Marder, A. Clowes, & J. George (eds.), *Hemostasis and thrombosis: Basic principles and clinical practice* (pp. 815-824). Philadelphia: Lippincott Williams & Wilkins.
7. McKeown, E. (1995). Undiagnosed hypercoagulable state: A case study. *Journal of Vascular Nursing 8*(4), 117-127.
8. Walker, I. (1998). Classification of bleeding disorders. In J. Ginsberg, C. Kearon, & J. Hirsch (eds.), *Critical decisions in thrombosis and hemostasis* (pp. 330-338). Hamilton, Ontario: Decker.
9. Fahey, V. (1995). Heparin induced thrombocytopenia. *Journal of Vascular Nursing 8*(4), 112-116.
10. Geerts, W.H., Heit, J.A., Clagett, G.P., Pineo, G.F., Colwell, C.W., Anderson, Jr., F.A., et al. (2001). Prevention of thromboembolism. *Chest 119,* 132S-175S.
11. Kurgan, A., & Nunnelee, J.D. (1995). Upper extremity venous thrombosis. *Journal of Vascular Nursing 13(1),* 21-23.
12. Bick, R. (1992). *Disorders of thrombosis and hemostasis.* Chicago: ASCP Press.
13. Crowther, M., & Ginsberg, J. (1998). Screening for thrombophilic states. In J. Ginsberg, C. Kearon, & J. Hirsch (eds.), *Critical decisions in thrombosis and hemostasis* (pp. 123-131). Hamilton, Ontario: Decker.
14. Andrew, M., David, M., & Adams, M. (1996). Venous thromboembolic complications (VTE) in children: Analysis of the Canadian Registry of VTE. *Blood 83,* 1251-1257.
15. Schmidt, B., & Andrew, M. (1995). Neonatal thrombosis: Report of a prospective Canadian and international registry. *Pediatrics 96,* 939-943.
16. Andrew, M., Paes, B., & Johnston, M. (1990). Development of the hemostatic system in the neonate and young infant. *American Journal of Pediatric Oncology 12,* 95-104.
17. Nunnelee, J. (2000). Henoch-Schonlein purpura—a review of the literature. *Clinical Excellence for Nurse Practitioners 18,* 6-10.
18. Colman, R., Clowes, A., George, J. Hirsch, J., & Marder, V. (2001). Overview of hemostasis. In R. Colman, J. Hirsch, V. Marder, A. Clowes, & J. George (eds.), *Hemostasis and thrombosis: Basic principles and clinical practice* (pp. 3-16). Philadelphia: Lippincott Williams & Wilkins.
19. Hoerl, H., Tabares, A., & Kottke-Marchang, K. (1996). The diagnosis and clinical manifestations of activated protein C resistance, a case resport and review of the literature. *Vascular Medicine 1,* 275-280.
20. Stenflo, J. (1984). Structure and function of protein C. *Seminars in Thrombosis and Hemostasis 10,* 104-109.
21. Lubetsky, A., Seligsohn, U, Ezra, D., & Halkin, H. (1992). The effect of the plasma levels of proteins C&S on the prediction of warfarin maintenance dose requirements. *Clinical Pharmacology and Therapeutics 52,* 42-49.
22. Khamashta, M., Cuadrado, M., Mujic, F., Taub, N., Hunt, B., & Hughes, G. (1995). The management of thrombosis in the antiphospholipid-antibody syndrome. *New England Journal of Medicine 332*(15), 993-997.
23. Fowler, W., Fretto, L., Hamilton, K. (1985). Substructure of human von Willebrand factor. *Journal of Clinical Investigation 76,* 4468-4471.
24. Langemo, D. (1999). Venous ulcers: Etiology and care of patients treated with human skin equivalents. *Journal of Vascular Nursing 17*(1), 6-11.
25. Nunnelee, J.D., & Spaner, S.D. (1997). An investigation of the explanatory model of illness in venous disease: A pilot study. *Journal of Vascular Nursing 15*(4), 131-133.
26. Nunnelee, J.D., & Spaner, S.D. (2000). The explanatory model of chronic venous disease in the rural Midwest-A factor analysis. *Journal of Vascular Nursing 18*(1), 6-10.
27. Anderson, L. (1999). Ischemic venous thrombosis: Its hidden agenda. *Journal of Vascular Nursing 17*(1), 1-5.
28. Okajima, K., Abe, H., & Binder, B. (1995). Endothelial cell injury induced by plasmin in vitro. *Journal of Laboratory and Clinical Medicine 126,* 377-384.
29. Mohanty, D., Al Hassan, H., Neglen, P.L, Eklof, B., & Das, K. (1995). Protein C deficiency in Kuwait. *Journal of Laboratory Clinical Medicine 126,* 373-376.
30. Griffin, J. (1984). Clinical studies on protein C. *Seminars in Thrombosis and Hemostasis 10,* 162-165.

31. Diefenderfer, S., Matula, P., & Niznik, C. (1994). Protein S deficiency: A case study. *Journal of Vascular Nursing 12*(3), 68-72.
32. Van den Belt, A., Sanson, B., Siminioni, P., Prandoni, P., Buller, H., Girolami, A., et al. (1997). Recurrence of venous thromboembolism in patients with familial thrombophilia. *Archives of Internal Medicine 157,* 2227-2232.
33. Brandt, J., Triplett, D., Alving, B., & Scharrer, I. (1995). Criteria for the diagnosis of lupus anticoagulants: An update. *Thrombosis and Hemostasis 74*(4), 1185-1190.
34. Nunnelee, J.D. (1996). Decision making in prevention and treatment of arterial ulcers: Use of patho-flow diagramming. *Journal of Vascular Nursing 14,* 72-78.
35. Nunnelee, J., & Kurgan, A. (1993). Interruption of the inferior vena cava for venous thromboembolic disease. *Journal of Vascular Nursing 11*(3), 80-82.
36. Warner, M., & Kelton, J. (1998). Approach to the patient with thrombocytopenia. In J. Ginsberg, C. Kearon, & J. Hirsch (eds.), *Critical decisions in thrombosis and hemostasis* (pp. 338-348). Hamilton, Ontario: Decker.
37. Warkentin, T. (1998). Diagnosis and treatment of disseminated intravascular coagulation. In J. Ginsberg, C. Kearon, & J. Hirsch (eds.), *Critical decisions in thrombosis and hemostasis* (pp. 322-329). Hamilton, Ontario: Decker.
38. Pabinger, J., Brucker, S., Kyrle, P., Schneider, B., Korninger, H., Niessner, H., et al. (1992). Hereditary deficiency of antithrombin II, protein C and protein S: Prevalence in patients with a history of venous thrombosis and criteria for rational patient screening. *Blood Coagulation and Fibrinolysis 3,* 547-553.
39. Amaragiri, S.V., & Lees, T.A. (2002). Elastic compression stockings for prevention of deep vein thrombosis (Cochrane Review). In: *The Cochrane Library,* Issue 4. Oxford: Update Software.
40. Handoll, H.H.G., Farrar, M.J., McBirnie, J., Tytherleigh-Strong, G., Milne, A.A., Gillespie, W.J. (2002). Heparin, low molecule weight heparin, and physical methods for preventing deep vein thrombosis and pulmonary embolism following surgery for hip fractures. (Cochrane Review). In: *The Cochrane Library,* Issue 4. Oxford: Update Software.
41. Estrada, C.A., Mansfield, C.J., & Heudebert, G.R. (2000). Cost-effectiveness of low-molecular weight heparin in the treatment of proximal deep vein thrombosis. *Journal of General Internal Medicine 15,* 108-115.
42. Nunnelee, J. (1997). Low molecular weight heparin. *Journal of Vascular Nursing 15,* 94-97.
43. Hirsch, J., Kearon, C., & Ginsberg, J. (1997). Duration of anticoagulant therapy after first episode of venous thrombosis in patients with inherited thrombophilia. *Archives of Internal Medicine 157,* 2174-2177.
44. Pulmonary Embolism Prevention (PEP) Trial Collaborative Group. (2000). Prevention of pulmonary embolism and deep vein thrombosis with low dose aspirin: Pulmonary Embolism Prevention (PEP) trial. *Lancet, 355,* 1295-1302.
45. Schulman, S., Rhedin, A.S., Lindmarker, P., Carlsson, A., Larfars, G., Nicol, P., et al. (1995). A comparison of six weeks with six months of oral anticoagulant therapy after a first episode of venous thromboembolism. Duration of Anticoagulation Trial Study Group. *New England Journal of Medicine 332,* 1661-1665.
46. McSweeney, J. (1993). Explanatory models of a myocardial event: Linkages between perceived causes and modified health behaviors. *Rehabilitation Nursing Research 2*(1), 40-50.
47. Nunnelee, J. (1999). The explanatory model of illness in chronic venous disease: A confirmatory factor analysis. [Unpublished doctoral dissertation.] University of Missouri–St. Louis.
48. Ansell, J.E., Weitz, J.I., Comerota, A.J., (2002). Advances in therapy and management of antithrombotic drugs for venous thromboembolism. *Hematology, 1,* 266-284.

CHAPTER 19 Impaired Sleep

KATHRYN A. LEE

DEFINITION

In healthy adults, normal sleep should consist of falling asleep 5 to 10 minutes after turning out the light, sleeping for 7 to 8 hours, and awakening feeling rested and ready to perform activities of daily living. Remaining alert and energetic throughout the day is an excellent indicator of a good night's sleep. A good night's sleep is often taken for granted until sleep becomes impaired and requires intervention strategies to manage the impairment.

What constitutes normal sleep varies across the life span and across cultures. Healthy infants have more sleep periods throughout the day and night, sleeping 40% to 50% of the 24-hour day.[1] Adolescents sleep about 10 hours at night but often have difficulty waking up in the morning, whereas elderly persons often sleep less than 6 hours and complain of awakening too early in the morning. In many cultures, napping in the afternoon is commonplace, particularly in warmer, tropical climates. Young children in the United States are often encouraged to nap once during the day, whereas an adult nap is often viewed as a sign of illness or laziness. For most North Americans, falling asleep during the day, whether voluntarily, as in a nap, or involuntarily, is seen as a symptom of either acutely impaired sleep the previous night or chronically impaired sleep.

Impaired sleep can be categorized as either sleep deprivation resulting from an inadequate amount of sleep or sleep disruption resulting from fragmented sleep during the night. As indicated in Figure 19-1, sleep deprivation is often a result of lifestyle or developmental issues, whereas sleep disruption is often a result of health-related conditions. Both sleep deprivation and sleep disruption result in sleep loss and potential adverse health outcomes. Impaired sleep in the form of sleep deprivation is easily recognized, because it can be quantified as reduced sleep time. Lifestyle behaviors, such as going to bed too late or getting up too early, drinking caffeinated beverages in the evening, and juggling work and family roles are examples of inadequate sleep resulting from sleep deprivation. This type of acute sleep loss, although still having detrimental consequences on mood and performance during the day, does not represent a pathological state. It is of less concern to health care providers, because it is a behaviorally induced sleep impairment that is easily treated by getting more sleep the following night. Other reasons for inadequate amounts of sleep include work schedules, such as working evenings or night shifts, and developmental adaptations, when sleep patterns are likely to change as a result of puberty, pregnancy, retirement, or old age.

The focus of this chapter is on impaired sleep that is more pathological and difficult to recognize and treat. Sleep disruption, or fragmented sleep, often results from physical or mental health problems or lifestyles with ongoing, chronic, poor health habits. What makes this type of impaired sleep more difficult to recognize is that it often goes unperceived by the person doing the sleeping and can only be documented by an alert bed partner or by objective monitoring.

PREVALENCE AND POPULATIONS AT RISK

Impaired sleep varies in its prevalence across the life span. In children, the most common forms of impaired sleep occur within the category of parasomnias. A parasomnia is a form of maintenance insomnia in which arousals from sleep occur during deep sleep stages. These arousals manifest as sleep talking, sleep walking, enuresis (bed wetting), bruxism (teeth grinding), and sleep terrors. There is often no memory of the arousal, which can be quite dramatic to parents who witness the event, and effects on daytime activity, such as school performance, fatigue, or sports, are not well known. Parasomnias affect between 3% (sleep terrors) and 30% (enuresis) of children. It has been estimated that bruxism can persist into adulthood for between 35% and 86%[2] of the population. Although it is rare for those with impaired sleep from a childhood parasomnia to have

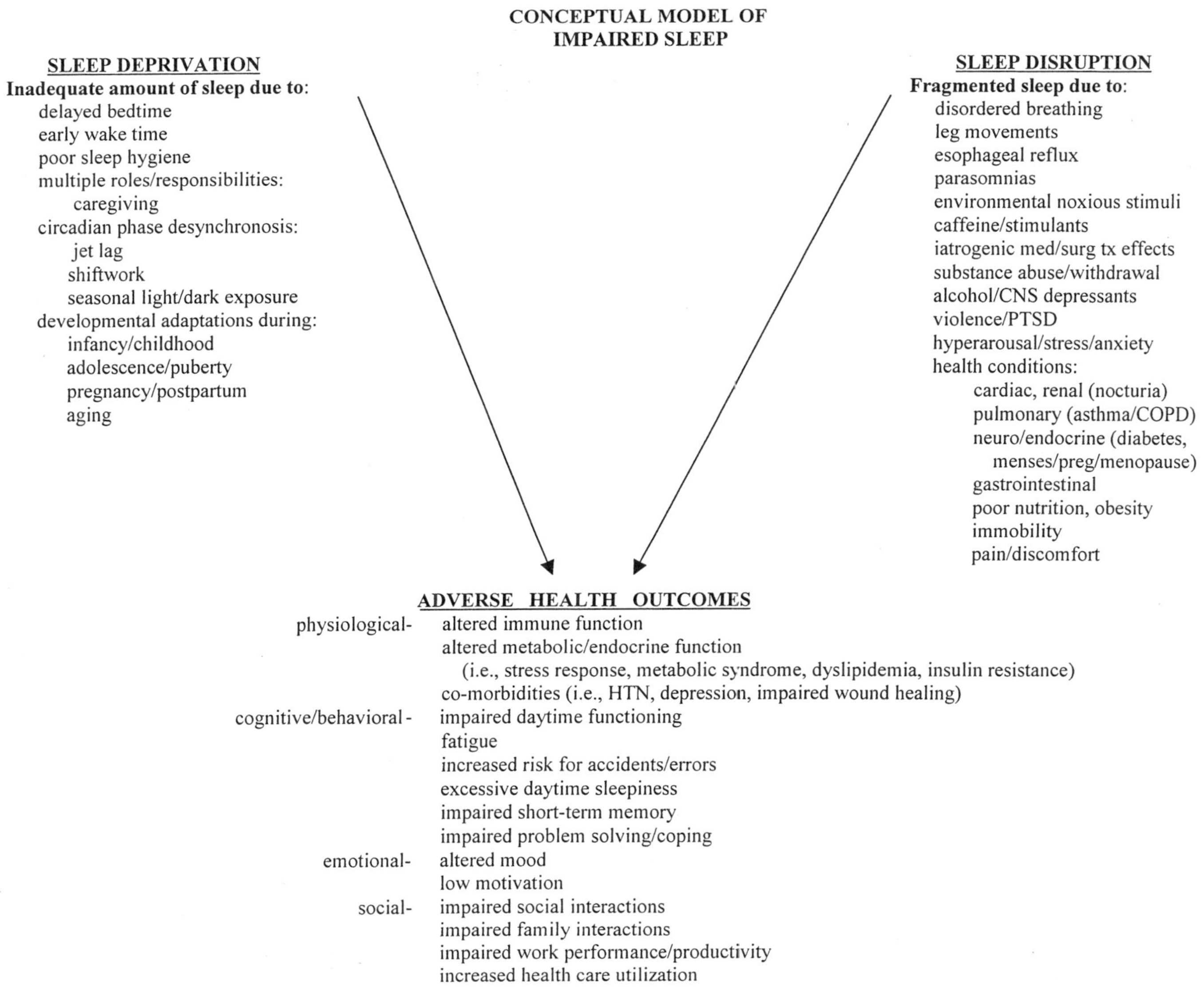

CONCEPTUAL MODEL OF
IMPAIRED SLEEP
SLEEP DEPRIVATION
Inadequate amount of sleep due to:
delayed bedtime
early wake time
poor sleep hygiene
multiple roles/responsibilities:
caregiving
circadian phase desynchronosis:
jet lag
shiftwork
seasonal light/dark exposure
developmental adaptations during:
infancy/childhood
adolescence/puberty
pregnancy/postpartum
aging
SLEEP DISRUPTION
Fragmented sleep due to:
disordered breathing
leg movements
esophageal reflux
parasomnias
environmental noxious stimuli
caffeine/stimulants
iatrogenic med/surg tx effects
substance abuse/withdrawal
alcohol/CNS depressants
violence/PTSD
hyperarousal/stress/anxiety
health conditions:
cardiac, renal (nocturia)
pulmonary (asthma/COPD)
neuro/endocrine (diabetes,
menses/preg/menopause)
gastrointestinal
poor nutrition, obesity
immobility
pain/discomfort
ADVERSE HEALTH OUTCOMES
physiological-
altered immune function
altered metabolic/endocrine function
(i.e., stress response, metabolic syndrome, dyslipidemia, insulin resistance)
co-morbidities (i.e., HTN, depression, impaired wound healing)
cognitive/behavioral -
impaired daytime functioning
fatigue
increased risk for accidents/errors
excessive daytime sleepiness
impaired short-term memory
impaired problem solving/coping
emotional-
altered mood
low motivation
social-
impaired social interactions
impaired family interactions
impaired work performance/productivity
increased health care utilization

Figure 19-1 Conceptual model of impaired sleep. (Courtesy Kathryn Lee, Chair, Nursing Sleep Curriculum Task Force, 2002.)

the same parasomnia continue into adulthood, longitudinal studies are lacking in this population, and long-term outcomes are unknown.

Adolescents experience impaired sleep related to circadian rhythm, rather than to a specific form of insomnia. During this time in development, adolescents are likely to have an alteration in their circadian rhythm in which it is difficult or impossible to fall asleep at a previously routine earlier bedtime and then equally as difficult to arouse from sleep in the morning. This phenomenon is called *delayed sleep phase syndrome.* Carskadon et al.[3] noted that it is most likely biological factors (such as timing of melatonin or sex hormone secretions) rather than social factors (such as peer group influences or lack of parental control) that result in adolescent delayed sleep phase syndrome. Schools that impose early class start times for adolescents often create difficulty for the students and their parents, yet long-term consequences remain unknown.

Delayed sleep phase syndrome can often continue into adulthood as the more familiar "night owl" phenomenon, with poor sleep hygiene lifestyle habits persisting in futile efforts to cope with this syndrome. Employers who expect workers to begin functioning in the early morning hours often have performance issues with those who have delayed sleep phase. Given longer commute times from home to work and society's expectations of work hours and school hours between 8:00 AM and 5:00 PM, this type of circadian rhythm disorder often manifests as impaired sleep because of the person's great difficulty in initiating sleep early enough to obtain sufficient hours of sleep before arriving at the work site the next morning. It is estimated that between 5% and 10% of insomniacs who seek treatment actually have a circadian rhythm disorder,[4] but actual prevalence estimates for delayed sleep phase is unknown. It may be unknown because human beings are very adaptable and can find alternative, albeit unhealthy and ineffective, ways to cope with this disorder. (Circadian rhythms and treatments for delayed sleep phase syndrome were discussed in Chapter 3.)

During adulthood, the prevalence of impaired sleep varies by gender and health status. Women's menstrual cycles, pregnancy, motherhood, and menopausal transition are well known periods of high prevalence for impaired sleep in women.[5-7] In the general population, national surveys estimate that the complaint of general insomnia is more prevalent among women (42.4%) than men (32.5%), even though there was no difference in the average hours of sleep (7 hours) each night.[8] It is estimated that 32% of adults have excessive daytime sleepiness, despite their perception that nighttime sleep is adequate.[9] Relationships with family members and co-workers inevitably lead to stress in our lives; this is cited as a major reason for impaired sleep. (Impaired sleep associated with stress is discussed further under Risk Factors.)

For both men and women, advanced age brings with it chronic health conditions, such as obesity, heart disease, inflammatory disease, and mental health problems, that lead to impaired sleep. Healthy older adults often experience impaired sleep related to long-term poor health habits, poor nutrition, or lack of physical activity. The National Institute on Aging conducted a multisite epidemiological study of the elderly that included more than 9000 men and women over 65 years of age and found that more than 50% of these subjects reported impaired sleep most of the time. Older women reported more difficulty falling asleep and midsleep awakenings, whereas men complained more of daytime sleepiness. These complaints are often confounded by chronic health problems and medication side effects,[10,11] and prevalence can be much higher in nursing home facilities. As discussed in Chapter 3, exposure to adequate periods of sunlight and darkness is essential for healthy sleep patterns. For older adults, melatonin secretion during darkness is already reduced significantly from the melatonin values measured in young adults, but elderly persons are also less likely to be exposed to light. Many are institutionalized, and many more have visual problems or experience social isolation that predisposes them to advanced sleep phase syndrome, in which they might still obtain the same amount of sleep but, in sharp contrast with adolescents, elders get sleepy earlier in the evening and awaken earlier in the morning.

In addition to advanced sleep phase syndrome, maintenance insomnia is common in the elderly, either because of periodic leg movements or nocturnal myoclonus, or because of urinary frequency, arthritic pain, or other health conditions. The sleeper is aware of the awakenings for bladder emptying but is often unaware of myoclonus. The jerks or kicks occur about every 30 seconds in clustered episodes throughout the night, and about 45% of healthy community-dwelling elderly persons experience periodic leg movements.[10]

The most prevalent specific cause of impaired sleep in adult men and women is sleep-disordered breathing, which encompasses a continuum from mild snoring to severe obstructive sleep apnea. Prevalence increases with age, from 10% of men and 5% of women between 30 and 40 years of age to 20% for men and 15% of women between 50 and 60 years of age.[12] The prevalence also increases with obesity and alcohol use, as well as genetic predisposition, perhaps because of inherited facial structures or vulnerability to airway collapse.[13] There are also ethnic differences in the prevalence of this sleep-disordered breathing, with higher prevalence among Hispanics (16.3%) compared with Whites (4.9%) in a San Diego population[14] and higher prevalence among Blacks at an earlier age compared with Whites.[15] Both craniofacial structure (i.e., more retropositioned mandible and smaller posterior airway space) and soft tissue characteristics (soft palate length and tongue volume) are inherited genetic risks for obstructive sleep apnea.

RISK FACTORS

Environmental, Personal, and Developmental Factors

Risk factors for impaired sleep include all of the factors responsible for sleep deprivation and sleep disruption depicted in Figure 19-1. These risk factors fall into three primary categories: environmental, personal, and developmental. External environmental factors known to impair sleep by fragmentation include unexpected noise and light during the night that results in arousals from sleep and thus maintenance insomnia. Although small children may have the capacity to sleep through loud noises and bright daylight, it is a different scenario for older adults and elderly persons, who have less-deep sleep stages than do younger adults and children. Fragmented sleep patterns are more frequent for adults when the noise at night is unexpected, such as in crowded urban settings with automobile traffic, airports, and noisy neighbors. Inpatient hospital settings can be so disruptive of sleep from light and noise that the patient's need for uninterrupted sleep results in premature hospital discharge. More common and expected noises within the home, such as a crying infant or snoring bed partner, are just as disruptive of sleep, yet the brief arousals and maintenance insomnia may or may not be consciously perceived. Nevertheless, sleep is impaired as a result of these external environmental factors, whatever their source and regardless of conscious perception, because of the resulting sleep loss and adverse health outcomes.

Personal risk factors for impaired sleep can be conceptualized as the internal environmental milieu that provides a balance of neuroendocrine functioning within the central nervous system. The internal environment is influenced by the physiological and psychological stressors that result from poor nutrition, a situational crisis, either inadequate or very strenuous physical activity, a disease process, or medical treatments such as surgery, radiation, chemotherapy, or surprisingly, prescription hypnotic agents. For example, anemic conditions result in inadequate oxygenation and may lead to a syndrome known as *restless legs*.[16] Persons with restless legs syndrome experience initiation insomnia because of a neurosensory sensation described as an uncontrollable need to move their legs[17] just as they try to relax to fall asleep.

Fragmented sleep, or frequent arousals from sleep during the night is also known as maintenance insomnia. This form of impaired sleep can result from frequent urination, diarrhea, or nausea and vomiting associated with disease processes or iatrogenic treatment effects. The impaired sleep that results from any of these internal personal factors is detrimental to daytime functioning and may be more detrimental to quality of life, resulting in more adverse health outcomes than the disease process itself.[8]

The major risk factor for impaired sleep among healthy adults is a stressful lifestyle. Stressful life events and chronic stress are major causes of impaired sleep, particularly when emotions and ruminating thoughts prevail and prevent initiating sleep. The classic stress response involves release of glucose to mobilize energy, increase cardiovascular tone, and sharpen the senses, which make sleep all but impossible. Because of the stimulatory effects of stress on the hypothalamic-pituitary-adrenal axis, sleep patterns are directly affected by both acute and chronic stress. Acute stress and situational crises are usually self-limiting, and therapeutic use of hypnotic agents is indicated in these brief situations. Acute stress can activate the immune system, but chronic stress can inhibit immune response and the cytokines involved in regulation of sleep.[18] This is discussed further in the section on mechanisms of impaired sleep. It is chronic stress that requires more challenging behavioral and cognitive interventions to promote sleep. Although it may be tempting to intervene with prescription hypnotic medications, they have significant adverse effects (discussed later in the chapter). Rather than a hypnotic agent, stress-reducing exercises during the daytime and relaxation strategies at bedtime are most beneficial for chronic life stressors.

Another common personal risk factor for impaired sleep in the adult population is working evening or night schedules or traveling rapidly across time zones and experiencing jet lag. Both situations are forms of circadian rhythm disturbances and result in sleep deprivation (discussed in depth in Chapter 3).

Developmental risk factors for impaired sleep consist of chronic unhealthy lifestyle behaviors that develop in young adulthood. These behaviors often develop in response to stressful life situations or undiagnosed sleep disorders, such as delayed sleep phase syndrome or narcolepsy. In addition to poor diet and lack of adequate exercise, other aspects of one's lifestyle increase the risks for chronically impaired sleep. Drinking caffeinated beverages in the evening, watching late-night television while in bed, or drinking alcoholic beverages in an attempt to fall asleep are all examples of poor sleep hygiene practices that develop in an attempt to self-treat stressful life situations or undiagnosed sleep disorders. For instance, drinking hot chocolate at bedtime may be relaxing and promote the onset of sleep, but the stimulating effects of the chocolate will cause brief arousals during sleep, particularly at its peak effect. Others may be drinking an herbal tea on a nightly basis, not realizing that a particular tea is high in caffeine, even though it is an herbal product. The consumer may not even be aware of the maintenance insomnia that ensues, yet will complain of not feeling rested in the morning and feeling irritable and fatigued the next day. This then perpetuates a cycle of drinking more caffeinated beverages to stay awake and maintain peak performance during the day. (For further discussion of caffeine, see Clinical Management.)

MECHANISMS OF NORMAL AND IMPAIRED SLEEP

The physiological mechanisms for normal sleep are poorly understood and still under investigation by many researchers involved in both animal models as well as human brain mapping and genetics. Until such time as the mechanisms for normal sleep are understood, the function of sleep or the purpose for sleep will remain a mystery, as will the pathological consequences of impaired sleep.

The mechanisms for normal sleep and wake cycles surely involve the suprachiasmatic nuclei in the anterior hypothalamus, an area known as the internal clock. Damage to this area of the brain results in impaired wake/sleep cycles. As discussed in Chapter 3, light and dark are the most powerful stimuli, operating through the retinohypothalamic pathway, that allows for wake to alternate with sleep in a predictable 24-hour pattern. Persons with retinal damage and blindness, or lack of exposure to environmental light and dark such as may occur in some institutionalized settings or intensive care environments, also have impaired sleep because they cannot stay entrained to a 24-hour day length. Melatonin, secreted only at night, is the brain's internal signal for darkness. Rhythmic melatonin secretion at night begins to occur at 2 to 3 months of age, peaks at 5 years of age, and a major decrease occurs at puberty, with a final decrease by 50% in the fourth decade of life and very low levels in old age.[19]

In addition to exposure to darkness, melatonin secretion requires the ability of cells in the pineal gland and other tissues to convert tryptophan to serotonin, in the presence of vitamin B_6, and then finally to melatonin. Low-dose tricyclic antidepressants, often prescribed for initiation insomnia, are sympathomimetic agents that stimulate melatonin secretion,[20] whereas beta-blockers used in treatment of hypertension suppress melatonin production.[21] Melatonin's ability to induce sleep directly may be related to its ability to reduce core body temperature, activate GABA neurons in the brain, or raise the threshold for cortical arousal.[22]

Recent efforts to discover the cause of narcolepsy, a sleep disorder discussed later, have brought to light the role of hypocretins, a class of neuropeptides found in lateral hypothalamic neurons that project to the cortex, limbic system, and brainstem. This neurotransmitter may prove to be directly involved in the "sleep gene."[23]

In addition to the internal clock for distinguishing day from night, increasing the threshold for arousal is necessary in order to initiate sleep. The role of the reticular activating system in the brain and its effect on level of arousal and consciousness is detailed in Chapter 8. Once arousal threshold is elevated, sleep onset can occur, and normal sleep begins, with cycles of light sleep, deep sleep, and REM sleep. As seen in Figure 19-2, there is a progression from awake and drowsiness (alpha waves) and very light sleep (theta waves) and slow rolling eye movements (stage 1) to light sleep (stage 2) and appearance of sleep spindles on the EEG. Then an episode of deep sleep (stages 3 and 4, slow EEG waves or delta sleep) occurs before the first appearance of a short REM period at about 90 minutes after the onset of sleep. The progression through these sleep stages across the night is more clearly depicted in the sleep hypnograms presented in Figure 19-3.

Healthy adults spend about 50% to 55% of their sleep time in light sleep, about 20% in deep sleep,

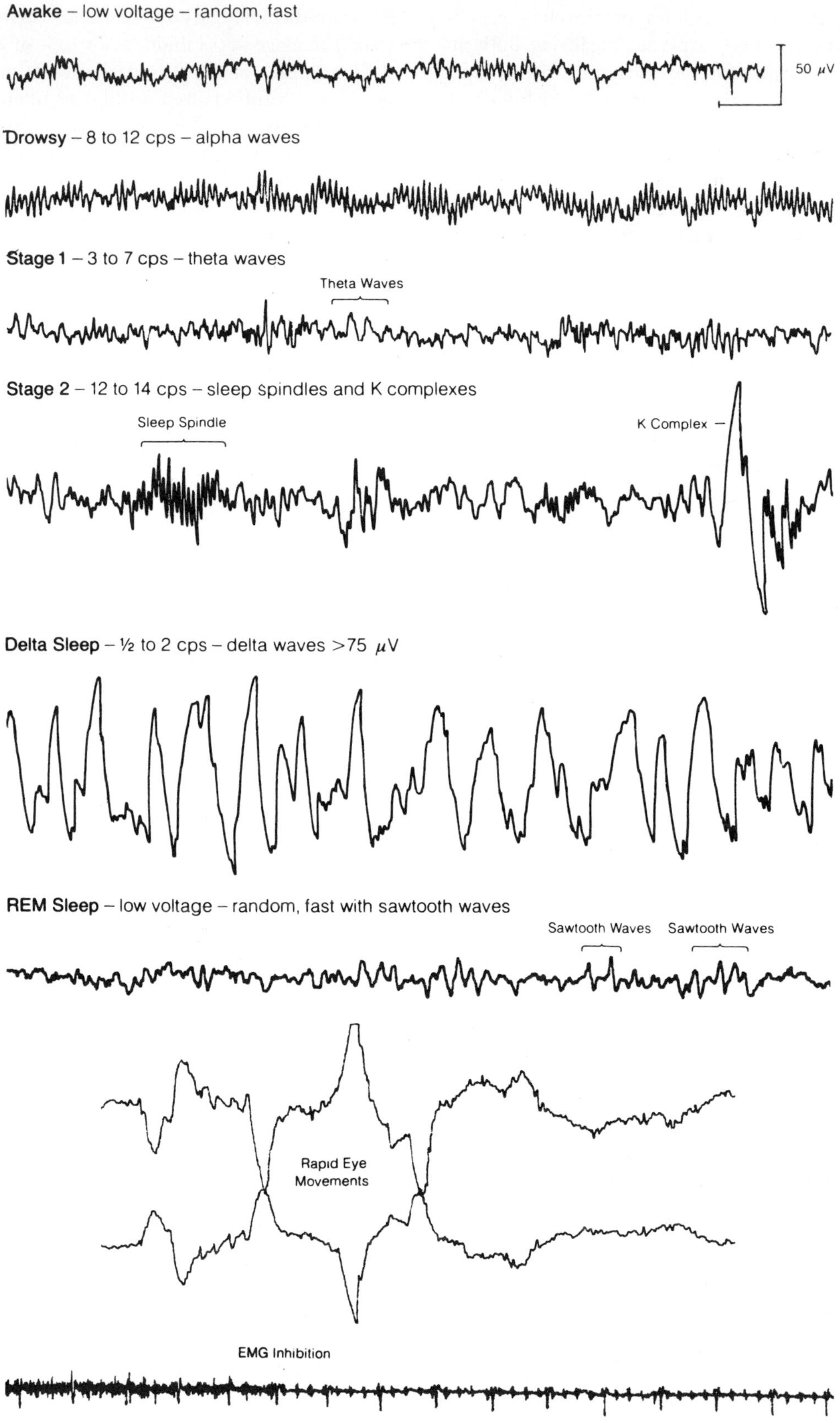

Figure 19-2 Polysomnographic depiction of stages of sleep. (From Hauri, P. [1992]. *Sleep disorders.* Pharmacia, Peapack NJ.)

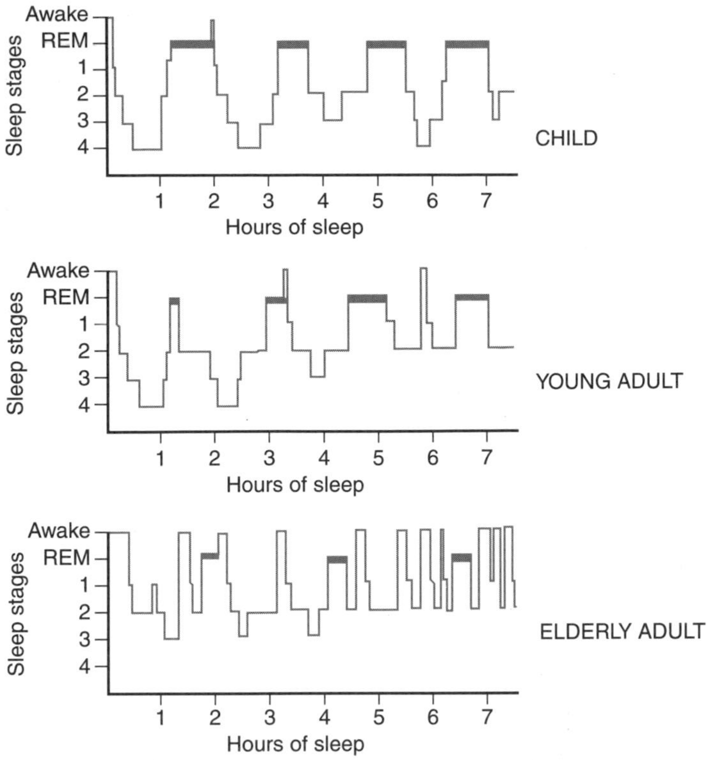

Figure 19-3 Hypnogram representation of typical progression through sleep stages during the night according to developmental age groups. (From Lee, K. [1999]. In C. Lindeman, & M. McAthie [eds.], *Fundamentals of contemporary nursing practice.* Philadelphia: W.B. Saunders.)

and about 25% in REM sleep, with less than 5% awake time during the night. In sharp contrast, young infants spend about 50% to 80% of their sleep time in REM and have very little light sleep or awake time, while the elderly have primarily light sleep stages 1 and 2, and may have as little as 5% deep sleep during the night (Figures 19-3 and 19-4). During non-REM light and deep sleep stages, muscle tone is greatly diminished, there is a fall in body temperature, and heart rate, respirations, and blood pressure are low and steady while thermoregulation is maintained.[24]

During REM sleep, however, there are noticeable heart rate and respiratory irregularities, small muscle twitches particularly in the face, a complete loss of skeletal muscle tone, and an inability to regulate body temperature. This may cause the patient monitored in intensive care environments to appear very unstable and in need of medical intervention. Often REM sleep is suppressed by opiates and other central nervous system depressants prescribed during hospitalization, and it is not until the drug is withdrawn that REM rebound occurs, with unstable cardiovascular responses.

The specific stages of sleep are regulated by brainstem mechanisms that involve orchestration of specific neurotransmitters and projections to the forebrain as well as spinal motoneurons. These specific stages of sleep have a circadian rhythm as well. As seen in Figure 19-3, deep sleep (stages 3 and 4, delta sleep) occurs primarily during the first third of the night and rapid-eye-movement (REM) sleep occurs primarily during the last third of the night. This is also the case in naps, where late afternoon and evening naps consist primarily of deep sleep while morning naps consist primarily of REM sleep. In the elderly, however, REM sleep loses its circadian rhythm and becomes more evenly distributed across the night.[25]

Both REM sleep and non-REM deep sleep are crucial to health and well-being, yet sleep deprivation studies would indicate that deep sleep is preferentially restored before REM sleep. There is very clear evidence for the role of serotonin in preparing the brain for slow wave sleep by acting on multiple receptors known to inhibit arousal. Non-REM deep sleep is induced soon after sleep onset by serotonergic mechanisms in the raphe nuclei in the brainstem

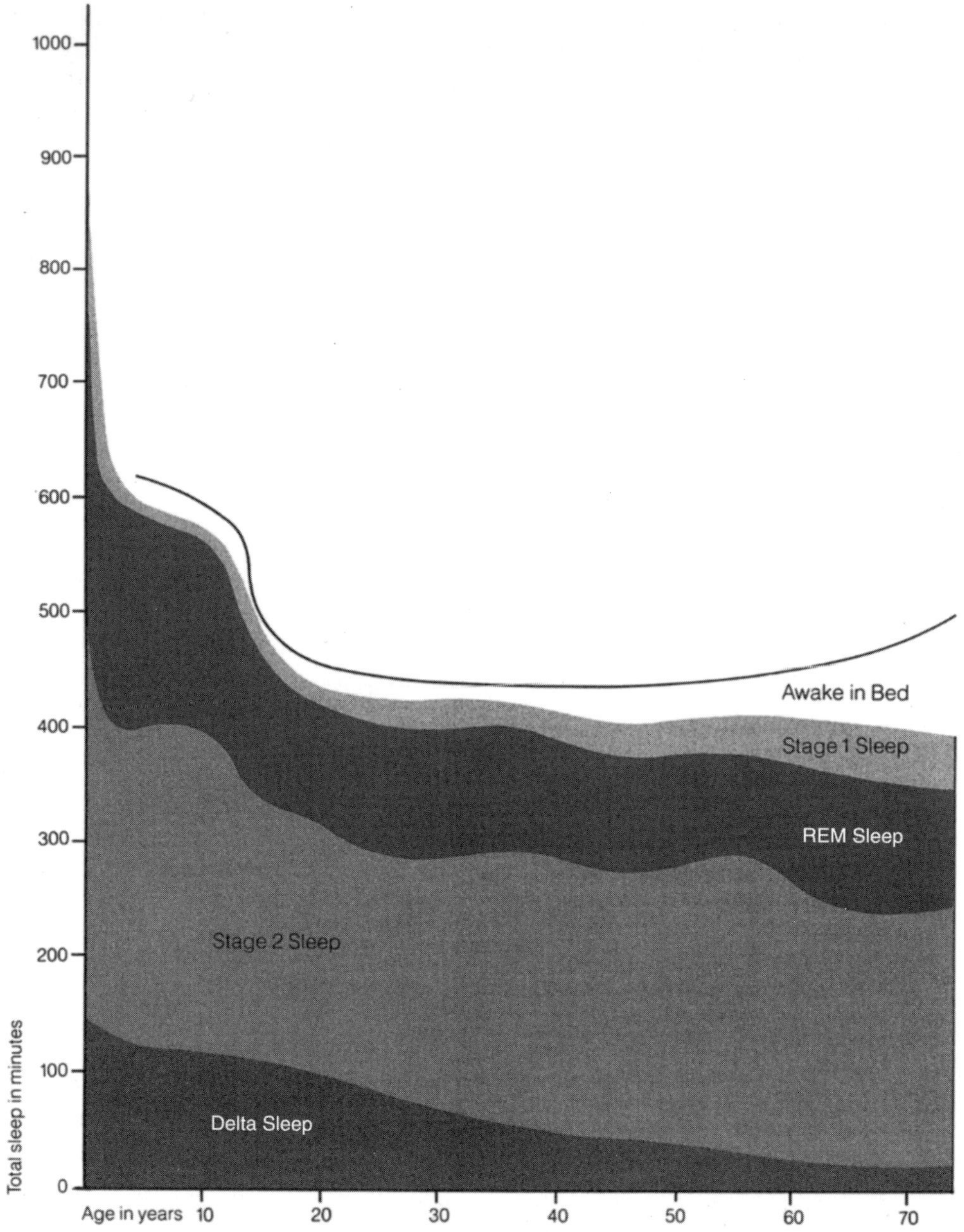

Figure 19-4 Changes in sleep time and stages of sleep across the life span. (From Hauri, P. [1992]. *Sleep disorders.* Kalamazoo: Upjohn.)

which inhibit cholinergic neurons responsible for cortical arousal. There is also evidence that gamma-aminobutyric acid (GABA), a major inhibitory neurotransmitter in the brain, plays a role in deep sleep. GABA-rich neurons in the thalamic reticular nucleus, cortex, hypothalamus, and basal forebrain are activated during initiation and maintenance of slow wave deep sleep.[26] In fact, benzodiazepines, a major class of sedative/hypnotic medication, act by binding to GABA receptors in the brain, thus increasing the level of GABA in the brain and enhancing postsynaptic action of GABA.[26] Some herbal products marketed for impaired sleep actually contain valerian, kava-kava or chamomile, compounds with properties and adverse effects similar to benzodiazepines[27] and other CNS depressants.[28]

Deep sleep, seen as slow waves or large delta waves on the EEG is thought to be the restorative component of sleep, because those deprived specifically of deep sleep in a sleep laboratory complain of feeling tired and not fully rested the next day. It is also the first cycle of deep sleep that contains the highest level of growth hormone secretion. Even growth hormone releasing factor, produced in the hypothalamus is thought to have a role in inducing slow wave sleep as well as the surge of growth hormone that occurs during the first cycle of deep sleep.

When monitored by EEG, the brainwave activity during REM sleep is remarkably similar to the brainwave activity seen while awake (see Figure 19-2). However, there are mechanisms within the brainstem that produce the characteristic pattern of REM sleep that cannot be replicated while awake. The area of the brainstem most active during REM sleep is the pons, with REM-on cells in the locus coeruleus that are responsive to GABA and acetylcholine, and REM-off cells in the raphe nuclei that are responsive to epinephrine and serotonin. It has been demonstrated in animal models that cholinergic stimulation of the pons specifically triggers REM sleep onset.[26] However, GABA, an inhibitory amino acid, is increased in both the raphe nucleus and the locus coeruleus during REM sleep, and injections of GABA into the serotonergic raphe nuclei in animal models result in increased REM sleep. Table 19-1 summarizes the neuroanatomical sites and neurotransmitters thought to be responsible for stimulating wakefulness, non-REM sleep, and REM sleep.

It is the visibly apparent rapid eye movements witnessed during REM sleep that gave it its name. These eye movements consist of horizontal saccades (see Figure 19-2) resulting from pontine signals to the abducens nuclei at the floor of the fourth ventricle. These particular eye movements, controlled by the abducens cranial nerve, are impossible to perform while awake. In addition to these rapid eye movements, REM sleep involves loss of muscle tone, or atonia, which results from pontine signals to the spinal motoneurons to inhibit anti-gravitational muscles, leaving only the diaphragm and small facial and eye muscles active during REM sleep. Noradrenergic cells in the locus coeruleus release glutamate during REM sleep, which simultaneously suppresses muscle tone and activates twitching and rapid eye movements. Occasionally persons who awaken directly from REM sleep experience sleep paralysis, a frightful phenomenon in which it takes a few seconds to be able to move after awakening, but has no lingering effects.

Dreaming does occur during non-REM sleep stages, but the vivid dreams reported on awakening from REM sleep are likely the result of intense activation of the amygdala in the forebrain during REM sleep. REM sleep is thought to be involved in cognitive processing and memory. From studies of specifically depriving humans of REM sleep, it has been shown that cognitive processes and memory are impaired. One current hypothesis for the function of REM sleep is that its periodic episodes during sleep prevent desensitization of aminergic

TABLE 19-1 Brain Anatomical Sites and Associated Neurotransmitters for Wakefulness, Non-REM Sleep, and REM Sleep

	ANATOMICAL SITES	NEUROTRANSMITTERS
Wakefulness stimulated by:	Brainstem	
	Oral pontine	Norepinephrine
	Midbrain reticular formation	Acetylcholine
	Caudal diencephalon	
	Posterior hypothalamus	Histamine
	Subthalamus	Acetylcholine
	Ventral thalamus	Glutamate
	Basal forebrain	Acetylcholine
Non-REM sleep stimulated by:	Brainstem raphe nuclei	Serotonin
	Anterior hypothalamus	GABA
	Preoptic area	Serotonin
	Basal forebrain	GABA
REM sleep stimulated by:	Ventral pons:	Acetylcholine
	Medial reticular formation (eye movements)	
	Pedunculopontine nuclei (EEG activation)	
	Paraabducens nucleus (eye movements)	
	Laterodorsal tegmentum (atonia)	
	Basal forebrain	Acetylcholine

neuroreceptors that are continuously activated during wakefulness.[29]

PATHOLOGICAL CONSEQUENCES

When the brain is functioning normally and receives adequate nutritional support and amino acids to maintain serotonergic pathways and other neurotransmitters, natural consequences include reduced arousal as darkness descends in the evening, and controlled sleep onset when the individual reclines in bed. There is one disorder of brain function, a genetic disorder known as *narcolepsy,* that results in unpredictable REM sleep onset during the daytime. Although it is found in less than 2% of the general population, a first-degree relative is between 10 and 40 times more likely to have narcolepsy. Narcolepsy in dogs (especially Dobermans and Labradors) was recently identified as an actual genetic mutation in the hypocretin-2 receptor gene, which is localized within the lateral hypothalamus and projects to REM-on cells in the dorsal raphe and pontine cholinergic nuclei.[23] In response to sudden external environmental stimuli (such as loud noise or bright lights), or strong emotional feelings (such as joy or crying), an individual with narcolepsy goes into REM sleep and experiences the muscle atonia (cataplexy) of REM sleep as well (Figure 19-5).

Pathological conditions of the pulmonary, gastrointestinal, or neuromuscular systems can also impair sleep by frequent arousals that prevent the sleeper from ever getting beyond light sleep to enter deep sleep or REM sleep. The reduction in muscle tone during light sleep can be just sufficient to reduce the diameter of the airway and create snoring sounds, or totally obstruct the airway so that arousal is necessary to resume breathing. This pathological state of disordered breathing during sleep sets up a cascade of cardiopulmonary events that severely impact health and well-being. Even snoring without significant obstructive apnea causes episodes of increased blood pressure that lead to chronic hypertension. In a sample of more than 500 adults, Young et al.[30] demonstrated that both diastolic and systolic blood pressure were increasingly higher in patients with simple snoring and severe sleep apnea compared with nonsnorers. Their findings indicate that simple snoring is a risk for hypertension and cardiovascular disease, even when controlling statistically for age, gender, and body mass index.[30] Efforts to treat an obstructive airway during sleep include dental appliances that alter jaw occlusion[31] and nasal continuous positive pressure that either forces the airway to remain open or stimulates the tissue to maintain its tone.[32] More invasive and dramatic surgical procedures range from laser surgery to uvulo-palato-pharyngoplasty (UPPP) and tracheostomy.

The reduced muscle tone that begins with the onset of light non-REM sleep can impact an already compromised esophageal sphincter and create gastric reflux during sleep that cause microarousals from sleep, and hence maintenance insomnia. The individual may be aware of an acidic taste on awakening. Milder forms can be self-treated by elevation of the head during sleep. This disorder is common during the third trimester of pregnancy when the esophageal sphincter is repositioned because of the gravid uterus, and when smooth muscle tone is greatly diminished because of high progesterone levels.

Although pathological processes that fragment sleep may not necessarily be perceived by the sleeper, a bed partner is often well aware of the sleep disorder, indeed, is often hit or injured from the thrashings that the sleeper involuntarily initiates in an attempt to arouse from sleep, whether from impaired breathing, esophageal reflux, or the periodic leg movements or kicks. Thus it is the bed partner who can often provide the best patient history for the health care provider. Without a bed partner, the sleeper may have a clue to the pathological condition by observing the bed linens in total disarray in the morning from leg movements, by awakening in unusual positions in an effort to breathe, by sensations of choking, or by having an acidic taste on awakening.

Regardless of these nighttime sleep behaviors that can be quite irritating to bed partners and family members, the adverse health outcomes of these frequent arousals from sleep can be life-threatening. Because the sleeper with disordered breathing, esophageal reflux, or periodic leg movements is aroused so frequently that deep sleep and REM sleep are diminished or absent, the result is excessive sleepiness during the day, impaired cognitive performance, and other adverse outcomes outlined in Figure 19-1. Initially, the sleepiness may be manifested by falling asleep easily at night, just when the "head hits the pillow." As the pathological condition progresses and sleep deprivation becomes chronic, the individual can easily fall asleep while conversing, while driving an automobile, or while operating hazardous machinery. People with obstructive sleep apnea are two to three times more likely to be involved in automobile accidents than are the general population.[33] Unfortunately, it is often an episode of falling asleep at the wheel of a car that brings the person into health care for treatment of his or her sleep disorder.

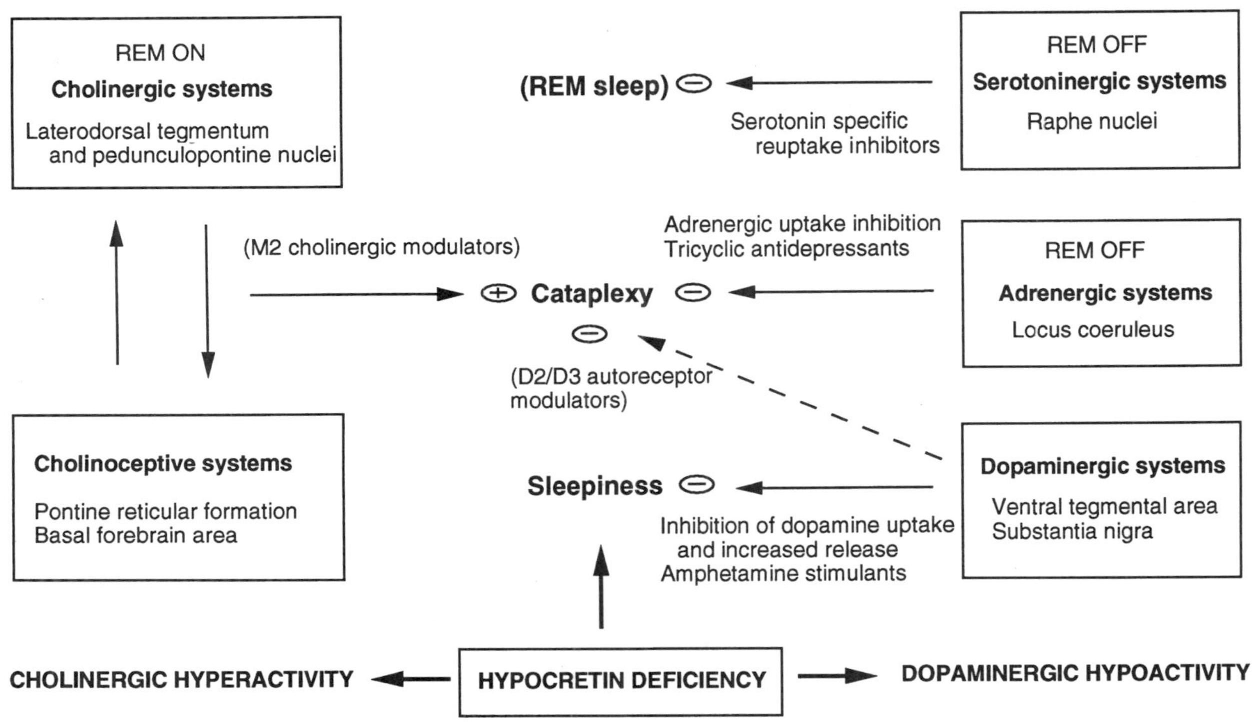

Figure 19-5 Brain mechanisms hypothesized in generating REM sleep and the cataplexy associated with narcolepsy and treatments to promote wakefulness. (From Kryger, M.H., Roth, T., & Dement, W.C. [2000]. *Principles and Practice of Sleep Medicine* [3rd ed., p. 668]. Philadelphia: W.B. Saunders.)

RELATED PATHOPHYSIOLOGICAL CONCEPTS/DIFFERENTIAL DIAGNOSIS

There are many pathophysiological concepts related to impaired sleep, a few of which are included as chapters in this book (circadian rhythm disorders, impaired immunity, and fatigue). Altered immune function, altered stress response, medication usage, posttraumatic stress disorder, and depression will be discussed in this section.

Altered Immune Function

Normal sleep and impaired sleep are the result of complex interactions between neurotransmitters in the brain, and environmental and developmental factors. Adding to the complexity of health care implications of impaired sleep is recent knowledge about the role of the immune system and cytokines in healthy sleep, and the effects of impaired sleep on immune function. In addition to the motoneuron innervation from the brainstem, sympathetic nerve fibers also innervate lymphoid tissues.[34] Interleukin-1, for instance, fluctuates on a circadian basis, activates serotonergic systems in the hypothalamus, and interacts with GABA receptors important for inducing deep sleep.[18] During experimental studies of sleep deprivation, young men had a higher rate of upper respiratory infection and reduced NK cell activity that returned to normal after recovery from their sleep deprivation.[35] Other researchers, however, have demonstrated an increase in NK activity in response to sleep deprivation, with no complaints of infection after completing the study.[36] It has been concluded from recent animal studies that immunosuppression can result from chronic sleep loss, with accumulation of antigen in lymph nodes and no fever in response to the opportunistic infection.[37] These results need to be replicated in other animal models and human research. Although research findings conflict, there are indications that cytokines have a role in promoting sleep as a normal mechanism of sleep induction and that impaired sleep does interfere with the circadian secretion of cytokines.

Medication Usage and Adverse Health Effects

With advanced age comes chronic illnesses and medical treatments that include pharmacological interventions. It is estimated that 90% of elderly persons take at least one prescription medication.[10] Because many of these medications have stimulating or depressing effects, with longer metabolic actions, the risk for impaired sleep is increased. Many older individuals also have developed a lifestyle habit that involves consuming alcohol or taking over-the-counter sleep medications in the evening to facilitate sleep. Tolerance to these substances develops over time, and REM suppression is common with many CNS depressants. Sudden withdrawal from these substances can induce a REM rebound effect. This can mean an increase of up to 300% in REM sleep and frequent arousals from sleep so that the person experiences very restless sleep and nightmares as well as fatigue and impaired daytime functioning, which prompt continued use of the substance.[38]

Posttraumatic Stress Disorder

Posttraumatic stress disorder (PTSD) includes disturbed sleep as part of its diagnosis. Hypothesized as a hyperarousal disorder that results from experiencing a traumatic event, PTSD victims have abnormal noradrenergic production and function and frequently complain of impaired sleep, restless sleep, and nightmares regardless of whether the traumatic event was recent or many years ago.[39,40] In a study reported by Lavie et al.,[41] initiating sleep took about 9 minutes longer and wake time was doubled (12%) in war veterans compared with control subjects (6%). The increased wake time may be related to the documented increase in body movements during sleep, particularly leg movements and parasomnias such as sleep talking and sleep walking in children or adults.[42]

Aside from a few studies of hurricane or robbery victims, most laboratory studies of PTSD involve male war veterans, and very little is known about women's experiences of PTSD and sleep complaints. Women who survive abuse by intimate male partners complain of impaired sleep. Whether this is because of the frequency with which the abuse occurs during the night or is a form of PTSD remains to be studied.[43] Women who experience a pregnancy loss can then experience a type of PTSD with a subsequent pregnancy.[44] Some of the sleep stage changes documented on polysomnography may be indirectly related to depression that results from the trauma experience rather than being directly related to the traumatic event. There appears to be no significant differences in stages of sleep, particularly REM sleep, or daytime sleepiness as a result of PTSD; some victims may have a distorted perception about time to initiate sleep rather than having actual impaired sleep.[45] Dream content is more likely to be anxiety related, with a vivid, nightmare quality and hostile, threatening content.[39]

Major Depressive Illness and Winter Depression

A major risk factor for disturbed sleep is depressive illness, which includes sleep disturbance and fatigue as major manifestations. Those diagnosed with major depression complain of initiation insomnia as well as maintenance insomnia, but also exhibit a characteristic REM sleep pattern when physiologically monitored in a laboratory setting. The first REM sleep episode usually begins earlier than expected, and there is more REM sleep than expected, spread equally across the night's sleep. Antidepressants have an immediate effect on the brain wave patterns monitored during sleep, but it may be a few weeks before individuals perceive any improvement in their mood, physical symptoms, or daytime functioning. In addition to the chronic sleep loss associated with resulting major depression, either from inadequate amounts of sleep or fragmentation of nightly sleep, sleep loss itself can alter metabolic and endocrine function in such a manner that depressive symptoms become a comorbid condition of impaired sleep.

In northern climates, the long period of darkness in the winter months and the long period of light during the summer months can affect melatonin secretion and circadian rhythms. This is often called *winter depression,* or *seasonal affective disorder,* and sleep deprivation is a major complaint. Although it is temporary, it does increase risk for all the adverse health outcomes associated with sleep loss from other etiologies outlined in Figure 19-1. (This disorder was discussed in greater detail in Chapter 3.)

MANIFESTATIONS AND SURVEILLANCE

The primary manifestation of impaired sleep is either difficulty falling asleep, difficulty arousing in the morning, daytime fatigue, daytime sleepiness, poor daytime performance, or misuse of hypnotics and other substances to manage the impaired sleep. An example of questions often used to assess patients for impaired sleep can be found in Box 19-1. If daytime sleepiness is evident from the patient's history, further assessment is warranted. Box 19-2 provides specific questions to assess some of the more common causes of daytime sleepiness. In the remainder of this section, objective and subjective measures to capture the extent of the impaired sleep will be discussed, with strengths and limitations of each.

The most valid and reliable objective measure of impaired sleep is polysomnography (PSG), which consists of multiple channels to record electrical activity (see Figure 19-2; electrooculography [EOG]) that includes: electroencephalography (EEG) from surface areas over the brain to obtain the rolling eye movements as sleep onset occurs and to document the rapid eye movements of REM sleep; electromyogram (EMG) of a small facial muscle under the chin or on the mandible; respiratory movements; oxygen saturation; anterior tibialis leg muscle movements; and even time-linked video-recorded body position during sleep.[46] PSG is the gold standard for impaired manifestations of sleep, and it must be carried out by technicians trained in the standardized protocol for monitoring and analyzed according to criteria for scoring the various stages of sleep. For the sleeper, who may already have impaired sleep, this method often requires a night to adapt to sleeping in a strange sleep clinic bed with electrodes on the scalp and face before a night of valid sleep can be measured. Home monitoring equipment is also available, but persons who complain of poor sleep may or may not experience the problem when actually monitored, and subjective reports of difficulty falling asleep or staying asleep may or may not correlate with the objective criteria established by sleep experts.[47]

To ascertain daytime sleepiness, a version of the PSG, called the *multiple sleep onset latency test,* can be conducted in the clinic setting. In addition to stages of sleep, this clinical evaluation includes measures of the length of time it takes to fall asleep every 2 hours during the day while resting in a reclined position. This is often used to distinguish narcolepsy from other disorders of excessive daytime sleepiness.[48]

Motion actigraphy, useful for continuously monitoring a person's movement, usually from the wrist, has developed as a method for estimating sleep and distinguishing it from wakeful, purposeful movements.[49,50] Although easily used in the person's own home, it does not allow for assessment of specific stages of sleep and at best provides an objective indication of awakenings during the night, particularly when individuals are less reliable in self-reported number of awakenings or amount of time spent awake. When used with an event marker, actigraphy can also provide an estimate of time to fall asleep, total sleep time, and nap time. Wrist actigraphy, however, can underestimate sleep in active sleepers like children, and overestimate sleep in sedentary individuals and the elderly.

Self-report measures are many, but fall into two categories and an example of each will be provided. The first category of measures involves self-report for a history of impaired sleep. The best known instrument is the 19-item Pittsburgh Sleep Quality

BOX 19-1 Assessing Patients for Impaired Sleep

Sleep clinicians often use the acronym BEARS as a format to organize the five domains of a thorough sleep history:

B Bedtime problems
E Excessive daytime sleepiness
A Awakenings during the night
R Regularity and duration of sleep
S Sleep disordered breathing

Age-specific types of questions, particularly questions for children at different stages of development, can be found at the American Academy of Sleep Medicine website located at www.aasmnet.org/MEDSleep.

The following questions are examples that can be used to obtain an adult's sleep history to evaluate for impaired sleep:

Have you noticed any change in your sleep patterns lately?
Describe your typical sleep period. When do you go to bed and get up on work days? On days off?
How long does it usually take you to fall asleep?
Do you take anything to help you fall asleep?
How often do you have trouble sleeping?
How often do you take naps?
How often do you travel by airplane?
Does your work involve night shifts or rotating schedules?
How many caffeinated beverages (cola, coffee, chocolate, tea, etc.) do you drink on a typical day? Do you drink caffeine to help stay awake?
How much alcohol do you drink on a typical day? Do you drink alcohol to help you fall asleep?
What medications are you taking routinely? Have you recently stopped taking a medication?
How often do you find yourself waking up during your sleep period? What do you think wakes you up?
What do you do when you wake up in the middle of the night?
How often do you wake up too early and can't get back to sleep?
Why do you think you are waking up so early?
Are you able to carry out your normal daytime activities without feeling exhausted or taking a nap?

Index, which asks the respondent to consider the past month and responses can be analyzed as a global sleep disturbance score or as seven components of impaired sleep: subjective sleep quality; sleep latency (initiation insomnia); sleep duration; habitual sleep efficiency; sleep disturbance; use of sleeping medication; and daytime dysfunction.[51] There is also a section in which the bed partner can provide information about the client's sleep, however, this section is not used in scoring. After many manipulations of the person's responses to the 19 items, which can be done more rapidly with computer scoring, a global score is calculated and can range from 0 to 21. In psychiatric patients, a score above 5 indicates severe sleep disturbance. Because the cut-off score is not clearly established for varying patient populations,[52] it is recommended that this tool be used for descriptive or screening purposes for referral to an accredited sleep clinic, rather than used for diagnostic purposes. Because it lacks sensitivity to detect small changes over time, the Pittsburgh Sleep Quality Index is less useful for research purposes and more useful as an assessment guideline for clinical practice.

Another subjective measure of sleep quality that is more sensitive to changes over time is the 21-item General Sleep Disturbance Scale[53] in which respondents are asked to indicate how frequently in the past week they have experienced difficulty falling asleep, staying asleep, daytime sleepiness, and taking medications for sleep. Although it may be useful to assess the *frequency* of impaired sleep, it is less informative about the *severity* of the sleep impairment. The Epworth Sleepiness Scale or Stanford Sleepiness Scale are often used as a self-report indicator of excessive daytime sleepiness, which is just one component of adverse health outcomes related to impaired sleep.[54]

In addition to excessive daytime sleepiness, major manifestations of impaired sleep also include injury or accidents, cognitive impairment, and reduced quality of life. Leger et al.[55] surveyed a representative sample from the French population and categorized impaired sleepers as those with difficulty initiating or maintaining sleep, those with impaired daytime

BOX 19-2 Assessing for Common Causes of Daytime Sleepiness

Sleep Apnea

Has anyone recently told you that you snore loudly?
Has anyone ever told you that you stop breathing when you sleep?
Do you wake up suddenly coughing or choking?
Do you have difficulty staying awake during the day?
If so, under what circumstances?
- Sitting in front of the television?
- While reading a book?
- While eating a meal?
- While working at your desk?
- While in the middle of a physical activity?
- While driving?

Myoclonus

Has anyone ever told you that your legs jerk while you are sleeping?

Esophageal Reflux

Do you wake up suddenly coughing or choking?
Do you frequently awaken suddenly with an acid taste in your mouth?

Narcolepsy

Do you fall asleep suddenly during the day in response to loud noises, bright lights, or strong emotional experiences?
Do you ever fall asleep during the day without deliberately lying down to take a nap?

functioning, or those with nonrefreshing sleep at least three times a week for at least 1 month. When those with severe insomnia were matched with cases of mild insomnia or no insomnia, there were no differences in age, gender, occupation, marital status, or socioeconomic status. In a subsequent survey the researchers assessed nine dimensions of quality of life (using a French version of the Medical Outcomes Study, Short Form-36), and after those with psychiatric disorders (anxiety and depression) were eliminated from each of the three groups, the severe and mild insomniacs were significantly worse in all aspects of quality of life, including physical functioning, social functioning, and mental health. These results are not totally surprising, given the selection criteria for severe insomnia, which included impaired daytime performance. Nevertheless, as indicated in Figure 19-1, these results support the need for assessing cognitive/behavioral, emotional, and social outcomes related to the manifestation and treatment of impaired sleep.[54]

In addition to the more obvious manifestations of impaired sleep that include complaints of initiating sleep, maintaining sleep, or daytime sleepiness, long-term use of hypnotics, over-the-counter sleep aids, or herbal remedies results in a manifestation often overlooked by health care professionals. Prescriptions are written for long-term hypnotic use at astonishing levels, despite consensus reports from the Institute of Medicine in 1979 and FDA guidelines that have been in effect since the early 1980s that hypnotics have questionable benefits for impaired sleep and are useful only for the treatment of short-term sleep impairment.[56] Tolerance to hypnotics develops within 1 to 2 weeks, setting up a response for the impaired sleeper to take higher dosages over time, while feeling less and less satisfied about sleep outcomes. It is estimated that 65% of total hypnotic use in the United States is by persons who take the medication on a nightly basis, with nearly half the users over 60 years of age and taking hypnotics for 5 years or more.[14] Prescription hypnotics are addictive and have adverse side effects, including daytime sleepiness as well as other impaired cognitive/behavioral functioning. In addition, there is a risk of death from overdose.

CLINICAL MANAGEMENT

The management of impaired sleep begins with an accurate diagnosis. When the diagnosis is made from an accredited sleep clinic using 1 or 2 nights of polysomnography in the clinic or home environment, then appropriate treatment can be initiated. Sleep problems such as sleep apnea syndrome, narcolepsy, esophageal reflux, restless legs syndrome, and periodic leg movements can be fairly easy to diagnose by polysomnography. Management includes medications such as stimulants or muscle relaxants, or mechanical devices to maintain a patent airway such as nasal CPAP or dental appliances.[57] Although diagnosis and management strategies are fairly well developed, the clinician is then faced with issues of long-term patient adherence to these management strategies.

For others with complaints of impaired sleep, there may be no obvious physical cause that can be documented by polysomnography. Clinical management for these individuals primarily rests with a set of educational, behavioral, and cognitive strategies known as sleep hygiene. A meta-analysis of treatments for impaired sleep found that these strategies can be more effective and more satisfying, in the long-term, to patients than hypnotics.[58,59] In treating patients for impaired sleep, health care providers must be challenged to not only educate patients on beneficial sleep hygiene behaviors, discussed in the next section on clinical management, but also to reduce the numbers of prescriptions for hypnotics by helping patients to slowly taper their withdrawal from the medication to prevent REM rebound effects experienced as restlessness, nightmares, and fragmented sleep.

Sleep hygiene principles vary in specifics and range from 11 to as many as 22. Patients and clinicians remember these principles more easily when they are organized according to the acronym *Sleep* BETTER. The acronym includes attending to the external environmental factors of light, noise, and temperature in the *B*edroom, *E*xercising during the day, reducing *T*ension and learning to relax in the evening before bed, and limiting *T*ime in bed to sleep or nap and getting up if not sleeping. *E*ating adequate protein and carbohydrates to maintain healthy sleep-related neurochemical processes, consuming noncaffeinated beverages after 6 PM or even earlier in older persons, and evaluating use of other CNS stimulants and depressants is a major component of sleep hygiene principles. Finally, paying attention to *R*hythm is very important. Going to bed and getting up at the same time each day, every day of the week, including vacations and days off from work or school is one way to train the body to stay in a 24-hour rhythm. (See Chapter 3.)

Limit Bedroom Light and Noise. As discussed earlier, light is a stimulus for arousal and blocks the secretion of melatonin. Rather than turning on bright lights to get out of bed during the night, a low-level night light or flashlight at the bedside is safe but provides less stimulation in the darkness. In a hospital environment, where lights are essential to safe health care, patients may want to consider wearing a comfortable eye mask, such as that provided to airline passengers on overseas flights, to shield their eyes from the light.

Intermittent noises, in the hospital or in the home, can be masked by white noise.[60,61] In most hospital rooms, monotonous background noise from motors in ventilation systems ranges from 32 to 38 dBA and serves as a source of continuous low-level white noise.[62] The Environmental Protection Agency[63] recommends a limit of 35 dBA to preserve the restorative process of sleep. However, Woods and Falk[64] found noise in the acute care setting to fluctuate between 53 and 60 dBA on the night shift; Hilton[65] found that noise above 70 dBA occurred about every 9 minutes during 24 hours of recording in a critical care unit. Ventilators produce about 70 dBA, a cardiac alarm registers about 78 dBA, and a flushing toilet results in about 74 dBA.[66] Patients in the hospital and elderly persons may find earplugs useful in muffling nighttime noises. White noise machines may also be useful. Sanchez and Bootzin[67] studied college students exposed to white noise at 63 dBA by earphones. After 2 hours of sleep from 7 PM to 9 PM, subjects in the white noise group had higher sleep maintenance (86%) compared with the no-sound group (54%).

Promote Exercise. Physical activity may also improve sleep, probably by increasing body temperature and enhancing circadian rhythm for temperature.[60,68] Exercise increased deep sleep 2 to 5 minutes and total sleep time by 10 minutes in physically fit persons.[69] A walking program instituted for cancer patients was successful in reducing self-reported sleep problems.[70] Whether exercise itself is the therapeutic agent or whether it is the exposure to light while exercising, the release of cytokines during the physiological stress of exercise, or the elevated body temperature that promotes sleep remains to be studied.

Reduce Tension and Stress. Tension and stress alter sleep patterns. Anxiety can result in a delayed onset of sleep and less REM sleep.[71] Meditation has been shown to improve sleep in patients with fibromyalgia, with 51% having moderate to marked improvement.[72] Others may find a warm bubble bath, hot milk, herbal decaffeinated tea, or Ovaltine (high in tryptophan and vitamin B_6) to be relaxing. In the hospital situation, a nurse's evening back massage for the patient remains an important stress-reduction strategy to facilitate sleep.

Limit Time in Bed. The time spent in bed can be either too long or too short, but in general the time should be restricted so that a person does not associate the bedroom and bed with lying awake trying to sleep; a person should stay in bed only long enough to obtain the necessary sleep to maintain wakefulness during the day. Not everyone requires 8 hours of sleep, or even 6 hours, to accomplish that goal. Persons complaining of insomnia tend to stay in bed too long and only achieve nonrestorative light sleep with many awakenings.[60] They actually can feel more tired when they try to "sleep in" later than usual. Many elderly persons are under a false impression that they must sleep 8 hours, yet the more one tries to sleep, the more anxious one becomes and the less able to sleep. Watching the illuminated clock only contributes to the light in the bedroom and anxiety at not sleeping. If a person is alert and not sleepy during the day, the time spent asleep at night was an adequate amount of time.

When an individual has difficulty falling asleep at night, there should be an assessment of daytime napping behavior. A nap during the day can disrupt circadian wake/sleep cycles and result in delaying sleep onset at night. On the other hand, if someone complains of daytime sleepiness, a scheduled nap in a controlled environment is preferable to falling asleep in a hazardous environment, and one or two scheduled naps during the daytime should be part of the strategy to control daytime sleepiness.

In the case of narcolepsy, in which daytime sleep episodes are a part of the pathological state, treatment largely consists of prescription stimulants and tricyclic antidepressants, which inhibit the reuptake of serotonin and also drastically suppress REM sleep. Modafinil (Provigil), a new amphetamine-like compound, is showing some promise, with fewer stimulant side effects, but a program of scheduled naps during the day and avoidance of unpredictable stimulation can be quite effective in reducing these REM attacks.[73]

Assess Eating, Drinking, and Drug Use. There are dietary influences on sleep. There is an increased need for sleep, particularly deep sleep stages, in catabolic states such as during severe dieting.[74,75] Foods high in protein induce sleep more rapidly and without distorting sleep stages. Protein foods contain L-tryptophan, the amino acid precursor of serotonin. Clinical studies indicate that L-tryptophan's effect on sleep is limited to only 1 or 2 nights[76] and higher doses can cause liver dysfunction. A light protein snack at bedtime may promote sleep by stimulating digestive hormones that have a sedative effect.[60]

Medications can have profound effects on sleep. Sedative-hypnotics lower the level of arousal (increase arousal threshold) by deactivating the reticular activating system to allow more rapid onset of sleep. However, suppression of REM sleep can occur with drugs such as barbiturates, amphetamines and opiate derivatives, L-dopa, alcohol, tricyclic antidepressants, monoamine oxidasein-hibitors, anticholinergics, and marijuana. Individuals may report better sleep the first few nights, but tolerance increases and these REM-suppressant drugs tend to lose their effect after about 2 weeks. If these REM-suppressant drugs are abruptly withdrawn after long-term usage, REM rebound (a marked increase in REM sleep) occurs. This rebound may last several days. In addition to increased REM, patients often complain of nightmares, restlessness, anxiety, depression, and dirupted sleep.[77,78]

Short-acting benzodiazepines (triazolam [Halcion]) and nonbenzodiazepines (zolpidem) are widely prescribed for complaints of disturbed sleep. Their ability to induce sleep is thought to result from their enhancing effect on GABA.[79] These drugs may increase total sleep time, but they suppress deep sleep and REM sleep, have a wide variation in rate of onset and elimination times, and cause a rebound effect of increased daytime anxiety.[80] Therefore only short-term, intermittent hypnotic use is recommended.[81]

Xanthine derivatives, such as caffeine, can be potent central nervous system stimulants. An 8-oz cup of coffee can vary between 50 and 150 mg of caffeine, chocolate has 15 to 30 mg/oz, and a cup of cocoa can have up to 30 mg. A cup of tea has between 40 and 125 mg, with some herbal teas having a very high content of caffeine. Carbonated drinks vary in caffeine content, from as low as 37 mg in a 12-oz can of Pepsi or 39.6 mg in a can of Dr Pepper, to as high as 45.6 mg in a can of Coca-Cola, and 55 mg in a 12-oz can of Mountain Dew. The amount of caffeine is the same whether the beverage is diet or regular. Jolt, a popular carbonated beverage among teenagers, has 120 mg of caffeine and caffeinated bottled waters are becoming popular. At the time of its peak effect, caffeine increases mental alertness, but also causes restlessness and elevates blood pressure and heart rate. Over-the-counter caffeine preparations are especially high in caffeine (NoDoz has 100 mg and Vivarin has 200 mg, according to the National Soft Drink Association).

Maintain a Consistent Wake/Sleep Rhythm. Exposure to light and dark influences nocturnal sleep. Light is a powerful alerting stimulus for wakefulness and suppresses melatonin. Studies of shift workers indicate that light of sufficient magnitude (greater than 150-lux light exposure) can alter the circadian timing of many physiological processes.[82] Advanced sleep phase syndrome, often seen in the elderly who go to bed early and awaken early, is best managed by reinforcing regular meal times and daytime activities, but bright light exposure (2500 lux) in the late afternoon or melatonin supplements may also be an effective strategy.[83] However, over-the-counter preparations of melatonin often contain therapeutic levels of vitamin B_6 rather than therapeutic levels of melatonin.

CONCEPTUAL MODELS

Many models of sleep have developed over time, with some attending to functions of sleep and others attending to mechanisms of sleep. In less evolved animals, the brain is always sensing input from the environment and the animal is never truly sleeping but can be considered resting. More evolved animals, such as dolphins, may sleep, but sleep occurs in only one hemisphere at a time. Only animals with highly developed brains actually sleep, wherein the brain remains active but does not effectively process any sensory input. Any valid model must consider all of the animal kingdom's sleep patterns and mechanisms for sleep.

Freud theorized that sleep was the ego's opportunity to rest from its control over the id. Based on knowledge gained from sleep deprivation studies, sleep has been conceptualized as an energy conservation mechanism for coping with the coldest hours of night, as a protective mechanism against predators, and as an opportunity to reorganize the day's experiences into memory.

Hobson,[84] however, discussed the function of sleep from both its homeostatic role in energy and thermoregulation and its heteroplastic (changing) role for development, learning, change, and adaptation. The heteroplastic role involves REM sleep and observations that REM sleep increases during animal training, whereas REM deprivation results in poor learning of tasks. In addition to incorporating new information into memory, Crick and Mitchison[85] hypothesized that REM sleep actually removes unnecessary details from the day's experience so that the brain does not become clogged with data. Krueger et al.[86] summarized research on human and animal sleep to present a more current, unified theory that sleep facilitates adaptation to continually changing internal and external environments.

Overall, the phenomenon of impaired sleep can be conceptualized for nursing practice as the sleep loss that results from sleep deprivation (lack of sufficient amount of sleep) or sleep disruption (fragmented sleep). Regardless of the mechanism, both place individuals at risk for excessive daytime sleepiness and poor quality of life (see Figure 19-1). As seen in the model, impaired sleep, regardless of the cause, affects many dimensions of one's overall health, including physiological processes involving immune and metabolic functions, cognitive/behavioral manifestations of impaired functioning, emotional well-being, and social interactions. It is these adverse health outcomes that need to be assessed when evaluating the effect of the impaired sleep on an individual, and it is these same outcomes that can be prevented or minimized with effective nursing interventions.

CASE STUDIES

CASE STUDY 1: SLEEP-RELATED BREATHING DISORDER

Ms. C, a 54-year-old single mother with three teenage children, was referred by her gynecologist to the sleep clinic for excessive daytime sleepiness. She was hypertensive and obese, with a body mass index of 34. Ms. C was taking antihypertensive medication. Her children complained that they were too embarrassed to have friends visit during the day or at night because of their mother's snoring and falling asleep in the living room. She had recently started looking for a job closer to home, because she found herself falling asleep while waiting at red-light intersections during her 15-minute commute.

In the sleep clinic, Ms. C fell asleep while the electrodes were being glued to her scalp for the polysomnography. While asleep, she repeatedly stopped breathing, averaging about 12 times/hour. Six of these apneic episodes lasted for longer than 75 seconds. She never had more than 3 or 4 minutes of uninterrupted sleep. Oxygen saturation levels fell below 50% during several of these apneic events. In the morning, she reported having awakened two or three times, but felt just as tired as when she went to bed.

Ms. C returned the following night for a trial of nasal continuous positive airway pressure (CPAP). Once the proper pressures were established during her sleep, apneic events disappeared. She remarked in the morning that she had more energy than she'd experienced since before she was pregnant with her first child. She was discharged home with nasal CPAP and instructed to return in 4 weeks for follow-up evaluation. At this follow-up visit, it is expected that her weight and blood pressure will be falling and her antihypertensive medication dosage will need to be adjusted. It is also expected that her level of daytime functioning will be greatly improved and that she and her children will be more socially interactive.

CASE STUDY 2: INITIATION INSOMNIA

Mr. S is a 33-year-old computer executive who started his own company about a year ago, after successfully achieving his goals with a former company and establishing an adequate client base. He has been meeting financial projections and, because he is single without family obligations, his financial resources are adequate. He recently bought a sailboat so that he could relax on the weekends. When first seen, he looked tired and thin, and his sentences were slurred and spoken with great effort. He had no trouble staying awake during the physical assessment and his chief complaint was lying awake at night listening to the noise from the neighbor's yard, where a dog was often barking and another neighbor who had the habit of washing his car at 1 or 2 AM. He was obviously angry about the neighbors and spoke of moving, but he felt too tired to do anything about it right now. He revealed that he had always been a light sleeper and used earplugs often, especially when he traveled and slept in hotel rooms.

Rather than schedule him for a diagnostic polysomnography, it was decided that he should keep a sleep/activity log for 2 weeks to document the extent of his problem and then return to the clinic. After careful review of his sleep/activity log, it was apparent that he lacked any exercise or recreational activity, drank 4 or 5 cups of coffee during the day, ate dinner at 9 or 10 PM, and typically drank 2 or 3 glasses of wine or 1 or 2 bottles of beer with his meal. The meal was always followed by a "night-cap" that, on questioning, he said he had been drinking since adolescence, because it always helped him to fall asleep.

Sleep hygiene principles, particularly focused on caffeine and alcohol, were then reviewed with Mr. S so that he could understand factors that can affect sleep in general. Then a plan of action was agreed on. First, he would begin to reduce the amount of coffee during the day by either alternating with a cup of decaffeinated coffee or by mixing half regular and half decaffeinated coffee. Then he wouldn't feel so "wired" in the evening, and the wine and beer with the evening meal could be reduced by half. Once he understood that alcohol is a CNS depressant, which of course can make one sleepy, but then acts to fragment sleep and causes frequent arousals, he agreed to make efforts to reduce his alcohol intake. This lifestyle habit may be the most difficult for him to break, but gradually cutting back on his daily intake of alcohol should improve his sleep and provide him with the positive feedback to continue limiting his alcohol intake.

Mr. S's noise issue was addressed next. Because the alcohol was most likely keeping him from getting deep sleep stages, he was easily aroused from light sleep. Although earplugs were somewhat useful in his experience, the nurse discussed with him how white noise may be an added measure to further ensure muffling of intermittent loud noises, such as barking dogs and moving traffic, and a few commercial products were recommended. He agreed to try these changes for 2 weeks and to return with the sleep/activity log to document his use of these principles and their effect on his sleep problem. Two weeks later, he cancelled his appointment, saying to the receptionist that he had "cured himself," and there was no need for him to return for a follow-up evaluation.

SELECTED RESEARCH

Nurses first began research on sleep in the early 1970s, with studies of intensive care patients after cardiac surgery.[87-89] These early studies, often in an attempt to understand the phenomenon of ICU psychosis, were descriptive and used actual observations of patients to estimate sleep quality and quantity. Technological advances in the past two decades now allow for more valid and reliable measures of sleep parameters in both in-patient and out-patient settings.[90]

Weaver et al.[91] conducted a study to describe the use of nasal CPAP during the first nine weeks of patient treatment for obstructive sleep apnea. A microprocessor embedded in the CPAP machine documented hours of usage each night and number of nights that CPAP was used in 32 patients. By the fourth day of treatment, these nurse researchers were able to distinguish patients as adherent or nonadherent. About half (N = 17) were adherent, using the CPAP over 90% of the nights and at least 6 hours each night. The nonadherent group, however, skipped many days and used CPAP for only about 3.5 hours at night. The nonadherent group continued to complain of daytime sleepiness and a lower level of daytime functioning. They noted discomfort from the nasal mask as a primary complaint and possible reason for not adhering to the therapy.[90]

Lentz et al.[92] recruited and enrolled 12 healthy women for a sleep laboratory study in which they were deprived specifically of deep, slow-wave sleep for 3 nights. Baseline data were collected using the Profile of Mood States (POMS) to establish levels of fatigue, vigor, depression, anger, confusion, and tension. They used an 85-dB tone every time deep sleep was seen on the polysomnography recording. This was a way to model the type of sleep disturbance (alpha/delta sleep patterns) seen in women with fibromyalgia and musculoskeletal pain. After 3 nights, these healthy women had increased fatigue and less vigor, without a change in tension, anger, depression, or confusion. What was even more intriguing was the increase in pain threshold by self-report on a 35-item bodily feelings questionnaire.[92]

Humphreys et al[43] studied 50 women living in shelters for battered women. Women in these settings often complain of poor sleep as a result of the battering, which can lead to PTSD, and also as a result of trying to sleep in a crowded, noisy shelter. After women had been in the shelter at least 3 weeks, those who agreed to and signed informed consent were asked to wear a wrist actigraphy monitor for 48 hours and complete the Pittsburgh Sleep Quality Index as well as participate in an open-ended interview. These women took, on average, 11 minutes to fall asleep, but 22% of them could be classified as having initiation insomnia, taking more than 20 minutes to fall asleep. The more people in the room trying to sleep, the longer it took for the subject to fall asleep. Many (44%) had their children with them, requiring the family to sleep in the same room. One third of the sample (34%, N = 17) spent at least 20% of their time awake during the night, and 42% indicated that their sleep was poor. The median score on the Pittsburgh Global Sleep Quality Index score was 9 on a scale of 0 to 21, with 70% scoring greater than 5, the cut-off score that indicates impaired sleep.[51] The number of awakenings, recorded objectively with the wrist actigraph, was significantly related to morning and evening fatigue level, but not correlated with the subject's perception of number of awakenings. Those with children, regardless of whether the children were in the shelter or not, experienced worse sleep than those who were not mothers. With these descriptive data, interventions can begin to be developed and targeted to improve sleep for persons living in all types of shelter environments.

Most recently, Lee et al.[49] completed a sleep study on 100 women with HIV/AIDS to further understand their symptom experience. Persons with HIV/AIDS often complain of impaired sleep and fatigue, but women may be especially vulnerable because of their multiple roles as wife, employee, mother, and caregiver. Using wrist actigraphy for 48 hours of continuous recording, it was found that sleep averaged only 6.5 hours. Those with lower CD4 cell counts had more awakenings during the night, and as a group they were awake 25% of the night. Amount of sleep was not related to marital status or having children in the home. However, those who experienced high fatigue also self-reported higher frequency of depressive symptoms, slept more during the day, and took longer to fall asleep at night. Results indicate that sleeping during the day is not a useful strategy for relieving fatigue, sleeping during the day may result in difficulty falling asleep at bedtime, and depressive symptoms are closely linked to impaired sleep patterns.[49]

QUESTIONS FOR FUTURE STUDY

Published research and metaanalysis studies that provide an integrative review of nonpharmacological interventions for impaired sleep consistently conclude that nonpharmacological interventions are better at long-term improvement in sleep compared with the results from use of medications. In addition, patient satisfaction in long-term follow-up is better with nonpharmacological intervention strategies that give patients control of their sleep behaviors.[58,59]

What is unfortunate, however, is that all these studies excluded persons with chronic illness or diagnosed medical conditions when subjects were being recruited and randomized to these nonpharmacological and hypnotic drug treatment studies. As health care providers, nurses deal primarily with persons who have chronic illness, and findings from these nonpharmacological intervention studies are only generalizable to essentially healthy insomniacs. Studies of this kind need to be replicated in patient populations with chronic illness and be tested for effectiveness and efficacy before incorporating them into practice. Many of these nonpharmacological interventions may also need to be gender specific. It is not clear that what works for men will work equally well for women.

As is true of all patient care strategies to improve health and well-being, there is little research on adherence issues. What we prescribe for patients to help them sleep must fit within their lifestyle and cultural sleep practices, and changes must be made slowly. Finally, there is increased attention to research on why adults delay seeking treatment for symptoms of myocardial infarction or asthma, but very little attention is given to why adults delay seeking treatment for excessive daytime sleepiness, a major cause of divorce, job loss, and traffic accidents and fatalities in the United States. It is often the automobile accident that prompts a referral to a sleep disorders center, but it is often too late to improve quality of life and family relationships.

REFERENCES

1. Sadeh, A. (1997). Sleep and melatonin in infants: A preliminary study. *Sleep 20,* 185-191.
2. Hublin, C., Kaprio, J., Partinen, M., & Koskenvuo, M. (1998). Sleep bruxism based on self-report in a nationwide twin cohort. *Journal of Sleep Research 7,* 61-67.
3. Carskadon, M.A., Vieira, C., & Acebo, C. (1993). Association between puberty and delayed phase preference. *Sleep 16,* 258-262.
4. Campbell, S.S., Murphy, P.J., van den Heuvel, C.J., Roberts, M.L., & Stauble, T.N. (1999). Etiology and treatment of intrinsic circadian rhythm sleep disorders. *Sleep Medicine Reviews 3,* 179-200.
5. Lee, K.A., Zaffke, M.E., & McEnany, G. (2000). Parity and sleep patterns during and after pregnancy. *Obstetrics & Gynecology 95,* 14-18.
6. Lee, K.A., & Taylor, D.L. (1996). Is there a generic midlife woman? The health and symptom experience of midlife women. *Menopause 3,* 154-164.
7. Shaver, J., Giblin, E., Lentz, M., & Lee, K. (1988). Sleep patterns and stability in perimenopausal women. *Sleep 11,* 556-561.
8. Baldwin, C.M., Griffith, K.A., Nieto, F.J., O'Connor, G.T., Walsleben, J.A., & Redline, S. (2001). The association of sleep-disordered breathing and sleep symptoms with quality of life in the sleep heart health study. *Sleep 24,* 96-105.
9. National Sleep Foundation. (2000). *Omnibus Sleep in America Poll.* Washington, D.C. Accessed from www.sleepfoundation.org.
10. Ancoli-Israel, S., Poceta, J.S., Stepnowsky, C., Martin, J., & Gehrman, P. (1997). Identification and treatment of sleep problems in the elderly. *Sleep Medicine Reviews 1,* 3-17.
11. Ancoli-Israel, S., & Roth, T. (1999). Characteristics of insomnia in the United States: Results of the 1991 National Sleep Foundation Survey. *Sleep 22*(Suppl 2), S327-S353.
12. Lindberg, E., & Gislason, T. (2000). Epidemiology of sleep-related obstructive breathing. *Sleep Medicine Reviews 4,* 411-433.
13. Redline, S., Tischler, P.V., Hans, M.G., Tosteson, T.D., Strohl, K.P., & Spry, K. (1997). Racial differences in sleep-disordered breathing in African-Americans and Caucasians. *American Journal of Respiratory and Critical Care Medicine 155,* 186-192.
14. Kripke, D.F., Klauber, M.R., Wingard, D.L., Fell, R.L., Assmus, J.D., & Garfinkel, L. (1998). Mortality hazard associated with prescription hypnotics. *Biological Psychiatry 43,* 687-693.
15. Redline, S., & Tishler, P.V. (2000). The genetics of sleep apnea. *Sleep Medicine Reviews 4,* 583-602.
16. Lee, K., Zaffke, M., & Barette-Beebe, K. (2001). Restless legs syndrome and sleep disturbance during pregnancy: The role of folate and iron. *Journal of Women's Health & Gender-Based Medicine 10,* 335-341.
17. Rijsman, R.M., & de Weerd, A.W. (1999). Secondary periodic limb movement disorder and restless legs syndrome. *Sleep Medicine Reviews 3,* 147-158.
18. Dickstein, J.B., Moldofsky, H. (1999). Sleep, cytokines and immune function. *Sleep Medicine Reviews 3,* 219-228.
19. Kennaway, D.J., Gable, F.C., & Stamp, G.E. (1996). Factors influencing the development of melatonin rhythmicity. *Journal of Clinical and Endocrinological Metabolism 81,* 1525-1532.
20. Skene, D.J., Bojkovski, C.J., & Arendt, J. (1994). Comparison of the effects of acute fluvoxamine and desipramine administration on melatonin and cortisol production in humans. *British Journal of Clinical Phar macology 37,* 181-186.
21. Brismar, K., Hylander, B., Eliasson, K. (1988). Melatonin secretion related to side-effects of beta-blockers from the central nervous system. *Acta Medica Scandinavica 223,* 525-530.
22. Luboshizsky, R., & Lavie, P. (1998). Sleep-inducing effects of exogenous melatonin administration. *Sleep Medicine Reviews 2,* 191-202.
23. Nishino, S., Okura, M., & Mignot, E. (2000). Narcolepsy: Genetic predisposition and neuropharmacological mechanisms. *Sleep Medicine Reviews 4,* 57-99.
24. Glotzbach, S.F., & Heller, C. (2000). Temperature regulation. In M.H. Kryger, T. Roth, & W.C. Dement (eds.), *Principles and practice of sleep medicine* (3rd ed., pp. 289-304). Philadelphia: W.B. Saunders.
25. Bliwise, D. (2000). Normal aging. In M.H. Kryger, T. Roth, & W.C. Dement (eds.), *Principles and practice of sleep medicine* (3rd ed., pp. 26-42). Philadelphia: W.B. Saunders.
26. Jones, B.E. (2000). Basic mechanisms of sleep-wake states. In M.H. Kryger, T. Roth, & W.C. Dement (eds.), *Principles and practice of sleep medicine* (3rd ed., pp. 134-154). Philadelphia: W.B. Saunders.
27. Garges, H.P., Varia, I., & Doraiswamy, P.M. (1998). Cardiac complications and delirium associated with valerian root withdrawal. *Journal of the American Medical Association 280,* 1566-1567.
28. Gyllenhaal, C., Merritt, S.L., Peterson, S.D., Block, K.I., & Gochenour, T. (2000). Efficacy and safety of herbal stimulants and sedatives in sleep disorders. *Sleep Medicine Reviews 4,* 229-251.
29. Siegel, J.M. (2000). Brainstem mechanisms generating REM sleep. In M.H. Kryger, T. Roth, & W.C. Dement (eds.), *Principles and practice of sleep medicine* (3rd ed., pp. 112-133). Philadelphia: W.B. Saunders.
30. Young, T., Finn, L., Hla, K.M., Morgan, B., & Palta, M. (1996). Snoring as part of a dose-response relationship between sleep-disordered breathing and blood pressure. *Sleep 19,* S202-S205.
31. Petitjean, T., Chammas, N., Langvin, B., Philit, F., & Robert, D. (2000). Principles of mandibular advancement device applied to the therapeutic of snoring and sleep apnea syndrome. *Sleep 23*(Suppl 4), S166-S171.
32. Douglas, N.J., & Engleman, H.M. (2000). Effects of CPAP on vigilance and related functions in patients with the sleep apnea/hypopnea syndrome. *Sleep 23*(Suppl 4), S147-S149.
33. Findley, L.J., Fabizio, M., Thommi, G., & Surratt, P.M. (1989). Severity of sleep apnea and automobile crashes. *New England Journal of Medicine 320,* 868-869.
34. Felten, D.L., Felten, S.Y., Bellinger, D.L., Carlson, S.L., Ackerman, K.D., Madden, K.S., Olschowki, J.A., & Livnat, S. (1987). Noradrenergic sympathetic neural interactions with the immune system: Structure and function. *Immunological Reviews 100,* 225-260.
35. Irwin, M., Mascovich, A., Gillin, J.C., Willoughby, R., Pike, J., & Smith, T.L. (1996). Partial sleep deprivation reduces natural killer cell and cellular immune responses in humans. *FASEB Journal 10,* 643-653.
36. Dinges, D.F., Douglas, S.D., Zaugg, L., Campbell, D.E., McMann, J.M., Whitehouse, W.G., et al. (1994). Leukocytosis and natural killer cell function parallel neurobehavioral fatigue induced by 64 hours of sleep

deprivation. *Journal of Clinical Investigation 93,* 1930-1939.
37. Everson, C.A., & Toth, L.A. (1997). Abnormal control of viable bacteria in body tissues during sleep deprivation in rats. *Sleep Research 26,* 613.
38. Roehrs, T., Zorick, F.J., & Roth, T. (2000). Transient and short-term insomnias. In M.H. Kryger, T. Roth, & W.C. Dement (eds.), *Principles and practice of sleep medicine* (3rd ed., pp. 624-632). Philadelphia: W.B. Saunders.
39. Pillar, G., Malhotra, A., & Lavie, P. (2000). Post-traumatic stress disorder and sleep—what a nightmare! *Sleep Medicine Reviews 4,* 183-200.
40. Woodward, S.H., Friedman, M.J., & Bliwise, D.L. (1996). Sleep and depression in combat-related PTSD inpatients. *Biological Psychiatry 39,* 182-192.
41. Lavie, P., Katz, N., Pillar, G., Zinger, Y. (1998). Elevated awaking thresholds during sleep: Characteristics of chronic war-related posttraumatic-stress disorder patients. *Biological Psychiatry 44,* 1060-1065.
42. Glod, C., Teicher, M.H., Hartman, C.R., & Harakal, T. (1997). Increased nocturnal activity and impaired sleep maintenance in abused children. *Journal of the American Academy of Child and Adolescent Psychiatry 36,* 1236-1243.
43. Humphreys, J.C., Lee, K.A., Neylan, T.C., & Marmar, C.R. (1999). Sleep patterns of sheltered battered women. *Image: Journal of Nursing Scholarship 31,* 139-143.
44. Turton, P., Hughes, P., Evans, C.D., & Fainman, D. (2001). Incidence, correlates and predictors of post-traumatic stress disorder in the pregnancy after still-birth. *British Journal of Psychiatry 178,* 556-560.
45. Hurwitz, T., Mahowald, M., Kuskowski, M., & Engdahl, B. (1998). Polysomnographic sleep is not clinically impaired in Vietman combat veterans with chronic posttraumatic stress disorder. *Biological Psychiatry 44,* 1066-1073.
46. Steriade, M. (2000). Brain electrical activity and sensory processing during waking and sleep states. In M.H. Kryger, T. Roth, & W.C. Dement (eds.), *Principles and practice of sleep medicine* (3rd ed., pp. 93-111). Philadelphia: W.B. Saunders.
47. Spielman, A.J., Yang, C., & Glovinsky, P.B. (2000). Assessment techniques for insomnia. In M.H. Kryger, T. Roth, & W.C. Dement (eds.), *Principles and practice of sleep medicine* (3rd ed., pp. 1239-1250). Philadelphia: W.B. Saunders.
48. Mitler, M.M., Carskadon, M.A., & Hirshkowitz, M. (2000). Evaluating sleepiness. In M.H. Kryger, T. Roth, & W.C. Dement (eds.), *Principles and practice of sleep medicine* (3rd ed., pp. 1251-1257). Philadelphia: W.B. Saunders.
49. Lee, K.A., Portillo, C., & Miramontes, H. (2001). The influence of sleep and activity patterns on fatigue in women with HIV/AIDS. *Journal of the Association of Nurses in AIDS Care 12*(Suppl), 19-27.
50. Redeker, M.S., Mason, D.J., Wykpisz, E., & Glica, B.W. (1995). Sleep patterns in women after coronary artery bypass surgery. *Applied Nursing Research 9,* 115-122.
51. Buysse, D.J., Reynolds, C.F., Monk, T.H, Berman, S.R., & Kupfer, D.J. (1989). The Pittsburgh sleep quality index: A new instrument for psychiatric practice and research. *Psychiatry Research 28,* 193-213.
52. Carpenter, J.S., & Andrykowski, M.A. (1998). Psychometric evaluation of the Pittsburgh sleep quality index. *Journal of Psychosomatic Research 45,* 5-13.
53. Lee, K. (1992). Self-reported sleep disturbances in employed women. *Sleep 15,* 493-498.
54. Weaver, T.E. (2001). Outcome measurement in sleep medicine practice and research. Part I: Assessment of symptoms, subjective and objective daytime sleepiness, health-related quality of life and functional status. *Sleep Medicine Reviews 5,* 103-128.
55. Leger, D., Scheuermaier, K., Philip, P., Paillard, M., & Guilleminault, C. (2001). SF-36: Evaluation of quality of life in severe and mild insomniacs compared with good sleepers. *Psychosomatic Medicine 63,* 49-55.
56. Kripke, D.F. (2000). Chronic hypnotic use: Deadly risks, doubtful benefit. *Sleep Medicine Reviews 4,* 5-20.
57. Hoffstein, V. (2000). Snoring. In M.H. Kryger, T. Roth, & W.C. Dement (eds.), *Principles and practice of sleep medicine* (3rd ed., pp. 813-826). Philadelphia: W.B. Saunders.
58. Morin, C.M., Colecchi, C., Stone, J., Sood, R., & Brink, D. (1999). Behavioral and pharmacological therapies for late-life insomnia. *Journal of the American Medical Association 281,* 991-999.
59. Murtagh, D.R.R., & Greenwood, K.M. (1995). Identifying effective psychological treatments for insomnia: A meta-analysis. *Journal of Consulting and Clinical Psychology 63,* 79-89.
60. Hauri, P. (1992). *Sleep disorders* (p. 13). Kalamazoo: Upjohn.
61. Dornic, S., & Laaksonen, T. (1989) Continuous noise, intermittent noise, and annoyance. *Perceptual and Motor Skills 68,* 11-18.
62. Vallet, M., & Mouret, J. (1984). Sleep disturbance due to transportation noise: Ear plugs vs oral drugs. *Experientia 40,* 429-437.
63. U.S. Environmental Protection Agency. (1974). *Information on levels of environmental noise requisite to protect public health and welfare with an adequate margin of safety.* EPA 550/9-74-004. Washington, D.C.: Author.
64. Woods, N.F., & Falk, S.A. (1974). Noise stimuli in the acute care area. *Nursing Research 23,* 144-150.
65. Hilton, B. (1985). Noise in acute patient care areas. *Research in Nursing and Health 8,* 283-291.
66. Topf, M., Bookman, M., & Arand, D. (1996). Effects of critical care unit noise on the subjective quality of sleep. *Journal of Advanced Nursing 24,* 545-551.
67. Sanchez, R., & Bootzin, R.R. (1985). A comparison of white noise and music: Effects of predictable and unpredictable sounds on sleep. *Sleep Research 14,* 121.
68. Shapiro, C.M., Warren, P.M., Trinder, J., Paxton, S.J., Oswald, I., Flenley, D.C., & Catterall, J.R. (1984). Fitness facilitates sleep. *European Journal of Applied Physiology 53,* 1-4.
69. Kubitz, K.A., Landers, D.M., Petruzello, S.J., & Han, M. (1996). The effects of acute and chronic exercise on sleep: A meta-analytic review. *Sports Medicine 21,* 277-291.
70. Mock, V., Dow, K.D., Meares, C.J., Grimm, P.M., Dienemann, J.A., Haisfield-Wolf, M.E., Quitasol, W., Mitchell, S., Chakravarthy, A., & Gage, I. (1997). Effects of exercise on fatigue, physical functioning, and emotional distress during radiation therapy for breast cancer. *Oncology Nursing Forum 24,* 991-1000.
71. Monroe, S.M., Thase, M.E., & Simons, A.D. (1992). Social factors and the psychobiology of depression: Relations between life stress and rapid eye movement sleep latency. *Journal of Abnormal Psychology 101,* 528-537.
72. Kaplan, K.E., Goldenberg, D.L., & Galvin-Nadeau, M. (1993). The impact of a meditation-based stress reduction program on fibromyalgia. *General Hospital Psychiatry 15,* 284-289.
73. Rogers, AE, & Aldrich, MS. (1993). Do regularly scheduled naps reduce sleep attacks and excessive daytime sleepiness associated with narcolepsy? *Nursing Research 42,* 111-117.

74. Evans, F.J. (1983). Sleep, eating, and weight disorders. In R.K. Goodstein (ed.), *Eating and weight disorders* (pp. 147-156). New York: Springer.
75. Schneider-Helmert, D. (1986). Nutrition and sleeping behavior. *Bibliotheca Nutritio et Dieta 38,* 87-93.
76. Sallanon, M., Janin, M., Buda, C., Jouvet, M. (1983). Serotoninergic mechanisms and sleep rebound. *Brain Research 268,* 95-104.
77. Nicholson, A.N., Bradley, C.M., & Pascoe, P.A. (1994). Medications: Effect on sleep and wakefulness. In M.H. Kryger, T. Roth, & W.C. Dement (eds.), *Principles and practice of sleep medicine* (3rd ed., pp. 364-372). Philadelphia: W.B. Saunders.
78. Hartmann, E. (1994). Nightmares and other dreams. In M.H. Kryger, T. Roth, & W.C. Dement (eds.), *Principles and practice of sleep medicine* (3rd ed., pp. 407-410). Philadelphia: W.B. Saunders.
79. Gaillard, J.M. (1994). Benzodiazepines and GABA-ergic transmission. In M.H. Kryger, T. Roth, & W.C. Dement (eds.), *Principles and practice of sleep medicine* (3rd ed., pp. 349-354). Philadelphia: W.B. Saunders.
80. Ashton, H. (1984). Benzodiazepine withdrawal: An unfinished story. *British Medical Journal 288,* 1135-1140.
81. Walsh, J.K., & Fillingim, J.M. (1990). Role of hypnotic drugs in general practice. *American Journal of Medicine 88*(Suppl 3A), 34S-38S.
82. Rosa, R.R., Bonnet, M.H., Bootzin, R.R., Eastman, C.I., Monk, T., Penn, P.E., Tepas, D.I., & Walsh, J.K. (1990). Intervention factors for promoting adjustment to nightwork and shiftwork. *Occupational Medicine: State of the Art Reviews 5,* 391-414.
83. Dowling, G.A., & Mastick, J.M. (2001). Melatonin secretion in Parkinson's disease: A 2.5 year follow-up. *Sleep 24* (Suppl 1), A368.
84. Hobson, J.A. (1989). *Sleep.* New York: W.H. Freeman and Company.
85. Crick, F., & Mitchison, G. (1983). The function of dream sleep. *Nature 304,* 111-114.
86. Krueger, J.M., Obal, Jr, F., & Fang, J. (1999). Why we sleep: A theoretical view of sleep function. *Sleep Medicine Reviews 3,* 119-129.
87. Woods, N., & Giblin, E. (1972). Patterns of sleep in post-cardiotomy patients. *Nursing Research 21,* 347-352.
88. Hilton, B.A. (1976). Quantity and quality of patient's sleep and sleep disturbing factors in a respiratory intensive care unit. *Journal of Advanced Nursing 1,* 453-468.
89. McFadden, E., & Giblin, E (1979). Sleep deprivation in patients having open heart surgery. *Nursing Research 20,* 249-254.
90. Colling, E., Mastick, J., Schmedlen, L., Dowling, G., Carter, J., Singer, C., & DeJongh, E. (2001). Wrist actigraphy as a method of sleep detection in Parkinson's disease. *Sleep 24*(suppl 1), A413.
91. Weaver, T.E., Kribbs, N.B., Pack, A.I., Kline, L.R., Chugh, D.K., Maislin, G., et al. (1997). Night-to-night variability in CPAP use over the first three months of treatment. *Sleep 20,* 278-283.
92. Lentz, M.J., Landis, C.A., Rothermel, J., & Shaver, J.L.F. (1999). Effects of selective slow wave sleep disruption on musculoskeletal pain and fatigue in middle aged women. *Journal of Rheumatology 26,* 1586-1592.

SECTION V

Alterations in Motion

Motion is defined as the act or process of changing place, referring to the whole human body, its structures and parts, or its internal components. Thus movement of the body from one place to another, changing the position or arrangement of the body or its parts, and the movement of ions, molecules, and substances from one side of a cell membrane to the other are all processes encompassed by this definition.

Examples of concepts related to motion include mobility, immobility diffusion, transudation, circulation, contraction, extension, flexion, osmosis, and flow. The pathological alterations related to motion can cause a variety of abnormalities, such as joint dislocations, muscle sprains, stasis of blood flow, remodeling of joint tissues, stasis of pulmonary secretions, cardiac deconditioning, skeletal muscle atrophy, hemorrhage, effusions, edema formation, fluid and electrolyte imbalances, and third space volume syndromes.

The two chapters in this section represent somewhat different perspectives on motion; Chapter 20 addresses the effects of immobility on skeletal muscle size, strength, and endurance, as seen with skeletal muscle atrophy, and Chapter 21 considers edema, the excess accumulation of fluid in tissues in response to altered hydrostatic or oncotic pressures or vascular permeability. The result of either of these alterations in motion is impaired functional status. Skeletal muscle atrophy results in decreased functional capacity and ability to perform activities of daily living. Edema can impede joint mobility, cause pain, impair gas exchange, or result in serious neurological deficits. Both of these phenomena are very prevalent in patients with acute or chronic illness and are encountered in a wide variety of clinical states and medical diagnoses.

These phenomena affect a wide variety of systems, such as cardiac, pulmonary, renal, musculoskeletal, and neurological, and are central concepts to nursing care of affected patients. Maintenance of normal body motion is traditionally viewed as an important function; considerable nursing effort is spent in prevention of the effects of immobility and in support of tissues that have become immobilized. However, the efficacy of many nursing actions related to these goals remains unknown. Nursing research has shown that periods of quiet chair-sitting or ambulation to the bathroom have important effects on preventing skeletal muscle atrophy and orthostatic hypotension and in reducing plasma volume losses in patients who otherwise stay in bed. Nursing research focusing on edema includes study of the effects of various nursing activities and body positions on intracranial pressure in patients with cerebral edema. More research on concepts relevant to alterations in motion is necessary to provide the empirical evidence as a basis for professional nursing practice.

CHAPTER

20 Skeletal Muscle Atrophy

CHRISTINE E. KASPER

DEFINITION

Skeletal muscle atrophy is defined as the decrease in the mass and cross-sectional area of a skeletal muscle that occurs when the average activities of daily living (ADLs) of an individual are decreased below their normal levels (Box 20-1). Current research has demonstrated that atrophy of skeletal muscle is a major sequela of most pathophysiological phenomena, such as fatigue. The phenomenon of skeletal muscle atrophy occurs across the entire age span of humans. The earliest onset could occur as early as the first month of life and can extend throughout advanced ages. In elderly persons, it is a predictor of disability and mortality.[1]

Skeletal muscle function depends on intact proprioceptive activity, motor innervation, mechanical load, and mobility of joints.[2-6] If one of these factors is changed, the muscle then adapts to a new functional set point, which depends on its average daily level of activity. When either movement or weight-bearing is decreased, skeletal muscle adapts by decreasing its mass and cross-sectional area.

Decreased movement (hypokinesia) and/or decreased weight-bearing (hypodynamia) can cause decreased contractile activity. Together they are referred to as *unloading* of muscle. In the more extreme forms of decreased activity, a muscle may lose up to 50% of its mass in 3 weeks.[7] Following a period of decreased contractile activity, subjects have impaired functional capacity and a reduced ability to perform their normal daily activities because of a loss of skeletal muscle mass.[8]

Decreased protein synthesis and increasing protein degradation decreases skeletal muscle mass.[9,10] Myofibrils are lost, resulting in decreased muscle size. A prolonged decrease in contractile activity, as seen as decreased movement and weight-bearing, is the principal stimulus for the occurrence of skeletal muscle atrophy.[11]

PREVALENCE AND POPULATIONS AT RISK

All hospitalized patients, bedfast and ambulatory, are subjected to some form of restricted mobility despite reduced duration of hospital stay. Patients with activity restriction are a major portion of both the short-term and long-term inpatient-based nursing caseload. The hospital environment structures the amount of functional activity that a fully mobile patient is capable of performing and effectively decreases their level of daily activity. The incidence of

BOX 20-1 Causes of Skeletal Muscle Atrophy

- Disuse
  - ↓ Activities of daily living
  - ↓ Weight-bearing motion
  - Bed rest
  - Microgravity
  - Mechanical ventilation
  - Psychiatric
    - Depression
    - Schizophrenia
  - Physiological aging
- Immobility
  - Orthopedic
    - Casting
    - Traction
    - Joint immobilization
  - Paralysis
  - Pathological
    - Paralytic poliomyolytis
    - Guillain-Barré syndrome
    - Various muscular dystrophies
- Pharmacological
  - Glucocorticoids
    - Chemotheraputic agents
    - Nucleosides (e.g., AZT)
    - Antiproteolytics

disuse atrophy is not limited to the inpatient setting. In recent years, ambulatory ill persons in community settings whose mobility is decreased by illness or pain, fatigue, and dyspnea have dramatically increased, leading to a higher potential for disuse atrophy.

The major losses of skeletal muscle mass and contractile proteins occur during the first 3 to 13 days of inactivity.[12] It is important to note that this time frame is the same as that of the average days of restricted activity (14.2 days per person) resulting from chronic or acute illness or injuries.[13] Therefore nearly all patient populations, regardless of the treatment location, are at risk for skeletal muscle atrophy resulting from decreased levels of activity (Table 20-1).

Despite 50 years of continuous research and evidence to the contrary,[14,15] bed rest is still prescribed for a large number of medical conditions. A recent systematic survey of the literature concluded: "We cannot assume any efficacy for bed rest … and … further studies need to be done to establish evidence for the benefit or harm of bed rest as a treatment."[16]

RISK FACTORS

Decreasing activity during periods of illness is an adaptive and protective mechanism. It is during these periods of conservation of movement that skeletal muscle structure and function adapt to the new lower level of activity. Such interventions as range of motion exercises and ambulating may decrease the rate and magnitude of the atrophy to a small extent, but only activities that match the duration and intensity of prior daily activity will prevent the onset of disuse atrophy.[17-19] Unfortunately, it is

TABLE 20-1 High Risk for Skeletal Muscle Atrophy

HIGH-RISK POPULATIONS	HIGH-RISK FACTORS
Intensive care patients	Restriction of mobility as a result of bed rest
Orthopedic patients Fractures Traction Pinning of joints	Immobilization; diminished muscle contraction
Chronic low back pain	Pain; guarding of site; restriction of mobility
Elderly patients	Diminished mobility, restriction to chairs, surgical restriction of movement; medications, social isolation, depression
Neurological disorders Closed head injury Cerebrovascular accident Spinal injury Neuromuscular disorder	Diminished or restricted movement and weight-bearing
Nutritional deficiencies Anorexia Cachexia	Catabolism of lean body mass; diminished force generation
Astronauts	Weightlessness, decreased load on skeletal muscle and cardiovascular system; diminished weight-bearing
Patients with a psychogenic disorder Depression Schizophrenia Organic brain syndrome	Decreased mobility and possible immobility
Postoperative patients	Altered mobility as a result of fatigue and pain
Pregnancy	High-risk pregnancies; antitocolytics therapy; bed rest
Cancer patients	Fatigue; diminished mobility; medication; pain
Respiratory	
Mechanical ventilation	Severe restriction of mobility; diminished contraction of respiratory muscles; drug induced paralysis, dyspnea
Emphysema	Diminished mobility as a result of insufficient tissue perfusion of oxygen
Patients receiving corticosteroids	Drug-induced atrophy of skeletal muscle
Patients with unrelieved pain	Guarding of site results in restriction of movement

often beyond the ability of a patient who is functionally limited by illness to maintain a high level of activity. The patient's movement, weight-bearing, and general activity can only be increased within the constraints of his or her pathological process. With the gap between these two different ADL levels in mind, the nurse can plan activities appropriate to the patient's recovery.

Skeletal muscle atrophy can be caused by three major conditions: inactivity, also known as *disuse*, immobilization (see Box 20-1), and pharmacological interventions. Inactivity and immobilization are better understood as existing on a continuum of impaired mobility. Inactivity or disuse atrophy is defined as atrophy resulting solely from decreased movement and weight-bearing. The muscles in question have not been subjected to immobilization, denervation, or other pathological states.

The severity of skeletal muscle atrophy is directly related to two key variables: the duration of decreased activity and the magnitude of the restriction of activity.[8] These variables affect the majority of patients, regardless of diagnostic category, and vary in predominance in different patient populations (see Table 20-1). This variation in predominance is directly related to the duration and magnitude of restriction of movement and weight-bearing. For example, a postoperative patient has more mobility and less atrophy than a patient in bilateral leg traction has.

The risk for skeletal muscle atrophy may be specific to one muscle group or involve the total body muscle mass. It is the additive effect of the duration of decreased movement, decreased weight-bearing, and the individual's pathological condition that determine the severity of skeletal muscle atrophy. The risk of involving other organ systems, such as the cardiovascular system, is linearly related to the total percentage of skeletal muscle mass involved. For example, a highly mobile patient whose right arm is casted is only at risk for atrophy of the affected limb. Conversely, a ventilator-assisted patient for whom total bed rest has been ordered and who is receiving glucocorticoids is at very high risk for severe skeletal muscle atrophy, as well as all of the associated organ system sequelae.

In addition to restriction of mobility and movement, the pathological condition itself may exacerbate the magnitude of skeletal muscle protein loss. For example, certain cancer cells excrete tumor necrosis factor (TNF), which has been found to lyse skeletal muscle cells and produce severe forms of degeneration and atrophy.[20] This form of atrophy may contribute to the fatigue experienced by oncology patients.[21]

Alternate environments also may place certain populations at risk. It is currently rare for nurses to care for patients after prolonged microgravity exposure; however, this environment causes atrophy by removing the force of gravity or load from skeletal muscle and causes atrophy. The microgravity of space flight produces atrophy of skeletal muscle that is as severe as that produced by casting. The mass of astronauts' leg muscles was reported to atrophy 11% during the Skylab missions.[22,23]

Other clinical conditions are linked with skeletal muscle atrophy. However, these are not usually the result of the "disuse" type of phenomenon. For example, The "low CG syndrome" (cystine and glutamine) exists with HIV infection, sepsis, ulcerative colitis, chronic fatigue syndrome, and cancer.[24] In this syndrome, a combination of abnormally low plasma cystine and glutamine levels, low natural killer (NK) cell activity, skeletal muscle wasting, muscle fatigue, and increased rates of urea production defines this complex.

Pharmacological intervention is a common cause of skeletal muscle atrophy (Table 20-2). The development of skeletal muscle weakness and atrophy is a well-known complication of the administration of exogenous glucocorticoids,[25,26] protease inhibitors,[27,28] and chemotheraputic agents.[21,29,30] Glucocorticoids primarily inhibit protein synthesis and result in generalized atrophy of the muscles.[31-33] Specifically, it is the fluorinated glucocorticoids (triamcinolone, betamethasone, and dexamethasone) that cause this form of clinical myopathy.[31,34] In addition, altered levels of cytokines are now associated with increased levels of fatigue.[35,36] Therefore it is possible that increased levels of skeletal muscle atrophy in patients with cancer may be potentiated by a cytokine-induced decrease in activity in addition to atrophy induced by chemotheraputic agents.

Decreased protein synthesis reduces muscle size by decreasing the volume and density of myofibrils and is manifested as weakness resulting from atrophied muscles, especially in the leg and thigh. Long-term glucocorticoid therapy and Cushing's disease result in the preferential atrophy of type II (fast-twitch fiber) groups, whereas type I (slow-twitch oxidative) fibers are not as severely affected.[37,38] The characteristic type II atrophy is opposite that of atrophy resulting from disuse or immobilization, in which type I fibers are preferentially affected. Losses of muscle tissue in these patients can approach 30%,

TABLE 20-2 Effects of Glucocorticoids on Skeletal Muscle Protein Synthesis

MUSCLE	DRUG	DURATION (DAYS)	CHANGE (%)
Soleus	Dexamethasone (25 mg/kg)	5	−7
Gastrocnemius White	Dexamethasone (100 mg/kg)	2	−29
		4	−52
		8	−33
Gastrocnemius Red	Dexamethasone (100 mg/kg)	2	−25
		4	−34
Soleus	Cortisol acetate (100 mg/kg)	5	No change
Gastrocnemius, whole	Cortisol acetate (100 mg/kg)	5	−55
EDL	Cortisol acetate (100 mg/kg)	3	−42

Data from references 28, 30-33, 125, 155.

compared with muscle tissue in a normal population.[39] The loss of type II fibers affects the ability to maintain contractile force in this patient population, especially during anaerobic activity.

Developmental Factors

Movement is fundamental to the development of mature skeletal muscle during the neonatal period.[40,41] Restriction of normal patterns of movement may alter the growth and development of skeletal muscle.[42] Immobilization of neonatal muscles in the shortened position decreases the longitudinal growth of the involved muscle. Studies have demonstrated that reduced longitudinal growth results from the myofibrils failing to develop sarcomeres in series; that is, at the ends of the muscle. Skeletal muscle is able to recover to normal resting lengths following a period approximately equal to the duration of immobilization and occurs by the addition of sarcomeres in series to the ends of myofibrils.[42]

Clinically, adaptation of muscle length is seen after tendon transplantation. If the length of a muscle is increased because of tendon transplantation of the distal end, the muscle will adapt to the new functional length within a few weeks.[43] Unlike developing muscle, the adult muscle has a remarkable ability to adapt to changes in length. If immobilized in the lengthened position, a muscle will add 25% of its sarcomeres in series within 2 to 3 days. When the immobilization is removed, sarcomere length is recovered within 1 week.

Muscle cells are more susceptible to the modifying influences of reduced activity in the neonatal period.[43,44] Specifically, the 14- to 21-day postnatal period appears to be a critical period in the differentiation of the different fiber types and occurs just after the establishment of single innervation of the fibers and normal locomotion and weight-bearing. For example, if the weight-bearing muscles of the leg are prevented from normal movement during this period, they are unable to develop normal contractile characteristics and normal enzymatic properties.[45] The long-term consequences of these alterations are not yet known.[44] Additionally, changes are also occurring at the neuromuscular junction, where in the latter part of the second postnatal week the fibers lose their polyinnervation and become innervated by a single motorneuron.[46,47] Therefore infants who are restrained or placed in traction or plaster casts for any prolonged period are at risk for developing alterations in skeletal muscle function. An example of restraint in this population would be Spika casts or long-term restraint imposed on premature infants.

During early development, the action of insulin and growth hormones stimulates skeletal muscle growth and maturation. In the absence of these hormones, there is abnormal development and growth. Testosterone has been shown to have a direct effect on skeletal muscle growth.[48] In adolescent males, continued muscle growth is stimulated by testosterone. When insufficient testosterone is present during adolescence, skeletal muscle growth will be severely limited. Therefore skeletal muscle growth will vary with the normal or abnormal variations in hormone levels of individuals.

Aging

During the process of aging, there is a progressive loss of lean body mass as a result of the gradual loss of the total number of muscle fibers. Between the ages of 30 and 80, a person gradually loses 40% of lean body mass, with an associated increase in the spread of fiber sizes.[49] This loss of muscle mass is reflected in a decreased cross-sectional area of the muscle and parallels a drop in muscular strength.[49-51]

Isometric and dynamic maximal strength also functionally declines beyond age 50.[52] Aging and inactivity exert similar deleterious effects on skeletal muscle function; however, the rate of atrophy resulting from inactivity is far more rapid than that of aging. When inactivity or immobilization is superimposed on aging muscle, the resulting atrophy may be more severe and require a longer period of recovery. The impact of disuse atrophy on elderly persons is largely one of altered function and is not necessarily caused by a larger magnitude of atrophic loss of muscle mass. [53-55]

A significant factor in the recovery of skeletal muscle following atrophy is the satellite cell.[56] Satellite cells are found between the sarcolemma and basal lamina of all skeletal muscle fibers; they are responsible for the regeneration of muscle. They are crucial in the regeneration of aging muscle, because their ability to mitotically divide is finite. The ability of a damaged or atrophied aged skeletal muscle to regenerate is impaired as a result of a decreased capacity of the satellite cells to divide and proliferate.[57-59] Recent studies have been able to recruit additional satellite cells to aging muscle by the use of IL-1 in an animal model. Further studies are needed to determine whether this is a useful model in the aging human.[60]

The neuromuscular system is also capable of changing its structure to reflect altered function. During the human life span, the neuromuscular junction (NMJ) undergoes morphological remodeling from early development through maturity. Exercise and decreased activity are important mediators of this effect before new perturbations in the NMJ are added as a result of aging.[56] Aged NMJs have greater nerve terminal areas, branch numbers, and sprouts than young NMJs do. The presence of significant morphological changes after only 5 days of subtotal disuse indicate that the NMJ is capable of a rapid anatomical remodeling in response to altered activity. It has been suggested that the simple increase in these structural parameters must underlie increased release of the acetylcholine transmitter in soleus muscle during aging. Acute inactivity also affects the morphological changes of the NMJ, creating an increase in neurotransmitter (ACh) release.

The structural and functional changes that occur in muscle during the process of aging place an inactive geriatric patient at very high risk. Although the magnitude of atrophy may not be more severe,[54] the ability of the individual to recover from atrophy can often be limited.[61,62] If geriatric patients are subjected to cycles of atrophy and recovery, it is hypothetically possible that they will reach a point beyond which they can no longer recover skeletal muscle mass and function, resulting in confinement to a wheelchair and bed. Further research is needed to clarify this phenomenon.

MECHANISMS

Skeletal muscle is "plastic" or adaptable and alters its structure, mechanical properties, and energy metabolism rapidly to adapt to an activity pattern.[63] Skeletal muscle atrophy caused by inactivity or immobilization primarily effects the antigravity muscles of the leg and back; however, all muscles of the body may be involved if their functional demands in the form of activity and muscle load are decreased (Figure 20-1). Restriction of movement and the amount of weight-bearing or load on a muscle regulate the rate and magnitude of skeletal muscle atrophy.[64]

Mass. The immobilization of limbs has been shown to lead to muscular atrophy, diminished muscular strength, and increased fatigue. Decreased loading of the weight-bearing muscles of the leg, especially the soleus, also produces a rapid loss of muscle mass. Three days following the start of hypodynamia, there is a decrease of 7% in the muscle mass with a further decline of 20% after 5 days.[69] Others have reported losses as high as 35% in the first 7 days; 45% by 2 weeks;[70] and 55% after 42 days of unloading.[71]

Muscle atrophy begins rapidly; the greatest losses are found early in the period of inactivity or immobilization. The onset of atrophy begins with rapid protein degradation, beginning within 6 hours of diminished activity.[72] Absolute losses of muscle mass and protein are greatest during days 3 to 7 of a period of inactivity or immobilization. The process of protein degradation results in a 14% to 17% decrease in fiber and muscle size following the initial 72 hours.[72,73]

It is possible to calculate the rate at which a muscle or group of muscles will atrophy by the following equation:

$$t_{1/2} = \frac{\text{In}2}{kd}$$

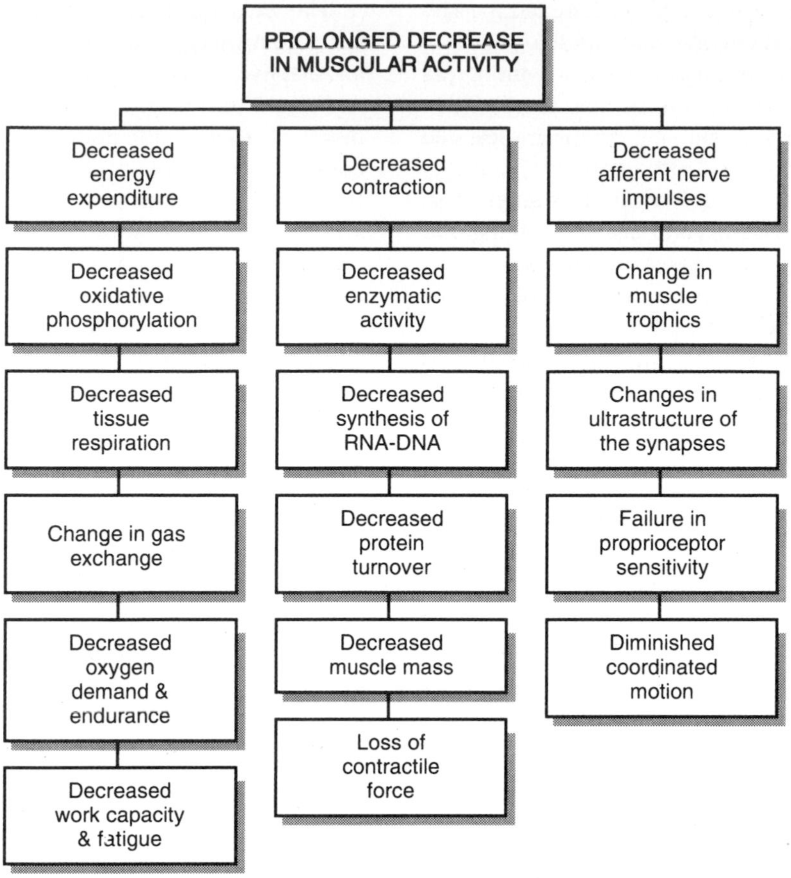

Figure 20-1 Adaptation to decreased skeletal muscle activity.

where $t_{1/2}$ is the half life, In2 the natural logarithm of 2, and kd the first-order rate constant for protein degradation.[74]

It remains unclear at this time which molecular mechanisms are responsible for the regulation of protein synthesis and degradation in response to activity levels.[10,75] It has been observed that changes in protein synthesis correlate with changes in RNA content in skeletal muscle following alterations in activity level, and changes in the phosphorylation state of eukaryotic initiation factor 2 (eIF_2) have been proposed as the regulatory site.[76]

CONTRACTILE AND BIOCHEMICAL PROPERTIES

The loss of muscle mass results in a decreased cross-sectional area of muscle. The total cross-sectional area of a muscle comprises bundles of individual muscle fibers. These fibers are normally 50 to 100 μm in diameter and during atrophy fiber diameter significantly decreases. The volumetric change in the muscle is caused by changes in fiber volume which first occur by decreasing the size and later the number of the myofibrils within each fiber. During the initial weeks, skeletal muscle volume will decrease by 25% to 30% from decreased activity and 75% to 80% in the same time period as a result of total denervation.[77] There is clear evidence that atrophy occurs in the first few months without a loss in the total number of fibers in the muscle.

The ability of a muscle to produce force is directly proportional to its cross-sectional area. When the process of atrophy reduces the cross-sectional area, the ability of a muscle to produce force is decreased. A muscle 1 cm^2 in cross-section can maximally contract a load of 3 or 4 g; therefore an individual's strength depends on the cross-sectional area of his or her muscles. When the cross-sectional area decreases as a result of atrophy, a person's strength and ability to produce force decreases. Fatigue is a sequela of the process of atrophy and is seen as a limitation in the force generating capacity or the inability to maintain the required force[2,78] (see Figure 20-1).

Decreased contractile activity has two characteristic components: decreased mechanical loading and decreased movement. Mechanical loading occurs when the patient stands and increases the load of a muscle or bears weight. The decreased weight-bearing or mechanical loading component of disuse is known as hypodynamia (HD).[79] Decreased movement or range of motion of the limb causes decreased contractile activity and is known as hypokinesia (HK). Patients may be subject to only one or both of these limitations.

The majority of human muscles can be characterized as fast- or slow-twitch muscles. The differences in the contractile speeds of these muscles are a function of the population of individual fibers of which these muscles are composed. For example, the classic slow-twitch muscle is the soleus, which contains predominantly slow fibers. The extensor digitorum longus (EDL) and the flexor digitorum longus (FDL) are faster muscles.

Slow and fast muscles are designed for different functions. Slow muscles are used for postural support and weight-bearing; whereas fast muscles are for rapid movement. Their functional uses also reflect two different forms of energy supply. Slow-contracting muscles use ATP at a slow rate and have endurance capacities over long periods (Table 20-3). Conversely, fast muscle is used for rapid movements, burns ATP at a high rate, and is rapidly fatigued.[80] The energy sources for these two types of muscle are also different. Slow muscles depend on ATP synthesis associated with a good oxygen supply and mitochondria. This is known as the *oxidative system.* However, fast muscle depends on anaerobic phosphorylation and glycogen.

Characteristically slow fibers within a muscle contain relatively high numbers of large mitochondria. Slow fibers are classified slow oxidative (SO) or type I fibers (see Table 20-3). Within the fast (type II) fibers there are subclassifications: the fast-twitch, oxidative-glycolytic (FOG) or type IIA, and the type IIB or fast-twitch, glycolytic (FG) fibers. The type IIA fibers are intermediate fibers and contain fast contraction speeds with aerobic and anaerobic energetics, and the type IIB or FG fibers have greater capacities.[81] There is a lower total mitochondrial content because of unloading resulting in a loss of absolute skeletal muscle endurance.[82,83] In the case of paralysis or spinal cord injury, although atrophy also occurs as a result of unloading, there are fewer mitochondria per unit volume of contractile protein.[84] This lessened aerobic capacity is demonstrated in lowered fatigue resistance following spinal cord injury.[85]

Alterations in the speed of contraction of an atrophic muscle can be linked to shifts in the regulatory proteins of the muscle. The myosin heads contain ATPase and the actin-binding characteristics of myosin. There is a switch in protein composition during inactivity so that the amount of fast myosin isozymes relative to slow myosin increases markedly in slow muscle.[86] In fast muscle there is an increase in the slow myosin isozymes. These changes in the myosin heavy chain regulatory proteins create a "regression toward the mean" effect. Slow-contracting endurance muscles become less able to sustain long-term aerobic activity, because inactivity has altered the muscles' function to act more like a fast-contracting muscle. The fast-contracting muscle also changes its speed and function to become more like a slow-twitch muscle.

The result of these shifts in contractile speed is that the original function of the muscle has been altered. Postural muscles, such as the soleus and medial gastrocnemius, are primarily endurance muscles. After inactivity and atrophy, the changes

TABLE 20-3 Classification of Muscle Fibers Based on Physiological, Biochemical, and Histochemical Properties

PROPERTY	GROUP I	GROUP II	
Twitch contraction time	Slow	Fast	Fast
Fatigability	Low	Intermediate	High
Oxidative enzymes	High	Moderate	Very low
Glycolytic enzymes	Very low	Moderate	High
Myosin ATPase activity	Low	High	High
Histochemical type	I	IIA	IIB

From St. Pierre, B.A., Kasper, C.E., & Lindsey, A.M. (1992). Fatigue mechanisms in cancer patients: TNF and exercise effects on skeletal muscle factors. *Oncology Nursing Forum 19*(3), 419-432.

in their contractile proteins cause them to fatigue easily, because they are no longer predominantly aerobic muscle.[86]

PATHOLOGICAL CONSEQUENCES

The adaptations that occur to skeletal muscle during inactivity and immobilization are not pathological by themselves. They appear to represent a normal attempt of the homeostatic mechanisms to adapt to altered movement and decreased metabolic needs. Altered insulin resistance and injury are two consequences of skeletal muscle atrophy. The lack or recognition of these changes by the health care professionals creates the potential for iatrogenesis.

Skeletal Muscle Injury

Injury to skeletal muscle recovering from atrophy is a potential problem. Recent evidence has shown that running causes the degeneration of large segments of postural skeletal muscle. It appears that during the first 3 to 5 days after a period of decreased weight-bearing, strenuous exercise should not be done.[87-89] Heavy exercise, such as weight-lifting or running, places a load in excess of the ability of the atrophied muscle to contract against. When contracting against the increased load, the muscle responds by "ripping" the myofibrils and degenerating.[90,91] The injured muscle will recover from this damage within 14 days in the absence of continued active exercise.[87]

Atrophic skeletal muscle is especially sensitive to eccentric contraction-induced injury.[87,92] Eccentric contraction is defined as contraction of the muscle while stretched.[93] Running downhill and walking down stairs are examples of eccentric contraction.

Insulin Resistance. During inactivity, bed rest, and immobilization, skeletal muscle becomes characteristically diabetic-like. In other words, insulin is unable to stimulate glucose uptake and to activate glycogen synthase in human muscle. This insulin resistance occurs at the third day of inactivity and bed rest—and within 24 hours in casted patients who are immobilized. Clinical studies have demonstrated false-positive test results for glucose intolerance, and diabetes can occur in humans as a result of inactivity and immobilization.[45,94]

The administration of an oral glucose load following 3 days of inactivity or bed rest may cause hyperinsulinemia and hyperglycemia, which is indicative of altered carbohydrate metabolism. It has been demonstrated that the longer the period of inactivity and immobility, the greater the altered glucose tolerance responses.[45,94] As previously discussed with other organ systems, the reduction in carbohydrate tolerance is directly proportional to the amount of restriction of activity.[95] Daily range of motion or other exercise decreases but does not eliminate this response. Following a period of inactivity, it takes approximately 7 to 14 days to recover normal carbohydrate tolerance.[96] If mild exercise is done during this recovery period, only 7 days are needed to recover plasma glucose levels to normal.[45]

Previous studies indicated that some responses to insulin in unloaded muscle differ from those in denervated muscle.[97] Denervated muscle showed insulin resistance of both 2-deoxyl[1,2-^{3}H] glucose and a-[methyl-^{3}H] aminoisobutyric acid uptake, whereas unloaded muscle showed an increased or normal response, respectively.[98] The inhibition of protein degradation and the stimulation of protein synthesis by insulin are less in denervated muscle than in unloaded muscle.[98]

RELATED PATHOPHYSIOLOGICAL CONCEPTS

Decreased activity and immobilization are known to cause alterations in every major organ system. They are the cause of a series of physiological adaptations that ultimately contribute to a deteriorating cardiovascular work capacity.

Cardiovascular Function

Intravascular fluid volume losses and changes affect cardiovascular function in cardiac contractility. Parameters within the intravascular compartment that are affected during inactivity and immobilization include blood and plasma volume, hemoglobin and hematocrit levels, and red blood cell volume. Adaptation in the structure of conduit arteries to unloading is also a factor. Chronic changes in activity patterns can influence arterial structure.[99]

Plasma Volume. The most significant changes in the vascular fluid compartment are reductions in plasma and blood volumes. Blood and plasma volume is influenced by body position. The horizontal recumbent position leads to a decrease in the plasma volume of approximately 500 ml or 7% of the body weight during the first 24 to 48 hours. Blood pools in the thorax rather than in the lower extremities and creates a cephalic shift of blood volume (Figure 20-2). The movement of blood into the thorax increases the venous volume, resulting in distention of the central veins and a stimulation of central blood volume receptors that trigger a

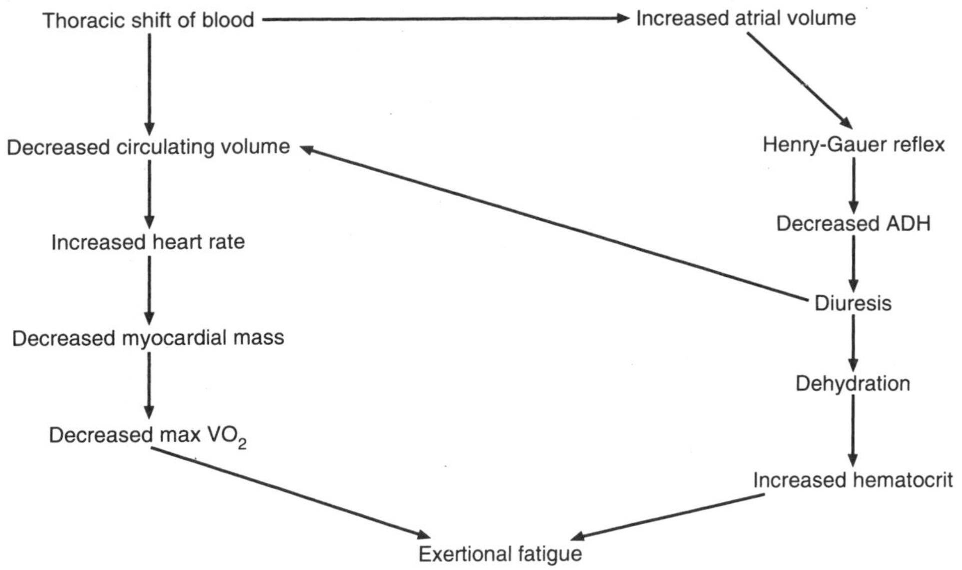

Figure 20-2 Cardiovascular adaptations to decreased activity.

decrease in ADH secretion.[45,100] Increases in central blood volume induce inhibition of ADH release through left atrial receptors and aldosterone through the right atrial receptors. Inhibition of ADH and aldosterone results in diuresis of salt and water. Fortunately, ADH production follows a pattern of diurnal circadian variation; therefore normal sleep patterns with the same thoracic pooling of blood do not cause a significant increase in the free water clearance. With at least 2 days of bed rest, there is a significant decline in thcsc volumes. These fluid volume losses are progressive over time, with the greatest drop beginning with the second and reaching its nadir at the twentieth day of inactivity.[45,100-102]

Vascular fluid volume loss also depends on the magnitude of the restriction of movement. Uncomplicated inactivity causes a plasma volume loss of 220 ml and blood volume loss of 340 ml in humans.[101,102] Severe losses of fluid volume were reported as a result of a 200-day period of confinement. This study reported plasma volume losses of 600 ml at 70 days, 900 ml at 105 days, and 1000 ml from 180 to 200 days of continued bed rest.[103,104] Recovery of plasma and blood volume is approximately 1.25 times the duration of inactivity.

Normal values for plasma volume are 42 ml/kg for adult men. Blood volume has a normal value of 64 to 69 ml/kg. A 10% to 20% decrease in these values, accompanied by increased hematocrit level and hemoglobin concentration, would present a suspicious picture to the attending medical and nursing staff of any hospital. It has been observed that patients admitted for conditions that require decreased activity resulting in confinement to bed are often the first to demonstrate signs of dehydration and have abnormal laboratory values. Current practice dictates that these changes are uniformly followed by the regulation of intake and output along with intravenous infusion. The sudden and unexplained drop in hematocrit and hemoglobin that occurs 3 days after inactivity begins may also lead to unnecessary medication and treatment being prescribed.

Red Blood Cell Volume. As the plasma and blood volumes decrease during a period of horizontal inactivity, there is a corresponding increase in hemoglobin concentration and hematocrit. Small increases in hematocrit and hemoglobin, usually not significant, occur during the bed rest period. However, after a period of inactivity and immobilization has ended, a significant drop in hemoglobin and hematocrit occurs in the first week of recovery.[45,105,106] Hemoglobin decreases 1.7 g/100 ml or 12% at the third day after bed rest begins.[105,106] The decrease in these values does not coincide with the return of plasma volume.

Cardiac Output and Stroke Volume. Cardiac output and stroke volumes are dependent on alterations in plasma volume and heart rate and are also affected by changes in body position. Movement from the upright to the supine position increases the cardiac output 25% to 30%, whereas stroke volume is increased by 40%.[104,107,108] Conversely, when the position is changed from supine to standing or sitting, there is a decrease in the end-diastolic size of the heart and a decrease in stroke volume.

The stroke volume of the heart is affected by various factors; venous return to the heart, distensibility of the ventricles, and force of contraction in relation to pressure in the aorta or pulmonary arteries. Therefore, when the extracellular fluid is decreased by clinical states such as bed rest, a decrease in cardiac output may also occur[104,107,108] (see Figure 20-2). Maximal cardiac output was 20.0 l/min before and 14.8 l/min after bed rest.[105] Also, it was found that bed rest produces a marked decrease in stroke volume from 103 ml before bed rest and 86 ml after bed rest; in the sitting position the stroke volume decreased 25%.

In a normal individual in the recumbent position, the left ventricular stroke volume, as determined angiographically, is approximately 60% to 70% of upright volumes in control subjects. Increased contractility may increase the ejection fraction and the stroke volume by producing a decreased end-systolic volume (ESV), with the end-diastolic volume (EDV) either decreasing or remaining the same. The heart compensates for the change in stroke volume by decreasing EDV 13% and increasing ESV 13%.[104] An increased stroke volume can also be produced by an increase in venous return, which increases the end-diastolic fiber length of the atria and ventricles. After prolonged supine bed rest, the ability to increase the venous return is unlikely because of the decrease in plasma volume plus the tendency for blood to pool in the legs when the subject is in the upright position.

Heart Rate. As stroke volume and cardiac output decrease with inactivity or immobilization, the ability of the cardiovascular system to return blood to the heart is decreased. Heart rate increases to compensate, which is one of the simplest and most effective ways of increasing cardiac output. It is the most important and most frequently used mechanism for effecting rapid changes in cardiac output, particularly in untrained persons under conditions of moderately increased demands. An increase in heart rate by itself increases cardiac output threefold.

Resting supine heart rate can increase 2 to 5 beats/min over 1 week of inactivity.[101,104,109,112] Heart rate averages an increase of 0.5 beats/min per day of decreased activity and immobilization.[101,112]

Increased heart rate on rising from a horizontal position is indicative of orthostatic intolerance, and this phenomenon can be attributed to adaptation of the peripheral vasculature to the removal of hydrostatic pressure during supine bed rest.[101,112] The lack of hydrostatic pressure on lower body vasculature causes the smooth muscle to lose its tone; thus these lower body blood vessels are unable to constrict, and they restrict the volume of blood that is delivered when the person returns to an upright position.[101,112]

Pulmonary Function

Pulmonary function is also reduced after inactivity or immobilization. Secondary to decreased function is an impedance of maximal ventilatory gas exchange which may be one of the mechanisms that causes Vo_2 max and exercise capacity to diminish following inactivity. Previous studies have demonstrated that the generalized effects of deconditioning did not change total lung capacity, forced vital capacity, 1-second forced expiratory volume or residual lung volume. Decreased activity and bed rest did decrease mean minute ventilation; however, this variable is directly correlated to changes in the Vo_2 max.[113,114]

Physical Work Capacity

For the skeletal muscle system, reuse damage and insulin resistance are significant conditions that contribute to the symptoms of deconditioning, weakness, and physiological fatigue. These symptoms originate not only with atrophy of skeletal muscle but also with changes in the cardiovascular, respiratory, and skeletal organ systems.

Deconditioning, weakness, and fatigue are the consequences of an altered ability to perform physical work. There are many factors that affect the relationship between work load and work capacity, such as (1) *physical work,* the ability to work, and the faculty of performing work is defined as the term *power;* (2) *capacity* is the maximum power output of the individual; and (3) *load* is the burden placed on the individual or the rate at which work is being performed. The ability to perform work depends on the ability of the muscle cell to transform energy into contractile force. If the system is altered by decreased oxygen or energy delivery, work capacity will decrease.[45,82,101,113]

Deconditioning

Deconditioning is a decrease in work capacity and is caused by a loss of Vo_{2max}, lean body mass, and endurance. Each of these components contributes to the ability of an individual to perform work or exercise. Because the oxygenation of the patient has been compromised by lowered oxygen uptake, circulating fluid volume, and cardiac output following inactivity, bed rest, and immobilization, the skeletal muscle is limited in its capacity to perform work. The skeletal muscle is also limited in its ability to perform work by contracting against a load with smaller muscles.[114] Because the strength of a muscle is directly related to its size, decreases in size will decrease its strength. The "weakness" or "fatigue" perceived by the patient is due to a decrease in strength resulting from atrophy.

Alterations in Calcium Metabolism

In addition to alterations in the cardiovascular system, diminished weight-bearing has a significant effect on the skeleton. The absence of longitudinal weight-bearing on the skeleton during inactivity produces bone demineralization and calcium loss.

Inactivity and immobilization are associated with alterations in bone formation and reabsorption, which lead to a net negative calcium balance.[115] The magnitude of bone demineralization and calcium depletion is related to the duration and severity of the removal of weight-bearing.[116] Recently it has been shown that loss of weight-bearing in the growing rat decreases bone formation, osteoblast numbers, and bone maturation in unloaded bones. These responses suggest an impairment of osteoblast proliferation and differentiation.[117] These losses destabilize the skeleton and place the patient at risk for fracture.

Urinary calcium losses during inactivity and bed rest are not related to the amount of calcium intake. Calcium is released from the skeleton during periods of inactivity and excreted.[115,118]

Patients remain in negative calcium balance even after ambulation has resumed. The duration of the recovery period is approximately equal to the duration of the decrease in weight-bearing.[118,119] The return to positive calcium balance is time dependent and is related to the amount of activity. Exercise has been shown to speed the recovery from negative calcium balance.[115] Weight-bearing exercise is more effective in restoring calcium retention after a period of inactivity than a sedentary mode of recovery. Following a 28-day period of inactivity, exercise has been demonstrated to decrease the duration of recovery of calcium levels from 25 days to 5 days.[115]

Cellular and Molecular Mechanisms of Atrophy

Much has been reported in the past 10 years relating to the mechanistic changes which occur at the level of the cell and drive the process of skeletal muscle atrophy. It is known that denervation or hindlimb suspension both decrease the content of rRNA, alpha-actin mRNA, and cytochrome C mRNA in adult rat skeletal muscle.[120] However, at this time a mechanism has not been found. The multiple intracellular systems are known to include those of RNA transcription and translation,[121,122] cytoskeletal elements,[123] and myonuclei.[124,125]

Various functional and pharmacological interventions have been attempted to prevent the onset of atrophy; some have been unsuccessful and some promising. In one study, the association between local insulin-like growth factors I (IGF-I) overexpression and atrophy were studied in skeletal muscle. It was hypothesized that endogenous skeletal muscle IGF-I mRNA expression would decrease with hindlimb unloading (HU) in mice, and that transgenic mice overexpressing human IGF-I (hIGF-I) specifically in skeletal muscle would exhibit less atrophy after HU.[126] However, it was found that high local expression of hIGF-I mRNA and peptide in skeletal muscle alone could not attenuate unloading-induced atrophy of fast-twitch muscle in mice.[126]

In another study, the effects of intermittent weight-bearing on aged animals during unloading were examined as a potential intervention. At the cellular level, inactivity significantly altered the contractile properties of single fibers isolated from aged mammalian soleus skeletal muscle.[127] It was found that weight-bearing attenuated the detrimental effects induced by inactivity in the SOL. However, this weight-bearing protocol did not attenuate the inactivity-induced alterations in aged mammalian GAS skeletal muscle.[127]

MANIFESTATIONS AND SURVEILLANCE

Skeletal muscle atrophy produces a wide range of manifestations, depending on the severity and duration of inactivity or immobilization. The primary alterations that occur with skeletal muscle atrophy are decreased strength, decreased exercise capacity, and fatigue.

Strength

Muscular strength is defined as the maximum forces or tension generated by a muscle or group of muscles. Human skeletal muscle is capable of generating 3 to 4 k of force per cm^2 of muscle cross-section irrespective of sex.[128] Muscles with the greatest cross-sectional areas exert the greatest forces. Therefore an early sign of skeletal muscle atrophy is patient report of weakness and fatigue as cross-sectional area decreases.[129] Because these signs may also be attributed to medication or pathology, they are difficult for the nurse to use in the assessment of strength without further objective data. Quantitative information may be obtained using: (1) tensiometry, (2) dynamometry, or (3) computer-assisted force and work output determinations.

Cable tensiometers are a simple and portable method of measuring the strength of large muscle groups. This tool measures the pulling force of a limb during a static or isometric contraction when there is no change in the muscle's length. Batteries of strength tests have been developed using this device to measure the static force of the hand, fingers, thumb, wrist, forearm, elbow, shoulder, trunk, neck, hip, knee, and ankle.[130] These tests enable the nurse to evaluate the strength decrement as a result of skeletal muscle atrophy. These tests are highly reproducible on repeated evaluations. The tensiometer may also be used to evaluate strength during various phases of movement and may give a more accurate assessment of patient weakness or strength than other methods.[131]

Handgrip is also used for the determination of patient strength. These devices work on the principle of compression.[131,132] When force is applied to the handle of the dynamometer, a steel spring is compressed and moves a needle on a gauge. The resulting number is reflective of the strength applied.

Muscle strength may also be monitored using computerized dynamometers, which provide a rapid method of accurately quantifying muscular forces generated during movement. Dynamometers (e.g., Cybex II) assess strength by measuring isokinetic movement. The torque movement of muscle force is recorded during limb extension and flexion at maximal effect and constant angular velocity. This test permits a functional measurement of strength.[132]

Muscle Volume. Different methods have been used to quantify atrophy (see Table 20-3). CT scans and MRIs permit the visualization of the actual cross-sectional and volumetric areas of a muscle.[85,89] Both of these methods also permit measurement of the extremities to determine changes in leg volume and muscle size following skeletal muscle atrophy.[85] Edema and increases in connective tissue that occur in conjunction with atrophy, even when MRI or CT scans are used, may conceal muscle atrophy.[133] Methods have not yet been developed to account for the contribution of edema and increased connective tissue when assessing atrophy. Because this method of assessing skeletal muscle atrophy is expensive, it should only be used in cases of severe, unexplained atrophy that occurs with complaints of extreme fatigue. These measures can help to distinguish symptoms of fatigue resulting from atrophy from those originating with the concurrent pathological process. MRI and CT scans can also be used in conjunction with laboratory analyses that monitor skeletal muscle protein losses. Measured 24-hour urine for creatinine loss directly correlates muscle protein loss with creatinine output in the urine.[134]

Work Capacity. The loss of skeletal muscle mass correlates with decreased exercise capacity of the patient. Clinical observation indicates that patients who have decreased their mean ADLs because of inactivity or immobility are less able to respond to the challenge of a given level of muscular exercise than a normal ambulating person. Their ability to perform work will depend on the severity of restriction of mobility and the duration of decreased activity. Maximal oxygen uptake (Vo_{2max}) is the accepted standard by which the functional or work capacity, of the cardiovascular and respiratory system is measured.[135,136]

The ability to perform work or exercise is measured by the Vo_{2max}. Maximal oxygen uptake is defined as the greatest oxygen uptake an individual can achieve during a given exercise at an intensity that can be sustained for at least 2.5 to 3 minutes but will cause complete exhaustion after 5 to 10 minutes. The highest levels of VO_{2max} are attained with work that uses the largest groups of muscles.[135,136]

During training, physical adaptations occur which allow the body to adequately respond to various exercise loads. Following inactivity, bed rest, or immobility, patients are detrained and respond to an exercise challenge with great effort. They are unable to maintain that effort without fatigue.[135] The trained individual responds to the same stress with less effort and can maintain the activity for a much longer period before fatigue begins.

Submaximal oxygen uptake also decreases after prolonged inactivity or immobilization. There is a high correlation between the cardiac output during exercise and oxygen uptake (in liters $\cdot$ min^{-1}); therefore counting the heart rate during exercise is all that is needed for the evaluation of exercise capacity.[135,136] During submaximal testing, the individual acts as his or her own control, and oxygen uptake can be predicted from the external power to which the person is subjected.

Inactivity in the form of chair rest has also been used in studies of oxygen uptake. In chair rest, patients are placed in the high Fowler's position in regular or cardiac chairs. This differs from the majority of bed rest studies where patients were placed in the supine position in bed for the entire day. Following 30 days of chair rest, a 7% decrease in maximal oxygen uptake was found. The large decrease was found by Saltin et al[100] who observed an average reduction in maximal oxygen uptake of 26% in healthy men who exercised following 20 days of supine bed rest. It should be pointed out, however, that these subjects underwent 55 days of training before their confinement in bed.

In most studies the maximal work capacity tests were performed with the subjects in the upright position. When exercise tests are performed immediately after supine bed rest and in the upright position, the resultant orthostatic hypotension may result in a variable decrease in the maximal working time and Vo_{2max}. Vo_{2max} is approximately 15% lower in the supine position than during the sitting position. Therefore study subjects performing exercise tests in the supine position should have lower results in Vo_{2max}.

A significant correlation exists between changes in body cell mass determined from isotope dilution and changes in the exercise capacity of large muscle masses. These are important considerations, because the major loss of protein during periods of stress and starvation is from skeletal muscle, thus depleting body cell mass and degrading function (exercise capacity).[137] Commonly used intravenous nutritional regimens have been shown to affect the functional status of skeletal muscle and cause a form of disuse atrophy.[137]

SURVEILLANCE AND MEASUREMENT

A professional nurse is responsible for monitoring a patient's physiological parameters and behavioral changes, as previously discussed. In addition, the nurse must monitor changes in the patient's functional status over time, which is important in determining the development, progression, and recovery of atrophic skeletal muscle from periods of decreased activity, bed rest, or immobility. It is also crucial that the nurse evaluate initial activity status as well as the severity of the restriction of mobility. Specific surveillance parameters such as urinary excretion of creatinine and 3-methylhistidine (3-MH) may be used to monitor skeletal muscle atrophy. The laboratory standards for these excretion rates in patient populations have been previously described.[138,139]

Alterations in heart rate, blood pressure, and orthostatic intolerance can be monitored during the standard daily vital signs checks. The staff would require education on the trends to follow that would indicate a deteriorating condition, such as increased heart rate at a rate of 1 beat/min/day of bed rest, and symptoms of orthostatic intolerance with standing. Routine laboratory analysis could be used to monitor the classic trends, such as increased hematocrit and hemoglobin concentrations, that result from prolonged inactivity or immobility. These trends are gradual and can be differentiated from those of the existing pathological condition.[139] It must be remembered that some diseases will mask these trends.

Behavioral indicators of atrophy may precede the physiological parameters. The timing of behavioral alterations resulting from inactivity or immobilization has not been well defined in the literature. The predominant symptoms are those associated with sensory deprivation, such as altered visual and auditory perception and time perception. These behavioral alterations have been found to be closely linked to confinement and isolation from normal social contact.[140] Intervention should focus on prevention of social isolation, and increasing visual and auditory stimulation. Patients on strict bed rest should be placed in multiple patient rooms near the nursing station. When possible, meals should be taken in group settings.

Prevention of severe skeletal muscle atrophy is most effective when there is an early recognition of potential decrement of activity. Early recognition will enable the professional nurse to plan a schedule of ADLs that will permit the patient to maintain the highest activity level possible. Patient education is also essential to enlist the cooperation of the patient in the plan of activity. Current research in the area of skeletal muscle atrophy has focused on normal adult populations; therefore data describing the course of atrophy in individual pathophysiological processes are not available.

Additional research data are needed about the time course of skeletal muscle atrophy in disease processes. The rate and magnitude of the behavioral components of inactivity, bed rest, and immobility are also needed. However, the research base of skeletal muscle atrophy and its sequelae in normal human populations is extensive and provides clear direction for nursing research. The role of the nurse is the continued monitoring of activity levels and the patient's ability to perform selfcare activities.

After the nurse has identified a patient at risk for skeletal muscle atrophy, key parameters must be assessed at least twice per day. These parameters include active and passive range of motion, antropometric measurements, weight changes, changes in upper and lower extremity strength, work capacity, fatigue, and related biochemical measurements (see Manifestations and Surveillance). In addition, the monitoring of patient activity levels over time and range of motion must always be compared with initial assessments and be projected to the levels of activity that will be needed when the patient is discharged to a skilled nursing facility or the home setting. These observations will enable the nurse to respond and provide appropriate interventions and therapy.

CLINICAL MANAGEMENT

Decreases in the regular ADLs produce dramatic adaptations in both the skeletal muscle and the cardiovascular system. The alteration in the composition of skeletal muscle is most pronounced in the weight-bearing muscles of the legs and postural muscles of the torso. The primary clinical goal is to encourage as much physical activity as is reasonable for the individual patient. Simple activities, such as performing self-care, eating in a group setting, and watching television in an activity room, encourage the patient to move from his or her room and exercise. The patient may participate in setting goals for walking the unit halls or simply increasing the time that he or she is able to bear weight at the bedside. The maintenance of activity is an effective method of diminishing the effects of disuse atrophy even under the extreme conditions of orthopedic traction and weightlessness. The maintenance of muscle strength by maintaining ADLs and movement assists in the support of the capacity of the cardiovascular system to defend against orthostatic hypotension following inactivity.

The simple countermeasures of chair rest and standing have shown promise for clinical use in the care of patients with cardiovascular alterations.[34,143] These methods have also been successful in treating conditions of aged muscles.[54,79,144] The simple method of placing a subject in a chair for 8 hours a day was found to slow the rate of decrease in orthostatic tolerance and work capacity. It has been found that the rate of decrease in work capacity was less rapid when chair rest was instituted than in supine bed rest. Birkhead et al[34] compared the effects of supine bed rest and sitting exercise with quiet sitting on the circulatory and metabolic consequences of 24 days of bed rest. Supine exercises did not prevent but diminished the decrease in orthostatic intolerance and work capacity. Sitting exercise (1 hour of bicycle ergometer exercise per day) minimized the effects in one of two groups. In the final comparison, it was found that 8 hours daily of quiet sitting in combination with 16 hours of supine bed rest resulted in only minor decreases in work capacity. Eight hours of quiet sitting per day for 21 days prevented orthostatic intolerance and insignificantly decreased work capacity. In a classic study of inactivity, Birkhead et al[34] demonstrated 3 hours per day of quiet standing during supine bed rest to be an effective rehabilitative measure for reversing bed rest induced orthostatic hypotension and hypercalciuria in normal populations.

One intervention did impede the reduction of plasma volume with restricted activity. Vogt[143] found that 12 hours of quiet sitting activity in conjunction with 12 hours of bed rest reduced plasma volume loss to the insignificant amount of 95 ml in patients. Birkhead et al[34] concurred, reporting that no significant change in plasma volume occurred during 42 days of unrestricted chair rest. Subjects in this study, normal adult men (age 18–35), were restricted to quiet chair sitting for 8 hours per day.

Quiet chair rest is contraindicated in few instances in the hospital. At the present time, standard nursing procedure attempts to place most patients in a chair for some portion of every day. The length of time spent in the chair is very subjective and is controlled by the discretion of the primary nurse. The risk in implementing a procedure to maintain patients in a chair for timed duration would be small, because this is already used in clinical practice.[45,114]

Studies of patients have shown that the pattern of deconditioning and its associated loss of Vo_{2max}, lean body mass, and endurance are similar to the studies performed on healthy subjects. Most of these studies used orthopedic and surgical populations.[107,145] One of the factors that may influence these vascular fluid volume losses is the amount of activity that persons perform during bed rest. When the supine position is maintained without periodic upright positioning, significant plasma volumes and blood volume losses of approximately 15% and 10% occur, respectively.[107,145,146] By contrast, when a supine bed rest patient is granted bathroom privileges and/or can sit in a chair for 10 to 15 minutes per day, the plasma volume and blood volume losses are almost half less than if that person had been on restricted bed rest.[147] This change in posture may temporarily halt or slow down the deconditioning process, because sitting or standing even for a short period causes some gravitational force to be exerted on the lower body.

Thus the effect on intravascular fluid volumes is minimized.

Fatigue in patients with skeletal muscle atrophy may be severe and is a result of the combined effects of decreased muscle mass, Vo_{2max}, and circulating plasma volume. Patient report of fatigue will vary with the individual and may begin within one day of decreased ADLs. Fatigue will increase however when the patient attempts increased mobilization and self-care activities. Slowly increasing activity in the atrophied patient will minimize the fatigue. Research is needed to determine the rate of remobilization that will minimize severe fatigue.

Another therapy that is used at present is electrical muscle stimulation (EMS).[148-151] EMS of skeletal muscle is increasingly employed in both research and clinical settings as a therapeutic method to increase skeletal muscle size and strength. Because there is a progressive loss of muscle mass and strength with aging resulting in loss of mobility, many have proposed and are currently using EMS in an attempt to recover these age related losses of skeletal muscle strength, mass, and size. Because strength is directly related to the cross-sectional area of a muscle, it is assumed that increasing contractile activity by EMS will increase the mass, and cross-sectional area yielding increased strength.

EMS was originally used as a physiological research tool to drive adaptation of contractile proteins, biochemical content, and speed of contraction by invasive stimulation of specific muscles in animal models. In rat models, implanted electrodes are used to directly stimulate nerve and muscle, and generally stimulation is continuous for periods up to 24 hours. Although methods under current use in human populations do not methodologically resemble these animal studies, the data have been extrapolated to the human and used as the physiological justification for further application to the aged. Therefore further research is needed before its extensive use in humans.

CONCEPTUAL MODELS

The use of overarching conceptual models is not common in basic and applied science research. However, a model relating to alterations in function and their relation to the atrophic process has been previously discussed. The first model of this kind in relation to skeletal muscle atrophy was originally published by Kasper.[8] At the core of this model is the notion that the daily average frequency and magnitude of mechanical loading of skeletal muscle produces a set point to which altered levels of function are compared. Skeletal muscle function depends on intact proprioceptive activity, motor innervation, mechanical load, and mobility of joints. If one of these factors is altered, then the muscle adapts to a new functional set point, which depends on its mean daily level of activity. Therefore diminished contractile activity produced by altered ADLs directly triggers adaptation of the rate and magnitude of protein degradation in addition to limiting protein synthesis.

SELECTED RESEARCH

The promotion of mobility and maintenance of self-care activities has been recognized as one of the primary foci of nursing care. Skeletal muscle wasting has been a widely observed phenomenon in response to illness, decreased ADLs, and immobilization and bed rest. A better understanding of the process of skeletal muscle atrophy can serve as a substantive foundation for the development and testing of new approaches to the promotion of mobility. Therefore selected research in the area of skeletal muscle atrophy will be reviewed in this section.

Decreased motion (hypokinesia) and decreased weight-bearing (hypodynamia) have been implicated as causes of pathological conditions in nearly every mammalian organ system. Hypokinesia and hypodynamia cause skeletal muscle atrophy, increased fatigability, alterations in skeletal muscle contraction time, loss of plasma and blood volumes, orthostatic hypotension, and pulmonary atelectasis.[104,152-154] After prolonged hypokinesia or hypodynamia, subjects have an impaired functional capacity and a reduced ability to perform their normal daily activities.[154]

Skeletal muscle atrophy is manifested by the exponential loss of muscle mass, over time, caused by a decrease of the number of myofibrils in parallel, the number of fibers per muscle, and muscle cell (fiber) diameter as documented in rat skeletal muscle following hypokinesia.[155,156] Skeletal muscles with predominantly slowly contracting oxidative fibers (type I), such as the soleus, have been reported to atrophy to a greater extent than those with a high proportion of fast-contracting (type II) fibers.[157] Mussachia et al[70] reported losses of 35% in soleus mass by 1 week and 45% by 1 week of hypokinetic suspension, whereas in the predominantly type II plantaris muscle, suspension restraint induced a 22% loss of mass after 7 days. In both types of muscles, the onset of atrophy is rapid.

Disuse or nonneurogenic atrophy is commonly produced in a variety of experimental protocols, such as tenotomy and limb immobilization. Unlike tenotomy, limb immobilization allows the muscle to be fixed at resting length or other specified lengths. Resting length is the length of choice as it is less likely to produce contracture and maintains the normal passive load placed on the muscle throughout its tendons and skeletal attachments. Previous investigations immobilized the hindlimbs in bilateral casts at less than resting lengths,[158,159] or by rigidly fixing the joints by pinning.[160] These models are clinically appropriate for determining changes in immobile subjects, but not for the general case of a mobile subject whose level of activity and weight-bearing has been compromised by hypokinesia or hypodynamia.

Animal models of inactivity, such as hindlimb suspension, are important in the study of disuse atrophy, because they closely resemble the degree of movement and lack of weight-bearing that persons subjected to periods of bed rest and restricted activity experience.[161,162] Furthermore, these models allow one to study fiber type distribution in atrophied muscle in a manner that is impossible in humans. A number of suspension models have been employed to simulate an environment of weightlessness.[160,162] Most recently, a modification of Morey's model was introduced to examine the effects of hindlimb suspension on bone fracture healing.[163]

Slow-twitch fibers, predominant in the soleus and postural muscles, are recruited first during weight-bearing and have a tonic activity pattern that may be very sensitive to changes in their contraction frequency.[117,163,164] The functional weight-bearing role of these muscles is therefore significantly altered during suspension. Muscle mass rapidly declined during the first 7 days of suspension, continuing at a more gradual rate through the twenty-eighth day. This reflected an early atrophic response caused by a more rapid rate of protein degradation and to a simultaneous decrease in protein synthesis. [117,163,164] Previous studies of hindlimb suspension and bed rest have shown that loss of muscle mass is associated with the development of a negative nitrogen balance, attributed to muscle protein catabolism.[165]

Changes in muscle mass give an estimate of the atrophic response of a particular muscle; however, the degree of fiber atrophy may be concealed to some extent by edema.[166] Therefore measurement of fiber cross-sectional area is considered a more accurate procedure to identify the response of skeletal muscle to hypokinesia and/or hypodynamia.[166] During inactivity, there is a marked decrease in type I mean cross-sectional area in contrast to type IIA fibers where the cross-sectional area was maintained. Selective atrophy of soleus muscle type I fiber during a period of decreased activity is consistent in all previous reports using both bed rest and immobilization models.[40,54,167] If the sample areas randomly chosen for analysis of fiber size and muscle composition are representative of the entire cross-sectional area, then the changes in muscle composition produced by hindlimb suspension would seem to be similar although not as profound as seen with immobilization. Booth and Kelso,[168] using the myosin ATPase technique, observed a significant reduction in the percentage of fibers staining as slow-twitch fibers in muscles of immobilized hindlimbs. However, using fiber diameter as an estimate of fiber area, the postural muscle exhibits a type I selective atrophy in the soleus muscle, which is manifested as a progressive decrease in individual fiber cross-sectional area, and corresponding to the observed decrease in muscle mass during suspension.

Mild exercise or weight-bearing during the first 14 days of recovery from hypokinesia in rats produced skeletal muscle damage which appeared in the form of necrosis, the presence of phagocytosis and central nuclei, and fiber debris in the intrafascicular and interfibrillar spaces in postural muscles.[66,87] The cause of exercise induced muscle damage during recovery from hypokinesia is not known, although it most likely involves movement associated with exercise and an altered ability of the muscle fibers to bear the mechanical stress of external loads (weight-bearing). The functional load or tension per unit area required to maintain weight-bearing or exercise may exceed the reduced force generating capacity of the atrophied muscle and may result in reuse injury. However, cellular defects such as sarcomere length nonuniformities, dissociation of Z-lines, loss of mitochondria, accumulation of redundant basement membrane, relative increases in the surface areas of the membrane systems (sarcoplasmic reticulum and T system), and evidence of secondary lysosomes are also possible contributing factors.[169]

With regard to the latter possibilities, the relationship of tension that a muscle can produce in response to a given level of calcium ion (tension-pCa relationship) in normal muscle is altered at long sarcomere lengths (3.00 to 3.25 μm), such that the development of tension at low Ca^{2+} concentrations is increased. This provides structural stability during submaximal activations with Ca^{2+}, since weaker sarcomeres will be stretched by stronger sarcomeres to a sarcomere length at which tension generating capacity matches the functional load. Progressive alterations in the tension-pCa relation as a function of sarcomere length could lead to longitudinal instability and eventually to muscle damage as a result of increased tension generating capabilities along the fibers. For example, atrophy may alter the strength of Ca^{2+} binding to the low affinity sites on troponin C (TnC) in skeletal muscle during force generation, resulting in damage of fibers even when normal weight-bearing does not load the muscle beyond its capacity to generate force as estimated by cross-sectional area. The underlying interaction between the tension-pCa relationship of individual fibers and atrophic damage has not been explored, particularly with regard to the time course of the development and the reversal of cellular contractile defects in the major types of skeletal muscle fibers (type I, IIA, IIB).

Loss of strength and mass in the lower extremities following inactivity, bed rest, and immobility can be severe in the human. The observation that 2.5 hours of daily cycling exercise in the patient on bed rest does not adequately prevent skeletal muscle atrophy is a significant finding.[17] Loss of strength in the lower limbs is twice that of the arms during maximal voluntary isometric exercise.[18] The relationships between skeletal muscle atrophy and strength studies were done to examine force development following bed rest.[170] It was found that 30 days of inactivity significantly decreased the force output of the knee extensors of the leg, but not the knee flexors.[170] Significant decreases in total cross-sectional area of the thigh and lower leg were found and did account for the total loss of strength. However, skeletal atrophy was not the sole source of the loss of strength as the type or speed of the muscle action did not affect these changes.

Further research is needed to compare these findings from normal populations to human patient populations. As previous work has demonstrated, drug therapy and pathology may influence the mechanisms of atrophy. It may be hypothesized that the addition of the circumstances of the clinical environment may have an additional deleterious effect on the progression of patient populations.

CASE STUDY

GG, a 34-year-old accountant, had been an avid walker all of his adult life. Mr. G was hospitalized for repair of the right patella resulting from chronic chondromalacia. Before admission, the patient's daily activity was gradually decreased over a 4-week period because of knee pain. At the time of admission, Mr. G was unable to walk further than 50 feet at 10 meters/min. Following surgical repair, Mr. G commented that he was fearful of losing his ability to exercise and walk long distances as he experienced weakness, fatigue, and orthostatic hypotension when ambulating in the unit.

Following surgical repair, physical assessment revealed an increased heart rate when standing, decreased range of motion in the affected limb, and decreased force production in both legs as measured by an isokinetic dynamometer. Further studies revealed an increased hematocrit and dehydration. MRI and measurements of calf size revealed a 30% decrease in the size of the major weight-bearing muscle groups of the right leg, the gastrocnemius, soleus, extensor digitorum longus, and the plantaris.

A gradual program of increased exercise was devised for Mr. G. During the first 2 weeks: walk 100 feet at a pace of 10 m/min, rest, and repeat 3 to 4 times per day. While in bed, do bed exercises of gently rolling from side to side and lower extremity extension. Week 3: walk 100 feet at 15 m/min, rest, repeat 5 to 6 times. Week 4: walk 100 feet at 20 m/min, rest, repeat 5 to 6 times. Do bed exercises as above plus supine on elbows and unilateral straight leg raising. Also during the recovery period, Mr. G was instructed to sit in a chair as much as possible and do as many self-care tasks as was possible.

Mr. G recovered normal hematocrit and heart rate by week 4 and no longer experienced orthostatic hypotension. Functional strength sufficient for the conduct of ADLs was also recovered by week 4. Measurement of his lower extremities revealed the return of normal skeletal muscle mass. However, Mr. G required another 4 weeks of gradual increased activity and walking to return to his prior level of rapid daily walking. At week 5, he began a program of walking ¼ mile per day and ascending two flights of stairs. Weeks 6 and 7: walk ½ to 1 mile per day and ascend three flights of stairs. Ultimately, additional mileage and stair climbing were incorporated into his exercise program.

To design an appropriate individualized exercise recovery program, a detailed physical assessment is required. This assessment should evaluate the patient's strength, level of fatigue, range of motion deficits; and activities that cause pain, balance and gait difficulties. The nurse should observe if the assessment is causing fatigue for the patient. The plan should be structured to incorporate the individuals prior work history, leisure activities, and his perception of the activities that he is capable of performing. It is also important to determine how long the individual has participated in favorite activities without fatigue. All of this information provides a sound basis for nursing diagnosis and prescription of appropriate activities.

QUESTIONS FOR FUTURE STUDY

The vast majority of the research on disuse atrophy has been centered on the effects of total immobility or weightlessness. Given that the majority of patients are not totally immobile or recovering from long duration space flight, nursing research is needed to focus on the effects of decreased activities of daily living in patient populations specifically in relation to skeletal muscle atrophy, cardiovascular alterations, and physiological fatigue. Atrophy in the patient population is gradual and not as apparent as that seen in healthy individuals. Current clinical therapy is based on research done by the disciplines of kinesiology and sports medicine. Subjects in these studies are typically healthy athletic college males and the research is focused on increasing human performance in relation to sports.

The measurement of exercise capacity or maximal oxygen uptake is based on a person's ability to cycle on a bicycle ergometer or run on a treadmill. The ability to evaluate this parameter is based on a person's mobility and exercise ability. To date only one study has examined these parameters in a debilitated population—burned patients.[171] Therefore basic and applied research is needed to develop quantitative measures of exercise capacity in patient populations.

In addition, the effects of disuse atrophy need to be examined across the life span. Preliminary research has clearly demonstrated that the effects of restricted mobility on normal neonates and geriatric populations are vastly different. It is important for nurses to determine how the addition of a pathological condition to the adaptive process of atrophy affects patient outcomes.

The rate and magnitude of recovery from atrophy has only been briefly examined in animal and human populations. Further studies are needed to determine the rates of skeletal muscle recovery from atrophy that can be expected in various patient populations. Additionally, there are few data as to the ability of the systems to recover without permanent or irreversible damage. Current research has been based on designs that measure the effects of a single acute occurrence of hypokinesia. The chronically ill are often subjected to repeated bouts of hypokinesia. Research designs should incorporate cyclical bouts of hypokinesia to mimic chronic populations. These studies are imperative before the initiation of work to determine the most effective methods of exercise prevention before disuse occurs and those that are necessary to promote recovery.

Teach us to live that we may dread
Unnecessary time in bed.
Get people up and we may save
Our patients from an early grave.[172]

REFERENCES

1. Ferrucci, L., Harris, T.B., Guralnik, J.M., Tracy, R.P., Corti, M.C., Cohen, H.J., et al. (1999). Serum IL-6 level and the development of disability in older persons. *Journal of the American Geriatric Society 47*(6), 639-646.
2. Fell, R.D., Gladden, L.B., Steffen, J.M., & Mussachia, X.J. (1985). Fatigue and contraction of slow and fast muscle in hypokinetic/hypodynamic rats. *Journal of Applied Physiology 58*(1), 65-69.
3. Burke, R.E., & Edgerton, V.R. (1975). Motor unit properties and selective involvement in movement. In Tepjung, R.L. (ed.), *Exercise and sport science reviews* (pp. 31-81). New York: Academic Press.
4. Finol, H.J., Lewis, D.M., & Owens, R. (1981). The effects of denervation on contractile properties of rat skeletal muscle. *Journal of Physiology 319*, 82-92.
5. Fischbach, G.D., & Robbins, N. (1969).Changes in contractile properties of disused soleus muscles. *Journal of Physiology 201*(2), 305-320.
6. Salvatori, S., Damiani, E., Zorzato, F., Volpe, P., Pierobon, S., Quaglino, D., et al. (1989). Denervation-induced proliferative changes of triads in rabbit skeletal muscle. *Muscle & Nerve 11*, 1246-1259.
7. Boyes, G., & Johnston, I. (1979). Muscle fibre composition of rat vastus intermedius following immobilisation at different muscle lengths. *Pflugers Archiv 381*(3), 195-200.
8. Kasper, C.E. (1990). *Antecedent condition: Impaired physical mobility (disuse syndrome)*. In *Altered Functioning: Impairment and Disability.* Cincinnatti, Ohio: Sigma Theta Tau.
9. Booth, F.W., & Seider, M.J. (1979). Early change in skeletal muscle protein synthesis after limb immobilization of rats. *Journal of Applied Physiology: Respiratory, Environmental, and Exercise Physiology 47*(5), 974-977.
10. Tucker, K.R., Seider, M.J., & Booth, F.W. (1981). Protein synthesis rates in atrophied gastrocnemius muscles after limb immobilization. *Journal of Applied Physiology: Respiratory, Environmental, and Exercise Physiology 51*(1), 73-77.
11. Cardasis, C.A. (1983). Ultrastructural evidence of continued reorganization at the aging (11-26 months) rat soleus neuromusclar junction. *Anatomical Record 207*, 399-415.
12. Booth, F.W. (1977). Time course of muscular atrophy during immobilization of hindlimbs in rats, *Journal of Applied Physiology 43*(4), 656-661.
13. Statistics: National Center for Farmworker Health. (1989). *Vital and health statistics: National Hospital Discharge Survey: Annual summary.* Washington, D.C.: U.S. Department of Health and Human Services.
14. Dock, W. (1944). The evil sequelae of complete bedrest. *Journal of the American Medical Association 125*, 1083-1085.
15. Harrison, T.R. (1944). Abuse of rest as a therapeutic measure for patient with cardiovascular disease. *Journal of the American Medical Association 125*(16), 1075-1077.
16. Allen, C., Glasziou, P., & Del Mar, C. (1999). Bed rest: A potentially harmful treatment needing more careful evaluation. *Lancet 354*, 1229-1233.

17. Graham, S.C., Roy, R.R., West, S.P., et al. (1989). Exercise effects on the size and metabolic properties of soleus fibers in hindlimb-suspended rats. *Aviation, Space, and Environmental Medicine 60,* 226-234.
18. Greenleaf., J.E. (1982). Physiological consequences of reduced physical activity during bed rest. In Terjung, R.L. (ed.), *Exercise and sports sciences reviews* (Vol. 10, pp. 84-119). Philadelphia: Franklin.
19. Issekutz, B., Blizzard, J.J., Birkhead, N.C., & Rodahl, K. (1966). Effect of prolonged bed rest on urinary calcium output. *Journal of Applied Physiology 21,* 1013-1020.
20. Cannon, J.G., Fielding, R.A., Fiatrone, M.A., Orencole, S.F., Dinarello, C.A., & Evans W. J. (1989). Increased interleukin 1 beta in human skeletal muscle after exercise. *American Journal of Physiology 257*(2 Pt 2), R451-455.
21. Mock, V., Dow, K., Meares, C., Grimm, P.M., Dienemann, J.A., Haisfield-Wolfe, M.E., et al. (1997). Effects of exercise on fatigue, physical functioning, and emotional distress during radiation therapy for breast cancer. *Oncology Nursing Forum 24*(6), 991-1000.
22. Buchanan, P., & Convertino, V.A. (1989). A study of the effects of prolonged simulated microgravity on the musculature of the lower extremities in man: An introduction. *Aviation, Space, and Environmental Medicine 60,* 649-652.
23. Convertino, V.A., Doerr, D.F., Mathes, K.L., Stein, S.L., & Buchanan, P. (1989). Changes in volume, muscle compartment, and compliance of the lower extremities in man following 30 days of exposure to simulated microgravity. *Aviation, Space, and Environmental Medicine 60,* 653-658.
24. Droge,W., & Holm, E. (1997). Role of cysteine and glutathione in HIV infection and other diseases associated with muscle wasting and immunological dysfunction. *FASEB Journal 11*(13), 1077-1089.
25. Mastaglia, F.L. (1982). Adverse effect of drugs on muscle. *Drugs 24,* 304-321.
26. Müller, R., & Kugelberg, E. (1959). Myopathy in Cushing's syndrome. *Journal of Neurology, Neurosurgery, and Psychiatry 22,* 314-317.
27. Silva, M., Skolnik, P.R., Gorbach, S.L., Spiegelman, D., Wilson, I.B., Fernandez-DiFranco, M.G., et al. (1998). The effect of protease inhibitors on weight and body composition in HIV-infected patients. *AIDS 12*(13), 1645-1651.
28. Grinspoon, S., Corcoran, C., Rosenthal, D., Stanley, T., Parlman, K., Costello, M., et al. (1999). Quantitative assessment of cross-sectional muscle area, functional status, and muscle strength in men with the acquired immunodeficiency syndrome wasting syndrome. *Journal of Clinical Endocrinology and Metabolism 84*(1), 201-206.
29. Kumar, N., Khwaja, G.A., Gupta, M., & Sharma, S. (1993). Antiepileptic drug induced osteomalacic myopathy with hyperparathyroidism and nephrolithiasis. *Journal of the Association of Physicians of India 41*(11), 748-749.
30. Wright, R.A., O'Duffy, J.D., & Rodriguez, M. (1999). Improvement of myelopathy in Sjogren's syndrome with chlorambucil and prednisone therapy. *Neurology 52*(2), 386-388.
31. Ruff, R.L., Martyn, D., & Gordon, A.M. (1982). Glucocorticoid-induced atrophy is not due to impaired excitability of rat muscle. *American Journal of Physiology 243,* E512-E521.
32. Askari, A.P., Vignos, P.J., & Moskowitz, R.W. (1976). Steroid myopathy in connective tissue disease. *American Journal of Medicine 61,* 485-492.
33. Kelly, F.J., & Goldspink, D.F. (1982). The differing responses of four muscle types to dexamethasone treatment in the rat. *Biochemistry Journal 208,* 147-158.
34. Birkhead, N.C., Haupt, G.J., Issekutz, B.J., et al. (1966). *Effect of exercise, standing, negative trunk and positive skeletal pressure on bedrest-induced orthostasis and hypercalciuria.* Wright-Patterson Air Force Base, Aerospace Medical Research Laboratories.
35. LaManca, J.J., Sisto, S.A., Zhou, X.D., et al. (1999). Immunological response in chronic fatigue syndrome following a graded exercise test to exhaustion. *Journal of Clinical Immunology 19*(2), 135-142.
36. Vojdani, A., & Lapp, C.W. (1999). Interferon-induced proteins are elevated in blood samples of patients with chemically or virally induced chronic fatigue syndrome. *Immunopharmacology and Immunotoxicology 21*(2), 175-202.
37. Khaleeli, A.A., Edwards, R.H.T., Gohil, K., et al. (1983). Corticosteroid myopathy: A clinical and pathological study. *Clinical Endocrinology 18,* 155-161.
38. Pleasure, D.E., Walsh, G.O., & Engel, W.K. (1970). At atrophy of skeletal muscle in patients with Cushing's syndrome. *Archives of Neurology 22,* 18-125.
39. Horber, F.F., Hoppeler, H., Herren, D., Claassen, H., Howald, H., Gerber, C., et al. (1986). Altered skeletal muscle ultrastucture in renal transplant patients on prednisone. *Kidney International 30,* 411-416.
40. Jaspers, S.R., & Tischler, M.E. (1984). Atrophy and growth failure of rat hindlimb muscles in tail-cast suspension. *Journal of Applied Physiology 57*(5), 1472-1479.
41. McCully, K.K., & Faulkner, J.A. (1986). Characteristics of lengthening contractions associated with injury to skeletal muscle fibers. *Journal of Applied Physiology 61*(1), 293-299.
42. Williams, P.E., & Goldspink, G. (1973). The effect of immobilization on the longitudinal growth of striated muscle fibers. *Journal of Anatomy 116*(1), 45-55.
43. Adler, M., Hinman, D., & Dudson, C.S. (1992). Role of muscle fasciculation in the generation of myopathies in Mammalian. *29,* 179-187.
44. Vejsada, R., Palecek, J., Hnik, P., & Soukup, T. (1985). Postnatal development of conduction velocity and fibre size in the rat tibial nerve. *International Journal of Developmental Neuroscience 3*(5), 583-595.
45. Krasnoff, J., & Painter, P. (1999). The physiological consequences of bed rest and inactivity. *Advances in Renal Replacement Therapy 6*(2), 124-132.
46. Brown, M.C., Jansen, J.K.S., & van Essen, D.C. (1976). Polyneural innervation of skeletal muscle in new-born rats and its elimination during maturation. *Journal of Physiology 261,* 387-422.
47. van Essen, D.C. (1982). Neuromuscular synapse elimination. In Spitzer, N.C. (ed.), *Neuronal development,* New York: Plenum.
48. Meeuwsen, I.B., Samson, M.M., & Verhaar, H.J. (2000). Evaluation of the applicability of HRT as a preservative of muscle strength in women. *Maturitas 36*(1), 49-61.
49. Borkan, G.A., Hults, D.E., & Gerzof, S.G. (1983). Age changes in body composition revealed by computed tomography. *Journal of Gerontology 38,* 673-677.
50. Larson, L. (1978). Morphological and functional characteristics of ageing skeletal muscle in man. *Acta Physiologica Scandinavica* (Suppl)(457), 463-466.
51. Larson, L., Grimby, G., & Karlsson, J. (1979). Muscle strength and speed of movement in relation to age and muscle morphology. *Journal of Applied Physiology 46*(3), 451-456.

52. Kuta, I., Parizkova, J., & Dycka, J. (1970). Muscle strength and lean body mass in old men of different physical activity. *Journal of Applied Physiology 29*(2), 168-171.
53. Fisher, J.S., & Brown, M. (1998). Immobilization effects on contractile properties of aging rat skeletal muscle. *Aging 10*(1), 59-66.
54. Brown, M., & Hasser, E.M. (1996). Differential effects of reduced muscle use (hindlimb unweighting) on skeletal muscle with aging. *Aging 8*(2), 99-105.
55. Brown, M., & Hasser, E.M. (1996). Complexity of age-related change in skeletal muscle. *Journals of Gerontology, Series A: Biological Science and Medical Science 51*(2), B117-123.
56. Mauro, A. (1961). Satellite cell of skeletal muscle fibers. *Journal of Biophysics, Biochemistry, and Cytology 9,* 493-498.
57. Gibson, M.C., & Schultz, E. (1983). Age-related differences in absolute numbers of skeletal muscle satellite cells. *Muscle & Nerve 6,* 574-580.
58. Handel, S.E., Wang, S., Greaser, M.L., Schultz, E., Bulinski, J.C., & Lessard, J.L. (1989). Skeletal muscle myofibrillogenesis as revealed with a monoclonal antibody to titin in combination with detection of the alpha- and gamma-isoforms of actin. *Developmental Biology 132,* 35-44.
59. Schultz, E., & Lipton, B.H. (1982). Skeletal muscle satellite cells: Changes in proliferation potential as a function of age. *Mechanisms of Ageing and Development 20,* 377-383.
60. Chakravarthy, M.V., Davis, B.S., & Booth, F.W. (2000). IGF-I restores satellite cell proliferative potential in immobilized old skeletal muscle. *Journal of Applied Physiology 89*(4), 1365-1379.
61. Roth, S.M., Martel, G.F., Ivey, F.M., Lemmer, J.T., Tracy, B.L., Hurlbut, D.E., et al. (1999). Ultrastructural muscle damage in young vs. older men after high-volume, heavy-resistance strength training. *Journal of Applied Physiology 86*(6), 1833-1840.
62. Metter, E.J., Lynch, N., Conwit, R., Lindle, R., Tobin, J., & Hurley, B. (1999). Muscle quality and age: Cross-sectional and longitudinal comparisons. *Journal of Gerontology, Series A: Biological Science and Medical Science 54*(5), B207-218.
63. Booth, F.W., Tseng, B.S., & Fluck, M. (1998). Molecular and cellular adaptation of muscle in response to physical training. *Acta Physiologica Scandinavica 162(*3), 343-350.
64. Gamrin, L., Berg, H.E., & Essen, P. (1998). The effect of unloading on protein synthesis in human skeletal muscle. *Acta Physiologica Scandinavica 163*(4), 369-377.
65. Fitts, R.H., Widrick, J.J., & Romatowski, J.G. (1994). Effect of limb immobilization on single muscle fiber contractile function. *FASEB J, 8*(4), A10.
66. Kasper, C.E., McNulty, A.L., Otto, A.J., & Thomas, D.P. (1993). Alterations in skeletal muscle related to impaired physical mobility: An empirical model. *Research in Nursing & Health 16*(4), 265-273.
67. Zemkova, H., Teisinger, J., Almon, R.R., Vejsada, R., Hnik, P., & Vyskocil, F. (1990). Immobilization atrophy and membrane properties in rat skeletal muscle fibres. *European Journal of Physiology 416,* 126-129.
68. Kondo, H., Miura, M., & Itokawa, Y. (1991). Oxidative stress in skeletal muscle atrophied by immobilization. *Acta Physiologica Scandinavica 142,* 527-528.
69. Feller, D.D., Ginoza, H.S., & Morey, E.E. (1981). Atrophy of rat skeletal muscles in simulated weightlessness. *Physiologist 24*(Suppl), S9-S10.
70. Musacchia, X.J., Steffan, J.M., & Deavers, D.R. (1981). Suspension restraint: Induced hyokinesia and antiorthostasis as a simulation of weightlessness. *Physiology 24*(6 Suppl), S21-S22.
71. Herbison, G.J., Jaweed, M.M., & Ditunno, J.F. (1978). Muscle fiber atrophy after cast immobilization in the rat. *Archives of Physical Medicine and Rehabilitation 59,* 301-305.
72. Booth, F.W. (1987). Physiologic and biochemical effects of immobilization on muscle. *Clinical Orthopedics 219,* 15-20.
73. Lindboe, C.F., & Platou, C.S. (1984). Effect of immobilization of short duration on the muscle fiber size. *Clinical Physiology 4,* 183.
74. Schimke, R.T. (1975). Methods for analysis of enzyme synthesis and degradation in animal tissues. *Methods* in *Enzymology 40,* 241.
75. Watson, P.A., Stein, J.P., & Booth, F.W. (1984). Changes in actin synthesis and alpha-actin-mRNA content in rat muscle during immobilization. *American Journal of Physiology 247*(1 Pt 1), C39-44.
76. Jagus, R., & Safer, B. (1981). Activity of eukaryotic initiation factor 2 is modified by processess distinct from phosphorylation. *Journal of Biochemistry 256,* 1317-1323.
77. Nicks, D.K., Beneke, W.M., Key, R.M., & Timson, B.F. (1989). Muscle fibre size and number following immobilization atrophy. *Journal of Anatomy 163,* 1-5.
78. Hainaut, K., & Duchateau, J. (1989). Muscle fatigue, effects of training and disuse. *Muscle & Nerve 12,* 660-669.
79. Vandenborne, K., Elliott, M.A., & Walter, G.A. (1998). Longitudinal study of skeletal muscle adaptations during immobilization and rehabilitation. *Muscle & Nerve 21*(8), 1006-1012.
80. Gupta, R.C., Misulis, K.E., & Dettbarn, W.D. (1989). Activity dependent characteristics of fast and slow muscle: Biochemical and histochemical considerations. *Neurochemical Research 14*(7), 647-655.
81. Marsh, D.R., Campbell, C.B., & Spriet, L.L. (1992). Effect of hindlimb unweighting on anaerobic metabolism in rat skeletal muscle. *Journal of Applied Physiology 72*(4), 1304-1310.
82. Berg, H.E., Dudley, G.A. Hather, B., Tesch, A. (1993). Work capacity and metabolic and morphologic characteristics of the human quadriceps muscle in response to unloading. *Clinical Physiology 13,* 337-347.
83. Duchateau, J. (1995). Bed rest induces neural and contractile adaptations in triceps surae. *Medicine and Science in Sports and Exercise 27,* 1581-1589.
84. Martin T.P., Stein, R.B., Hoeppner, P.H,. Reid, D.C. (1992). Influence of electrical stimulation on the morphological and metabolic properties of paralyzed muscle. *Journal of Applied Physiology 72*(4), 1401-1406.
85. McColl, R.W., Fleckenstein, J.L., Bowers, J., Theriault, G., & Peshock, R.M. (1992). Three-dimensional reconstruction of skeletal muscle from MRI. *Computerized Medical Imaging and Graphics 16*(6), 363-371.
86. Reiser, P.J., Kasper, C.E., & Moss, R.L. (1987). Myosin subunits and contractile properties of single fibers from hypokinetic rat muscles. *Journal of Applied Physiology 63*(6), 2293-3000.
87. Kasper, C.E., White, T.P., & Maxwell, L.C. (1990). Running during recovery from hindlimb suspension induces transient muscle injury. *Journal of Applied Physiology 68*(2), 533-539.
88. Fielding, R.A., Manfredi, T.J., Ding, W., et al. (1993). Acute phase response in exercise III. Neutrophil and IL- accumulation in skeletal muscle. *American Journal of Physiology 265,* R166-R172.

89. Ploutz-Snyder, L., Tesch, P., Crittenden, D., et al. (1995). Effect of unweighting on skeletal muscle use during exercise. *Journal of Applied Physiology 79,* 168-175.
90. Ploutz-Snyder, L.L., Tesch, P.A., Hather, B.M., & Dudley, G.A. (1996). Vulnerability to dysfunction and muscle injury after unloading. *Archives of Physical and Medical Rehabilitation 77*(8), 773-777.
91. Clarkson, P.M., & Sayers, S.P. (1999). Etiology of exercise-induced muscle damage. *Canadian Journal of Applied Physiology 24*(3), 234-248.
92. McCully, K.K. (1986). Exercise-induced injury to skeletal muscle. *Federation Proceedings 45*(13), 2933-2936.
93. Stauber, W.T. (1989). *Eccentric action of muscles: Physiology, injury, and adaptation.* In Pandolf, K.B. (ed.), *Exercise and sport sciences reviews* (pp. 157-185). Baltimore: Williams & Wilkins.
94. Vissing, J., Ohkuwa, T., Ploug, T., & Galbo, H. (1988). Effect of prior immobilization on muscular glucose clearance in resting and running rats. *American Journal of Physiology 255*(EM18), E456-E462.
95. Lutwak, L., & Whedon, G.D. (1959). The effect of physical conditioning on glucose tolerance. *Clinical Research 7,* 143-144.
96. Lipman, R.L., Raskin, P., Love, T., Triebwasser, J., Lecocq, F.R., & Schnure, J.J. (1972). Glucose intolerance during decreased physical activity in man. *Diabetes 21,* 101.
97. Seider, M.J., Nicholson, W.F., & Booth, F.W. (1982). Insulin resistance for glucose metabolism in disused soleus muscle of mice. *American Journal of Physiology 242*(1), E12-18.
98. Tischler, M.E., Satarug, S., Eisenfeld, S.H., Henriksen, E.J., & Rosenberg, S.B. (1990). Insulin effects in denervated and non-weightbearing rat soleus muscle. *Muscle & Nerve 13,* 593-600.
99. Chew, H.G., Jr., & Segal, S.S. (1997). Arterial morphology and blood volumes of rats following 10-14 weeks of tail suspension. *Medicine and Science in Sports and Exercise 29*(10), 1304-1310.
100. Saltin, B., Blomqvist, G., Mitchell, J.H., Johnson, R.L., Jr, Wildenthal, K., & Chapman, C.B. (1968). Response to exercise after bed rest and after training. *Circulation 33*(5), VIIl-60.
101. Convertino, V.A., Bloomfield, S.A., & Greenleaf, J.E. (1997). An overview of the issues: Physiological effects of bed rest and restricted physical activity. *Medicine and Science in Sports and Exercise 29*(2), 187-190.
102. Greenleaf, J.E. (1984). Physiology of fluid and electrolyte responses during inactivity: Water immersion and bed rest. *Medicine and Science in Sports and Exercise 16*(1), 20-25.
103. Sandler, H., & Vernikos, J. (eds.). (1986). *Inactivity: Physiological effects* (pp. 1-8, 77-95). Orlando: Academic Press.
104. Sandler, H., Popp, R.L., & Harrison, D.C. (1988). The hemodynamic effects of repeated bed rest exposure. *Aviation, Space, and Environmental Medicine (59)* (11 pt 1), 1047-1054.
105. Greenleaf, J.E., Bernauer, E.M., & Juhos, L.T. (1977). Effects of exercise on fluid exchange and body compostion in man during 14-day bed rest. *Journal of Applied Physiology 43*(1), 126-132.
106. Greenleaf, J.E., Bernauer, E.M., Young, H.L., Morse, J.T., Staley, R.W., Juhos, L.T., et al. (1977). Fluid and electrolyte shifts during bed rest with isometric and isotonic exercise. *Journal of Applied Physiology 42,* 59-66.
107. Oberfield, R.A., Ebaugh, F.G., Jr., O'Hanlon, E.P., & Shoaf, M. (1968). Blood volume studies during and after immobilization in human subjects as measured by sodium radiochromate (chromium 51) technique. *Aerospace Medicine 39,* 10-13.
108. Parin, V.V. (1970). Principle changes in the healthy human body after 120 days bed confinement. In *Space, biology, and medicine.* Washington D.C.: National Aeronautics and Space Administration.
109. Allen, C., Glasziou, P., & Del Mar, C. (1999). Bed rest: A potentially harmful treatment needing more careful evaluation (see comments). *Lancet 354*(9186), 1229-1233.
110. Ferretti, G., Girardis, M., Moia, C., & Antonutto, G. (1998). Effects of prolonged bed rest on cardiovascular oxygen transport during submaximal exercise in humans. *European Journal of Applied Physiology 78*(5), 398-402.
111. Levine, B.D., Zuckerman, J.H., & Pawelczyk, V. (1997). Cardiac atrophy after bed-rest deconditioning: A nonneural mechanism for orthostatic intolerance. *Circulation 96*(2), 517-525.
112. Convertino, V.A. (1997). Cardiovascular consequences of bed rest: Effect on maximal oxygen uptake. *Medicine and Science in Sports and Exercise 29*(2), 191-196.
113. Convertino, V.A., Goldwater, D.J., & Sandler, H. (1986). Bedrest-induced peak VO_2 reduction associated with age, gender, and aerobic capacity. *Aviation, Space, and Environmental Medicine 57*(1), 17-22.
114. Gui, D., Tazza, L.G., Boldrini, G., Sganga, G., & Tramutola, G. (1982). Effects of supine versus sitting bedrest upon blood gas tensions, cardiac output, venous admixture and ventilation-perfusion ratio in man after upper abdominal surgery. *International Journal of Tissue Reaction 4*(1), 67-72.
115. Lutz, J., Chen, F., & Kasper, C.E. (1987). Hypokinesia-induced negative net calcium balance reversed by weight-bearing exercise. *Aviation, Space, and Environmental Medicine 58*(4), 308-314.
116. Dehority, W., Halloran, B.P., Bikle, D.D., Curren, T., Kostenuik, P.J., Wronski, T.J., et al. (1999). Bone and hormonal changes induced by skeletal unloading in the mature male rat. *American Journal of Physiology 276* (1 Pt 1), E62-69.
117. Kostenuik, P.J., Halloran, B.P., Morey-Holton, E.R., & Bikle, D.D. (1997). Skeletal unloading inhibits the in vitro proliferation and differentiation of rat osteoprogenitor cells. *American Journal of Physiology 273*(6 Pt 1), E1133-1139.
118. Evans, R.A., Bridgeman, M., Hills, E., & Dunstan, C.R. (1984). Immobilisation hypercalcemia. *Mineral and Electrolyte Metabolism 10,* 244-248.
119. Donaldson, C.L., Hulley, S.B., Vogel, J.M., Hattner, R.S., Bayers, J.H., & McMillan, D.E. (1970). Effect of prolonged bed rest on bone mineral. *Journal of Metabolism 19*(12), 1071-1084.
120. Babij, P., & Booth, F.W. (1988). Clenbuterol prevents or inhibits loss of specific mRNAs in atrophying rat skeletal muscle. *American Journal of Physiology 254*(5 Pt 1), C657-660.
121. Esser, K.A., & Hardeman, E.C. (1995). Changes in contractile protein mRNA accumulation in response to spaceflight. *American Journal of Physiology 268* (2 Pt 1), C466-471.
122. Booth, F.W., & Kirby, C.R. (1992). Changes in skeletal muscle gene expression consequent to altered weight bearing. *American Journal of Physiology 262*(3 Pt 2), R329-332.

123. Helliwell, T.R., Gunhan, O., & Edwards, R.H.T. (1989). Lectin binding and desmin expression during necrosis, regeneration, and neurogenic atrophy of human skeletal muscle. *Journal of Pathology 159,* 43-51.
124. Kasper, C.E., & Xun, L. (1996). Cytoplasm-to-myonucleus ratios following microgravity. *Journal of Muscle Research and Cell Motility 17*(5), 595-602.
125. Kasper, C.E., & Xun, L. (1996). Cytoplasm-to-myonucleus ratios in plantaris and soleus muscle fibres following hindlimb suspension. *Journal of Muscle Research and Cell Motility 17*(5), 603-610.
126. Criswell, D.S., Booth, F.W., DeMayo, F., Schwartz, R.J., Gordon, S.E., & Fiorotto, M.L. (1998). Overexpression of IGF-I in skeletal muscle of transgenic mice does not prevent unloading-induced atrophy. *American Journal of Physiology 275*(3 Pt 1), E373-379.
127. Alley, K.A., & Thompson, L.V. (1997). Influence of simulated bed rest and intermittent weight bearing on single skeletal muscle fiber function in aged rats. *Arch Phys Med Rehabil 78*(1), 19-25.
128. Ikai, M., & Fukunaga, T. (1968). Calculation of muscle strength per unit cross-sectional area of human muscle by means of ultrasonic measurement. *Int Z Angew Physiol 26*(1), 26-32.
129. Adolfsson, G. (1969). Circulatory and respiratory function in relation to physical activity in female patients before and after cholecystectomy. *Acta Chir Scand Suppl. 401,* 1-106.
130. Clarke, D.H. (1973). Adaptations in strength and muscular endurance resulting from exercise. *Exerc Sport Sci Rev 1,* 73-102.
131. Bandinelli, S., Benvenuti, E., Del Lungo, I., et al. (1999). Measuring muscular strength of the lower limbs by hand-held dynamometer: A standard protocol. *Aging (Milano) 11*(5), 287-293.
132. Lindle, R.S., Metter, E.J., Lynch, N.A., et al. (1997). Age and gender comparisons of muscle strength in 654 women and men aged 20-93 yr. *Journal of Applied Physiology 85*(5), 1581-1587.
133. McCully, K.K., Landsberg, L., Suarez, M., et al. (1997). Identification of peripheral vascular disease in elderly subjects using optical spectroscopy. *J Gerontol A Biol Sci Med Sci 52*(3), B159-B165.
134. Schutte, J.E., Longhurst, J.C., Gaffney, F.A., et al. (1981). Total plasma creatinine: an accurate measure of total striated muscle mass. *J Appl Physiol 51*(3), 762-766.
135. Bergh, U., Ekblom, B., & Astrand, P.O. (2000). Maximal oxygen uptake "classical" versus "contemporary" viewpoints [comment] [published erratum appears in *Med Sci Sports Exerc* 2000 Apr;32(4), 880]. *Med Sci Sports Exerc 32*(1), 85-88.
136. Astrand, I., & Astrand, P.O. (1978). Aerobic work performance,: A review. pp. 149-63. In: L.J. Folinsbee, et al., (eds.), *Environmental stress.* New York, Academic Press.
137. Wood, C.D., Glover, J., McCune, M., et al. (1989). The effect of intravenous nutrition on muscle mass and exercise capacity in perioperative patients. *Am J Surgery 158,* 63-67.
138. Winters, K.M., & Snow, C.M. (2000). Detraining reverses positive effects of exercise on the musculoskeletal system in premenopausal women. *J Bone Miner Res 15*(12), 2495-2503.
139. Heymsfield, S.B., Nunez, C., Testolin, C., & Gallagher, D. (2000). Anthropometry and methods of body composition measurement for research and field application in the elderly. *European Journal of Clinical Nutrition 54*(Suppl 3), S26-S32.
140. Simons-Morton, D.G., Hogan, P., Dunn, A.L., Pruitt, L., King, A.C., Levine, B.D., et al. (2000). Characteristics of inactive primary care patients: Baseline data from the activity counseling trial. *Preventive Medicine 31*(5), 513-521.
141. Bouchard, C. (1999). Physical inactivity. *Canadian Journal of Cardiology 15*(Suppl G), 89G-92G.
142. St. Pierre, D. (1987). The effects of immobilization and exercise on muscle function. *Physiotherapy Canada 39,* 24-36.
143. Vogt, F.B., & Johnson, P.C. (1967). Effectiveness of extremity cuffs or leotards in preventing or controlling the cardiovascular deconditioning of bedrest. *Aerospace Medicine 38,* 702-707.
144. Buchner, D.M. (1997). Preserving mobility in older adults. *Western Journal of Medicine 167*(4), 258-264.
145. Watenpaugh, D.E., Ballard, R.E., Schneider, S.M., & Hargans, A.R. (2000). Supine lower body negative pressure exercise during bed rest maintains upright exercise capacity. *Journal of Applied Physiology 89*(1), 218-227.
146. Iwasaki, K.I., Zhang, R., Zuckerman, J.H., Pawelczyk, J.A., & Levine, B.D. (2000). Effect of head-down-tilt bed rest and hypovolemia on dynamic regulation of heart rate and blood pressure. *American Journal of Physiology: Regulatory, Integrative, and Comparative Physiology 279*(6), R2189-R2199.
147. Friman, G. (1979). Effect of clinical bed rest for seven days on physical performance. *Acta Medica Scandinavica 205,* 389-393.
148. Kagaya, H., Sharma, M., Kobetic, R., & Marsolais, E.B. (1998). Ankle, knee, and hip moments during standing with and without joint contractures: Simulation study for functional electrical stimulation. *American Journal of Physical Medicine & Rehabilitation 77*(1), 49-66.
149. Endo, Y., Tabata, T., Kuroda, H., Tadano, T., Matsushima, K., & Watanabe, M. (1998). Induction of histidine decarboxylase in skeletal muscle in mice by electrical stimulation, prolonged walking and interleukin-1. *Journal of Physiology 509*(Pt. 2), 587-598.
150. Gaines, J.M., & Talbot, L.A. (1999). Isokinetic strength training in research and practice. *Biological Research in Nursing 1*(1), 57-64.
151. Oldham, J., & Howe, T. (1997). The effectiveness of placebo muscle stimulation in quadricaps muscle rehabilitation: A preliminary evaluation. *Clinical Effectiveness in Nursing 1,* 25-30.
152. Sandler, R.B., Burdett, R., Zaleskiewicz, M., Sprowls-Repcheck, C., & Harwell, M. (1991). Muscle strength as an indicator of the habitual level of physical activity. *Medicine and Science in Sports and Exercise 23*(12), 1375-1381.
153. Roberts, D., & Smith, D.J. (1989). Biochemical aspects of peripheral muscle fatigue: A review. *Sports Medicine 7,* 125-138.
154. Hung, J., Goldwater, D., Convertino, V.A., McKillop, J.H., Goris, M.L., & DeBusk, R.F. (1983). Mechanisms for decreased exercise capacity after bed rest in normal middle-aged men. *American Journal of Cardiology 51*(15), 344-348.
155. Faulkner, J.A., Niemeyer, J.H., Maxwell, L.C., & White, T.P. (1980). Contractile properties of transplanted extensor digitorum longus muscle of the cat. *Journal of Applied Physiology 238,* C120-C126.

156. Appell, H.J. (1986). Skeletal muscle atrophy during immobilization. *International Journal of Sports Medicine 7,* 1-5.
157. Booth, F.W., Seider, M.J., & Hugman, G.R. In Pette, D. (ed.), *Effects of disuse by limb immobilization on different muscle fiber types. Plasticity of muscle.* New York: Walter de Gruyter.
158. Holloszy, J.O., & Booth, F.W. (1976). Biochemical adaptations to endurance exercise in muscle. *Annual Review of Physiology 38,* 273-291.
159. Booth, F.W., & Kelso, J.R. (1972). Cytochrome oxidase of skeletal muscle: Adaptive response to chronic disuse. *Canadian Journal of Physiology Pharmacology 51,* 679-681.
160. Max, S.R. (1972). Disuse atrophy of skeletal muscle loss of functional activity of mitochondria. *Biochemi-cal and Biophysical Research Communications 46,* 1394-1398.
161. Shepard, R.J., Bouhlel, E., Vandewalle, H., et al. (1988). Muscle mass as a factor limiting physical work. *Journal of Applied Physiology 64*(4), 1472-1479.
162. Fitts, R.H., Metzger, J.M., Riley, D.A., & Unsworth, B.R. (1986). Models of disuse: A comparison of hindlimb suspension and immobilization. *Journal of Applied Physiology 60*(6), 1946-1953.
163. Morey-Holton, E.R., & Globus, R.K. (1998). Hindlimb unloading of growing rats: A model for predicting skeletal changes during space flight. *Bone 22*(5 Suppl), 83S-88S.
164. Globus, R.K., Bikle, D.D., & Morey-Holton, E. (1986). The temporal response to unloading. *Endocrinology, 118,* 733-742.
165. Musacchia, X.J., Steffen, J.M., & Deavers, D.R. (1983). Rat hindlimb muscle responses to suspension hypokinesia/hypodynamia. *Aviation, Space, and Environmental Medicine 54*(11), 1015-1020.
166. Maxwell, L.C., Hyatt, G.J., & Layman, D. (1974). Adaptation of growing skeletal muscle fibers to immobilization, tenotomy, and training. *Medicine and Science in Sport and Exercise 6,* 75.
167. Kasper, C.E., Maxwell, L.C., & White, T.P. (1996). Alterations in skeletal muscle related to short-term impaired physical mobility. *Research in Nursing & Health 19*(2), 133-142.
168. Booth, F.W., & Kelso, J.R. (1973). Effect of hind-limb immobilization on contractile and histochemical properties of skeletal muscle. *Pflügers Archiv 342,* 231-238.
169. Tidball, J.G. (1984). Myotendinous junction: Morphological changes and mechanical failure associated with muscle cell atrophy. *Experimental and Molecular Pathology 40,* 1-12.
170. Dudley, G.A., Duvoisin, M.R., Convertino, V.A., & Buchanan, P. (1989). Alterations of the in vivo torque-velocity relationship of human skeletal muscle following 30 days exposure to simulated microgravity. *Aviation, Space, and Environmental Medicine 60,* 659-663.
171. Black, S., Carter, G.M., Nitz, A.J., & Worthington, J.A. (1980). Oxygen consumption for lower extremity exercises in normal subjects and burned patients. *Physical Therapy 60*(10), 1255-1258.
172. Asher, R.A.J. (1947). The danger of going to bed. *British Medical Journal,* 967-968.

CHAPTER

21 Ischemia

CLAUDIA M. WEST & MICHELE M. PELTER

DEFINITION

Ischemia is the reversible cellular injury that occurs when tissue demand for oxygen exceeds the supply and when toxic metabolites accumulate. The imbalance in oxygen supply and demand is produced by a reduction or cessation of blood flow that results in tissue hypoxia, decreased energy substrate, and buildup of toxic metabolic wastes. These events result in identifiable derangements of cellular structure and function that are manifested by subsequent alterations in tissue function. Infarction is the inevitable outcome if perfusion is not reestablished in a timely fashion.[1,2]

The phenomenon of ischemia can be manifested in any or all tissues of the body, is caused by multiple conditions, and is seen frequently by nurses in all health care settings. Given this great breadth, myocardial ischemia is the prototype for examining the phenomenon of ischemia in most of this chapter. A more broad-based perspective on ischemia is presented in the section on mechanisms.

PREVALENCE AND POPULATIONS AT RISK

The prevalence of ischemia is hidden in the myriad diseases and conditions with which it is commonly associated, and it is difficult to estimate. Table 21-1 provides a comprehensive, although not exhaustive, list of the causes of ischemia and populations at risk. The prevalence of only those conditions related to myocardial ischemia is discussed here: coronary heart disease (CHD), angina, and myocardial infarction (MI). CHD is a clinical diagnosis of coronary atherosclerosis based on a patient's history and physical findings but before arteriographic confirmation of coronary artery disease (CAD). The term CHD is used in the early sections of the chapter to be consistent with how the epidemiologic literature reports diseases related to coronary atherosclerosis.

In 1998, an estimated 60.8 million Americans had one or more forms of cardiovascular disease, including 12.4 million with CHD. Of these, 6.4 million had angina pectoris and 7.3 million had MI.[3] The incidence of CHD in women lags behind that of men by 10 years and by 20 years for serious coronary events such as MI and death. Women after menopause have two to three times the incidence of CHD than women of the same age before menopause.[3]

Table 21-2 lists the age-adjusted (using 2000 standards) prevalence rates of CHD, MI, and angina pectoris by sex and race. The highest prevalence of CHD and MI is in the nonwhite ethnic groups, primarily in the men, although black women have the highest prevalence of CHD. These higher prevalence rates among nonwhite ethnic groups probably reflect poor access to and less effective health care and discrimination in allocation of health care resources.[4,5] The even higher prevalence of CHD in black women may reflect a higher prevalence of type 2 diabetes mellitus in black women than black men or whites.[6] In addition, black women with elevated lipoprotein (a) levels are at greater risk for CHD than black men and white women.[7]

The prevalence of CHD has increased with the increasing age of the population in this country. However, death rates from CHD have declined in all ethnic groups since 1965, although more so in white men than in white women and ethnic minorities.[8,9] This decline is attributable to modification of coronary risk factors, especially hypertension and dyslipidemia,[10,11] and improved medical treatment.[12,13] Despite this decline, CHD is the leading cause of death in the United States in both men and women, accounting for 459,841 deaths in 1998, or 1 out of every 5 deaths. Of these deaths, men accounted for 50.8% and women 49.2%.[3]

CHD is the leading cause of premature, permanent disability, accounting for 19% of all Social Security disability allowances. Two thirds of those who survive an MI do not return to their baseline health status, but 88% of those younger than 65 are able to return to their usual work.[3] In 2001, CHD cost $100.8 billion for hospital, physician and nursing care, medications, nursing home services, and

TABLE 21-1 Causes of Ischemia and Populations at Risk

CLINICAL STATES AND DIAGNOSES	POPULATION—PERSONS WHO EXPERIENCE
A. Decreased cardiac output (↓MAP)	
1. Hypovolemia	Motor vehicle or industrial accidents
	Burns
	Infants
	Elderly persons
2. Vasodilation	Gram-negative sepsis
	Primary infection with a gram-negative organism after instrumentation or surgery of the GU or GI tract
	Therapy with a potent vasodilator
3. Reduced pumping efficiency of the heart	Decreased left ventricular contractility due to
	Congenital valve disease or valve disease acquired from rheumatic fever, papillary muscle infarction, or bacterial endocarditis
	Myocardial infarction
	Ventricular septal defect
	Ventricular aneurysm
	Pericardial effusion and tamponade
	Supraventricular and ventricular arrhythmias
	Asystole
B. Increased vascular resistance	
1. Obstruction of blood vessels	
a. Atherosclerosis	Coronary heart disease and stroke
	Elderly persons
	Men older than 40, women after menopause
	Cigarette smoking
	Hyperlipidemia
	Hypertension
	Diabetes mellitus
	Family history of atherosclerosis
	Use of oral contraceptives and cigarette smoking and/or hypertension
	Obesity
	Sedentary lifestyle
	Negative affect
b. Thromboembolism	Increased blood viscosity
	Polycythemia
	Leukemia
	Severe hyperglycemia
	Dehydration
	Hypercoagulability
	Pregnancy, delivery, postpartum
	General anesthesia
	Immobility
	Estrogen replacement therapy
	Bacterial endocarditis
	Atrial fibrillation
	Sickle cell crisis
	DIC
	Septicemia
	Crush injury
	Transfusion reaction
	Burns
	Amniotic fluid embolism
	Placental abruption

TABLE 21-1 Causes of Ischemia and Populations at Risk—cont'd

CLINICAL STATES AND DIAGNOSES	POPULATION—PERSONS WHO EXPERIENCE
b. Thromboembolism (cont'd)	HELLP syndrome (severe preeclampsia)
	Air embolism
	Central venous or pulmonary artery catheter
	Mechanical ventilation with high peak airway pressure
	Fat embolism
	Long bone fractures
	Burns
	Contusion
	Childbirth
	Pump oxygenator
c. Vasospasm	Prinzmetal's angina
	Raynaud's disease and phenomenon
	Shock states
	Subarachnoid hemorrhage
	Cocaine use
d. Mechanical compression	Severe tissue edema
	Hypoproteinemia
	Lymphedema
	Cerebral edema
	Solid tumors
	Bedrest
	Decreased level of consciousness
	Elderly persons
	Fatigued
	Neuromuscular disability
	Surgical clamps
	Vascular bypass surgery
	Entrapment
	Thoracic outlet syndrome
	Compartment syndrome
c. Intraarterial catheters	Arterial pressure monitoring
2. Shunting of blood flow	
a. Decreased MAP	Major trauma with hemorrhage
	Large surgical blood loss
	Burns
	Septic shock
	Cardiogenic shock
	Dehydration
b. Increased metabolic demand	Vigorous aerobic exercise
	Mild to moderate exercise of a limb with atherosclerotic occlusive disease
c. AV anastomosis	Congenital
	Surgical
	Hemodialysis access
	Traumatic injury to blood vessels
3. Injury to blood vessels	Trauma or surgery
	Burns
	Leaking aneurysms
	Atherosclerosis
	Hypertension
	Vasculopathies
	Vasculitis
	HIV/AIDS

Continued

TABLE 21-1 Causes of Ischemia and Populations at Risk—cont'd

CLINICAL STATES AND DIAGNOSES	POPULATION—PERSONS WHO EXPERIENCE
4. Decreased capillary-tissue ratio	Severe tissue edema Lymphedema Hypoproteinemia Tissue hypertrophy Left ventricular hypertrophy

DIC, disseminated intravascular coagulation; *GI*, gastrointestinal; *GU*, genitourinary; *HELLP*, hemolysis, elevated liver enzymes, and low platelet count; *MAP*, mean arterial pressure.

lost productivity from disability and death.[3] In 1997, Medicare paid $10.8 billion to beneficiaries for CHD-related illnesses.

RISK FACTORS

Diseases and clinical states displayed in Table 21-1 are risk factors for ischemia.

Environmental Factors

Examples of environmental risk factors include traumatic injury, such as motor vehicle accidents, and instrumentation of the genitourinary tract (such as occurs with indwelling bladder catheterization and cystoscopy), which can increase the risk of gram-negative sepsis with resultant systemic vasodilation and reduced MAP.

Environmental tobacco smoke, or second-hand smoke, is a recently recognized risk factor for myocardial ischemia secondary to atherosclerosis.

TABLE 21-2 Prevalence of CHD, MI, and Angina Pectoris by Gender and Race

ETHNICITY	CHD (%)	MI (%)	ANGINA (%)
Non-Hispanic white men	6.9	5.2	2.6
Non-Hispanic white women	5.4	2	3.9
Non-Hispanic black men	7.1	4.3	3.1
Non-Hispanic black women	9	3.3	6.2
Mexican-American men	7.2	4.1	4.1
Mexican-American women	1.9	1.9	5.5

CHD, coronary heart disease; *MI*, myocardial infarction. Data from the National Health and Nutrition Evaluation Survey, Third Report (1988-1994) as cited in American Heart Association (AHA).[3]

The American Heart Association (AHA)[3] reported that 47% of nonsmoking working adults are exposed to second-hand smoke in their home or workplace. A recent meta-analysis[14] of 18 epidemiologic studies found a relative risk of CHD in nonsmokers exposed to second-hand smoke at home or in the workplace to be 1.25 (95% confidence interval [CI], 1.17-1.32; $p<0.001$) in all studies and 1.26 in the four studies that controlled for major CHD risk factors. There also was found to be a dose response relationship; as the duration or the level of exposure to second-hand smoke increased, the risk increased significantly.

Personal Factors

The classic personal risk factors for CHD are age older than 45 for men and postmenopausal status for women, family history of atherosclerosis, cigarette smoking, hypertension, elevated total cholesterol, elevated low-density lipoproteins (LDL), or reduced high-density lipoproteins (HDL).[3,15] A growing body of evidence indicates that elevated systolic blood pressure is more predictive of CHD, CHD deaths, and all cardiovascular deaths than elevated diastolic blood pressure.[16-18] The National High Blood Pressure Education Program of the National Heart, Lung, and Blood Institute issued an advisory statement[17] recommending that systolic blood pressure become the principal indicator for hypertension and effectiveness of treatment and that blood pressure be maintained less than 140/90 mm Hg and below 130/85 mm Hg in diabetics.

Total cholesterol levels of 240 mg/dL or higher are associated with a high risk of CHD.[3] In the third report of the National Cholesterol Education Program (Adult Treatment Panel), elevated low density lipoprotein cholesterol levels (LDL-C) continue as the primary target for identification and treatment. However, new categories of risk for graded intensities of treatment have been developed based on levels of LDL-C and the presence of other

CHD risk factors. The new classification of lipids and lipoproteins are (1) optimal LDL-C is less than 100 mg/dL, (2) an abnormal high-density lipoprotein cholesterol (HDL-C) level is less than 40 mg/dL (which was increased from 35 mg/dL in earlier guidelines), and (3) triglyceride values less than previously recommended, with moderate levels warranting earlier intervention.

The AHA recently declared diabetes mellitus an independent risk factor for CHD that is as important as cigarette smoking or hypertension as a cause of cardiovascular disease.[19] In fact, diabetes has a more profound effect on CHD mortality than does CHD alone.[19,20] The CHD mortality rate in women with diabetes is comparable to that of both diabetic and nondiabetic men. The relative risk of fatal CHD in diabetic women is 8.70 when compared with nondiabetic women.[20] Given this evidence, persons with diabetes have a high priority for early and aggressive risk factor modification.[19,20]

Obesity and sedentary life style are highly predictive of type 2 diabetes mellitus, which accounts for 90% of all diabetes in the United States. Evidence indicates that fasting blood sugar levels lower than previously believed increase the risk of CHD, which prompted the American Diabetes Association in 1997 to lower the diagnostic criterion for diabetes to 126 mg/dL or higher.[21]

Type A behavior pattern (TABP) was believed to be an independent risk factor for CHD,[22,23] but recent studies have demonstrated that the anger and hostility components of the global TABP are associated with the greatest risk for CHD.[24,25] The association of hostility with electron beam computed tomography evidence of coronary calcification has been seen even in young men and women and may be predictive of future CHD.[26] Negative affective states, such as depression, also have been independently linked with increased CHD risk and mortality after MI.[27-29]

Epidemiologic studies have shown a significant association between the occurrence of CHD and elevated serum levels of homocysteine and C-reactive protein.[30-32] Currently, however, there is insufficient data to use either of these biochemical markers as predictors of primary CHD.[33,34]

Another risk factor for CHD generating increasing attention is obstructive sleep apnea (OSA). OSA is prevalent in men and women with CHD and may be an independent risk factor for CHD because of its contribution to atherogeneis.[35] Cocaine may accelerate coronary atherogenesis[36] in addition to its other deleterious effects on the cardiovascular system, such as acute increases in heart rate and blood pressure, coronary vasospasm, and increased platelet aggregation with subsequent MI or stroke.[37]

Developmental Factors

Pregnancy and the postpartum period cause hypercoagulability of the blood and put women at increased risk for ischemia because of potential thromboembolic events such as MI or stroke.[38] Another risk factor for ischemia during pregnancy is a severe form of preeclampsia that results in vascular injury, intravascular coagulation, and significant end-organ damage.[39] This life-threatening condition results in hemolysis, elevated liver enzymes, and low platelet count (i.e., the HELLP syndrome) that classically occurs. HELLP occurs in 0.17% to 0.85% of all live births and appears on average between 32 and 34 weeks' gestation. Approximately 30% of cases occur in the postpartum period.[39]

Use of oral contraceptives (OCs) and concomitant cigarette smoking and/or hypertension greatly increase the risk of acute MI (AMI) and other CHD events.[40,41] A recent World Health Organization case-control study.[42] found that the attributable risk of AMI in users of OCs younger than 35 years old who smoked was 34.9 per 10^6 woman-years. In those older than 35 who smoked, their attributable risk of AMI was about 400 per 10^6 woman-years. Cigarette smoking in users of OCs of any age who also failed to have their blood pressure checked before beginning OCs had an odds ratio for an AMI of 71.4 (95% CI, 16.5–309).[42] Women who cannot quit smoking or have hypertension should be prescribed an alternative form of birth control.

The onset of menopause increases women's risk of CHD, so that by age 75 the prevalence of CHD is nearly identical in women and men.[3] Numerous observational studies supported the belief that estrogen conferred this cardioprotective effect in premenopausal women. This belief is consistent with the known physiologic effects of estrogen in the body, such as inhibition of atherosclerosis and decreasing blood pressure.[43,44] However, the results of several recent, large, randomized clinical trials found that estrogen plus progestin did not lower the risk of CHD deaths and nonfatal MI[45,46] or slow progression of coronary atherosclerosis[47] in postmenopausal women with or without known CHD. In fact, the Heart and Estrogen/progestin Replacement Study (HERS).[45] found a significant increase in CHD events and nonfatal MI in the hormone replacement (HRT) group in the first year after randomization. This increase was reversed in years 3 to 5 and a small but significant reduction in these events were reported, a finding that did not persist in the 2.7 years of follow-up of this cohort.[48] In the Women's Health Initiative study[46] of postmenopausal women (most without known coronary disease), CHD events, mostly as nonfatal MIs, also increased in the HRT group in the first year of the study but they continued to increase throughout the 5.2 years of follow-up. The investigators of these clinical trials recommended that HRT not be initiated or continued for postmenopausal women for the purpose of reducing their CHD risk.[45,46]

A large, international randomized clinical trial[49,50] is being conducted to study the effectiveness of raloxifene, a new selective estrogen receptor modulator, on reducing coronary deaths, nonfatal acute MI, and hospitalized acute coronary syndromes other than MI. Raloxifene has effects similar to estrogen in lowering LDL-C, while not raising triglyceride levels. It also does not stimulate the endometrium, so it does not require a concurrent progestin, which is known to counteract many of estrogen's favorable effects on CHD risk.[49]

MECHANISMS

Determinants of Blood Flow

Blood flow is directly related to driving pressure (mean arterial pressure minus central venous pressure) and inversely related to arteriolar resistance.[51] Factors influencing driving pressure include blood volume, myocardial contractility, and heart rate (which also determine cardiac output). Arteriolar resistance is dependent on the net effects of systemically circulating substances, such as catecholamines, angiotensin, and prostaglandins. Substances locally released in response to a tissue's changing oxygen and energy needs (autoregulation) include carbon dioxide, potassium, lactate, adenosine, and nitric oxide (formerly known as endothelium-derived relaxing factor).[51] In atherosclerotic arteries, nitric oxide synthesis is impaired, thus an important substance for physiologic control of arterial resistance is not operative when demand for oxygen and substrate exceeds the vessel's ability to respond.[51]

Tissue perfusion depends on a delicately regulated balance between cardiac output and vascular resistance. The etiologic factors that result in ischemia are those that reduce cardiac output or increase vascular resistance or both. The mechanisms by which these factors decrease tissue perfusion are discussed in the following sections.

Reduction in Cardiac Output

Any disease or clinical state that reduces cardiac output below a tissue's ability to compensate results in ischemia of that tissue. Because cardiac output is a major determinant of MAP, the MAP is also decreased, placing all tissues at risk for ischemia. Situations that result in reduced cardiac output are ones in which there is (1) a reduction in total blood volume (hypovolemia), (2) an increase in the vascular space secondary to systemic vasodilation, or (3) a reduction in the pumping efficiency of the heart.

Diseases or clinical states that compromise the pumping efficiency of the heart, such as congestive heart failure or ventricular arrhythmias, threaten systemic tissue perfusion. Also, because the heart is uniquely responsible for its own perfusion, a reduction in cardiac output propagates a vicious circle of events that can be difficult to halt: a reduction in coronary artery perfusion resulting in myocardial ischemia, which further decreases cardiac output and systemic perfusion, which further aggravates coronary artery perfusion, and so forth.

Increased Vascular Resistance

Factors that increase systemic or tissue vascular resistance cause a low-flow state that may result in a partial or complete cessation of blood flow to most body tissues or to a localized region. The causes of increased vascular resistance can be organized under the broad categories displayed in Table 21-1.

Obstruction of Blood Vessels. Ischemia resulting from obstruction of blood vessels occurs primarily on the arterial side of the circulation, that is, arteries, arterioles, and capillaries, which deliver oxygen and nutrients to the tissues. A large obstruction of the venous side of the circulation (e.g., deep vein thrombosis) can cause localized ischemia if there is massive tissue edema and compression of tissue capillaries.

It is possible to have concomitant processes causing arterial obstruction. For example, atherosclerotic coronary arteries seem to be hypersensitive to vasospastic stimuli such as cold environmental temperature.

Shunting of Blood Flow. Diminished cardiac output states or physiologic stress cause release of vasoactive substances that constrict peripheral vascular beds and shunt blood flow to the central circulation. Peripheral tissues, such as the kidneys and intestines, are vulnerable to ischemia.

Shunting also is the result of congenital arteriovenous (AV) malformations or traumatically or surgically created anastomoses. In the absence of collateral flow these types of shunt can result in significant loss of oxygen and nutrients to the tissue. In addition, AV malformations or anastomoses can cause pooling of blood within themselves and become a source of emboli. The malformation can also rupture, jeopardizing distal tissues. In the brain, an AV malformation can be a space-occupying lesion or can rupture and cause significant pressure and compression of other blood vessels, further compromising flow.

Injury to Blood Vessels. Any process that interrupts the integrity of nutrient blood vessels places the distal tissues at risk for ischemia. Traumatic laceration of an artery, surgical incision, chemical or thermal injury, dissection of an aneurysm, and inflammatory processes all result in interruption of the vessel wall and in abnormal hemodynamics, which compromise distal perfusion.

Decreased Capillary-Tissue Ratio. The normal number and distribution of capillaries are such that the diffusion distance for oxygen, nutrients, and waste products is optimal for the requirements of the individual tissues.[52] A reduction in capillary density can result when either the number of cells relative to the capillary supply increases, such as with hypertrophic cardiomyopathy, or tissue edema, which increases the distance between capillary and cell.

Energy Metabolism

Understanding the underlying pathophysiologic mechanisms and consequences of ischemia is predicated on a basic familiarity with the normal processes of energy production. Several basic concepts of normal energy metabolism are presented here and the reader is referred to other sources[51,53,54] for in-depth discussions of this topic.

Under aerobic conditions, amino acids, sugars, and fat derivatives produce energy in the form of adenosine triphosphate (ATP), with the Krebs citric acid cycle being the common final pathway for their metabolism (Figure 21-1).[51] Under anaerobic conditions, the metabolism of glucose via glycolysis is the only source of energy for the cell. Fatty acid and amino acid metabolism require oxygen and so do not produce energy under anaerobic conditions.[51]

Glycolysis results in the net production of 2 moles of ATP per mole of blood glucose.[51] Under aerobic conditions, the pyruvate formed via glycolysis enters the mitochondria and is converted to acetyl-coenzyme A (acetyl-CoA). Acetyl-CoA enters the Krebs citric acid cycle, through which ATP, hydrogen ions, and carbon dioxide are produced. The hydrogen ions enter the electron transport chain, where oxidative phosphorylation occurs (Figure 21-1). Various proteins (the flavoprotein-cytochrome system [FAD-FADH system]) act as electron (hydrogen) carriers until the electrons are accepted by oxygen, the last carrier in the series.[51] For each pair of hydrogen ions transferred from one protein to the next, 2 moles of ATP are generated. For every mole of glucose, a total of 38 moles of ATP are produced (i.e., 2 from glycolysis and 36 from oxidative phosphorylation). The ATP is then transported out of the mitochondria into the cytoplasm by means of a special carrier located in the membrane of the mitochondria. Once in the cytoplasm ATP becomes the most important source of high energy phosphate that is available to fuel the synthesizing and transporting functions of the cell.[51] Another source of high energy phosphate is creatine phosphate (CrP), which is found in muscle.

Cellular Events in Ischemia

Obstruction of an artery results in a regional decrease in blood flow to the tissue it subserves, whereas global ischemia results when blood flow to the entire organ has been interrupted, such as during harvesting and transport of an organ for transplantation or during a state of asystole. The experimental studies of ischemia often employ a model of complete occlusion of a critical artery resulting in total cessation of blood flow to the effected region. In clinical practice, however, it is unusual to have complete absence of blood flow to a tissue, because of collateral circulation. Consequently, it is likely that even small amounts of oxygen and energy substrate are available to the cells, allowing for a longer time before irreversible injury.

When perfusion to a tissue slows or completely stops, the resultant decreased oxygen and substrate delivery causes a reduction in oxidative phosphorylation and energy production. Anaerobic glycolysis produces more lactate than pyruvate with a concomitant decrease in pH. Figure 21-2 is a diagram depicting several of the major cellular events that occur in ischemia in all cells. A number of important reactions are summarized in this discussion, but for a more comprehensive review of these processes the reader is referred to other references.[53-56]

A drastic reduction in the amount of cellular energy, first CrP, then later ATP,[53] initiates a complex series of reactions that, if not checked, eventually result in irreversible injury, the so-called point of no return.[57] Reduced energy production decreases the

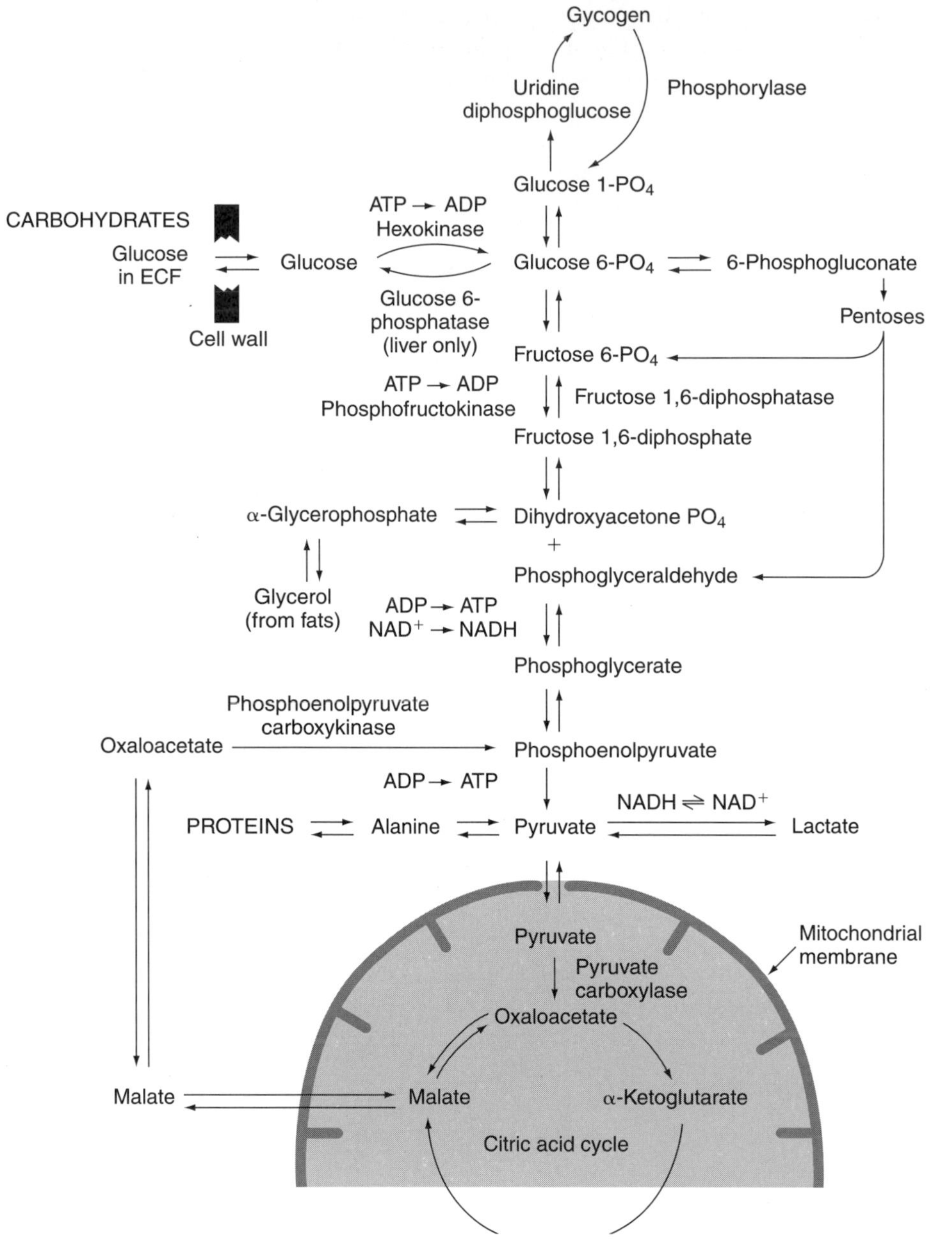

Figure 21-1 Glycolysis and the Krebs citric acid cycle. (From Ganong, W.F. [2001]. *Review of medical physiology* [20th ed.]. San Francisco: McGraw-Hill.[51] With permission.)

activity of the ATPase ion pumps that normally maintain specific concentrations of these ions in the cell. In the absence of these pumps, sodium (Na^+), chloride (Cl^-), calcium (Ca^{++}), and potassium (K^+) diffuse down their concentration gradients. The result is increased intracellular Na^+, Cl^-, and Ca^{++} and decreased intracellular K^+. With increased intracellular Na^+, intracellular water increases, causing the cell and most organelles to swell, a very early electron microscopic manifestation of ischemia.[56,57] As ischemia progresses, toxic metabolites accumulate in the cell and swelling increases.[55,56]

Alteration in K^+ flux may be responsible, in part, for arrhythmogenesis in myocardial ischemia. Other products of ischemia also are arrhythmogenic, such as free fatty acids (FFAs), catecholamines, prostaglandins, thromboxanes, and hydrogen ions.[58]

With the alterations in normal ion concentrations, the transmembrane potential changes, resulting in several important reactions, such as

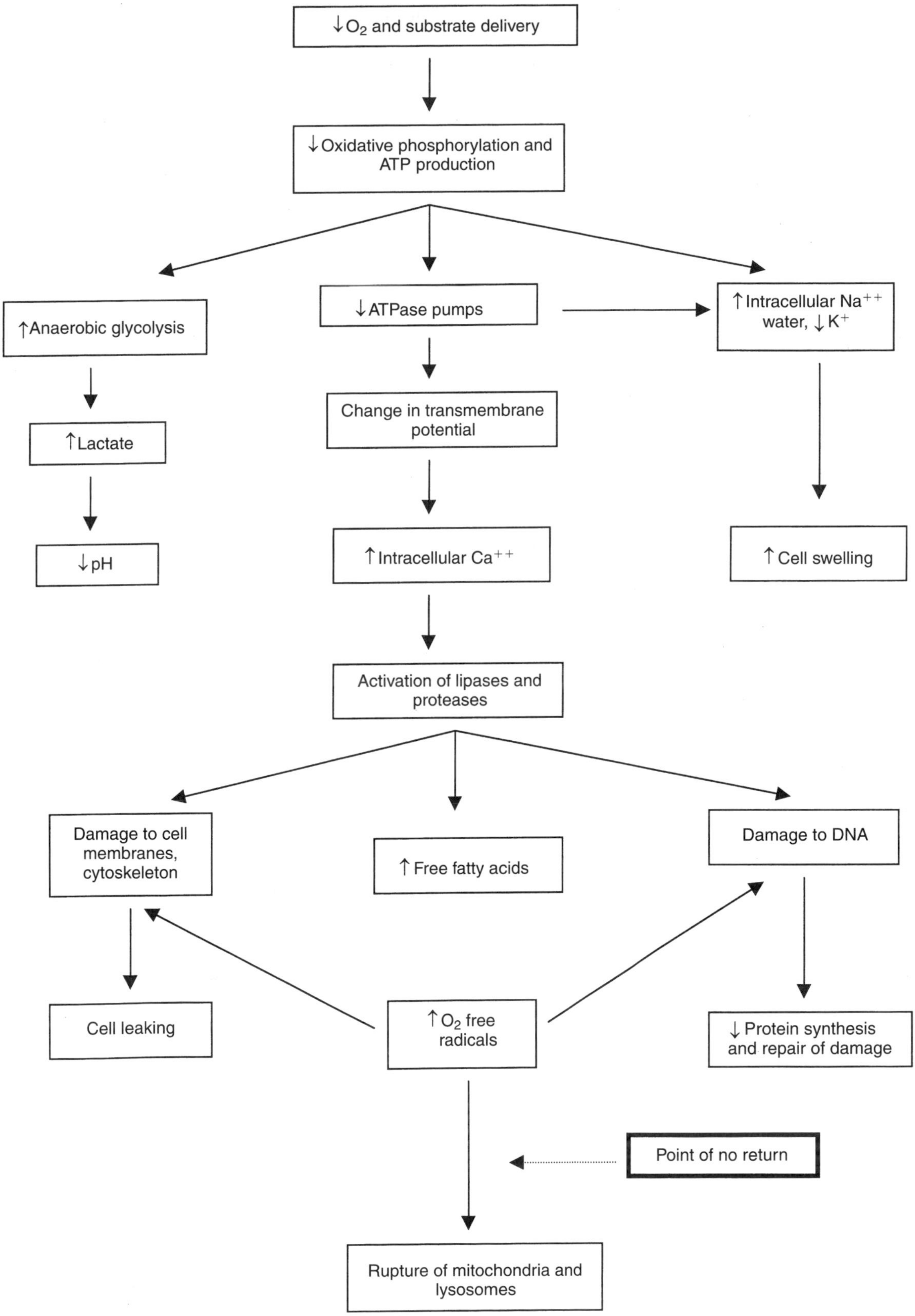

Figure 21-2 Diagram of several major cellular events that occur in ischemia.

opening of Ca^{++} channels in the cell membrane, the mitochondria, and endoplasmic reticulum, and further elevation in intracellular Ca^{++}.[53,54] Increased intracellular Ca^{++} is responsible for a number of injurious reactions that can ultimately lead to cell death and necrosis if perfusion is not reestablished (Figure 21-3). For example, Ca^{++} activates phospholipases and proteases, which cause the breakdown of cell and subcellular membranes and proteins.[53,54] This disruption of cell

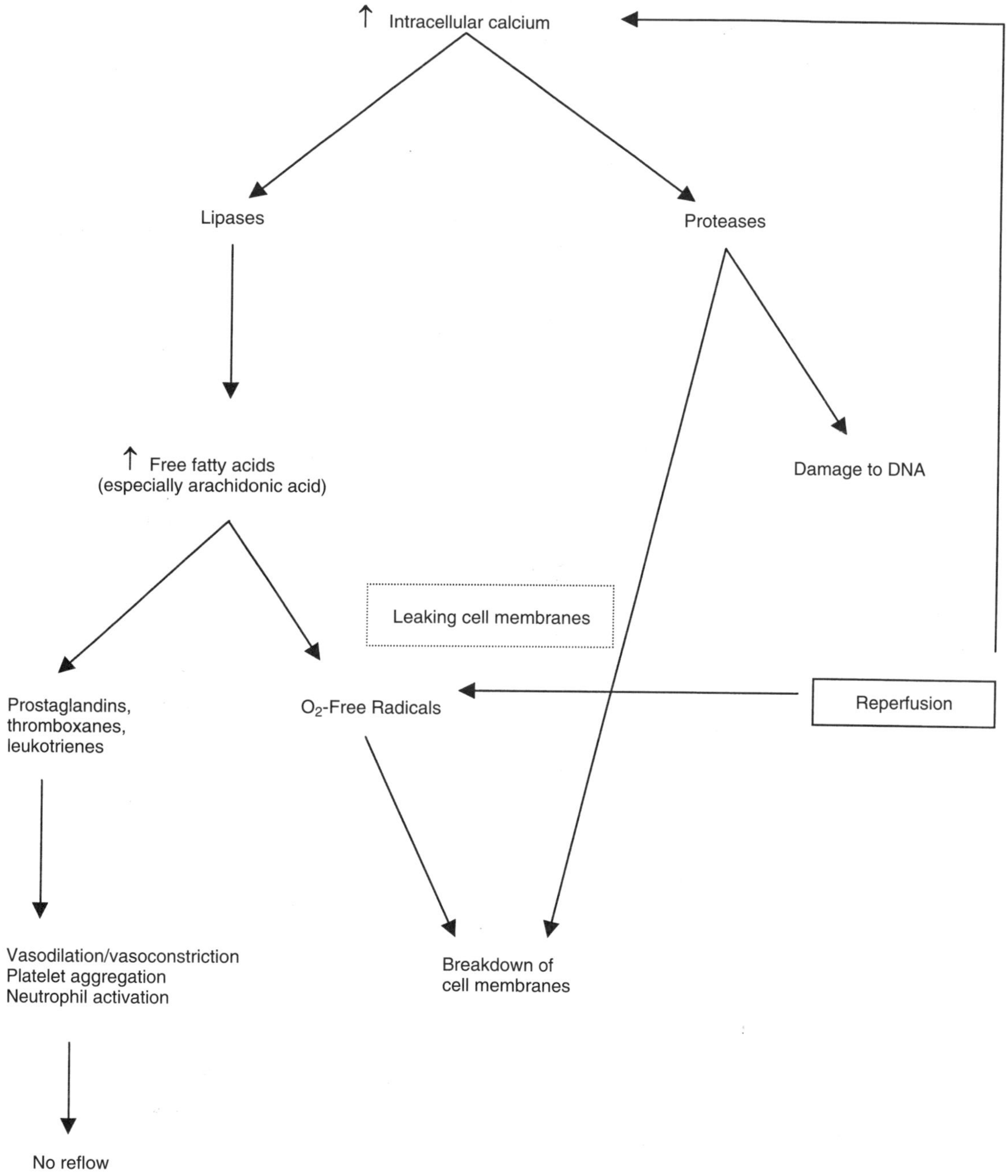

Figure 21-3 Calcium-mediated processes in ischemia and reperfusion injury. Ca^{++} activates lipases and proteases, ultimately resulting in the disruption of cell membranes and potentially irreversible damage. Reperfusion allows for delivery of oxygen and calcium resulting in further production of oxygen free radicals and damage to cell membranes. If perfusion is reestablished before the point of no return, damage to cell membranes and internal structures can be repaired.

membranes results in the release of FFAs, especially arachidonic acid. The products of arachidonic acid metabolism are prostaglandins, thromboxanes, and leukotrienes. These substances produce vasospasm and vasodilation in varying degrees in different vascular beds, platelet aggregation, increased neutrophil adhesion and clumping, reduced deformability of red blood cells, arteriolar and capillary endothelial leaking, and further disruption of cell membranes.[59,60]

Because there is likely to be a small amount of blood flow to the tissue, some oxygen and energy substrate is delivered. When oxygen is present, it is reduced by the FFAs released from cell membranes to form oxygen free radicals, superoxide ($\cdot O_2^-$), hydrogen peroxide (H_2O_2), and hydroxyl radical ($\cdot OH$). These are highly reactive products of oxygen metabolism that are toxic to many biologic substances. A missing electron from their outer orbits allows them to react with many substances within the cell, forming additional highly reactive free radical species that perpetuate multiple other cellular injuries.[53-56] Free radical scavengers that are normally produced by the cell to catabolize free radicals to harmless end products are rapidly depleted by the increased production of free radicals.[54,56]

Increased intracellular Ca^{++} also activates nucleases that damage deoxyribonucleic acid (DNA), which interferes with protein synthesis, repair of damaged cell membranes, and recovery of the tissue after reperfusion.[53,54,60] Concurrently, cellular pH drops quickly as the rate of glycolysis increases to provide energy. It was once believed that acidosis was responsible for much of the damage to protein structures and genetic material. It is now known that the pH becomes neutral or alkaline late in ischemia and that the cellular acidosis may delay irreversible injury by inhibiting enzymatic breakdown of cell membranes.[56]

As a result of these many alterations, the entire machinery of the cell becomes depressed or nonfunctional. The rate at which this occurs varies depending on several factors, such as the oxygen content of the blood, metabolic rate of the tissue, the amount of collateral flow, ability of the tissue to store oxygen, and temperature.[56,57,61,62]

As the point of irreversible injury is approached within the cell, there is increasing leakiness and eventual rupture of organelles. Swelling and rupture of mitochondria and lysosomes, in particular, are thought of as the final events signaling irrevocable cell injury.[56,57] When the lysosomes rupture, hydrolases that digest cellular contents and surrounding tissue are released. Other intracellular enzymes are released to the surrounding tissue as well, such as aspartate aminotransferase (AST), lactate dehydrogenase (LDH), creatine phosphokinase (CPK), and troponin I, which are used as clinical indicators of infarction.

Once autodigestion of the cell has begun, prostaglandins and other products of inflammation are released from the cells themselves and from capillary endothelium.[56] Polymorphonucleocytes accumulate in the area and phagocytize the remainder of the cellular structures.[56,57] Over time, fibrin and collagen fibers replace the infarcted tissue, and a scar is formed.

After brief periods of critically diminished blood flow (i.e., $\leq$15 minutes in the heart), reestablishment of perfusion results in fairly rapid resolution of the above derangements in cellular energy production, ion fluxes, and membrane injury.[53] Even after this brief period, however, reperfusion injury occurs when reestablished blood flow increases delivery of oxygen, calcium, sodium, water, and leukocytes to the ischemic tissue, causing acceleration of oxygen-free radical production, protease and phospholipase activation, and cell membrane damage.[53,56]

Myocardial Ischemia

Two types of myocardial ischemia have been identified: (1) "demand"-related ischemia and (2) "supply"-related ischemia. In general, demand-related ischemia is induced by situations such as exercise, tachycardia, or emotional stress that increase the myocardium's demand for oxygen beyond the flow capabilities of a coronary artery with a "stable" atherosclerotic plaque. A stable plaque usually has a thick fibrous cap over the lesion that typically often occludes 75% of the coronary vessel.[63] Demand-related ischemia is generally self-limiting and is observed in patients diagnosed with chronic stable angina. In addition, demand-related myocardial ischemia can occur with cardiomyopathies as a result of impaired myocardial perfusion because of increased thickness of the myocardial tissue, increased oxygen demand, and elevated filling pressures.[64]

Supply-related ischemia is induced by total obstruction of coronary blood flow and is believed to be responsible for the acute coronary syndromes of acute MI (both ST and non-ST elevation MI) and unstable angina. Supply-related ischemia in patients with CAD often results from rupture of a "vulnerable" atherosclerotic plaque. A vulnerable plaque is described as having a thin fibrous cap over the coronary lesion that is prone to rupture.[63] Interestingly, vulnerable plaques, unlike stable plaques, occlude the coronary vessel by no more than 50% to 70%.[65] The coronary processes believed to be responsible for supply-related ischemia in patients with CAD include vasospasm at the site of an atherosclerotic plaque, plaque fissure and/or rupture with resultant platelet stimulation, thrombus formation, and resultant coronary occlusion.[66-68] The major differences between the disorders of MI and unstable angina are the severity and duration of coronary occlusion. Coronary vasospasm can also occur in persons without CAD, usually at rest, and is not precipitated by exercise or emotional stress.[69,70]

PATHOLOGIC CONSEQUENCES OF ISCHEMIA

Acute and severe ischemia results in transient organ system failure and, if prolonged, eventual infarction and irreversible loss of tissue function. If the area of ischemia is large or in a critical tissue, such as the bundle of His in the heart, the alteration in tissue function could cause the death of the individual.

Chronic and less severe states of ischemia cause changes in the tissue that may be adaptive in that they allow the tissue to remain somewhat functional. Changes in the size of the affected tissue, such as hypertrophy or atrophy, are common adaptations to chronic states of absolute or relative reductions in perfusion.[56]

RELATED PATHOPHYSIOLOGIC CONCEPTS

A phenomenon closely related to ischemia is hypoxia. Hypoxia denotes a reduction in tissue oxygen, which can occur in the presence of adequate perfusion when arterial oxygen content is reduced. Energy substrate may still be delivered, and toxic metabolites may still be eliminated. As a result of lactate elimination, cellular acidosis occurs over a slower period, and glycolysis can proceed for a longer period than would be possible if perfusion were inadequate.[56,71] Reduced perfusion results in earlier and greater tissue injury than only lowering the tissue oxygen tension.[56] Experiments have shown that the ischemic heart is much more susceptible to ventricular fibrillation than hearts made hypoxic but continuously perfused.[72] In addition, the electrophysiologic abnormalities occurring within the initial 20 minutes of myocardial ischemia *in vivo* were eradicated when this same tissue was perfused *in vitro*.[73] Presumably, one or more substances accumulated during the period of ischemia that caused the arrhythmia and were washed out during perfusion. Support for this conclusion is found in studies in which venous blood from ischemic myocardium produced qualitatively similar electrophysiologic aberrations in isolated myocardium as those found in ischemic myocardium *in vivo*.[74]

MANIFESTATIONS AND SURVEILLANCE

Subjective Manifestations

The most common symptom associated with myocardial ischemia is angina. Typical angina descriptors include complaints of pressure, squeezing, crushing, or tightness in the chest that may radiate to the neck, jaws, or ulnar surface of one or both arms. Individuals may also experience anginal "equivalents," or symptoms of myocardial ischemia other than angina, which include dyspnea, faintness, or fatigue. In addition, studies show that atypical descriptors of angina, for instance anginal pain described as sharp, burning, stinging, or even indigestion, can occur in approximately 11% to 25% of persons with true myocardial ischemia.[75-77] These same studies showed that atypical angina is more prevalent among women, elderly persons, and in nonwhites compared with their white counterparts. Hence, angina symptoms can vary considerably among patients with myocardial ischemia.

Angina brought on by exertion or emotional stress (demand-related) that is relieved within minutes by rest or by the use of nitroglycerine is typically diagnosed as stable angina. Angina exhibiting the presence of one or more of the following features: (1) crescendo angina (i.e., increased severity, prolonged, or frequent), in patients with known stable angina; (2) new onset angina, which is brought on by minimal exertion; and (3) angina at rest, is characteristic of unstable angina (supply-related).[78] On the other hand, the pain of acute MI (supply-related) is severe and often prolonged, usually lasting for more than 30 minutes and, in most cases, several hours. It is not uncommon for patients who present for treatment of acute MI to have had symptoms suggestive of unstable angina days or weeks before hospital presentation. Although angina is the most common symptom associated with myocardial ischemia, it is sometimes difficult to distinguish from other types of chest discomfort, such as that resulting from mitral valve prolapse; esophageal reflux or spasm; peptic ulcer disease; or biliary, musculoskeletal, or pulmonary disease.

Interestingly, in over 50% of patients with ECG-detected ischemia, myocardial ischemia is clinically "silent," or occurs in the absence of angina.[79-82] Researchers have postulated a number of possible mechanisms for silent myocardial ischemia, such as an increased threshold and tolerance to pain in some individuals; neuropathy of sensory fibers (as may occur with diabetes mellitus); or irreversible injury to vagal and sympathetic afferent fibers from previous ischemia or infarction, a type of "autodenervation."[83]

Compelling evidence indicates that patients with silent myocardial ischemia detected with continuous ECG monitoring are at significant risk for subsequent MI and death at both short- and long-term follow-up periods compared with those without such events.[80,81,84,85] Thus angina is an unreliable indicator of myocardial ischemia that could result in potential misdiagnosis and treatment of those with noncardiac conditions or failure to detect myocardial ischemia when it occurs.

Objective Manifestations

Objective manifestations of myocardial ischemia may include clinical evidence of impaired myocardial contraction, arrhythmias, and ST-segment changes on the ECG. Patients with transient myocardial ischemia may not display overt signs and symptoms of impaired myocardial contraction because there may only be brief interruption of coronary blood flow. If myocardial ischemia is sustained or occurs in patients with impaired myocardial function resulting from heart failure or prior MI, physical findings may be observed, such as anxiety, shortness of breath, crackles, diffuse wheezing, heart rate changes (either bradycardia or tachycardia), and hypotension or hypertension. Overall, physical findings may or may not be helpful in identifying persons with ischemia.

The onset of myocardial ischemia produces electrical dysfunction of myocardial cells that may result in lethal ventricular arrhythmias (ventricular tachycardia, fibrillation). Changes in ion flux discussed previously and acidosis cause reduction of the transmembrane potential, enhanced automaticity in some tissues, and alteration of the refractory period. These physiologic events increase the susceptibility of the myocardium to lethal ventricular arrhythmias.

The only biomarker available for myocardial ischemia is serum lactate, but it must be obtained from the coronary sinus, making it too invasive and expensive for practical use.[86] The serum biomarkers used to detect MI are creatine kinase-myocardial band (CK-MB) and troponin I.

Treadmill stress testing is used to diagnose myocardial ischemia by increasing myocardial oxygen demand with either active exercise (i.e., treadmill or stationary cycling) or medications that provoke an increase in heart rate (e.g., dipyrida mole). The development of 100 microvolts (μV) (1 mm) of ST-segment depression measured at 60 to 80 msec past the J-point (the junction at which the QRS complex ends and the ST-segment begins) is considered an abnormal, or positive, stress test.

Noninvasive imaging techniques such as echocardiography and perfusion imaging (i.e., thallium and sestamibi or computed tomography [CT] scans) are used to identify myocardial wall motion abnormalities that may indicate the presence of acute myocardial ischemia. Coronary angiography is an invasive myocardial imaging technique that provides real-time imaging of blood flow through the coronary arteries and can be used to identify the site and nature of coronary lesions or occlusions. Importantly, although these imaging techniques are valuable screening and diagnostic tools for myocardial ischemia they provide only "snap-shot" information about the status of the myocardium. This is an important potential limitation, because of the dynamic, mostly silent, and unpredictable nature of myocardial ischemia.

Knowing whether unprovoked or spontaneous ischemia is occurring is essential in guiding treatment decisions. With this in mind, continuous monitoring of the ECG for ST-segment changes (either elevation or depression) provides the most reliable objective indicator of ischemia. Because ECG data can be obtained noninvasively and in a continuous manner, this method has important advantages for the assessment of transient myocardial ischemia.

The standard ECG diagnostic criteria for ischemia are 100 microvolts (μV) or more of ST-segment deviation (i.e., depression or elevation), 60 to 80 msec past the J-point, lasting for greater than 60 seconds (Figure 21-4).[87] The typical ECG ST-segment manifestation of demand-related ischemia is ST-segment depression (Figure 21-5). Demand-related ST-segment changes on the 12-lead ECG reflect ischemia of the subendocardial layer of the myocardium, or innermost aspect. Typically, the ST-segment changes associated with demand-related ischemia disappear when the supply and demand for myocardial blood flow are equalized (i.e., heart rate decreases).

The typical ECG ST-segment manifestation of supply-related ischemia, which is characterized by total coronary occlusion, is ST-segment elevation (Figure 21-6). The presence of this ECG pattern is

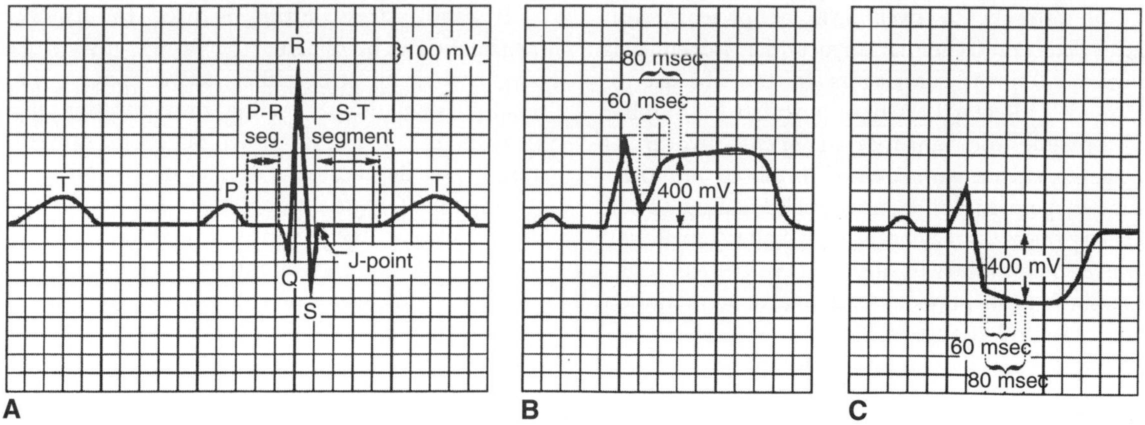

Figure 21-4 **These three panels illustrate the measurement points used to diagnose myocardial ischemia using the ECG. A, A normal ECG complex, with an isoelectric ST-segment. Typically, the PR segment serves as the isoelectric reference point from which to measure ST-segment deviation. ST-segment deviation is measured from the J-point, which marks the end of the QRS complex and the beginning of the ST-segment, at 60 or 80 milliseconds (msec) past the J-point. When the ECG instrument is programmed with the standard amplitude settings, 100 μV equals one small box (1 mm) on the ECG paper as shown in A. The 100 μV measurement value is illustrated. B, ST-segment elevation of 400 μV, measured 80 msec past the J-point. The 60 msec measurement point is also illustrated. C, ST-segment depression of 400 μV, measured 80 msec past the J-point. The 60 msec measurement point is also illustrated.** (Adapted from Tisdale, L.A., & Drew, B.J. [1993]. ST-segment monitoring for myocardial ischemia. *AACN Clinical Issues, 4*(1), 34-43,[164] with permission.)

diagnostic of acute ST elevation MI. Supply-related ischemia results in transmural ischemia, or ischemia of the entire thickness of the myocardium. Because the entire thickness of the myocardium is threatened, it is imperative that this condition be reversed immediately to prevent infarction. If infarction occurs, serum biomarkers (i.e., CK-MB, troponin I) will be positive and Q waves will develop on the ECG.

For all of its value in detecting myocardial ischemia, the ECG is not reliable in some patients. Up to 50% of those patients who are eventually diagnosed with acute MI do not meet the ECG criteria for an MI,[88] which is ST elevation in two or more contiguous leads of a standard 12-lead. The reasons for this include inaccurate, inconsistent, and noncontinuous electrode placement; failure of the electrodes to detect ischemia in the posterior regions of the heart; and the dynamic nature of coronary occlusion consisting of intermittent

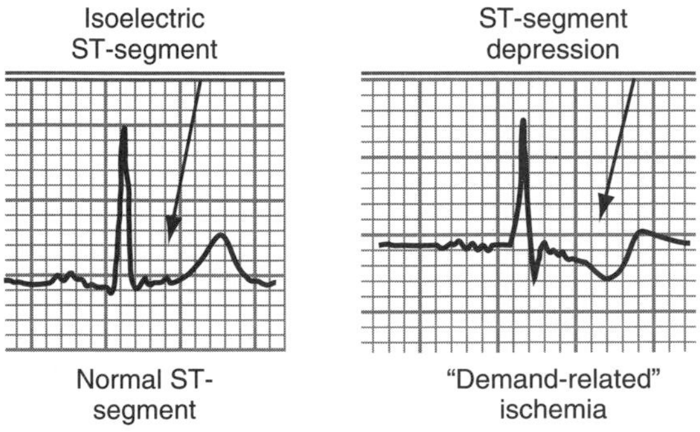

Figure 21-5 **Illustrates the typical ECG manifestations of "demand-related" myocardial ischemia, which is characterized by ST-segment depression.** (Courtesy the Ischemia Monitoring Laboratory, University of California San Francisco, School of Nursing.)

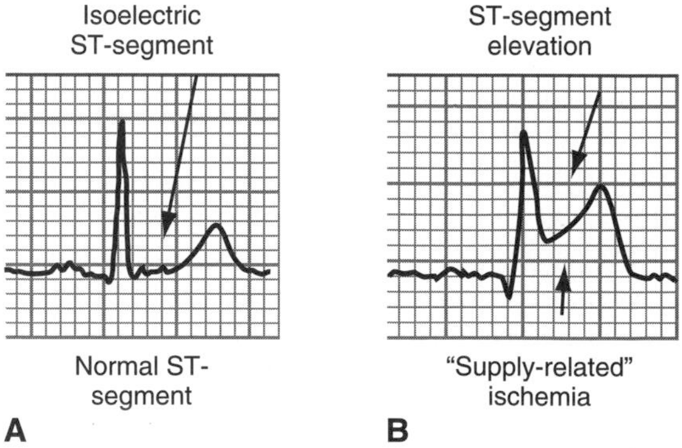

Figure 21-6 **A and B, Typical ECG manifestations of "supply-related" myocardial ischemia, which is characterized by ST-segment elevation. B Also illustrates the development of a Q-wave, which indicates that infarction has occurred.** (Courtesy the Ischemia Monitoring Laboratory, University of California San Francisco, School of Nursing.)

periods of obstruction and recanalization of the coronary artery.[89-95] Evidence from continuous ECG recordings obtained during percutaneous coronary interventions (PCIs) show that approximately 20% of patients do not exhibit ST-segment changes during balloon inflation.[96-98]

In the surveillance of myocardial ischemia the nurse must incorporate both subjective and objective assessments. Episodes of angina must be evaluated for location, intensity, nature, precipitating event, duration, and actions that may have relieved the episode. Angina severity can be assessed using a 0 to 10 numerical rating scale, with 0 being no pain and 10 being the worst pain imaginable. This scale can be used to determine the success or failure of treatment for acute ischemia and can enhance continuity of care if used across hospital (i.e., emergency department, coronary care unit [CCU], catheterization laboratory, telemetry unit) and outpatient settings.

A thorough history should be performed to identify risk factors for myocardial ischemia, a prior history of CAD or coronary procedures (i.e., percutaneous transluminal coronary angioplasty [PTCA], stent placement, or coronary artery bypass graft [CABG] surgery). In addition, the nurse should assess the patient for potential clinical signs of ischemia, such as anxiety, shortness of breath, crackles, diffuse wheezing, and changes in heart rate and blood pressure. It is important to consider that myocardial ischemia is often a transient event lasting only minutes, thus overt clinical signs and symptoms may not be exhibited.

In 1999, an international panel of physician and nurse experts in the field of ischemia monitoring developed a practice guideline that included a strategy for optimal ECG ST-segment monitoring in patients with acute coronary syndromes.[96] They recommended that when using the ECG to evaluate patients for the presence of myocardial ischemia, it is imperative to record the maximum amount of ECG information. This is because the pathophysiologic mechanisms (i.e., demand- vs. supply-related ischemia) may differ over time in individual patients with acute coronary syndromes resulting in distinctly different ECG patterns. This is a vital consideration in clinical practice because supply-related ischemia requires immediate and aggressive treatment to avoid acute infarction. For instance, although lead V_5 often shows maximal ST deviation during demand-related ischemia, it is not uncommon for diffuse ST changes to occur in multiple ECG leads. Accordingly, it is necessary to record all 12 ECG leads to accurately quantify ischemic burden in patients who experience demand-related ischemia. Measurement of ischemic burden using the ECG should incorporate (1) duration (number of ischemic episodes/24 hours multiplied by duration of each episode), (2) extent (number of ECG leads demonstrating ST-segment elevation and/or depression), and (3) severity (total sum of ST deviation amplitudes in all 12 ECG leads).

Unlike demand-related ischemia, ST-segment elevation caused by supply-related ischemia can be used to localize the area of the myocardium that is ischemic and in most cases identify the "culprit" artery responsible for ischemia. For example, ST-segment elevation in leads V_2 to V_4 reflects ischemia of the anterior portion of the myocardium, and most often indicates occlusion of the left anterior descending (LAD) coronary artery.[99] ST-segment elevation in leads III, aVF, and II reflects ischemia of the inferior portion of the myocardium, and most often indicates occlusion of the right coronary artery (RCA).[99] Finally, occlusion of the left circumflex (LCX) coronary artery may produce inferior, lateral, or posterior ECG patterns; thus no one ECG lead or leads has been found to be superior for detecting ischemia resulting from occlusion of the LCX.[100-102] However, it is possible to diagnose posterior ischemia, which is most often the result of LCX artery occlusion, using ST-segment depression in leads V_1, V_2, and V_3, because these ST-segment changes reflect the reciprocal, or mirror image, ST changes of posterior ischemia.[103]

CLINICAL MANAGEMENT

The primary clinical objective in patients with acute or ongoing myocardial ischemia is immediate identification of ischemia and restoration of blood flow to prevent or limit the extent of infarction. This concept is based on the open artery hypothesis,[104] which states that reperfusion to the myocardium must be immediate, complete, and sustained to reduce infarct size, preserve left ventricular function, and reduce morbidity and mortality. Therapies used to restore perfusion in the setting of acute or ongoing myocardial ischemia include (1) pharmacologic agents, (2) mechanical/surgical therapies, and (3) nonpharmacologic therapies (Table 21-3). In addition, risk factor modification can be implemented to prevent subsequent ischemic events.

Pharmacologic Therapies

Pharmacologic therapies are aimed at restoring blood flow to the myocardium, either by lowering

TABLE 21-3 Goals of Pharmacologic and Mechanical/Surgical Treatment Strategies Used to Treat Acute or Ongoing Ischemia

GOALS OF THERAPY	PHARMACOLOGIC	MECHANICAL AND SURGICAL	NONPHARMACOLOGIC
Reduce oxygen demand	Vasodilators Calcium antagonists Beta-blockers Antiarrhythmics ACE inhibitors		Rest Stress reduction Patient education
Increase oxygen supply	Fibrinolytics Vasodilators Antithrombins (heparin, LMWH) Antiplatelet agents (aspirin, clopidogrel, ticlopidine, GP IIb/IIIa receptor inhibitors) Antiarrhythmics Oxygen Red blood cell transfusion	PCI techniques PTCA Stent Atherectomy CABG surgery	

ACE, angiotensin-converting enzyme; *CABG*, coronary artery bypass graft; *GP*, glycoprotein; *LMWH*, low molecular weight heparins; *PCI*, percutaneous coronary intervention; *PTCA*, percutaneous transluminal coronary angioplasty.

the demand for oxygen or by increasing the supply of oxygen in the setting of coronary obstruction resulting from vasospasm or thrombus formation.

Compelling evidence demonstrates that fibrinolytic therapies aimed at abolishing ongoing ischemia can substantially improve outcomes in patients with acute MI. Large randomized clinical studies that used fibrinolytic therapy for treatment of AMI show that successful and sustained reperfusion of the infarct related artery improves left ventricular function and ultimately patient survival.[99,105-108] Moreover, studies show that the mortality rate is significantly higher in patients in whom reperfusion is not restored or when reocclusion of the infarct related artery occurs following an initial period of reperfusion, compared with patients who achieve and maintain reperfusion.[109,110]

Numerous adjunctive agents also are available and are typically used as combination therapies. Because myocardial ischemia may be the result of vasoconstriction and thrombus formation at the site of an atherosclerotic plaque, many antiischemic therapies are aimed at relaxation of vascular musculature and vasodilatation (i.e., angiotensin-converting enzyme [ACE] inhibitors, nitrates, beta-blockers, and calcium antagonists) and inhibition of thrombus formation (i.e., aspirin, heparin, glycoprotein IIb/IIIa platelet receptor inhibitors). Studies show that a combination of nitrates, beta-blockers, and calcium antagonists substantially reduce the number and duration of ischemic episodes and improve short- and long-term survival.[111-114] Clinical investigations in patients with unstable angina that compare placebo with the newest class of antiplatelet agents, Glycoprotein IIb/IIIa receptor inhibitors, show a significant reduction in the occurrence of MI, death, or urgent revascularization for refractory ischemia following administration of these agents.[115-117]

Mechanical and Surgical Therapies

Successful reperfusion of the infarct related artery in patients with AMI can be achieved using primary (emergency) PTCA and/or stent. This intervention is also available for use in patients with angina and unstable angina. The immediate success of PTCA and/or stent is greater than 90%, and most patients recover from interventional procedures without any untoward consequences. However, successful PTCA or stent results in intimal disruption, which has been described as a "crack," "tear," or "fracture" at the site of the atherosclerotic plaque where the PTCA procedure is performed.[118] This creates a potentially unstable area at the intervention site, which is susceptible to coronary artery spasm, thrombus formation, and coronary artery dissection.[119] The reported frequency of ischemia following PTCA ranges from 8% to 26%[79,102] and 33% following stent placement.[120] The frequency of ECG detected abrupt reocclusion, which is characterized by a total obstruction of the coronary artery, ranges from 4% to 9%[79,80] following PTCA and 3.5% to 6% following stent.[121,122]

There is evidence that primary PTCA and/or stent may provide more complete and sustained reperfusion of the infarct-related artery compared with fibrinolytic therapy. Primary PTCA resulted in earlier patency of the infarct related artery, smaller infarct size, improved left ventricular function, and lower mortality compared with thrombolytics for treatment of AMI.[123-128] Although these investigations suggest that primary PTCA may establish more complete myocardial perfusion compared with fibrinolytics, it should be emphasized that the success of primary PTCA and/or stent requires the institutional capability of performing emergency procedures (e.g., CABG surgery) 24 hours a day, 7 days a week. Because many hospitals are incapable of providing this type of clinical coverage, fibrinolytics remain an important and successful strategy in the management of AMI.

One final treatment option available for patients with acute coronary syndromes is CABG surgery. Clinical trials show that patients who have surgical revascularization experience more favorable long-term outcomes compared with patients who have medical treatment, including greater relief of angina, improved exercise performance, fewer antianginal medications prescribed following surgery, and decreased mortality.[129,130] CABG surgery may be indicated in patients with persistent angina unrelieved by aggressive medical management or in patients with serious side effects to medications used to treat ischemia. CABG surgery is also indicated in patients in whom PTCA and/or stent cannot be used (i.e., multivessel CAD).

Nonpharmacologic Therapies

The goal of nonpharmacologic therapies for treatment of ischemia is to reduce the oxygen demand. Approaches may include rest during the early acute hospital phase, progressive ambulation soon thereafter to prevent deconditioning, stress reduction, and patient education.

Early mobilization and shortened lengths of hospitalization have become the standard of care in patients with acute coronary syndromes. Many hospitals now admit patients with uncomplicated MI or angina to the telemetry units rather than the CCU.[131] Typically, patients are not maintained on strict bedrest in this environment. Several nurse and physician researchers have shown that various self-care activities including bathing, shaving, and sitting at the bedside do not result in significant physiologic changes (i.e., increased blood pressure, cardiac rhythm disturbances, altered left ventricular function) and thus are activities that most patients can perform without substantial consequence to myocardial function.[132-137] Without close observation, however, patients may engage in activities that increase the heart rate and lead to demand-related ischemia. Careful monitoring of patient activity level and its potential association with ischemia is an important nursing assessment.

Mental stress has been shown to increase adrenergic tone, reduce vagal activity, and increase blood pressure.[138] Anger has also been cited as a triggering event in AMI that leads to acute disruption of an atherosclerotic plaque[139] and arterial vasoconstriction.[140] Given these physiologic responses to stress it is important to relieve distress in patients by providing a calm professional environment and by explaining thoroughly medications, equipment, and treatments used.[141] Antianxiety medications may be necessary in some patients during the acute hospital phase. Among persons with severe stress or major depression, more aggressive psychologic counseling should be incorporated in the treatment plan as a long-term strategy.

Secondary Prevention

Currently, there is evidence that aggressive long-term management of multiple CAD risk factors can improve coronary endothelial function and halt or even reverse the progression of atherosclerotic plaques. The results are lower mortality, reduced rehospitalization, and ultimately lower costs of care.[142-146] Important risk factor modification should include smoking cessation, aggressive pharmacologic and nonpharmacologic (i.e., dietary) lipid management, physical activity (i.e., cardiac rehabilitation), and pharmacologic interventions aimed at improving and maintaining myocardial perfusion (i.e., ACE inhibitors, beta-blockers, and antiplatelet agents).

Smoking Cessation. Patients who continue to smoke following AMI or after CABG or PCI procedures are more likely to develop postprocedural angina or recurrent MI, require repeat revascularization, or die compared with nonsmokers or persons who stopped smoking.[147-150] Importantly, the risk of untoward outcomes declines rapidly in patients who discontinue smoking and within 3 years of cessation reaches that of patients who have never smoked.[142] Taylor et al.[151] showed that the smoking cessation rate in patients following acute MI was higher among patients enrolled in a nurse-managed intervention compared with patients in a control group (71% intervention vs. 45% control). The highest rate of success is achieved from both formal behavioral interventions and the use of adjunctive agents (i.e., oral or transcutaneous nicotine preparations).

Lipid Management. Investigations show that lowering serum lipids and using diet and/or lipid-lowering drugs results in stability, or regression of atherosclerotic plaques, and lowers the rate of subsequent cardiac events in patients with AMI. For example, in the Familial Atherosclerotic Treatment Study (FATS),[143] a randomized clinical trial using double-drug therapy, the coronary event rate among patients in the treatment group was 85% lower as compared with control patients after 6 months and 73% lower than controls over the 2-year treatment period. Subsequent studies using only one lipid-lowering drug have confirmed these findings.[152-156]

Additional studies in patients following CABG surgery show that aggressive lipid lowering, using statin drugs, leads to a reduction in the progression of atherosclerotic plaques,[144] as measured with angiography, risk of MI, cardiovascular death, or need for revascularization.[157] Interestingly, the benefits of lipid lowering in patients with documented CAD are appreciated even when cholesterol levels are only minimally elevated or even normal.[144,157]

Exercise. The benefits of aerobic exercise in patients with CAD include weight loss, decreased lipid levels, lowered blood pressure, reduced myocardial oxygen demand, and improved functional capacity.[145,158] Studies of cardiac rehabilitation programs show that fewer patients in structured cardiac rehabilitation programs die at 1 to 3 years compared with patients in control groups.[145,146] Additional benefits of exercise training include quicker return to work following MI or CABG surgery,[159] as well as improvement in activities of daily living, improved sexual function, and lessened feelings of fear and depression.[160]

CASE STUDY

The following case study illustrates the usefulness of ST-segment monitoring in detecting silent and non-silent myocardial ischemia and subsequent treatment.

Mr. W. is a 68-year-old man patient presenting with angina that has increased in frequency and intensity over the past week. The patient's history includes prior PTCA, hypercholesterolemia, and chronic obstructive pulmonary disease. Cardiac catheterization performed on admission revealed triple vessel CAD. The patient was then admitted to the telemetry unit and scheduled for "elective" CABG surgery, which was to be performed in 2 to 3 days. Figure 21-7 illustrates a 48-hour ST trend in lead V_4. This ST trend indicates that during the first 12 hours of ST monitoring, the patient's ST level remained stable. However, he then experienced a total of four ST events *(top panel)*, which were characterized by ST-segment depression *(bottom two figures)*. The first two ST events were clinically silent. The third event was accompanied by chest pain that occurred during ambulation to the bathroom and was rated as a 3/10. Subsequently, the patient was assisted back to bed and given sublingual nitroglycerine. Because the patient's chest pain was unrelieved following several doses of nitroglycerine, he was then transferred to the CCU for more aggressive medical management (i.e., intravenous nitroglycerine, heparin, and oxygen via nasal cannula).

Not long after transfer to the CCU, the patient experienced a fourth ST event, which he rated as an 8/10 in severity. The nitroglycerine drip was increased until his pain was relieved. The patient was then taken to the cardiac catheterization laboratory where an intraaortic balloon pump (IABP) was placed to improve coronary perfusion and to reduce left ventricular workload. Following IABP insertion, the ST level remained stable for approximately 12 hours (Figure 21-7, *top panel*). The following morning the patient was taken for CABG surgery. The serum troponin level was negative for infarction, which indicates that permanent myocardial damage had been averted, most likely because of aggressive medical management. Following an uneventful clinical course, the patient was transferred home and was scheduled for cardiac rehabilitation. In this case, the information obtained from ST-segment monitoring was valuable in the diagnosis of myocardial ischemia. In addition, ST-segment monitoring was useful for determining the outcome of the interventions used in this patient's care.

SELECTED RESEARCH

Drew and her group have conducted a number of important investigations related to the development of more sensitive and clinically feasible ECG technology, a few of which are reviewed here. An experimental 12-lead ECG method was developed to enhance the ECG detection of the varying ST-segment patterns that occur in different leads in the same individual. The method, first developed by Dower and associates (EASI Lead System, Philips Medical Systems, Andover, MA), derives all 12 ECG leads with only five ECG electrodes applied

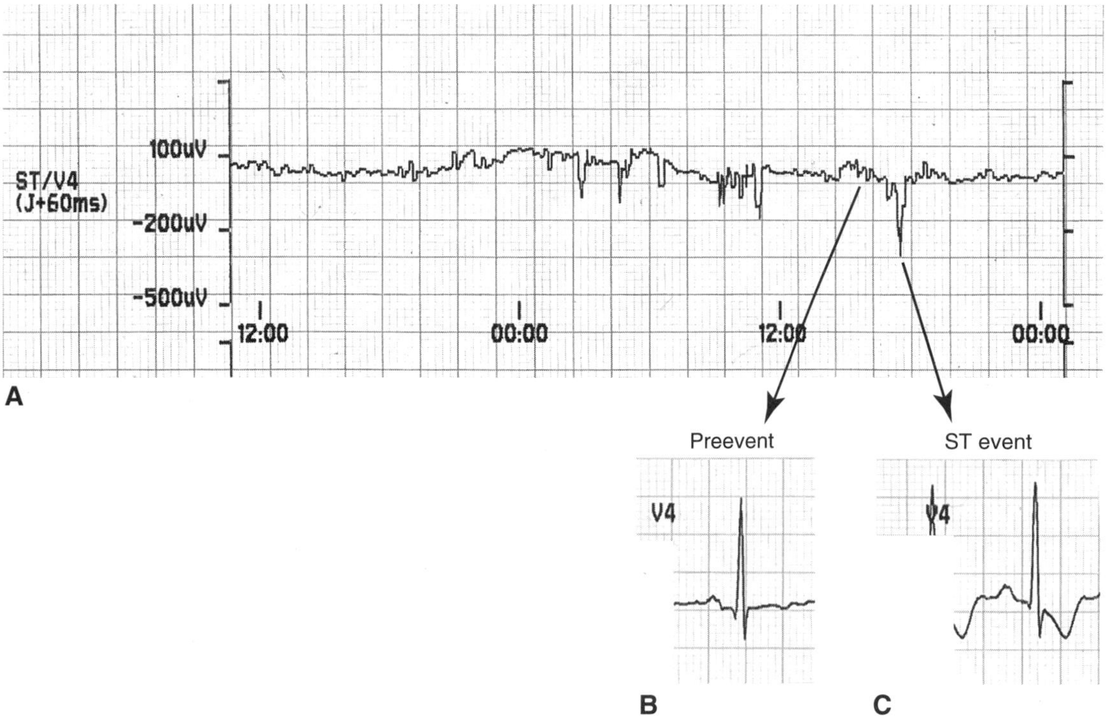

Figure 21-7 Case Study: **A, A 48-hour (X-axis) ST-segment trend in lead V4 obtained in a 68-year-old male patient admitted to the telemetry unit with progressive angina over the past week. The magnitude of ST-segment deviation is indicated along the Y-axis in microvolts (μV) measured at 60 milliseconds past the J-point. B, The patient's isoelectric ST-segment level in lead V4 before an acute ischemic event. C, Acute ST-segment depression (demand-related ischemia) in this same lead that occurred during continuous ST-segment monitoring.** (Courtesy the Ischemia Monitoring Laboratory, University of California San Francisco, School of Nursing.)

to the patient's chest (Figure 21-8). Preliminary studies in patients undergoing electrophysiologic procedure, or PCI procedures, showed that the derived 12-lead ECG was valuable for diagnosing various cardiac problems (i.e., prior MI, preexcitation, bundle branch block, and distinguishing supraventricular tachycardia with aberrant conduction from ventricular tachycardia) and PCI-induced ischemia.[161,162]

In the first study conducted in the CCU using this technology, Drew and co-workers[80] showed that the derived 12-lead ECG was superior to the routine monitoring lead V_1 or lead II for ischemia detection (100% sensitivity of derived vs. 40% sensitivity of leads V_1 or II). In a subsequent investigation,[96] these same investigators conducted a direct comparison of the derived ECG to the standard ECG in patients presenting for treatment of acute coronary syndromes. Patients were maintained on both ECG methods throughout their entire hospitalization (i.e., emergency department, CCU, cardiac catheterization laboratory, and cardiac telemetry unit). The findings revealed that the derived ECG demonstrated nearly perfect agreement compared with the standard 12-lead ECG when assessing various cardiac diagnoses, underlying cardiac rhythm, and ST-elevation pattern during acute MI and during transient ischemia.[96]

Currently, there is little information regarding the frequency or consequences of transient myocardial ischemia in patients admitted to the telemetry unit for treatment of acute coronary syndromes. This knowledge is important given the current trend for directly admitting these patients to the telemetry unit, rather than the CCU. Pelter[163] sought to determine the frequency and consequences of ischemia in 237 patients treated in the telemetry unit of a tertiary care medical center between 1997 and 2000. Continuous 12-lead ST-segment monitoring was maintained a mean of 28 hours. Ischemia was defined as 100 μV or greater

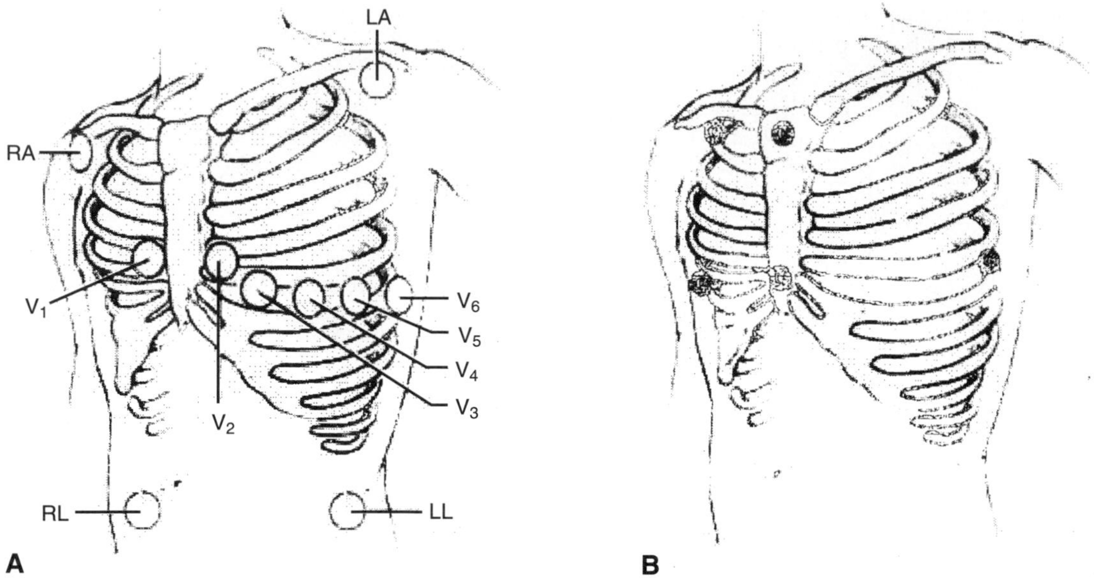

Figure 21-8 **A, ECG lead locations required to obtain a standard 12-lead ECG. B, The lead locations used to derive the 12-lead ECG.** (Courtesy the Ischemia Monitoring Laboratory, University of California, San Francisco, School of Nursing.)

ST change, compared with a baseline ECG, in one or more ECG leads, lasting 1 minute or longer.

The sample consisted of 178 (75%) patients initially admitted to the telemetry unit and 59 (25%) initially admitted to CCU then transferred to the telemetry unit. Of the 237 patients, 190 were admitted with angina and 47 had an MI, 39 (17%) had a total of 89 ischemic events, and 70 events (79%) were clinically silent. Of the 89 total ischemic events, only 27 (30%) were 100 μV or greater in V_1 or lead II, which are the two most commonly selected ECG leads for telemetry monitoring. In comparison with the patients who did not have myocardial ischemia, a greater number of those who had ischemia required transfer to the CCU (18% vs. 2%; $p < 0.001$); had an adverse outcome such as cardiogenic shock, pulmonary edema, major arrhythmia, acute MI, or death (41% vs. 9%; $p < 0.001$); and had longer hospitalizations (142 hours vs. 86 hours; $p < 0.001$). Pelter concluded that transient ischemia is not uncommon and largely silent in patients admitted to the telemetry setting for acute coronary syndromes. ST-segment-detected ischemia identified patients at increased risk for serious in-hospital complications.

QUESTIONS FOR FUTURE STUDY

Despite the explosion of knowledge in the area of myocardial ischemia research over the last decades, many gaps in our knowledge still exist and new questions are continually evolving. A few of them are presented here.

A compelling area for study is the need to develop and test new models of health care delivery that improve access to health care for nonwhite ethnic minorities. In addition, investigators must test ethnically appropriate strategies that educate and assist people to modify their risk factors.

Clarification is needed of the mechanisms of negative affective states in the evolution of atherosclerosis and CHD, as well as development and testing of effective cognitive-behavioral interventions to modify these risk factors. The roles of homocysteine and C-reactive protein as predictors and/or precursors of CHD need further study.

The randomized clinical trials exploring the role of HRT in primary and secondary prevention of CHD in postmenopausal women have left important questions unanswered. For example, could other forms of estrogen and progestin reduce the risk of CHD and acute MI? Or could one or more subgroups of women without known CHD show a differential reduction in CHD risk with HRT?

Work in the basic science of ischemia is needed to fully elucidate the complex processes involved in ischemic injury and recovery, identify the biochemical event(s) that signals irreversible injury, and continue to develop new interventions that minimize reperfusion injury.

The work that has been done with ST-segment monitoring has been primarily descriptive in nature. Prospective, randomized clinical trials need to be conducted to determine whether ST monitoring changes outcomes in patients with myocardial ischemia. The 12-lead ECG is the gold standard for detecting and diagnosing myocardial ischemia and infarction; however, its sensitivity and specificity can be limited in some patients. In this regard, two areas for further development and testing include improvements in the derived 12-lead ECG and development of a system to detect ischemia over the entire surface of the heart that is comfortable for patients and convenient for nurses to use.

REFERENCES

1. Astrup, J. (1982). Energy-requiring cell functions in the ischemic brain. *Journal of Neurosurgery, 56,* 482-497.
2. Velican, C., & Velican, D. (1989). *Natural history of coronary atherosclerosis.* Boca Raton, FL: CRC Press.
3. American Heart Association. (2000). *2001 Heart and Stroke Statistical Update.* Dallas, TX: American Heart Association.
4. Giles, W., Anda, R., Casper, M., Escobedo, L., & Taylor, H. (1995). Race and sex differences in rates of invasive cardiac procedures in US hospitals. Data from the National Hospital Discharge Survey. *Archives of Internal Medicine, 155,* 318-324.
5. Winkleby, M., Kraemer, H., Ahn, D., & Varady, A. (1998). Ethnic and socioeconomic differences in cardiovascular disease risk factors. *Journal of the American Medical Association, 280,* 356-362.
6. Harris, M., Flegal, K., Cowie, C., Eberhardt, M., Goldstein, D., Little, R., et al. (1998). Prevalence of diabetes, impaired fasting glucose, and impaired glucose tolerance in U.S. adults. *Diabetes Care, 21,* 518-524.
7. Dahlén, G., Srinivasan, S., Stenlund, H., Wattigney, W., Wall, S., & Berenson, G. (1998). The importance of serum lipoprotein (a) as an independent risk factor for premature coronary artery disease in middle-aged black and white women from the United States. *Journal of Internal Medicine, 244,* 417-424.
8. Gillum, R. (1993). Trends in acute myocardial infarction and coronary heart disease death in the United States. *Journal of the American College of Cardiology, 23,* 1273-1277.
9. Fang, J., Madhavan, S., & Alderman, M. (1996). The association between birthplace and mortality from cardiovascular causes among black and white residents of New York City. *New England Journal of Medicine, 335,* 1545-1551.
10. Burt, V.L., Cutler, J.A., Higgins, M., Horan, M.J., LaBarthe, D., Whelton, P., et al. (1995). Trends in the prevalence, awareness, and control of hypertension in the adult U.S. population: Data from the Health Examination Surveys, 1960-1991. *Hypertension, 26,* 60-69.
11. Johnson, C.L., Rifkind, B.M., Sempos, C.T., Carroll, M.D., Bachorik, P.S., Breifel, R.R., et al. (1993). Declining total serum cholesterol levels among U.S. adults: The National Health and Nutrition Examination Surveys. *Journal of the American Medical Association, 269,* 3002-3008.
12. Beller, G.A. (2001). Coronary heart disease in the first 30 years of the 21st century: Challenges and opportunities. *Circulation, 103,* 2428-2435.
13. Levy, D., & Thom, T. (1998). Death rates from coronary disease—Progress and a puzzling paradox. *New England Journal of Medicine, 339,* 915-917.
14. Jiang, H., Vupputuri, S., Allen, K., Prerost, M., Hughes, J., & Whelton, P. (1999). Passive smoking and the risk of coronary heart disease—A meta-analysis of epidemiologic studies. *The New England Journal of Medicine, 340,* 920-926.
15. Third Report of the National Cholesterol Education Program (NCEP) Expert Panel on Detection, Evaluation, and Treatment of High Blood Cholesterol in Adults (Adult Treatment Panel III). Executive Summary. (2001). *Journal of the American Medical Association, 285,* 2486-2497.
16. Benetos, A., Thomas, F., Bean, K., Gautier, S., Smulyan, H., & Guize, L. (2002). Prognostic value of systolic and diastolic blood pressure in treated hypertensive men. *Archive of Internal Medicine, 162,* 577-581.
17. Izzo, J., Levy, D., & Black, H. (2000). Importance of systolic blood pressure on older Americans. *Hypertension, 35,* 1021-1024.
18. Lloyd-Jones, D.M. (1999). Impact of systolic versus diastolic blood pressure level of JNC-VI blood pressure stage classification. *Hypertension, 34,* 381-385.
19. Grundy, S., Benjamin, I., Burke, G., Chait, A., Eckel, R., Howard, B., et al. (1999). Diabetes and cardiovascular disease: A statement for healthcare professionals from the American Heart Association. *Circulation, 100,* 1134-1146.
20. Hu, F., Stampfer, M., Solomon, C., Liu, S., Willett, W., Speizer, F., et al. (2001). The impact of diabetes mellitus on mortality from all causes and coronary heart disease in women. *Archives of Internal Medicine, 161,* 1717-1723.
21. Report of the Expert Committee on the Diagnosis and Classification of Diabetes Mellitus. (1997). *Diabetes Care, 20,* 1183-1197.
22. Friedman, M., & Rosenman, R.H. (1959). Association of specific overt behavior pattern with blood and cardiovascular findings. *Journal of the American Medical Association, 169,* 1286-1296.
23. Krantz, D.S., Contrada, R.J., Hill, D.R., & Friedler, E. (1988). Environmental stress and biobehavioral antecedents of coronary heart disease. *Journal of Consulting and Clinical Psychology, 56,* 333-341.
24. Miller, T.Q., Smith, T.W., Turner, C.W., Guijarro, M.L., & Hallet, A.J. (1996). A meta-analytic review of research on hostility and physical health. *Psychological Bulletin, 119,* 322-348.
25. Suinn, R. (2001). The terrible twos—Anger and anxiety. *American Psychologist, 56,* 27-36.
26. Iribarren, C., Sidney, S., Bild, D., Liu, K., Markovitz, J., Roseman, J., et al. (2000). Association of hostility with coronary artery calcification in young adults. *Journal of the American Medical Association, 283,* 2546-2551.
27. Anda, R., Williamson, D., Jones, D., Macera., C., Eaker, E., Glassman, A., et al. (1993). Depressed affect, hopelessness, and the risk of ischemic heart disease in a cohort of U.S. adults. *Epidemiology, 4,* 281-283.
28. O'Connor, C., Gurbel, P., & Serebruany, V. (2000). Depression and ischemic heart disease. *American Heart Journal, 140,* S63-S69.
29. Musselman, D.L., Evans, D.L., & Nemeroff, C.B. (1998). The relationship of depression to cardiovascular disease:

Epidemiology, biology, and treatment. *Archives of General Psychiatry, 55,* 580-592.
30. Christen, W., Ajani, U., Glynn, R., & Hennekens, C. (2000). Blood levels of homocysteine and increased risks of cardiovascular disease: Causal or casual? *Archive of Internal Medicine, 160,* 422-434.
31. Eichholzer, M., Lüthy, J., Gutzwiller, F., & Stähelin, H. (2001). The role of folate, antioxidant vitamins and other constituents in fruit and vegetables in the prevention of heart disease: The epidemiological evidence. *International Journal for Vitamin and Nutrition Research, 71,* 5-17.
32. Friso, S., Jacques, P., Wilson, P., Rosenberg, I., & Selhub, J. (2001). Low circulating vitamin B_6 is associated with elevation of the inflammation marker C-reactive protein independently of plasma homocysteine levels. *Circulation, 103,* 2788-2791.
33. Delanghe, J., Langlois, M., De Bacquer, D., Mak, R., Capel, P., Van Renterghem, L., et al. (2002). Discriminative value of serum amyloid A and other acute-phase proteins for coronary heart disease. *Atherosclerosis, 160,* 471-476.
34. Levinson, S.S., & Elin, R.J. (2002). What is c-reactive protein telling us about coronary artery disease? *Archives of Internal Medicine, 162,* 389-392.
35. Peker, Y., Kraiczi, H., Hedner, J., Löth, S., Johansson, Ä., & Bende, M. (1999). An independent association between obstructive sleep apnoea and coronary artery disease. *European Respiratory Journal, 13,* 179-184.
36. Wilson, L. (1998). Rapid progression of coronary artery disease in the setting of chronic cocaine abuse. *Journal of Emergency Medicine, 16,* 631-634.
37. Pitts, W., Lange, R., Cigarroa, J., & Hillis, D. (1997). Cocaine-induced myocardial ischemia and infarction: Pathophysiology, recognition, and management. *Progress of Cardiovascular Diseases, 40,* 65-76.
38. Ros, H., Lichtenstein, P., Bellocco, R., Petersson, G., & Cnattingius, S. (2001). Increased risks of circulatory diseases in late pregnancy and puerperium. *Epidemiology, 12,* 456-460.
39. Rath, W., Faridi, A., & Dudenhausen, J. (2000). HELLP syndrome. *Journal of Perinatal Medicine, 28,* 249-260.
40. Burkman, R.T. (2000). Cardiovascular issues with oral contraceptives: Evidenced-based medicine. *International Journal of Fertility and Women's Medicine, 45,* 166-174.
41. Heinemann, L.A. (2000). Emerging evidence on oral contraceptives and arterial disease. *Contraception, 62*(Suppl.), 29S-36S.
42. WHO Collaborative Study of Cardiovascular Disease and Steroid Hormone contraception. (1997). Acute myocardial infarction and combined oral contraceptives: Results of an international multicentre case-control study. *Lancet, 349,* 1202-1209.
43. Mosca, L., Collins, P., Herrington, D., Mendelsohn, M., Pasternak, R., Robertson, R., et al. (2001). Hormone replacement therapy and cardiovascular disease: A statement for healthcare professionals from the American Heart Association. *Circulation, 104,* 499-503.
44. Rosano, G.M., & Panina, G. (1999). Cardiovascular pharmacology of hormone replacement therapy. *Drugs and Aging, 15,* 219-234.
45. Hulley, S., Grady, D., Bush, T., Furberg, C., Herrington, D., Riggs, B., et al. (1998). Randomized trial of estrogen plus progestin for secondary prevention of coronary heart disease in postmenopausal women. *Journal of the American Medical Association, 280,* 605-613.
46. Writing Group for the Women's Health Initiative Investigators. (2002). Risks and benefits of estrogen plus progestin in healthy postmenopausal women. Principal results from the Women's Health Initiative randomized controlled trial. *Journal of the American Medical Association, 288,* 321-333.
47. Herrington, D.M., Reboussin, D.M., Brosnahan, B., Sharp, P.C., Shumaker, S.A., Snyder, T.E., et al. (2000). Effects of estrogen replacement on the progression of coronary artery atherosclerosis. *New England Journal of Medicine, 343,* 522-529.
48. Grady, D., Herrington, D, Bittner, V., Blumenthal, R., Davidson, M., Hlatky, M., et al. (2002). Cardiovascular disease outcomes during 6.8 years of hormone therapy. Heart and Estrogen/progestin Replacement Study follow-up (HERS II). *Journal of the American Medical Association, 288,* 49-57.
49. Mosca, L, Barrett-Connor, E, Wenger, N.K., Collins, P., Grady, D, Kornitzer, M., et al. (2001). Design and methods of the Raloxifene Use for The Heart (RUTH) study. *American Journal of Cardiology, 88,* 392-395.
50. Wenger, N.K., Barrett-Connor, E., Collins, P., Grady, D., Kornitzer, M., Mosca, L., et al. (2002). Baseline characteristics of participants in the Raloxifene Use for The Heart (RUTH) trial. *American Journal of Cardiology, 90,* 1204-1210.
51. Ganong, W.F. (2001). *Review of Medical Physiology* (20th ed.). San Francisco: McGraw-Hill.
52. McCluskey, R.S. (1982). Microcirculation: Basic considerations. In R.A. Cowley & B.F. Trump (Eds.), *The pathophysiology of shock, anoxia, and ischemia* (pp. 156-164). Baltimore: Williams & Wilkins.
53. Kloner, R., & Jennings, R. (2001). Consequences of brief ischemia: Stunning, preconditioning, and their clinical implications. *Circulation, 104,* 2981-2989.
54. White, B., Grossman, L., O'Neil, B., DeGracia, D., Neumar, R., Rafols, J., et al. (1996). Global brain ischemia and reperfusion. *Annals of Emergency Medicine, 27,* 588-594.
55. Collard, C.D., & Gelman, S. (2001). Pathophysiology, clinical manifestations, and prevention of ischemia-reperfusion injury. *Anesthesiology, 94,* 1133-1138.
56. Cotran, R.S., Kumar, V., & Collins, T. (1999). Cellular pathology 1: Cell injury and cell death. In R.S. Cotran, V. Kumar, & T. Collins (Eds.), *Robbins pathologic basis of disease* (6th ed., pp. 1-29). Philadelphia: W.B. Saunders.
57. Trump, B.F., Berezesky, L.K., & Cowley, R.A. (1982). Cellular and subcellular characteristics of acute and chronic injury with emphasis on the role of calcium. In R.A. Cowley & B.F. Trump (Eds.), *The pathophysiology of shock, anoxia, and ischemia* (pp. 6-46). Baltimore: Williams & Wilkins.
58. Oliver, M. (2002). Metabolic causes and prevention of ventricular fibrillation during acute coronary syndromes. *American Journal of Medicine, 112,* 305-311.
59. Forman, M.B., Puett, D.W., & Virmani, R. (1989). Endothelial and myocardial injury during ischemia and reperfusion: Pathogenesis and therapeutic implications. *Journal of the American College of Cardiology, 13,* 450-459.
60. Krause, G.S., White, B.C., Aust, S.D., Nayini, N.R., & Kurvar, K. (1988). Brain cell death following ischemia and reperfusion: A proposed biochemical sequence. *Critical Care Medicine, 16,* 714-726.
61. Kloner, R.A., Przyklenk, K., & Patel, B. (1989). Altered myocardial states: The stunned and hibernating myocardium. *American Journal of Medicine, 86,* 14-22.

62. Safar, P., Behringer, W., Böttiger, B.W., & Sterz, F. (2002). Cerebral resuscitation potentials for cardiac arrest. *Critical Care Medicine, 30*(Suppl.), S140-S144.
63. Libby, P. (1995). Molecular basis of the acute coronary syndromes. *Circulation, 91,* 2844-2850.
64. Maron, B.J. (1989). Hypertrophic cardiomyopathy. *Current Problems in Cardiology, 18,* 639-645.
65. Kullo, I.J., Edwards, W.D., & Schwartz, R.S. (1998). Vulnerable plaque: Pathophysiology and clinical implications. *Annals of Internal Medicine, 129,* 1050-1060.
66. DeWood, M.A., Spores, J., Notske, R., Mouser, L.T., Burroughs, R., & Golden, M.S. (1980). Prevalence of total coronary occlusion during the early hours of transmural infarction. *New England Journal of Medicine, 303,* 897-902.
67. Ambrose, J.A., Winters, S.L., & Arora, R.R. (1985). Coronary angiographic morphology in myocardial infarction: A link between the pathogenesis of unstable angina and myocardial infarction. *Journal of the American College of Cardiology, 6,* 1233-1238.
68. Terrosu, P., Ibba, G.V., Contini, G.M., & Franceschino, V. (1984). Angiographic features of the coronary arteries during intracoronary thrombolysis. *British Heart Journal, 52,* 154-163.
69. Prinzmetal, M., Kennamer, R., Merliss, R., Wada, T., & Bor, N. (1959). A variant form of angina pectoris. *American Journal of Medicine, 27,* 375-388.
70. Maseri, A., Severi, S., deNes, M., L'Abbate, A., Chierchia, S., Marzilli, M., et al. (1978). Variant angina: One aspect of a continuous spectrum of vasospastic myocardial ischemia. *American Journal of Cardiology, 42,* 1019-1035.
71. Braunwald, E., & Sobel, B.E. (1988). Coronary blood flow and myocardial ischemia. In E. Braunwald (Ed.), *Heart disease. A textbook of cardiovascular medicine* (3rd ed., pp. 1191-1221). Philadelphia: W.B. Saunders.
72. Bagdonas, A.A., Stucky, J.H., Piera, J., Amer, N.S., & Hoffman, B.F. (1961). Effects of ischemia and hypoxia on the specialized conducting system of the canine heart. *American Heart Journal, 61,* 206-218.
73. Ten Eick, R.E., Singer, D.H., & Solberg, L.E. (1976). Coronary occlusion: Effect on cellular electrical activity of the heart. *Medical Clinics of North America, 60,* 49-67.
74. Downar, E., Janse, M.J., & Durrer, D. (1977). The effect of "ischemic" blood on transmembrane potentials of normal porcine ventricular myocardium. *Circulation 55,* 455-462.
75. Summers, R.L., Cooper, G.J., Carlton, F.B., Andrews, M.E., & Kolb, J.C. (1999). Prevalence of atypical chest pain descriptions in a population from the southern United States. *American Journal of the Medical Sciences, 318,* 142-145.
76. Kannel, W.B., & Abbott, R.D. (1984). Incidence and prognosis of unrecognized myocardial infarction. An update on the Framingham study. *New England Journal of Medicine, 311,* 1144-1147.
77. Clark, L.T., Adams-Campbell, L.L., Maw, M., Bridges, D., & Kline, G. (1989). Clinical features of patients with acute myocardial infarction presenting with and without typical chest pain: An inner city experience. *Journal of the Association for Academic Minority Physicians, 1*(1), 29-31.
78. Braunwald, E. (1989). Unstable angina. A classification. *Circulation, 80,* 410-414.
79. Krucoff, M.W., Jackson, Y.R., Kehoe, M.K., & Kent, K.M. (1990). Quantitative and qualitative ST-segment monitoring during and after percutaneous transluminal angioplasty. *Circulation, 81*(Suppl. IV), IV-20-IV-26.
80. Drew, B.J., Adams, M.G., Pelter, M.M., & Wung, S.F. (1996). ST-segment monitoring with a derived 12-lead electrocardiogram is superior to routine cardiac care unit monitoring. *American Journal of Critical Care, 5*(3), 198-206.
81. Gottlieb, S.O., Weisfeldt, M.L., Ouyang, P., Mellitis, E.D., & Gerstenblith, G. (1986). Silent ischemia as a marker for early unfavorable outcomes in patients with unstable angina. *New England Journal of Medicine, 314,* 1214-1218.
82. Klootwijk, P., Meij, S., Melkert, R., Lenderink, T., & Simoons, M. (1998). Reduction of recurrent ischemia with abciximab during continuous ECG-ischemia monitoring in patients with unstable angina refractory to standard treatment (CAPTURE). *Circulation, 98,* 1358-1364.
83. Cohn, P. (2000). *Silent myocardial ischemia and infarction* (4th ed.). New York: Marcel Dekker.
84. Goodman, S.G., Cohen, M., Bigonzi, F., Furfinkel, E.P., Radley, D.R., Le Iouer, V., et al. (2000). Randomized trial of low molecular weight heparin (enoxaparin) versus unfractionated heparin for unstable coronary artery disease: One-year results of the ESSENCE Study. Efficacy and Safety of Subcutaneous Enoxaparin in Non-Q Wave Coronary Events. *Journal of the American College of Cardiology, 36,* 693-698.
85. Langer, A., Freeman, M.R., & Armstrong, P.W. (1989). ST-segment shift in unstable angina: Pathophysiology and association with coronary anatomy and hospital outcome. *Journal of the American College of Cardiology, 13,* 1495-1502.
86. Gilard, M., Mansouratu, J., Etienne, Y., Larlet, J.M., Troung, B., & Boschat, J. (1998). Angiographic anatomy of the coronary sinus and its tributaries. *Pacing and Clinical Electrophysiology, 21,* 2280-2284.
87. Pepine, C., Singh, B., Gibson, R., & Kent, K. (1987). Recognition, pathogenesis, and management options in silent coronary artery disease. *Circulation Supplement, 75,* II-52-II-53.
88. Gibler, W.B., Runyon, J.P., Levy, R.C., Sayer, M.R., Kacich, R., Hattemer, C.R., et al. (1995). A rapid diagnostic and treatment center for patients with chest pain in the emergency department. *Annals of Emergency Medicine, 25,* 1-8.
89. Davies, G.J., Chieerchia, S., & Maseri, A. (1984). Prevention of myocardial infarction by very early treatment with intracoronary streptokinase. *New England Journal of Medicine, 311,* 1488-1492.
90. Hacket, D., Davies, G., Chierchia, S., & Maseri, A. (1987). Intermittent coronary occlusion in acute myocardial infarction. *New England Journal of Medicine, 317,* 1055-1059.
91. Krucoff, M.W., Croll, M.A., Pope, J.E., Pieper, K.S., Kanani, P.M., Granger, C., et al. (1993). Continuously updated 12-lead ST-segment recovery analysis for myocardial infarct arterial patency assessment and its correlation with multiple simultaneous early angiographic observations. *American Journal of Cardiology, 71,* 145-151.
92. Dellborg, M., Riha, M., & Swedberg, K. (1991). Dynamic QRS-complex and ST-segment monitoring in acute myocardial infarction during recombinant tissue-type plasminogen activator therapy. *American Journal of Cardiology, 67,* 343-349.
93. Kwon, K., Freedman, B., Wilcox, I., Allman, K., Madden, A., & Carter, G.S. (1991). The unstable ST-segment early after thrombolysis for acute infarction and its usefulness as a marker of recurrent coronary occlusion. *American Journal of Cardiology, 67,* 109-115.

94. Veldkamp, R.F., Green, C.L., Wilkins, M.L., Pope, J.E., Sawchak, S.T., Ryan, J.A., et al. (1994). Comparison of continuous ST-segment recovery analysis with methods using static electrocardiograms for noninvasive patency assessment during acute myocardial infarction. *American Journal of Cardiology, 73,* 1069-1074.
95. Langer, A., Krucoff, M.W., Klootwijk, P., Veldkamp, R., Simoons, M.L., Granger, C., et al. (1995). Noninvasive assessment of speed and stability of infarct-related artery reperfusion: Results of the GUSTO ST-segment monitoring study. *Journal of the American College of Cardiology, 25,* 1552-1557.
96. Drew, B.J., Pelter, M.M., Wung, S.F., Adams, M.G., Taylor, C., Evans, G.T., Jr., et al. (1999). Accuracy of the EASI 12-lead electrocardiogram compared to the standard 12-lead electrocardiogram for diagnosing multiple cardiac abnormalities. *Journal of Electrocardiology, 32*(Suppl. 2), 38-47.
97. Mizutani, M., Freedman, S. B., Barns, E., Ogasawara, S., Bailey, B. P., & Bernstein, L. (1990). ST monitoring for myocardial ischemia during and after coronary angioplasty. *American Journal of Cardiology, 66,* 389-393.
98. Drew, B.J., Adams, M.A., Pelter, M.M., & Wung, S.F. (1997). Comparison of standard and derived 12-lead electrocardiograms for diagnosis of coronary-induced myocardial ischemia. *American Journal of Cardiology, 79,* 639-644.
99. The GUSTO Investigators. (1993). An international trial comparing four thrombolytic strategies for acute myocardial infarction. *New England Journal of Medicine, 329,* 673-682.
100. Aldrich, H.R., Hinman, N.B., Hinohara, T., Jones, M.G., Boswick, J., Lee, D., et al. (1987). Identification of the optimal electrocardiographic leads for detecting acute epicardial injury in acute myocardial infarction. *American Journal of Cardiology, 59,* 20-23.
101. Bush, H.S., Ferguson, J.J., Angelini, P., & Willerson, J.T. (1990). Twelve-lead electrocardiographic evaluation of ischemia during percutaneous transluminal coronary angioplasty and its correlation with acute reocclusion. *American Heart Journal, 121,* 1591-1599.
102. Drew, B.J., & Tisdale, L.A. (1993). ST-segment monitoring for coronary artery reocclusion following thrombolytic therapy and coronary angioplasty: Identification of optimal bedside monitoring leads. *American Journal of Critical Care, 2,* 280-292.
103. Wagner, G.S. (1994). *Marriott's practical electrocardiology* (9th ed.). Baltimore: Williams & Wilkins.
104. Braunwald, E. (1989). Myocardial reperfusion, limitation of infarct size, reduction of left ventricular dysfunction, and improved survival. Should the paradigm be expanded? *Circulation, 79,* 441-444.
105. ASSENT-2 Investigators. (2000). Single-bolus tenecteplase compared to front-load alteplase in acute myocardial infarction: The ASSENT-2 double-blind randomized trial. *Lancet, 354,* 719-722.
106. International Joint Efficacy Comparison of Thrombolytics. (1995). Randomized, double-blind comparison of reteplase double-bolus administration with streptokinase in acute myocardial infarction (INJECT): Trial to investigate equivalence. *Lancet, 346,* 329-346.
107. The TIMI Study Group. (1985). The thrombolysis in myocardial infarction (TIMI) trial. *New England Journal of Medicine, 312,* 932-936.
108. The GISSI Study Group. (1986). Effectiveness of intravenous fibrinolytic treatment in acute myocardial infarction. *Lancet, 1,* 397-401.
109. Krucoff, M.W., Croll, M.A., Pope, J.E., Granger, C.B., O'Connor, C.M., & Sigmon, K.N. (1993). Continuous 12-lead ST-segment recovery analysis in the TAMI 7 study: Performance of a non-invasive method for real-time detection of failed myocardial reperfusion. *Circulation, 88,* 437-446.
110. Ohman, E.M., Calif, R.M., Topol, E.J., Candela, E.J., Abbottsmith, C., & Ellis, S. (1989). Consequences of reocclusion after successful reperfusion therapy in acute myocardial infarction. *Circulation, 82,* 781-791.
111. Deedwania, P.C., & Carbajal, E.V. (1990). Prevalence and patterns of silent myocardial ischemia during daily life in stable angina patients receiving conventional antianginal drug therapy. *American Journal of Cardiology, 65,* 1090-1096.
112. Knatterud, G.L., Bourassa, M.G., Pepine, C.J., Geller, N.L., Sopko, G., Chaitman, B.R., et al. (1994). Effects of treatment strategies to suppress ischemia in patients with coronary artery disease: 12-week results of the Asymptomatic Cardiac Ischemia Pilot (ACIP) study [see comments] [published erratum appears in *Journal of the American College of Cardiology* 1995;26:842]. *Journal of the American College of Cardiology, 24,* 11-20.
113. Pepine, C.J., Cohn, P.F., Deedwania, P.C., Gibson, R.S., Handberg, E., Hill, J.A., et al. (1994). Effects of treatment on outcome in mildly symptomatic patients with ischemia during daily life. The Atenolol Silent Ischemia Study (ASIST) [see comments]. *Circulation, 90,* 762-768.
114. Stone, P.H., Gibson, R.S., Glasser, S.P., DeWood, M.A., Parker, J.D., Kawanishi, C.T., et al. (1990). Comparison of propranolol, diltiazem, and nifedipine in the treatment of ambulatory ischemia in patients with stable angina. Differential effects on ambulatory ischemia, exercise performance, and anginal symptoms. The ASIS Study Group [see comments]. *Circulation, 82,* 1962-1972.
115. PURSUIT Trial Investigators. (1998). Platelet glycoprotein IIb/IIIa in unstable angina: Receptor suppression using integrilin therapy. *New England Journal of Medicine, 339,* 436-443.
116. The CAPTURE Investigators. (1997). Randomised placebo-controlled trial of abciximab before and during coronary intervention in refractory unstable angina: The capture study. *Lancet, 349,* 1429-1435.
117. PRISM-PLUS Investigators. (1998). Inhibition of the platelet glycoprotein IIb/IIIa receptor with tirofiban in unstable angina and non-Q-wave myocardial infarction. Platelet Receptor Inhibition in Ischemic Syndrome Management in Patients Limited by Unstable Signs and Symptoms (PRISM-PLUS) Study Investigators [see comments] [published erratum appears in *New England Journal of Medicine* 1998;339:415]. *New England Journal of Medicine, 338,* 1488-1497.
118. Waller, B.F. (1987). Pathology of transluminal balloon angioplasty used in the treatment of coronary heart disease. *Human Pathophysiology, 18,* 476-484.
119. Baim, D.S., & Ignatius, E.J. (1988). Use of percutaneous transluminal coronary angioplasty: Results of a current survey. *American Journal of Cardiology, 61,* 3G-8G.
120. Kathiresan, S., Jordan, M.K., Gimelli, G., Lopez-Cuellar, J., Madhi, N., & Jang, I. (1999). Frequency of silent myocardial ischemia following coronary stenting. *American Journal of Cardiology, 84,* 930-932.
121. Dabbs, A.D., Chambers, C.E., & Macauley, K. (1998). Complications after placement of an intracoronary stent: Nursing implications. *American Journal of Critical Care, 7,* 117-122.

122. Serruys, P.W., Jaegere, P., Kiemeneij, F., Macaya, C., Rutsch, W., & Heyndrickx, G. (1994). A comparison of balloon-expandable-stent implantation with balloon angioplasty in patients with coronary artery disease. *New England Journal of Medicine, 331,* 489-495.
123. Gibbons, R.J., Holmes, D.R., Reeder, G.S., Bailey, K.R., Hopfenspringer, M.R., & Gersh, B.J. (1993). Immediate angioplasty compared with the administration of thrombolytic agent followed by conservative treatment for myocardial infarction. *New England Journal of Medicine, 328,* 685-691.
124. Grines, C.L., Browne, K.F., Marco, J., Rothbaum, D., Stone, G.W., & O'Keefe, J. (1993). A comparison of immediate angioplasty with thrombolytic therapy for acute myocardial infarction. *New England Journal of Medicine, 328,* 673-679.
125. Lange, R.A., & Hillis, L.D. (1993). Immediate angioplasty for acute myocardial infarction [editorial; comment]. *New England Journal of Medicine, 328,* 726-728.
126. O'Neill, W., Timmis, G.C., Bourdillon, P.D., Lai, P., Ganghadarhan, V., Walton, J., Jr., et al. (1986). A prospective randomized clinical trial of intracoronary streptokinase versus coronary angioplasty for acute myocardial infarction. *New England Journal of Medicine, 314,* 812-818.
127. Ribeiro, E.E., Silva, L.A., Carneiro, R., D'Oliveira, L.G., Gasquez, A., Amino, J.G., et al. (1993). Randomized trial of direct coronary angioplasty versus intravenous streptokinase in acute myocardial infarction. *Journal of the American College of Cardiology, 22,* 376-380.
128. Zijlstra, F., de Boer, M.J., Hoorntje, J.C., Reiffers, S., Reiber, J.H., & Suryapranata, H. (1993). A comparison of immediate coronary angioplasty with intravenous streptokinase in acute myocardial infarction [see comments]. *New England Journal of Medicine, 328,* 680-684.
129. The VA Coronary Artery Bypass Surgery Cooperative Study Group. (1992). 18 year follow-up in the veterans affairs cooperative study of coronary artery bypass surgery for stable angina. *Circulation, 86,* 121-132.
130. Yusuf, S., Zucker, D., Peduzzi, P., Fisher, L.D., Takaro, T., Kennedy, J.W., et al. (1994). Effect of coronary artery bypass graft surgery on survival: Overview of 10-year results from randomized trials by the Coronary Artery Bypass Graft Surgery Trialists Collaboration [see comments] [published erratum appears in *Lancet* 1994;344:1446]. *Lancet, 344,* 563-570.
131. Pelter, M.M., Adams, M.G., & Drew, B.J. (2002). Association of transient myocardial ischemia with adverse in-hospital outcomes for angina patients treated in a telemetry unit or a coronary care unit. *American Journal of Critical Care, 11,* 318-325.
132. Rowe, M.H., Jelinek, M.V., Liddell, N., & Hugens, M. (1989). Effects of rapid mobilization on ejection fractions and ventricular volumes after acute myocardial infarction. *American Journal of Cardiology, 63,* 1037-1041.
133. Johnston, B.L., Watt, E.W., & Fletcher, G.F. (1981). Oxygen consumption and hemodynamic and electrocardiographic responses to bathing in recent post-myocardial infarction patients. *Heart & Lung, 10,* 666-671.
134. Magder, S. (1985). Assessment of myocardial stress from early ambulatory activities following myocardial infarction. *Chest, 87,* 442-447.
135. Quaglietti, S.E., Stotts, N.A., & Lovejoy, N.C. (1988). The effect of selected positions on rate pressure product of the postmyocardial infarction patient. *Journal of Cardiovascular Nursing, 2,* 77-85.
136. Winslow, E.H., Lane, L.D., & Gaffney, F.A. (1984). Oxygen uptake and cardiovascular response in patients and normal adults during in-bed and out-of-bed toileting. *Journal of Cardiac Rehabilitation, 4,* 348-354.
137. Winslow, E.H., Lane, L.D., & Gaffney, F.A. (1985). Oxygen uptake and cardiovascular response in control adults and acute myocardial infarction patients during bathing. *Nursing Research, 34,* 164-169.
138. Jiange, W., Hayano, J., & Coleman, E.R. (1993). Relation of cardiovascular responses to mental stress and cardiac vagal activity in coronary artery disease. *American Journal of Cardiology, 72,* 551-559.
139. Mittleman, M.A., Maclure, M., & Sherwood, J.B. (1995). Triggering of acute myocardial infarction onset by episodes of anger. *Circulation, 92,* 1720-1725.
140. Boltwood, M.D., Taylor, C.B., & Burke, M.B. (1993). Anger report predicts coronary artery vasomotor response to mental stress and atherosclerotic segments. *American Journal of Cardiology, 72,* 1361-1365.
141. Duryee, R. (1992). The efficacy of inpatient education after myocardial infarction. *Heart & Lung, 21,* 217-222.
142. Rosenberg, L., Kaufman, D.W., Helmrich, S.P., & Shapiro, S. (1985). The risk of myocardial infarction after quitting smoking in men under 55 years of age. *New England Journal of Medicine, 313,* 1511-1514.
143. Brown, B.G., Albers, J.J., Fisher, L.D., Schaefer, S.M., Lin, J.T., Kaplan, C.K., et al. (1990). Regression of coronary artery disease as a result of intense lipid-lowering therapy in men with high levels of apolipoprotein B. *New England Journal of Medicine, 323,* 1289-1298.
144. The Post Coronary Artery Bypass Graft Trial Investigators. (1997). The effect of aggressive lowering of low density lipoprotein cholesterol levels and low dose anti-coagulation on obstructive changes in saphenous-vein coronary artery bypass grafts. *New England Journal of Medicine, 336,* 153-162.
145. Haskell, W.L. (1994). Sedentary lifestyle is a risk factor for coronary heart disease. In T.A. Pearson, M.H. Criqui, & R.V. Leupker (Eds.), *Primer in preventive cardiology* (pp. 173-187). Dallas, TX: American Heart Association.
146. O' Connor, G.T., Buring, J.E., Yusuf, S., Goldhaber, S.Z., Olmstead, E.M., Paffenbarger, R.S., Jr., et al. (1989). An overview of randomized trials of rehabilitation with exercise after myocardial infarction. *Circulation, 80,* 234-244.
147. Taira, D.A., Seto, T.B., Ho, K.K., Krumholz, H.M., Cutlip, D.E., Berezin, R., et al. (2000). Impact of smoking on health-related quality of life after percutaneous coronary revascularization. [Comment in *Circulation* 2000;102:1340-1341]. *Circulation, 102,* 1369-1374.
148. Hasdai, D., Garratt, K.N., Grill, D.E., Lerman, A., & Holmes, D.R., Jr. (1997). Effect of smoking status on the long-term outcome after successful percutaneous coronary revascularization. [Comment in *American College of Physicians Journal Club* 1997;127:52]. *New England Journal of Medicine, 336,* 755-761.
149. Cameron, A.A., Davis, K.B., & Rogers, W.J. (1995). Recurrence of angina after coronary artery bypass surgery: Predictors and prognosis (CASS Registry). Coronary Artery Surgery Study. *Journal of the American College of Cardiology, 26,* 895-899.

150. Herlitz, J., Haglid, M., Albertsson, P., Westberg, S., Karlson, B.W., Hartford, M., et al. (1997). Short- and long-term prognosis after coronary artery bypass grafting in relation to smoking habits. *Cardiology, 88,* 492-497.
151. Taylor, C.B., Houston-Miller, N., Killen, I. D., & DeBusk, R.F. (1990). Smoking cessation after acute myocardial infarction: Effects of a nurse-managed intervention. *Annals of Internal Medicine, 113,* 118-123.
152. Scandinavian Simvastatin Survival Study. (1994). Randomized trial of cholesterol lowering in 4444 patients with coronary heart disease. *Lancet, 344,* 1383-1389.
153. Shepherd, J., Cobbe, S.M., Ford, I., Isles, C.G., Lorimer, A.R., MacFarlane, P.W., et al. (1995). Prevention of coronary heart disease with pravastatin in men with hypercholesterolemia. *New England Journal of Medicine, 333,* 1301-1307.
154. Byington, R.P., Jukema, W., Salonen, J.T., Pitt, B., Bruschke, A.V., Hoen, H., et al. (1995). Reduction in cardiovascular events during pravastatin therapy. Pooled analysis of clinical events of the pravastatin atherosclerosis intervention program. *Circulation, 92,* 2419-2425.
155. Yusuf, S., & Anand, S. (1996). Cost of prevention. The case of lipid lowering [editorial; comment]. *Circulation, 93,* 1774-1776.
156. Herd, J.A., Ballantyne, C.M., Farmer, J.A., Ferguson, J.J., Jones, P.H., West, M.S., et al. (1997). Effects of fluvastatin on coronary atherosclerosis in patients with mild to moderate cholesterol elevations (lipoprotein and coronary atherosclerosis study [LCAS]). *American Journal of Cardiology, 80,* 278-286.
157. Sacks, F.M., Pffeffer, M.A., Moye, L.A., Rouleau, J.L., Rutherford, J.D., Cole, T.G., et al. (1996). The effects of pravastatin on coronary events after myocardial infarction in patients with average cholesterol levels. *New England Journal of Medicine, 335,* 1001-1009.
158. Laslett, L., Paumer, L., & Amsterdam, E.A. (1987). Exercise training in coronary artery disease. *Cardiology Clinics, 5,* 211-225.
159. Rechnitzer, P.A., Pickard, H.A., Paivio, A.U., Yuhasz, M.S., & Cunningham, D. (1972). Long-term follow-up study of survival and recurrence rates following myocardial infarction in exercising and control subjects. *Circulation, 45,* 853-857.
160. Wenger, N.K. (1986). Rehabilitation of the coronary patient: Status 1986. *Progress in Cardiovascular Diseases, 29*(3), 181-204.
161. Drew, B.J., Koops, R.R., Adams, M.G., & Dower, G.E. (1994). Derived 12-lead ECG: Comparison with the standard ECG during myocardial ischemia and its potential application for continuous ST-segment monitoring. *Journal of Electrocardiology, 27,* 249-255.
162. Drew, B.J., Scheinman, M.M., & Evans, G.T. (1992). Comparison of a vectorcardiographically derived 12-lead electrocardiogram with the conventional electrocardiogram during wide QRS complex tachycardia, and its potential application for continuous bedside monitoring. *American Journal of Cardiology, 69,* 612-618.
163. Pelter, M.M., Drew, B.J., Engler, M.M., & Slaughter, R.E. (2001). What are the frequency and consequences of transient myocardial ischemia in the telemetry unit setting detected with continuous 12-lead electrocardiographic monitoring? (Doctoral Dissertation; University of California, San Francisco, Vol. 1). Ann Arbor, MI: Bell & Howell.
164. Tisdale, L.A., & Drew, B.J. (1993). ST-segment monitoring for myocardial ischemia. *AACN Clinical Issues, 4*(1), 34-43.

Index

Page numbers followed by "t" indicate tables; those followed by "f" indicate figures; those followed by "b" indicate boxes

D

I

Q

R

S

X

Y

Z